Thomas Erastus and the Palatinate

Brill's Series in Church History

VOLUME 48

Thomas Erastus and the Palatinate

A Renaissance Physician in the Second Reformation

By

Charles D. Gunnoe, Jr.

BRILL

LEIDEN • BOSTON
2011

On the cover: Portrait of Thomas Erastus by Tobias Stimmer (1582). Image courtesy of the Kunstmuseum Basel, Martin P. Bühler.

This book is printed on acid-free paper.

Library of Congress Cataloging-in-Publication-Data

Gunnoe, Charles D., 1963-
Thomas Erastus and the Palatinate : a Renaissance physician in the Second Reformation / by Charles D. Gunnoe, Jr.
p. cm. – (Brill's series in church history ; v. 48)
Includes bibliographical references (p.) and index.
ISBN 978-90-04-18792-4 (hardback : alk. paper)
1. Erastus, Thomas, 1524-1583. I. Title. II. Series.

BX9419.E72G86 2010
284'.2092–dc22

2010026553

Printed and bound in Great Britain by
CPI Antony Rowe, Chippenham and Eastbourne

ISSN: 1572-4107
ISBN: 978 90 04 18792 4

For Marji, Jake, Erik, & Katya

CONTENTS

PART II

CHURCH DISCIPLINE AND THE DESTRUCTION OF THE REFORMED CONSENSUS IN HEIDELBERG

PART III

NEW SCHOLARLY DIRECTIONS AFTER 1570

ACKNOWLEDGEMENTS

My first word of appreciation goes to my Doktorvater H.C. Erik Midelfort who helped me conceptualize this project and in all ways made it possible. Current and former faculty of the University of Virginia have made their mark on my academic progress in official and unofficial ways, and I thank Edward Ayers, Alon Confino, Carlos M.N. Eire, James D. Hunter, Thomas F.X. Noble, Duane J. Osheim, Gianfranco Poggi, and Heather Warren. I have profited from many academic godparents along my scholarly pilgrimage, including C. Edward Balog, James Bratt, Leo Graff, Jr., Carter Lindberg, George Thomas, and Retha Warnicke.

Many individuals and institutions have facilitated my research in Germany, Switzerland and the United States. The German Historical Institute's archive tour and paleography course (funded by the Volkswagen Foundation) and Center for Reformation Research paleography seminar put me in the position to undertake this project. The German Academic Exchange Service (DAAD) funded a year of research at the University of Heidelberg. My ongoing research also benefited from an NEH summer institute and a sabbatical leave granted by Aquinas College. I am indebted to Eike Wolgast's hospitality and guidance at the University of Heidelberg. Joachim Telle adopted me into his modern Paracelsus circle and has offered of immense assistance with bibliography and manuscripts. He also aided in editing the texts in Appendix B. Wolf-Dieter Müller-Jahncke generously shared materials in his private possession. The late Robert Walton breathed life into my project at a critical juncture. Christopher Burchill has been an extremely generous and stimulating Heidelberger in exile. Kurt Berends, Charlotte Lindner, and Sharon Lindner read the dissertation version of this study. I also thank J. Wayne Baker, Jordan Ballor, Jacob Baum, Amy Nelson Burnett, Scott Clark, Alex Clemens, Stephan Davis, Charles de Mooi, Peter Dykema, Fred Ehrman, Michael Graham, Randolph Head, Won Lee, Sven Limbeck, Bruce Moran, Michael Monheit, Richard Muller, Julian Paulus, Beth Plummer, Ryan Reeves, Jole Shackelford, Ann Tlusty, Arjan van Dijk and Frans van Liere for lending their technical expertise to selected topics covered here. Michael Walton, Gerhild Scholz Williams and the late Allen G. Debus have been encouraging mentors in early modern science. Lyle Bierma, Richard Muller, and Kate van Liere have helped me maintain contact with the sixteenth century in modern Grand Rapids. I am indebted to Karin Maag, Raymond Mentzer and the participants of the NEH institute "John Calvin and the Transformation of Religious Culture in Geneva, France, and Beyond" in 2004. Thanks as well to my academic fellow travelers Ty Buckman, Jason Duncan, Doug Howard, Tal Howard, Lew Klatt, Humphrey Mar, John Pinhiero, and Jeremy Venema.

I gratefully acknowledge the following institutions for allowing me to access their holdings: Öffentliche Bibliothek der Universität Basel; the Historical Division of the National Library of Medicine (Bethesda, Maryland); Staatsbibliothek Bern; Staats- und Universitätsbibliothek Bremen; Sächsisches Hauptstaatsarchiv (Dresden); Universitätsbibliothek Erlangen; Houghton Library, Harvard University; Universitätsbibliothek Heidelberg; Universitätsarchiv Heidelberg; Generallandesarchiv Karlsruhe, Landesbibliothek und Murhardsche Bibliothek der Stadt Kassel, Universitätsbibliothek Kassel; Lambeth Palace Library; Gemeinschaftliches Hennebergisches Archiv im Thüringishes Staatsarchiv Meiningen; Germanisches Nationalmuseum (Nuremberg); Stadtbibliothek Schaffhausen; Dibner Library, Smithsonian Institution, Washington, D.C; Herzog-August-Bibliothek Wolfenbüttel; Staatsbibliothek, Stadt und Heimatsarchiv Zofingen; Staatsarchiv des Kantons Zürich; Zentralbibliothek Zürich. Past and present staff of the Institut für schweizerische Reformationsgeschichte and the Bullinger-Briefwechsel-Edition have supplied generous assistance (especially Christian Moser and Kurt Jakob Rüetschi). In the United States, I have been aided by the libraries of Aquinas College (special thanks to Jeanine Weber and Shellie Jeffries), Arizona State University, Calvin College (especially Paul Fields and Ryan Noppen), the University of Maryland, the University of Michigan, and the University of Virginia.

I also extend my thanks for the patient and generous assistance of Wim Janse, the Brill Series in Church History editor, as well as to Arjan van Dijk, Peter Buschman, Ivo Romein, and the Brill staff. I acknowledge the collegial assistance of my American copy editor Laura Bennett-Kimble who greatly enhanced the literary quality of the manuscript. I also thank Andrew Giguere for his work developing maps of Erastus's correspondence network. (It was not possible to reproduce the maps in this volume though they should appear on a website soon.) I extend my sincere appreciation to Monica Edison whose generous assistance was of great help in pushing Erastus out the door.

Marco Neumaier supplied illustrations of early modern Heidelberg on behalf of the University of Heidelberg for the volume. The Basel

Kunstmuseum also permitted the reproduction of the oil painting of Thomas Erastus by Tobias Stimmer.

I remain deeply appreciative of European friends who supplied the human connection that made this project so rewarding: Verena, Daniel, Martin, Stephan, and Thomas Baumann, Oliver Behre, Johannes and Barbara Müller, Rudolf and Heidi Westerheide, Hans-Dieter and Rosemary Eicker, Bianca Bielig, Ulrik Krener and Käthy Shaery. Finally thanks go to my wife and family for enduring Erastus for so long. It is to them that this Erastian excursus is dedicated.

Ashgate Press, Truman State University Press, and the Franz Steiner Verlag have granted permission to reprint portions of previously published articles here. The works in question are cited in full in the respective chapters.

ABBREVIATIONS

ADB	*Allgemeine Deutsche Biographie*. Leipzig, 1875–1912.
ARG	*Archiv für Reformationsgeschichte*
Basel UB	Öffentliche Bibliothek der Universität Basel
BBG	Basler Beiträge zur Geschichtswissenschaft
BGLRK	Beiträge zur Geschichte und Lehre der Reformierten Kirche
BL	British Library, London
BN	Biographie Nationale, L'Académie Royale des sciences, des lettres et des beaux arts de Belgique. Brussels, 1876.
B.Pal.	Bibliotheca Palatina. See *Bibliotheca Palatina* [Textband]. Ed. Elmar Mittler. Heidelberg: Editions Braus, 1986; Stevenson, Enrico, ed. *Inventario dei Libri Stampati Palatino-Vaticani*. 3 vols. Rome, 1886–1891.
BSB	Bayerische Staatsbibliothek, Munich. See *Bayerische Staatsbibliothek Alphabetischer Katalog 1501–1840*. Munich: K.G. Saur, 1987. www.bsb-muenchen.de/
CB	*Correspondance de Théodore de Bèze*. Ed. Hippolyte Aubert, et al. Geneva: Librairie Droz, 1960–.
CH	Church History
CO	*Ioannis Calvini Opera Quae Supersunt Omnia*. Corpus Reformatorum, vols. 29–87. Ed. Wilhelm Baum, Eduard Cunitz and Eduard Reuss. Brunswick and Berlin, 1863–1900.
CR	*Philippi Melanthonis Opera quae supersunt omnia*. Corpus Reformatorum, vols. 1–28. Ed. K.G. Bretschneider and H.E. Bindseil. Halle and Brunswick, 1834–1860.
DSB	*Dictionary of Scientific Biography*. Ed. Charles Coulston Gillispie. New York: Scribner, [1970–1980].
EKO	Sehling, Emil, ed. *Die evangelischen Kirchenordnungen des XVI. Jahrhunderts*. Band 14, Kurpfalz, [ed. J.F. Gerhard Goeters]. Tübingen: J.C.B. Mohr (Paul Siebeck), 1969.
Er UB	Universitätsbibliothek Erlangen
FVB	*French Vernacular Books: Books published in the French Language before 1601*. Ed. Andrew Pettegree, et al. Leiden: Brill, 2007.
GHA	Gemeinschaftliches Hennebergisches Archiv im Thüringisches Staatsarchiv Meiningen
HAB	Herzog-August-Bibliothek, Wolfenbüttel
Hd UB	Ruprecht-Karls-Universität Heidelberg, Universitätsbibliothek
Leiden UB	Leiden, Bibliotheek der Rijksuniversiteit
NDB	*Neue Deutsche Biographie*. Berlin, 1953–.
n.d.	No date

n.y.	No year
NHJ	*Neue Heidelberger Jahrbücher*
NLM	National Library of Medicine, History of Medicine Division. Cf. Richard J. Durling. *A Catalogue of Sixteenth Century Printed Books in the National Library of Medicine*. Bethesda, Md.: NLM, 1967.
n.p.	No place of publication listed
n.y.	No year of publication listed
OER	Hillerbrand, Hans J. ed. *The Oxford Encyclopedia of the Reformation*. New York: Oxford University Press, 1996.
PI	Paracelsus [Theophrastus von Hohenheim]. *Theophrast von Hohenheim gen. Paracelsus, Sämtliche Werke. I. Abteilung: Medizinische, naturwissenschaftliche und philosophische Schriften*. 14 vols. Ed. Karl Sudhoff. Munich and Berlin: Oldenbourg, 1922–1933.
SBB	Staatsbibliothek zu Berlin, Preußischer Kulturbesitz
SB	Staatsbibliothek
SBPF	Salzburger Beiträge zur Paracelsusforschung
SCE&S	Sixteenth Century Essays and Studies
SCJ	Sixteenth Century Journal
SMRT	Studies in Medieval and Reformation Thought
SUB Bremen	Staats- und Universitätsbibliothek Bremen
SVRG	Schriften des Vereins für Reformationsgeschichte
StAZ	Staatsarchiv des Kantons Zürich
THR	Travaux d'humanisme et renaissance
UAH	Universitätsarchiv Heidelberg
UB	Universitätsbibliothek
UP	University Press
STC	English Short Title Catalog. http://estc.bl.uk/
Tü UB	UniversitätsBibliothek, Tübingen
VD 16	*Verzeichnis der im deutschen Sprachbereich erschienenen Drucke des XVI. Jahrhunderts*. Stuttgart: Anton Hiersemann, 1983–1995. www.vd16.de/
VD 17	*Das Verzeichnis der im deutschen Sprachraum erschienenen Drucke des 17. Jahrhunderts*. http://www.vd17.de/
Wing	Donald Wing. *A Short-Title Catalogue of Books Printed in England, Scotland, Ireland, Wales, and British America, and of English Books Printed in Other Countries, 1641 to 1700*. Data available at: http://estc.bl.uk/
WLB	Württembergische Landesbibliothek Stuttgart
Z	*Huldreich Zwinglis sämtliche Werke*. Corpus Reformatorum, vols. 88–101. Ed. E. Egli, et al Leipzig: Verlag von Martin Henius Nachfolger, 1905–1968.
ZBRG	Zürcher Beiträge zur Reformationsgeschichte
ZBZ	Zentralbibliothek Zürich

INTRODUCTION

Thomas Erastus was arguably the most important Reformed natural philosopher of the late sixteenth century. With a few notable exceptions, however, modern scholars have not found Erastus an attractive figure. Though he made a significant theological contribution, the fact that he opposed Calvinist ideas of church discipline has generally banished him from the Reformed faith's pantheon of heroes.[1] Likewise, his opposition to the German Hippocrates, Paracelsus, has earned him an ignominious place in the history of medicine. Add to these sins the fact that Erastus upheld the validity of the death penalty for witches, and there is little for a positivistic historian to hope for from our subject.

While much of the attention that Erastus's career has garnered has been negative, historians have not ignored Erastus. Two excellent monographs, one in French and one in German, have investigated his theory of the proper relationship between magistrate and church, "Erastianism."[2] Though his scientific contribution has received less sustained analysis, it has attracted the attention of Walter Pagel, Owsei Temkin,

---

[1] While this process was already underway in Heinrich Alting's *Historia de ecclesiis Palatinis*, the best example of this phenomenon was Karl Sudhoff's *C. Olevianus und Z. Ursinus*. Sudhoff presented Zacharias Ursinus and Caspar Olevianus as the leaders of the Heidelberg Reformed movement and took a negative stance toward Erastus and the anti-disciplinists, casting them as a morally suspect lot. Karl Sudhoff, *C. Olevianus und Z. Ursinus, Leben und ausgewählte Schriften der Väter und Begründer der reformierten Kirche*, vol. 8 (Elberfeld: R.L. Friedrichs, 1857); Heinrich Alting, *Historia de ecclesiis Palatinis* (Amsterdam, 1644); reprint in Menso Alting, *Mensonis Altingii ... Vita descripta per Ubbonem Emmium* (Groningen, 1728). N.B.: All references to Alting's *Historia de ecclesiis Palatinis* are to the 1728 Groningen reprint. (I thank R.S. Clark for sharing this edition with me.) See also Walter Hollweg, *Heinrich Bullingers Hausbuch: Eine Untersuchung über die Anfänge der reformierten Predigtliteratur* [*BGLRK* 8] (Neukirchen-Vluyn: Verlag der Buchhandlung des Erziehungsvereins, 1956), 261.

[2] Ruth Wesel-Roth, *Thomas Erastus: Ein Beitrag zur Geschichte der reformierten Kirche und zur Lehre von der Staatssouveränität* [Veröffentlichungen des Vereins für Kirchengeschichte in der evang. Landeskirche Badens 15] (Lahr/Baden: Moritz Schauenberg, 1954); Auguste Bonnard, *Thomas Éraste (1524–1583) et la Discipline Thomas Ecclésiastique* (Lausanne, 1894). See also Robert C. Walton, "Der Streit zwischen Thomas Erastus und Caspar Olevian über die Kirchenzucht in der Kurpfalz in seiner Bedeutung für die internationale reformierte Bewegung," *Monatshefte für Evangelische Kirchengeschichte des Rheinlandes* 37–38 (1988–1989): 205–246. The origin and meaning of the term "Erastian" are discussed in chapter 5 and the epilogue.

and Lynn Thorndike, three of the greatest scholars of the history of science and medicine of the twentieth century.[3] While from time to time Erastus has been ignored in works in which one would have expected to find him, more often than not he has been remembered in reference works and historical overviews.[4] Being the eponymous father of Erastianism, however, has been a dubious honor; scholars have applied his name to movements and people who had little affinity with his own thought. While he has become a signpost in the field of church history, his inclusion in the *Dictionary of Scientific Biography* suggests that he has also achieved canonical status in the history of science. Thus, to suggest that Erastus has languished in obscurity would be misleading. He has not been forgotten.

In all of this attention, however, there has been one major defect. Since almost everything that has been written on Erastus has focused narrowly on one or another aspect of his career, the scholarly world does not know one Erastus but many competing and mutually contradictory visions of Erastus. On the one hand, Erastus has sometimes been hailed as a man ahead of his time. For example, analyzing Erastus from the perspective of his theory of church-state relations, J. Neville Figgis cast him as a sixteenth-century "Aufgeklärter," and more recently Robert Dàn characterized him as a "freethinker" on the basis on his heretical associations and his opposition to the Calvinist disciplinarians.[5] He has also won intermittent praise in the history of science; for example, John Brooke portrayed Erastus as a sixteenth-century forerunner of Francis

[3] Walter Pagel, *Paracelsus: An Introduction to Philosophical Medicine in the Era of the Renaissance*, 2nd ed. (Basel: Karger, 1982), 332; Owsei Temkin, *The Falling Sickness: A History of Epilepsy from the Greeks to the Beginning of Modern Neurology*, rev. ed. (Baltimore: Johns Hopkins UP, 1971), 184–202; idem, "Fernel, Joubert, and Erastus on the Specificity of Cathartic Drugs," in *Science, Medicine and Society in the Renaissance*, ed. Allen G. Debus (New York: Science History Publications, 1972), 1:61–68; Lynn Thorndike, *A History of Magic and Experimental Science*, 8 vols. (New York: Columbia UP, 1923–1958), 5:652–667. See also Eberhard Stübler, *Geschichte der medizinischen Fakultät der Universität Heidelberg 1386–1925* (Heidelberg: Carl Winter, 1926), 45; Allen G. Debus, *The Chemical Philosophy: Paracelsian Science and Medicine in the Sixteenth and Seventeenth Centuries*, 2 vols. (New York: Science History Publications, 1977).

[4] For example, there is no article on him in the *Theologische Realenzyklopädie* (*TRE*) (Berlin, 1977–1990) and no discussion of his theories of church-state relations in J.H. Burns, ed., *The Cambridge History of Political Thought, 1430–1700* (Cambridge: Cambridge UP, 1991).

[5] J. Neville Figgis, "Erastus and Erastianism," *Journal of Theological Studies* 2 (1901): 68; Robert Dán, *Mathias Vehe-Glirius: Life and Work of a Radical Antitrinitarian with his Collected Writings* [Studia Humanitatis 4] (Leiden: E.J. Brill; Budapest: Akadémiai Kiadó, 1982), 14.

Bacon.[6] On the other hand, Erastus has also been characterized as a narrow-minded scholastic who was the opponent of nearly every positive intellectual trend of the sixteenth century, namely those represented by Paracelsus, Johann Weyer, and Petrus Ramus.[7] My goal has been to replace the multiple and often competing versions of Erastus in the historiography with a more unified, intelligible portrayal of Erastus; in short, to move from many Erastuses to one. I endeavor to do this by analyzing Erastus's career in the light of the Heidelberg context and by tracking salient themes across his written corpus.

The chief goal of this study is to present a coherent narrative of Erastus's life and work during his time in Heidelberg; put simply, how Erastus shaped the Heidelberg Reformation and the history of the German Reformed movement, and how his own work was in turn influenced by his times, struggles, enemies, and friends. While in Heidelberg, Erastus rarely experienced the tranquility of proverbial ivory tower isolation, and when he did, the results were not necessarily salutary. During the 1560s, as one of the fathers, if not the central ringleader, of the Palatine Reformed movement, he was blown from one theological controversy to another. His theological acumen and political skill helped him win Frederick III and the Palatinate for the Reformed cause and carried him to heights of influence. With his work on the church council and with his vernacular theological treatises, he had a decisive influence on the development of the Palatine Reformed Church—including a prominent role in the authorship of the Heidelberg Catechism. In the second half of the 1560s, Erastus went from the position of insider to dissenter by championing the resistance to the Calvinist-led effort to establish a church consistory, independent from state control, to control moral life. With the victory of his Calvinist rivals and the humiliation of his antidisciplinist partisans in an Antitrinitarian scandal, Erastus lost political clout in the Palatinate. Erastus's public humiliation and exile from church politics proved the watershed event of his career. Now forcibly silenced in the theological arena, Erastus would concentrate his efforts on

[6] John Hedley Brooke, *Science and Religion: Some Historical Perspectives* (Cambridge: Cambridge UP, 1991), 71. D.P. Walker also suggested this connection. D.P. Walker, *Spiritual and Demonic Magic from Ficino to Campanella* (London: Warburg Institute, 1958), 158.

[7] Johann Karcher, "Thomas Erastus (1524–1583), der unversöhnliche Gegner des Theophrastus Paracelsus," *Gesnerus* 14 (1957): 1–13. Thorndike, while favoring Erastus over the Paracelsians, likewise had little positive to say for Erastus. Thorndike, *History of Magic and Experimental Science*, 5:652–667.

natural philosophical pursuits. After 1570, his academic publishing career gained new momentum, weight, and acerbity. Upon the death of Frederick III in 1576, Erastus enjoyed a brief but frustrating return to favor in Heidelberg under the Lutheran Elector Ludwig VI, which lasted until 1580. Then, at the time of the adoption of the *Formula of Concord* in Heidelberg, Erastus moved to Basel, where he died in 1583.

This study focuses on the years from 1558 to 1580 when Erastus was a member of the faculty of the University of Heidelberg. The narrative that his surviving letters tell is primarily of an ecclesio-political struggle in Heidelberg. Although this is the best known of the many potential Erastus narratives, it has received little prior attention in English language scholarship. This study crosses disciplinary boundaries and turns over new ground, particularly in the setting of Erastus's anti-Paracelsianism and his controversy with Johann Weyer over the punishment of witches. Because Erastus's surviving correspondence illuminates the theological side of his career more thoroughly, I have chosen to focus primarily on the religious dimensions of the later controversies. This limiting strategy no doubt introduces a certain distortion of Erastus's larger worldview by the material I have chosen to cover in depth and, more significantly, by all that due to necessity has been left out.

Sources

This study is based chiefly on Erastus's correspondence and his printed works. Standing on the shoulders of Auguste Bonnard, Ruth Wesel-Roth, and Gustav Adolf Benrath, and with the help of Wim Janse and the editors of Heinrich Bullinger's correspondence, I have been able to construct a database of some five hundred letters of Erastus, the vast majority of which have not been printed (see Correspondence Register). While earlier studies drew heavily on Erastus's letters to Heinrich Bullinger and Johann Jakob Grynaeus, I have expanded this source base with use of Erastus's letters to Joachim Camerarius II, Rudolf Gwalther, Albert Hardenberg, Konrad Pellikan, Josias Simmler, Konrad Ulmer, and Theodor Zwinger. In the selections from Erastus's correspondence and other sources that follow in the footnotes, illegible or damaged spots in the manuscripts are denoted by brackets without text. In other cases, brackets are used to indicate plausible interpolations or to fill out conventional Latin abbreviations. It is my hope to make these transcriptions available to other scholars by means of a Website devoted to the correspondence of the Heidelberg Reformation. Likewise, I have had access to all of Erastus's printed works and to the works of the many early modern figures who engaged Erastus, though they are not all treated in detail here.

Much source material for Palatine history did not survive the multiple depredations of the Thirty Years' War or the wanton destruction by Louis XIV's armies.[8] A particular deficit exists in the church records from the era of the Reformation, which, when they do exist, are often divided among the many successor states of the Palatinate. Fortunately for this study, the most critical surviving church records concerning the Antitrinitarian affair were published by Hans Rott. After the Palatine Wittelsbachs inherited the throne of the duchy of Bavaria, the political records of the Palatine Wittelsbachs were removed to Munich; these records survive in the *Geheimes Staatsarchiv*. Since these sources do not directly concern Erastus's career and since Volker Press studied these records exhaustively, these sources have not been directly consulted in preparing this study. The archive of the University of Heidelberg preserves the records of the university senate from the late sixteenth century. These protocols, which document faculty appointments and remuneration and shed light on the various controversies between the court and the university, were of inestimable value. These named sources, along with other standard printed records from the period, make up the bulk of this study's source base.

Names

In general, I have sought to render the names of individuals and places in each subject's native language (e.g., "Ottheinrich" and "Girolamo Zanchi" as opposed to "Otto Henry" and "Jerome Zanchi" or "Hieronymus Zanchius"). When such figures are so well known as to have a common English language rendering of their name, however, I use the accepted form (e.g., John Calvin; Frederick III the Pious). I also break the rule of favoring the vernacular spellings when uncertain of the person's name in their original language (e.g., lesser known faculty of the University of Heidelberg) or in such cases where the person's nationality is debatable (particularly with Eastern Europeans and Netherlanders). In these cases, I have adopted the Latin spelling.

[8] See Henry J. Cohn, *The Government of the Rhine Palatinate in the Fifteenth Century* (Oxford: Oxford UP, 1965), 251–255.

CHAPTER ONE

PROLOGUE

The Palatinate before Erastus

Origins and Structure of the Palatinate

The Electoral Palatinate (*Kurpfalz*) was a German territory on the upper Rhine whose domains were clustered around Heidelberg and Mannheim. The Palatinate enjoyed a limited run on the stage of German history since it only emerged as a territorial unit in the high Middle Ages and it would be later dissolved into several neighboring territories in the imperial recess (*Reichsdeputationshauptschluß*) of 1803. There was some discussion of reviving the Kurpfalz after the Second World War, and the more recent mooting of combining Baden-Württemberg with Rheinland-Pfalz would at least present the opportunity for a possible reunion of the Palatine lands on the right and left of banks the Rhine.[1]

In the sixteenth century, the Palatinate was one of the leading states of the Holy Roman Empire in prestige, but not in actual power.[2] Its ruler,

[1] See Gerd Hepp, "Wiederherstellung der alten Kurpfalz? Zur Frage der Revision der Ländergrenzen im deutschen Südwesten zwischen 1945 und 1956," in *Zeitschrift für die Geschichte des Oberrheins* 137 (1989): 414–427.

[2] For simplicity in this work, "Palatinate" will denote the Electoral Palatinate (*Kurpfalz*), the territories ruled over by the elector palatine including both the Lower and Upper Palatinate. For the general contours of Palatine history, see Henry J. Cohn, *The Government of the Rhine Palatinate in the Fifteenth Century*; idem, "Territorial Princes in Germany's Second Reformation, 1559–1622," in *International Calvinism 1541–1715*, ed. Menna Preswich (Oxford: Oxford UP, 1985), 135–166; Charles D. Gunnoe Jr., "The Reformation of the Palatinate and the Origins of the Heidelberg Catechism, 1500–1562" in *An Introduction to the Heidelberg Catechism: Sources, History, and Theology*, Lyle D. Bierma et al. (Grand Rapids: Baker, 2005), 15–47; Volker Press, *Calvinismus und Territorialstaat: Regierung und Zentralbehorden der Kurpfalz 1559–1619* [Kieler Historische Studien 7] (Stuttgart: Ernst Klett Verlag, 1970); idem, "Die 'Zweite Reformation' in der Kurpfalz," in *Die reformierte Konfessionalisierung in Deutschland* [*SVRG* 195], ed. Heinz Schilling (Gutersloh, 1986) 104–129; Meinrad Schaab, *Geschichte der Kurpfalz*, 2 vols. (Stuttgart: Kohlhammer, 1988, 1992); Anton Schindling and Walter Ziegler, "Kurpfalz, Rheinische Pfalz und Oberpfalz," in *Die Territorien des Reichs im Zeitalter der Reformation und Konfessionalisierung: Land und Konfession 1500–1650*, vol. 5, Der Südwesten, ed. Anton Schindling and Walter Ziegler (Münster: Aschendorff, 1993), 8–49; Eike Wolgast, *Die*

the elector palatine, belonged to the highest echelon of princes in the imperial constitution as one of the seven electors (*Kurfürsten*) who had the right to cast a vote for the emperor.

The Palatinate was a rather artificial conglomeration of territories; indeed, many of the city districts of modern Heidelberg were not originally subjects of the elector palatine. The state was a political-dynastic construct, and not based on any ethnic, linguistic, or geographic principle. Likewise, it was not one of the German duchies associated with the settlement of an early Germanic tribe. The Palatinate's territorial incoherence was due to the fact that it was a state that had emerged around an office, rather than being a traditional county or duchy. The title, "count palatine" (Latin, *comes palatinus*; German, *Pfalzgraf*) preceded the Palatinate's territorial formation.

In the early Middle Ages, a count palatine had been an office of the Merovingian kingdom. While once there were four such counts, only the count palatine of Lorraine continued to employ this title into the high Middle Ages. In the twelfth century the count palatine of Lorraine established a territorial base along the upper Rhine and became the *Pfalzgraf bei Rhein*. In the thirteenth century, the *Pfalzgraf bei Rhein* gained both the privilege of participating in imperial elections and the ceremonial dignity of imperial steward (*Erztruchseß*). As imperial vicar (*Reichsvikar*), the elector palatine filled the emperor's role in the case of a vacancy of office.

After passing through the hands of the Hohenstaufens (1142–1195) and Welfs (1195–1213), the Wittelsbach dynasty, rulers of Bavaria, acquired the Palatinate in 1214 in the form of a grant from Emperor Frederick II. In the late Middle Ages, the Wittelsbachs were one of the leading houses of the empire, alongside the Luxemburgs and the Habsburgs, frequently putting up candidates for imperial election. Rivalries between the various branches of the Wittelsbach family, however, undermined their opportunity to achieve the dominant position of the aforementioned dynasties.

The Treaty of Pavia (1329) gave the count palatine control of the north Bavarian territory known as the Upper Palatinate (*Oberpfalz*), thus establishing the classic territorial configuration of the Palatinate in the late medieval period. The Golden Bull of Charles IV (1356) confirmed the

Universität Heidelberg 1386–1986 (Berlin: Springer, 1986); idem, *Reformierte Konfession und Politik im 16. Jahrhundert: Studien zur Geschichte der Kurpfalz im Reformationszeitalter* (Heidelberg: Universitätsverlag C. Winter, 1998).

count palatine's right to vote in imperial elections and nominally recognized the elector palatine as the first secular prince of the empire. The Golden Bull's provision that the elector's core territories were not partible gave the Palatinate a legal territorial unity independent from personal overlordship of the count palatine for the first time in the state's history.[3]

The most glorious moment in the history of the Palatine Wittelsbachs occurred with the election of Elector Ruprecht III to the office of king of the Romans in 1400. He served as sovereign of the empire until 1410 without being crowned emperor by the pope. The limited demographic and material resources of the Palatinate handcuffed Ruprecht's effectiveness in the imperial office and undermined the Palatine Wittelsbachs' opportunity to keep the imperial title in their dynasty.

In the fifteenth century, while the nucleus of the Palatine lands around Heidelberg remained in the elector's possession, others were divided among the count palatine's heirs, giving birth to the smaller states Pfalz-Mosbach, Pfalz-Neumarkt, Pfalz-Zweibrücken, Pfalz-Simmern, and later Pfalz-Veldenz, thus named for their residence cities.[4] The leaders of these cadet branches were also entitled to style themselves "counts palatine," while only the ruler of the Electoral Palatinate bore the more distinguished title "elector palatine."[5] After the Bavarian Succession War, a new state, Pfalz-Neuburg, was created primarily from Bavarian Wittelsbach lands.[6] Additional collateral lines such as Pfalz-Lautern and Pfalz-Sulzbach were spawned in the course of the sixteenth century.[7]

---

[3] Schaab, *Geschichte der Kurpfalz*, 1:96.

[4] Schaab, *Geschichte der Kurpfalz*, 1:145–160; Cohn, *The Government of the Rhine Palatinate*, 6–7. Simmern and Zweibrücken were originally one line which later split into two separate houses in 1453. Pfalz-Neumarkt and Pfalz-Mosbach returned to the domain of the Electoral Palatinate in 1499.

[5] The title holder actually bore the fuller designation (linked to the family's Bavarian heritage): "count palatine on the Rhine and duke in Bavaria." Cohn, *The Government of the Rhine Palatinate*, 7.

[6] This principality, which was a miniscule remnant of the former duchy of Bayern-Landshut, along with some lands from Bayern-München and the Oberpfalz, bore the title Pfalz-Neuburg, as its original rulers were from the Palatine Wittelsbach line in Heidelberg. Elizabeth von Bayern-Landshut, daughter and sole heir of the last duke of Bayern-Landshut, Georg der Reiche (1479–1503), married Ruprecht of the Palatinate, the third son of Elector Philipp der Aufrichtige (1476–1508). Their attempt to win the inheritance of Bayern-Landshut failed in the Bavarian War of Succession. While both husband and wife died in 1504, the new principality was carved out of Bayern-Landshut in the peace settlement as a compensation for their sons Philipp and Ottheinrich. Thus, Pfalz-Neuburg was a principality ruled by a branch of the Palatine Wittelsbach line detached from Bavarian Wittelsbach territory.

[7] To follow these complicated developments, see Schaab's excellent tables in *Geschichte der Kurpfalz*, 1:220–225 and 2:253–255.

In the sixteenth century, the Palatinate was made up of two territorial blocs: the Lower Palatinate (*Unterpfalz*)—the domains along the Rhine and Neckar rivers containing the districts of Alzey, Germersheim, Kaiserslautern, Heidelberg, and Neustadt—and the Upper Palatinate (*Oberpfalz*)—a territory in northern Bavaria bordering Bohemia with its administrative center in Neumarkt and later Amberg.[8]

The Lower Palatinate was in a region of particularly scattered lordship: the Palatine territories lay jumbled in a rather haphazard fashion alongside the lands of the nearby bishoprics of Worms and Speyer. Despite the fact that he was a relative latecomer to the region and that he even held most of his lands as fiefs from the local ecclesiastical lords, the elector palatine became the most powerful ruler in the vicinity and utilized claims of dominion over the Rhine and Neckar and the right of safe conduct (*Geleit*) on the regional highways to extend his dominion.[9] Indeed, in the early sixteenth century the bishoprics of Worms and Speyer could fairly be called satellites of the Palatinate. The Lower Palatinate remained something of an atypical territorial state, especially as it did not possess an assembly of estates. Most of the local nobility were free imperial knights, not direct vassals of the elector palatine, though members of these families often sought appointments at the Heidelberg court. When the elector desired a new tax, his administration negotiated directly with the individual towns. In the late sixteenth century, the militant commitment to the Reformed confession of the electors alienated much of the regional nobility, but a new bourgeois elite consisting of pastors and administrators would step into their place. Likewise, the move toward the Reformed faith would undermine the traditional Palatine satellite system.[10]

Unlike the Lower Palatinate, the Upper Palatinate was a more typical enclosed territorial state with a tradition of an assembly to represent the district's estates. On many occasions the elector's heir apparent would fill the post of governor (*Statthalter*) of the territory. Though the Upper Palatinate was considered an integral part of the elector's domains, at times the elector had difficulty imposing his will on it, par-

[8] The administration was moved from Neumarkt to Amberg in 1544. Volker Press, "Die Grundlagen der kurpfälzischen Herrschaft in der Oberpfalz 1499–1621," in *Verhandlungen des Historischen Vereins für Oberpfalz und Regensburg* (Regensburg: Verlag des Historischen Vereins, 1977), 43.

[9] Cohn, *The Government of the Rhine Palatinate*, 121.

[10] Press, "Die 'Zweite Reformation' in der Kurpfalz," 115–116; Schaab, *Geschichte der Kurpfalz*, 2:81.

ticularly in questions of religious policy. The Upper Palatinate remained a haven for Melanchthonian Lutheranism until the end of the sixteenth century.[11]

The Palatinate possessed bureaucratic machinery roughly similar to that of many sixteenth-century states. The key executive body was the high council (*Oberrat*), which generally met daily and worked in close cooperation with the elector—that is, if he was not off hunting, as was frequently the case with electors such as Frederick IV. Majority decisions of this body, with the elector's assent, established state policy. The procedural rules of the *Oberrat*, which had evolved over the previous decades, were codified in 1557. While individuals may have been called "privy councilor" (*Geheimrat*) on occasion, there is no evidence to suggest a privy council as such existed separately from the high council.[12] The highest officials of the Palatine government were the chief steward (*Großhofmeister*), the chancellor (*Kanzler*), and the marshal (*Marschall*). The "supreme court" of the Palatinate was the *Hofgericht*, and since the Palatine court possessed the privilege *de non appellando* according to the Golden Bull, external courts had strictly limited jurisdiction over subjects of the elector palatine. As parties outside of the elector's jurisdiction sometimes lodged cases in the Palatine *Hofgericht*, the court was another means of enhancing the elector's regional hegemony.

The economy of the Lower Palatinate was largely agrarian, though the territory was moderately urbanized by sixteenth-century standards. The fertile Rhine plane was the territory's most productive granary, although its comparatively dense population level held the standard of living of its residents in check. The Palatinate also possessed viniculture along the mountainous fringes of both sides of the Rhine valley.[13] Meinrad Schaab has estimated that the entire population of the Lower Palatinate numbered 180,000 in 1577.[14] This compared to a population of ca. 80,000 for the Upper Palatinate. Approximately twenty-nine percent of the population of the Lower Palatinate lived in cities, the largest of

[11] Press, "Die Grundlagen der kurpfälzischen Herrschaft in der Oberpfalz," 31–67.

[12] Press, *Calvinismus und Territorialstaat*, 34–36.

[13] Schaab, *Geschichte der Kurpfalz*, 2:97.

[14] This number includes the population of both Pfalz-Lautern and Pfalz-Simmern. Cohn has suggested that the population of the Palatinate in 1503 was closer to 200,000 than 100,000. This estimate would appear to be in basic harmony with Schaab's estimates. In 1439 the population of the city of Heidelberg was ca. 5,000, with its administrative district numbering ca. 21,000 occupants. Cohn, *The Government of the Rhine Palatinate*, 4; Schaab, *Geschichte der Kurpfalz*, 2:95–98.

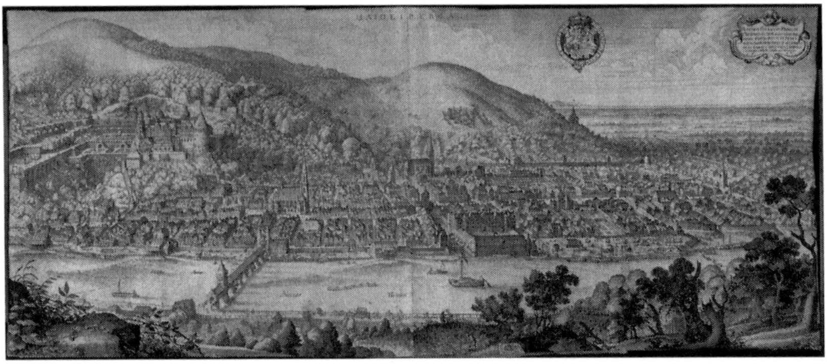

Engraving of Heidelberg by Matthaeus Merian, 1620.

which was far and away Heidelberg, with a population of approximately 7,000 residents in the late sixteenth century.[15] Konrad von Staufen, the brother of Frederick I. Barbarossa, founded a castle at the site of Heidelberg, and by the twelfth century a town had emerged in its vicinity as well. Heidelberg served as the administrative headquarters of the Palatinate until the Wittelsbachs moved their chief residence to Mannheim in 1720.[16] Its location on both east-west and north-south roads, as well as its position on the navigable Neckar with easy access to the Rhine, facilitated Heidelberg's commercial importance. However, Heidelberg could not be reckoned among the economic heavyweights of Southern Germany, like Augsburg and Nuremberg. The north-south road figured more prominently in Palatine trade than the east-west route, linking Heidelberg with Frankfurt and her fairs to the north as well as to Strasbourg and Basel farther up the Rhine.[17]

As the home to the third oldest university in the empire and, according to modern boundaries, the oldest university in Germany, Heidelberg has long possessed an intellectual standing far exceeding its political and economic status. Elector Ruprecht I founded the university in 1386 after the Great Schism made study in Paris unpalatable for students from the Holy Roman Empire who were loyal to the Roman pontiff.

[15] Schaab, *Geschichte der Kurpfalz*, 2:98, 223. The Heidelberg "suburbs" (especially Weinheim) were among the other larger settlements of the territory. Amberg, with a population numbering ca. 4,000, was the largest city in the Oberpfalz and the second largest city in the entire Kurpfalz.

[16] The Heidelberger Schloß had been turned into a ruin by the armies of Louis XIV in 1689 and 1692. Schaab, *Geschichte der Kurpfalz*, 2:151–153, 174.

[17] Schaab, *Geschichte der Kurpfalz*, 1:57; 2:81–108, passim.

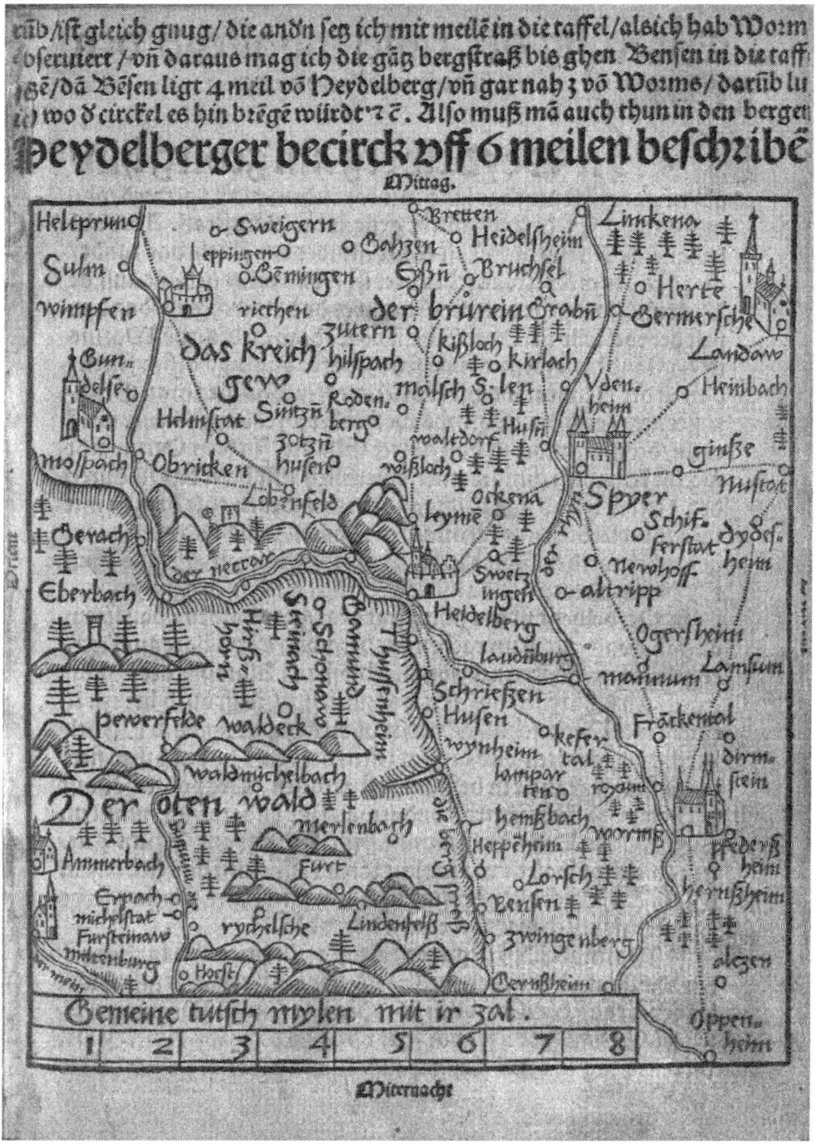

Heydelberger becirck uff 6 meilen beschribe[n], from in Sebastian Münster, *Erklerung des newen Jnstruments der Sunnen, nach allen seinen Scheyben und Circkeln*, Oppenheim 1528.

The electors were also noteworthy for being the most important patrons of early humanism in Germany. Late medieval Heidelberg reached its cultural apogee in the last decades of the fifteenth century, with the electoral court serving as a base for humanists such as Jacob Wimpfeling, Johann von Dalberg, Rudolf Agricola, Johannes Reuchlin, Johannes Trithemius, and Conrad Celtis.[18] The presence of such luminaries made Heidelberg, according to Henry Cohn, "the paramount center in Germany for humanist activities between 1484 and the end of the century."[19] The impact of this humanist circle on the university was ambivalent. On the one hand, Cohn has suggested that the university was not resistant to humanist impulses and noted that humanists like Wimpfeling also taught at the university.[20] On the other hand, Eike Wolgast has concluded that this early phase of humanism passed without making a lasting impression on the style or content of teaching at the university.[21]

The fifteenth and early sixteenth centuries also witnessed important Gothic and Renaissance building in the Palatinate, including the *Heiliggeistkirche* (1348–1544) and major additions to the Heidelberg castle, the apex of which was the *Ottheinrichs Bau*, whose ruin stands as a great example of German Renaissance architecture. The political decline of Heidelberg in the early years of the sixteenth century brought a concomitant decline in intellectual and cultural life. Only later during the reign of the openhanded Elector Ottheinrich (r. 1556–1559) would Palatine intellectual and cultural life begin to approach its former glory.

Ludwig V and Frederick II

The late fifteenth century witnessed the apogee both of Palatine cultural achievement and political influence. It was a time of territorial aggrandizement as Frederick the Victorious (1449–1476, Friedrich I *der Siegreiche*) made a play to become a dominant power in Southern Germany. The defeat of the Palatinate, however, in the *Landshuter Krieg* (Bavarian Succession War, 1503–1504) set a limit on Palatine territorial expansion. As the sixteenth century opened, the Palatinate was not in a position to take a leading role in the political affairs of the empire.

When Martin Luther posted his "Ninety-Five Theses" in 1517, Elector Ludwig V (1508–1544), together with his brother Frederick II, who served as governor in the Upper Palatinate, ruled the Palatinate. The Pala-

[18] Henry J. Cohn, "The Early Renaissance Court in Heidelberg," *European Studies Review* 1 (1971): 295–322.

[19] Cohn, "The Early Renaissance Court in Heidelberg," 312.

[20] Cohn, "The Early Renaissance Court in Heidelberg," 302–303.

[21] Wolgast, *Die Universität Heidelberg*, 23.

tine Wittelsbachs enjoyed close personal relations with the Habsburg family at this juncture and demonstrated their loyalty by supporting Charles V's imperial election in 1519. Charles rewarded Ludwig by confirming the Palatinate's extra-territorial privileges. Their threatened position in the empire, living in competition with the neighboring prince-bishops while simultaneously warding off their Bavarian relatives who were envious of the Palatinate's right to vote in the imperial elections, was a leading factor behind the electors' ambivalent reaction to the Reformation during the first half of the sixteenth century.[22] Ludwig enjoyed a measure of success in reinvigorating the Palatine satellite system, and by 1529 he had been able to place his brothers in the episcopal sees of Speyer and Worms. Although Luther made a significant impression on a number of young Upper German humanists at the Heidelberg Disputation (1518), and thus had a lasting impact on Upper German Protestantism, Luther's appearance bore little immediate fruit in the Palatinate itself. Ludwig took part in the famous Diet of Worms, but did not vote to place Luther under the imperial ban due to Ludwig's close tie to the Saxon Elector Frederick the Wise.[23]

While Ludwig's early reaction to the Reformation was noncommittal, he began to move into the anti-Protestant camp after having to take up arms to suppress both the Knights' Revolt (1523) and the Peasants' War (1525). Ludwig took the Knights' Revolt personally, since it was led by his own former councilor Franz von Sickingen, and Ludwig took part in besieging Sickingen's castle. The Peasants' War proved an even more serious threat to the Southwestern German princes. The south German "Twelve Articles" served as the program of the social revolutionaries who aspired to remake society according to "God's law." In one of his finest moments, Ludwig acted decisively to disband the hordes that rose on Palatine territory, primarily on the left bank of the Rhine. This rising was noteworthy in that it was ended by a feast thrown by the elector

[22] The rarely amicable relations between the Wittelsbach dynasties are charted in Volker Press, "Bayerns wittelsbachische Gegenspieler—Die Heidelberger Kurfürsten 1505–1685," in *Um Glauben und Reich: Kurfürst Maximilian I.*, ed. Hubert Glaser (Munich: Hirmer Verlag, 1980), 24–48.

[23] Wolfgang Eger, "Kurfürst Ludwig V. der Friedfertige (von Wittelsbach), Pfalzgraf bei Rhein," in *Der Reichstag zu Worms von 1521: Reichspolitik und Luthersache* (Worms, 1971), 352–368. See also Walter Müller, *Die Stellung der Kurpfalz zur lutherischen Bewegung von 1517 bis 1525* (Heidelberg: Carl Winter's Universitätsbuchhandlung, 1937). For the early reception of Protestant ideas in the Palatinate and environs, see Walter Henss, "Frühe Spuren der Reformation in der Kurpfalz," *Blätter für pfälzische Kirchengeschichte und religiöse Volkskunde* 50 (1983): 5–42.

rather than by mass bloodshed. On another occasion, other peasants rose to put down the rebellion.[24] After quashing the revolt at home largely by peaceful means, the elector's forces also took part in suppressing the revolt in the bishoprics of Speyer and Würzburg.

While these experiences strengthened Ludwig's public identification with the Catholic cause, he never became a zealous anti-Protestant partisan. Rather, he sought to play a mediating role between the increasingly antagonistic Protestant and Catholic factions in imperial politics. While maintaining official adherence to Catholicism, Protestantism put down extensive roots in Palatine territory. A host of distinguished Protestants lectured at the university in the 1520s, including Theobald Billicanus, Johannes Brenz, and Martin Frecht.[25] However, by the end of the decade, most of the prominent Protestants had moved on to other posts. The university suffered both from low salaries and competition from the emerging Protestant universities in Wittenberg, Marburg, and Tübingen, which drew away students. Nevertheless, numerous evangelical pastors worked in Palatine parishes during Ludwig's reign. The papal nuncio Peter Paul Vergerio considered the region surrounding Heidelberg to be "one of the most Lutheran in Germany."[26] This ambiguous situation—official Catholicism with wide tolerance of Protestants—is perhaps best reflected in the career of Heinrich Stoll, a conciliatory Protestant minister who maintained the favor of the Wittelsbach family, attended the second session of the Council of Trent, and survived long enough to experience the formal adherence of the Palatinate to the evangelical confession in the 1540s.[27]

The Palatinate briefly became an officially Protestant territory during the reign of Ludwig's starry-eyed brother Frederick II (1544–1556). Frederick made the confession public in the Lower Palatinate by authorizing the Lutheran celebration of the Eucharist and by allowing priests to publicly marry. The Church Order (1546) codified these changes. This commitment was not a new development for Frederick, since he already had moved toward Protestantism while governor of the Upper Palatinate in Amberg, where he called Lutheran preachers and celebrated commu-

[24] Schaab, *Geschichte der Kurpfalz*, 2:17–18. See also Günther Franz, *Der deutsche Bauernkrieg*, 11th ed. (Darmstadt, 1984).

[25] Wolgast, *Die Universität Heidelberg*, 26; Press, *Calvinismus und Territorialstaat*, 174.

[26] Wolgast, *Reformierte Konfession und Politik im 16. Jahrhundert*, 18.

[27] Gustav Adolf Benrath, "Heinrich Stoll (Stolo) aus Diebach (1489 bis 1557), Pfarrer und Professor in Heidelberg," *Monatshefte für Evangelische Kirchengeschichte des Rheinlandes* 16 (1967): 273–285.

nion in both kinds. Both Frederick and his nephew and heir Ottheinrich communicated with Martin Bucer, and Bucer advised the Heidelberg reform movement at crucial junctures.[28] Frederick II's passion for political and dynastic intrigue exceeded his religious devotion, though his various schemes, which included attempts to win the hand of a Habsburg princess and claim the Danish throne, produced little fruit. He was fundamentally trapped between his lifelong bond with the Habsburgs and his rather tenuous, if genuine, commitment to the Protestant faith.

The Schmalkaldic War (1546) ended the first round of the Palatinate's experiment with a state-sponsored Lutheran Reformation, though the setback was only temporary. As a close ally of Charles V and something of an outsider among the leaders of the Protestant Schmalkaldic league, Frederick's loyalties were severely strained in the conflict, and the Electoral Palatinate took only the limited step of supplying a small cohort to aid the defense of their regional ally Duke Ulrich of Württemberg. The defeat of the Protestant forces in the Schmalkaldic War—without significant involvement of the Palatinate—nevertheless brought imperial wrath down on the Palatine Wittelsbachs. Spanish troops sacked Neuburg, the residence of the future Elector Ottheinrich, and restored his territory (Pfalz-Neuburg) to the Catholic faith.[29] While Ottheinrich endured defeat with equanimity, Frederick submitted to his lord lest he be deprived of his lands and titles as well. This included a distasteful scene in which the Emperor Charles berated Frederick, a boyhood friend of his father Philip the Fair and former military leader of the imperial forces in Hungary, for his disloyalty. Unwilling to risk incurring Charles's wrath again, Frederick dutifully imposed the conditions of the Interim (1548) on his territories, which included the reintroduction of Catholic services, though the Interim conceded the cup to the laity and clerical marriage as a provisional compromise. While the imperial defeat in the Princes' Revolt (1552) allowed Protestant territorial lords to determine the religion of their territories once again, Frederick remained cautious and did not officially restore Protestantism.[30]

Unfortunately, we do not possess adequate sources to track the progress of the Reformation in the parishes under Frederick II. Hans Rott has

[28] Hans Rott, *Friedrich II. von der Pfalz und die Reformation* (Heidelberg: Carl Winter's Universitätsbuchhandlung, 1904), 56–57, 142–150.

[29] Schaab, *Geschichte der Kurpfalz*, 2:26.

[30] See Adolf Hasenclever, *Die kurpfälische Politik in den Zeiten des schmalkaldischen Krieges (Januar 1546 bis Januar 1547)* (Heidelberg: Carl Winter's Universitätsbuchhandlung, 1905); Albrecht Pius Luttenberger, *Glaubenseinheit und Reichsfriede: Konzeptionen*

suggested through his investigation of the district of Germersheim that pastoral turnover as a result of the Interim likely was not heavy; many of the evangelical pastors who flourished under Frederick II still held the same positions during the reign of Ottheinrich. Likewise, the majority of Frederick II's civil servants were Protestants. These individuals provided another avenue for the survival of Protestant religious life in the outlying parishes through their halfhearted implementation of the Interim's injunctions.[31] Between Ludwig V's only marginal commitment to the old faith and his tolerance for evangelicals in his territory and Frederick II's timid embrace of the Reformation and even less committed compliance with the Interim, the Protestant movement had been able to put down extensive roots in the Palatinate. It is therefore more accurate to speak of the continuous progression of Protestantism rather than an absolute new beginning under Ottheinrich. Likewise, the popularity of the peasants' uprising in the countryside along with the enthusiastic reception of the evangelical message in the cities and among the Palatine bureaucracy suggests that the populace of the Palatinate eagerly supported the Reformation more than the princes ever did. Though the evidence is perhaps thin, it may not be premature to speak of the success of the "Reformation from below" in the case of the Palatinate.

Ottheinrich

After the false start under Frederick II, the Reformation came in earnest to the Palatinate with the ascension of the Elector Ottheinrich in 1556. The colorful Ottheinrich has passed into history as a prime example of a German Renaissance prince; he patronized the arts, built a lavish new wing on the Heidelberg Castle, sponsored alchemical experiments, and happily collected books and manuscripts. Ottheinrich was also the first elector palatine with an uncompromising commitment to the Protestant faith. Before his accession to the electoral office, Ottheinrich had ruled Pfalz-Neuburg, a poor rump of his ancestor Georg the Rich's lower Bavarian patrimony, and introduced Lutheranism into his small territory in the early 1540s. Ottheinrich's expensive tastes had led to financial ruin and the territorial estates forced him into exile in 1544 with

und Wege konfessionsneutraler Reichspolitik 1530–1552 (Kurpfalz, Jülich, Kurbrandenburg) [Schriftenreihe der Historischen Kommission bei der Bayerischen Akademie der Wissenschaften 20] (Göttingen: Vandenhoek & Ruprecht, 1982).

[31] Rott, *Friedrich II*, 124–125.

a carrot: the estates agreed to assume his debts if he would depart. He took up residence near Heidelberg at that point and waited to claim his more lucrative inheritance. Although he possessed unquestioned Protestant convictions, it has been a commonplace observation that Ottheinrich was not acquainted with the finer points of theology—especially in comparison to his Bible-reading successor Frederick III. This theological naïveté did not deter his political espousal of the evangelical cause, and during his reign the Palatinate first emerged as a leading Protestant power on the imperial stage. The Palatine Reformation under Ottheinrich possessed a distinctive Upper German flavor. Württemberg's church order, composed by Johannes Brenz, and Melanchthon's *Examen Ordinandorum* strongly influenced the Palatine *Kirchenordnung* of 1556.[32] Brenz's *Landescatechismus* and Luther's *Small Catechism* were used until the adoption of the Heidelberg Catechism in 1563. Johann Marbach, the Lutheran president of the Strasbourg church conventicle, headed the first systematic visitation of the Palatine church and issued a list of recommendations for advancing Evangelical doctrine and practice.[33] Although Ottheinrich attempted to win Marbach for the Heidelberg church on two occasions, Marbach refused the invitation, citing his commitment to Strasbourg. Another characteristic of Ottheinrich's Reformation that mirrored the Upper German tradition was state-mandated iconoclasm. Here the image of Ottheinrich the art patron conflicts with his reputation as a reformer. His love of art and monuments aside—he even left instructions for the dusting of his own memorial—Ottheinrich was adamant in his desire to deliver the common folk from idolatry. In the three short years of his reign, Ottheinrich's officials largely cleared the Palatinate of the material artifacts of late medieval piety.[34]

[32] Printed in *EKO*, 14:113–220. See J.F.G. Goeter's introduction to the same, in which he discusses the various theories that have been entertained regarding the antecedents of the 1556 Church Order (pp. 23–26). See also Bard Thompson, "The Palatinate Church Order of 1563," *Church History* 23 (1954): 339–343.

[33] Walther Koch, "Johann Marbach in seiner Bedeutung für die Pfälzische Kirchengeschichte," *Blätter für pfälzische kirche und religiöse Volkskunde* 22 (1962): 119–120. Marbach's recommendations are printed in C. Schmidt, *Der Antheil der Strassburger an der Reformation in Churpfalz: Drei Schriften Johann Marbach's mit einer geschichtlichen Einleitung* (Strasbourg, 1856).

[34] Hans Rott, "Kirchen- und Bildersturm bei der Einführung der Reformation in the Pfalz," *Neues Archiv für die Geschichte der Stadt Heidelberg* 6 (1905): 229–254. The order to bring Catholic services to an end (which included instructions regarding the abolition of images, vestments, etc.) is printed in *EKO*, 14:111–113.

Ottheinrich undertook his most lasting contribution to the Palatine reformation through his promotion of the University of Heidelberg. He initiated a wide ranging "reformation" of the university in 1558, relying on the advice of the Palatine native son Philipp Melanchthon. Not only did he augment the financial basis of the university and enhance its library (both often at the expense of local monasteries), he also attracted many leading scholars to Heidelberg. Ottheinrich's university reflected a wide range of Protestant theological opinion betraying either his lack of appreciation for theological subtleties or his preference for professional reputation over confessional correctness—or, perhaps, both. Alternatively, Ruth Wesel-Roth has suggested that Lutheran misrepresentations of Huldrych Zwingli's theology may have made in-the-flesh Zwinglians unrecognizable to such casual observers as Ottheinrich.[35] The end result was clear, as Eike Wolgast has noted: "Ottheinrich had certainly recruited Protestant intellectuals of most varying theological orientations to Heidelberg: Gnesio-Lutherans, Philippists, Zwinglians, and Calvinists—conflicts were therefore unavoidable."[36] In 1558, Ottheinrich acquired a special prize for his university with the appointment of the humanist physician Thomas Erastus to the second chair of medicine.

Erastus before the Palatinate

Origins and Early Education

So little is known about Erastus's early life that even into this century confusion has reigned as to whether he was born in Baden in the modern canton of Aargau in Switzerland or in the Margraviate of Baden in Southwestern Germany (in modern Baden-Württemberg). While Eras-

[35] Wesel-Roth, *Thomas Erastus*, 18.

[36] Wolgast, *Die Universität Heidelberg*, 37: "Allerdings hat Ottheinrich evangelische Gelehrte unterschiedlichster theologischer Richtungen nach Heidelberg geholt: Gnesiolutheraner, Philippisten, Zwinglianer, Calvinisten—Auseinandersetzungen waren damit unausbleiblich." Regarding Ottheinrich's religiosity, see Press, *Calvinismus und Territorialstaat*, 205–206. See also Heinrich Bornkamm, "Kurfürst Ottheinrich von der Pfalz," in *Das Jahrhundert der Reformation: Gestalten und Kräfte* (Göttingen: Vandenhoek & Ruprecht, 1961), 253–262; Barbara Kurze, *Kurfürst Ott Heinrich: Politik und Religion in der Pfalz, 1556–1559* (Gütersloh, C. Bertelsmann, 1956); Georg Poensgen, ed., *Ottheinrich: Gedenkschrift zur vierhundertjährigen Wiederkehr seiner Kurfürstenzeit in der Pfalz (1556–1559); Ruperto Carola Sonderband* (1956); and Joachim Telle, "Kurfürst

tus nearly always referred to himself as Swiss (*Helvetius*)[37] and his Basel professors remembered him as a Swiss Badener,[38] a seductively detailed tradition developed that held that he was from the town Auggen in the nearby German province of Baden. That this tradition enjoyed such longevity was partially due to the fact that it was picked up in Zedler's *Universal-lexicon* and even mysteriously found its way into an eighteenth-century printed list of the rectors of the University of Heidelberg.[39] The various ways in which Erastus identified his place of origin throughout his life, however, all suggest Swiss Baden over Baden in Germany, and modern scholars have accepted Swiss Baden as Erastus's actual birthplace.[40] Erastus certainly thought of himself as Swiss, and most of

---

Ottheinrich, Hans Kilian und Paracelsus: Zum pfälzischen Paracelsismus im 16. Jahrhundert," in *Von Paracelsus zu Goethe und Wilhelm von Humboldt* [*SBPF* 22] (Vienna: Verband der wissenschaftlichen Gesellschaften Österreichs, 1981), 130–146.

[37] E.g., Gustav Toepke, *Die Matrikel der Universität Heidelberg von 1386 bis 1662* (Heidelberg, 1886), 2:14: "Thomas Erastus, Helvetius, medicinarum doctor, Badensis, diocesis Constantiensis, 3a May." (The fact that he listed himself as being from the diocese of Constance does not settle the question since both of the proposed birthplaces, Swiss Baden and German Baden, were within the diocese.) He signed the introductory epistle of his first publication with "Thomas Erastus Helvetius." *Astrologia Confutata* (Schleusingen: Hermann Hamsing, 1557), fol. Avr. His epitaph also referred to him as "Helvetius Aquensis Thomas Erastus." Melchior Adam, *Vitae Germanorum Medicorum* (Heidelberg: Johannes Georg Geyder, 1620), 244 (http://www.uni-mannheim.de/mateo/camenaref/adam/adam2/s276.html).

[38] Rudolf Thommen noted the letter from Bonifacius Amerbach to his son Basilius, who was then studying in Bologna, in which Bonifacius remarked, "The one who returns these [letters] to you is Thomas Lüber born in Baden of the Swiss (Qui has tibi reddit, Thomas Luberus est Badae Helvetiorum ... natus)." Rudolf Thommen, *Geschichte der Universität Basel, 1532–1632* (Basel, 1889), 280.

[39] J.H. Zedler and C.G. Ludovici, *Grosses vollständiges Universal-Lexicon aller Wissenschaften und Künste* (Halle, 1732–1750), 8:1471–1472. Zedler recounts: "Erastus (Thomas) ein Medicus, wurde zu Auggenen, einem in der Herrschafft Badenweiler, drey meilen von Basel gelegenen Flecken, an. 1523 von geringen Eltern geboren. Sein Teutscher Geschlechts-Namen hiesse Lieber." The rector list is the seventh appendix of Toepke's *Die Matrikel der Universität Heidelberg*, 2:619. Erastus is here listed as "Thomas Erastus al[ias] Liebler de Auggen." This list is the synthetic work of the editor and does not reflect an actual sixteenth-century roster.

[40] This question was addressed as early as 1778 when the editors of the *Athenae rauricae* wrote: "Thomas Erastus (Liebler, s. Lüber) natus est d. 7. Sept. 1524. non, ut quidam perhibent, in Auggen, vico ditionis Badenweiler, Marchionatus Badensis, sed in oppido helvetico Baden, unde & Aquensis dicebatur. Badensem certe ipse se vocavit in matricula Rectoris academiae Basil. & in ejus epitaphio, Basileae exstante, itidem Helveto Aquensis vocatur." *Athenae rauricae sive catalogus professorum Academiae Basiliensis ab anno 1460 ad annum 1778* (Basel, 1778), 427–430. See also "Schlußbemerkung über Thomas Erastus," *Argovia* 12 (1881): 69–70; Thommen, *Geschichte der Universität Basel, 1532–1632*, 280. A. Schumann solidified this point in an errata volume of the *ADB*,

his close friends were Swiss. As we shall see below, he became the chief contact for Swiss students in Heidelberg, keeping an eye on and sometimes boarding students from many cantons, especially Basel, Zurich, and Schaffhausen. In later years after his standing in Heidelberg deteriorated, he would express a certain sentimentality for his homeland, saying that he would prefer to work in Switzerland for 150 florins per annum as opposed to remaining in Heidelberg for three hundred florins, and he later made repeated requests of his friend Johann Jakob Grynaeus to procure a colored rendition of all the crests of the Swiss territories.[41] Almost certainly by birth and definitely at heart, Erastus was an *Eidgenosse*.[42]

The question of his place of birth holds a potential key to understanding Erastus's early religious experience, about which we know very little. When Erastus was a child in the 1520s and early 1530s, Switzerland attained its modern confessional configuration with the confederation split rather evenly between Catholicism, which predominated in the rural, Alpine Cantons, and the Reformed faith, which was eventually embraced by the more urban and affluent cantons like Zurich, Bern, and Basel less than a decade after Zwingli initiated his own brand of the Reformation in Zurich.

Though the city of Baden is located in the modern canton of Aargau, in the early sixteenth century this territory, which had been wrested from Habsburg control in 1415, was divided into three major sectors.[43] The western half, including the city of Aarau, was administered directly by Bern. The eastern half was splintered into various jurisdictions that were considered common lordships (*Gemeine Herrschaften*) of the Swiss Confederation. The southern lands sandwiched between Lucerne, Zurich, and Zug were known as the Free-bailiwicks (*Freie-Ämter*). The northern section of the eastern half of modern Aargau was known as County of Baden (*Grafshaft Baden*), which was somewhat ironic since it was a

29:774. See also Bonnard, *Thomas Éraste*, 201–202; Wesel-Roth, *Thomas Erastus*, 2; Gustav Adolf Benrath, "Die Korrespondenz zwischen Bullinger und Thomas Erastus," in *Heinrich Bullinger 1504–1575: Gesammelte Aufsätze sum 400. Todestag* [*ZBRG* 8], ed. Ulrich Gäbler and Erland Herkenrath (Zurich: Theologischer Verlag, 1975), 2:87–88.

[41] Benrath, "Die Korrespondenz zwischen Bullinger und Thomas Erastus," 110–111; Erastus to Grynaeus, April 23, (15)78, Basel, Öffentliche Bibliothek der Universität Basel, MS G II 4, fol. 227.

[42] Literally an "oath-taker," commonly rendered "confederate" or as simply "Swiss."

[43] The number would increase to four if one includes the Fricktal region, which remained in the hands of the Habsburgs as part of Vorderösterreich in the early modern period.

county without a count.[44] The complication does not end here, since the towns of Bremgarten, Mellingen, and Baden itself were not technically part of the "*Grafschaft*," as they were chartered towns with their own liberties and privileges stemming from their prehistory of Habsburg rule.[45]

Thus, when Erastus identified himself as a "Badener," one might plausibly question whether he had the town or the larger county in mind. The political-religious situation in Erastus's home region was similarly complicated during his youth. Friction between the Catholic forest cantons and the more urban Protestant cantons concerning the religious policy of the common lordships was one of the main factors leading to the Kappel wars. The town of Baden had been the location of the famous Baden Disputation of 1526 in which the Catholic theologian Johann Eck scored perhaps his greatest debating victory over the Protestants represented by Basel's Johannes Oecolampadius. Though Zurich continued to encourage evangelical pastors in the common lordships, Grafschaft Baden ultimately remained predominately Catholic. Thus, despite the fact that Erastus was born after the coming of the Reformation in Switzerland, his early religious experience was more than likely within the old church. Another hint that Erastus began his life as a Catholic can be seen in his Christian name "Thomas," which was becoming an uncommon Protestant baptismal name by this juncture. In any event, the young Erastus would have experienced the existence of rival Protestant and Catholic confessions in close proximity as a settled fact already in the 1530s.[46]

Although it is not really an issue of scholarly controversy, Erastus's name has also been variously rendered in different historical accounts. In every surviving record before 1549 Erastus gives his name as "Thomas

[44] In the specific case of the Grafschaft Baden, the common lordship was exercised jointly by the eight ruling cantons (*VIII Orte*: Zurich, Bern, Lucerne, Unterwalden, Schwyz, Glarus, Zug, and Uri).

[45] See Christophe Seiler and Andreas Steigmeier, *Geschichte des Aargaus: Illustrierter Überblick von der Urzeit bis zur Gegenwart* (Aarau: AT Verlag, 1991) 38–43; Walter Schaufelberger, "Spätmittelalter" in *Handbuch der Schweizer Geschichte*, 2nd ed. (Zurich: Buchverlag Berichthaus, 1980), 1:280–285. I am indebted to Randolph Head of the University of California, Riverside for assisting me with the thorny issues of Swiss territorial organization.

[46] Alternatively Wesel-Roth alleged, "Die Kindheit und Jugend unseres Schweizers liegt völlig im Dunkeln, nur daß er einmal bekennt, von Jugend auf in der reformierten Lehre erzogen worden zu sein." However, she offered no documentation for this remark. Wesel-Roth, *Thomas Erastus*, 2.

Lüberus."[47] While a student in Italy, Erastus graecized his name to "Erastus," a rough translation of the German "Lieber," meaning "lover."[48] Around the year 1550 Erastus went through a period of transition and would sign his name with combinations like "Thomas Lüber or Erastus."[49] While his surname was uniformly given as "Lüber" in the early records, he did once refer to a relative named "Conrad Lüber or Lieber," which suggests that the name, not surprisingly, did not have a fixed spelling.[50] From time to time his German name has also been given as "Liebler" in secondary literature, though this phenomenon likely stems from the re-translation of "Erastus" into German and does not reflect Erastus's own usage. In recent days a second generation over-correction "Lieb" has crept into the literature. For those who aspire to hyper-correctness, "Lüber" is the only German name that is well-documented, though Erastus himself did not use this name after 1552 and it did not appear on any of his publications (in Latin *or German*) or in the records of the University of Heidelberg. "Erastus" was *not* his penname; it was his complete identity to the same degree that a certain orphan from Rotterdam was known as "Erasmus" or the Palatinate's most famous son, Philipp Schwartzerdt, was known as "Melanchthon." Thus, the current fashion of referring to him as "Thomas Lüber" would appear to be a subtraction rather than an addition to knowledge, unless we are prepared to go the entire distance and likewise re-christen his theory of church-state relations "Lüberanism."[51]

---

[47] Hans Georg Wackernagel, ed., *Die Matrikel der Universität Basel* (Basel: Verlag der Universitätsbibliothek, 1956), 30: "Thomas Lüberus Badensis—nihil." Also relevant here are the letters from Erastus to Konrad Pellikan and Oswald Myconius. See the Correspondence Register.

[48] The name is graecized with a Latin spelling. One rarely sees the Greek "Ἐραστος" in his writings, and he naturally opted for the Latinate "Erastus" over the strict transliteration "Erastos." He never used the potential Latin translation "*amator*" to my knowledge. He did not invent the name "Erastus," as it is found in ancient literature and in the New Testament, and though the name is rare in German-speaking lands, it has had some currency as a Christian name in the English-speaking world.

[49] The first letter to clearly attest to this change comes from 1549. Erastus to Pellikan, July 9, 1549, Zurich, Zentralbibliothek (Simmlersche Sammlung), MS S 70, no. 168: "Thomas Lüber seu quod idem est Erastus." It should be noted, however, that since the majority of these early letters are copies rather than autographs, it is difficult to observe this transition with great confidence.

[50] The etymological origin of the name is also murky. See J.K. Brechenmacher, ed., *Etymologisches Wörterbuch der Deutschen Familiennamen* (Limburg a. d. Lahn: C.A. Starke, 1960–1963) 2:186.

[51] E.g., the contradictory editorial policy of the *OER*. Whereas Erastus is exclusively referred to as Lüber in the work (which will render most of these references meaningless

We are quite poorly informed about the Lüber clan. Presumably the family was of peasant stock from central Switzerland. The name survives in Switzerland in a band from St. Gallen to Bern, with the highest concentration in Zurich, as well as in the German districts of Baden-Württemberg adjacent to the Swiss border.[52] Erastus's biological relatives rarely come up in his correspondence, and when they do, we lack sufficient background information to make the passages fully intelligible. In 1557, for example, we find Erastus asking Konrad Gessner to convey letters to his unnamed brother, who was apparently in the inner canton of Schwyz. Erastus does not give much identifying information, but it must be assumed that Gessner's and Erastus's relatives were well enough acquainted that they easily make the connection.[53] This must be the same brother whose name is later given as "Conrad Lüber" in Erastus's correspondence to Heinrich Bullinger. Conrad Lüber was evidently a cutler from Schwyz and a good friend to a merchant relative of Gessner's who occasionally traveled to the Frankfurt fair. The Schwyz connection raises interesting speculative questions. For example, given that Erastus apparently had an artisan brother with some property in Schwyz, this might suggest that the Lüber family originated there. While we do not know the definitive origin of Erastus's family, the geographical distribution of his immediate relatives evidences some straddling of confessional boundaries. In any event, Conrad Lüber had passed away by 1567,[54] and Erastus employed a more distant, and apparently less affluent, cousin, Johann Lüber, to settle Conrad's estate in Schwyz.[55] Johann Lüber would lodge

to those who do not chance to look up Lüber), Erasmus's birth name is not even given in the biographical entry dedicated to him.

[52] Prior to 1800 the name was most common in the canton of St. Gallen. *Familiennamenbuch der Schweiz* (Zurich: Polygraph, 1940).

[53] Erastus to Gessner, April 11, (1557), Zurich, Staatsarchiv des Kantons Zürich, MS E II 361, fol. 56: "Dabo operam ut mittantur, cum primum facultas certi nobis alicuius hominis dabitur. Inclusas literas velim perferri Suitiam ad fratrem. Id commodissime fiet, si Gesnero agnatorum tuorum [iri] reddendas curaveris. Nomen hominis mihi excidit, (puto Henrici esse) sed cognosces ex eo inditio, quod uxorem habet, quae Suitiae olim habuit [recto] maritum, quo tempore frater meus apud eius maritum habitavit."

[54] Wesel-Roth suggests that the death probably was between 1557 and 1560, since Erastus speaks of him in the past tense in 1560. Wesel-Roth, *Thomas Erastus*, 2.

[55] Erastus to Bullinger, July 13, 1567, StAZ, E II 361, fol. 11: "Mitto meum agnatum Johannem Lüber/ cuius pater et ego patrueles fuimus, ut Suiciae, quae frater meus reliquit, exigat, et iis pro suo arbitrio utatur. Quamvis autem credo, aut non multum superesse, aut saltem quae in ei debebantur, non posse facile exigi (Die mögen nit leiden, das ein Landtman einen frembden etwas gebe, das aus dem landt kome. Novi eorum mores.) nolui tamen non tentare. Si quid obtinebit, lucrum erit: si nihil, nihil prodiderit."

with Erastus in Heidelberg in 1576, and Erastus advanced a modest sum to him in 1580.[56] While Erastus remained in close contact with Swiss intellectuals, familial connections with his biological relatives apparently played little role in his adult life.

Unlike his name and his place of birth, we are less confident in the dates of Erastus's life. While there is no controversy concerning the date of his death on December 31, 1583 (Julian calendar), even this fact is complicated because the last year of his life fell in the period of the early stages of the transition from the Julian calendar to the Gregorian calendar from 1582—but only gradually in Protestant lands. Since Erastus likely only experienced the Julian calendar, we are spared great confusion.[57] Likewise, since his epitaph gave his death date in the Roman fashion as falling on the first of the calends of January 1583, a plausible interpretation of his epitaph in isolation could lead one to conclude that he died on December 31, 1582.[58] However, unless the works that Erastus composed in 1583 were literally "ghost-written," it would seem safe to assume that he lived through the year 1583.[59]

While it is an accepted fact that Erastus died of pneumonia on December 31, 1583, it is unlikely that such certainty can be attained regarding the date of his birth. Various sources suggest that he was born in 1520, 1523, or 1524.[60] The 1520 date is derived from a letter to Bullinger from 1570 in which Erastus said that he was nearing his fiftieth year.[61] Since Erastus was not speaking in precise terms, however, but merely waxing philosophical about the wisdom of age, this off-hand remark lends little weight to accepting 1520 as his precise birth year. Likewise, if his epitaph, which stated he died a "*sexagenarius*," were taken literally, we would assume he was born in 1523. Finally, an eighteenth century his-

[56] See letters from Erastus to Grynaeus: Jan. 27, (15)76, Basel UB, G II 4, fol. 195; Feb. 3, (15)76, Basel UB, G II 4, fol. 196; March 7, (15)76, Basel UB, G II 4, fol. 194; and April 24, (15)80, Basel UB, G II 4, fol. 311.

[57] All sixteenth century dates will be given according to the Julian calendar. The central European custom of dating the change of the year from Jan. 1 also spares us further potential confusion.

[58] Printed in Bonnard, *Thomas Éraste*, 206: "AN. SAL. MDXXCIII PRID. KAL. IAN."

[59] E.g., Erastus to Theophil Mader, Jan. 12, 1583, Bremen, Staats- und Universitätsbibliothek, MS 8, fol. 253. Indeed, since Johann Jakob Grynaeus wrote Rudolf Gwalther and Konrad Ulmer in early January 1584 to inform them of Erastus's death, there can be no controversy here. Wesel-Roth, *Thomas Erastus*, 11, notes. See also discussion in Bonnard, *Thomas Éraste*, 207.

[60] Wesel-Roth, *Thomas Erastus*, 2.

[61] Erastus to Bullinger, Jan. 1, (15)70, StAZ, E II 361, fol. 17: "et iam incipio ad .50. annum accedere." I would translate this as, "And now as I begin to approach my fifties."

tory of the faculty of the University of Basel (*Athenae rauricae*) listed his birth date with enticing precision as September 7, 1524—though without providing documentation.[62] Alternatively, Erastus's earliest biographer, Johannes Oporinus, only remarked that he was born "around 1524," which agrees with notation on Erastus's portrait by Tobias Stimmer that he was 58 in early 1582.[63] Recent scholarship has opted for the 1524 date without pushing the issue further.[64] The preponderance of the evidence suggests that at least Erastus thought he was born in 1524, although no confirmation can be offered for the September birthdate.

Beyond the odd comment in his later correspondence, our primary source for Erastus's early life is a one-page biographical portrait published in the third volume of Heinrich Pantaleon's *Biographies of Heroes and Illustrious Men of all of Germany*, which was composed by the famous humanist printer Johannes Oporinus, who had also served as the amanuensis of Paracelsus as a young man. Since Erastus would spend much of his mature career refuting the magical world view of Germany's greatest medical prophet, it is a profound irony that Oporinus should serve as the most important biographical source for both Erastus and Paracelsus. Since Oporinus's account of Erastus's life to 1565 is of primary importance, a complete translation of it is offered here:[65]

[62] *Athenae rauricae*, 427–430. See Wesel-Roth, *Thomas Erastus*, note, p. 125.

[63] See discussion and translation of Oporinus below. The text on Erastus's portrait (Kunstmuseum Basel, reproduced on the cover) reads "Anno 1552. die April 24. Aetatis 58."

[64] Benrath, "Die Korrespondenz zwischen Bullinger und Thomas Erastus," 87–88; Ruth Wesel-Roth, "Thomas Erastus," in *Neue Deutsche Biographie* (Berlin, 1953–), 4:1560.

[65] Heinrich Pantaleon, *Prosopographia Heroum Atque Illustrium Virorum Totius Germaniae* (Basel: In officina haeredum Nicolai Brylingeri, 1565–1566), 3:545: Thomas Erastus Medicus Heidelbergensis [Title]. Thomas natus est Badenis Helvetiorum anno circiter 1524. Ibi cum prima literarum rudimenta didicisset, sese anno millesimo quingentesimo quadragesimo ad Basiliensem Academiam contulit, atque artibus & linguis praeclaram operam navavit. Cum etiam dextrae manus usum minus expeditum haberet, sinistra omnia scripsit atque eum habitum sibi comparavit, ut praeceptorum dictata celeriter exciperet, & suos commilitones plerunque superaret. Tum etiam sacris literis incubuit atque earum assidua lectione verae religionis fundamenta feliciter iecit. Eo in loco nos commilitones literarum fuimus, atque nunquam inter-morituram familiaritatem inivimus. Quoniam autem sumptus ij, qui ad studia requiruntur, ipsi deessent, post tertium annum commode accidit ut patronum aliquem nactus in Italiam sese receperit, atque Bononiae magna assiduitate Philosophos differentes per aliquot annos audiverit. Ubi etiam talem rerum cognitionem adeptus est, ut merito doctissimis Philosophia connumeretur. Postea quoque Medicinae Studium coniunxit atque sua eruditione effecit, ut

Thomas Erastus, Physician of Heidelberg

Thomas Erastus was born in Baden, Switzerland around the year 1524. Having already learned the first rudiments of letters there, he moved to the Basel academy in 1540 and did excellent work in arts and letters. Since he was less adept with his right hand, he always wrote with the left, and having challenged himself in this state, he clearly matched the dictations of the teachers and surpassed most of his comrades. In those days he also directed his attentions to theology, and by assiduous reading, he successfully laid the foundations of true religion. In this place we were comrades in learning, and we never approached a jaded familiarity. Since he did not possess the funds needed to continue his studies, after the third year at university it fortunately happened that he secured a certain patron born in Italy, and for some years he studied with different philosophers in Bologna with great vigor. There also he was adept in many subjects, so that he was justifiably reckoned among the most learned philosophers. Later he undertook the study of medicine, and by his erudition he achieved such success that he obtained his doctorate by universal acclamation. Then he practiced medicine for some years, and likewise, having been instructed in every type of learning, he returned to Germany from Italy after about ten years.

After Thomas had returned to Germany, he attended for some time the illustrious family of the counts of Henneberg and became well known to the entire medical community. This was well known to the most illustrious Prince Frederick, Elector Palatine, who especially prized [Erastus] among

suprema Doctorum insignia omnium acclamatione impetrarit. Deinde per aliquot annos Medicinam exercuit, atque tandem, post decennium quasi, ex Italia in Germaniam, omni genere literarum instructus rediit.

Cum in Germaniam Thomas redisset, aliquandiu illustri familiae comitum Hennenbergensium adfuit, & arte Medica omnibus doctis innotuit. Id cum illustrissimus princeps Fredericus Elector Palatinus cognovisset, eum Heydelbergae inter professores receptum plurimum dilexit, suum Medicum constituit, atque etiam, ob raram prudentiam & vitae integritatem, inter consiliarios adoptavit. Eam functionem Thomas suscepit, atque Heydelbergensem Academiam plurimum decoravit. Nec tantum Philosophica & Medica, verum etiam Theologica ea eruditione tractavit & explicavit, ut ad omnes quaestiones enodandas esset promptissimus. Itaque cum contentio illa de Coena Domini in Germania reviresceret, ipse sese Lutheranis opposuit, atque in verbis Domini, una cum Zuinglio, tropum subesse significavit, quae sententia etiam Heidelbergae plurimorum consensu invaluit. Hoc modo Thomas etiamnum in ea Academia pergit, atque de hac quaestione libellis aliquo editis, non modo Germanis, verum etiam exteris nationibus plurimum innotuit. Ioan[nes] Opor[inus].

The woodcut illustration which accompanies the text of a physician holding a urine flask has been mistakenly reproduced on occasion as a picture of Erastus. The same woodcut was also used in this work as an illustration for the physicians Achilles Pirmin Gasser, Johann Winther von Andernach, and Giulio Alessandrini, among others. See also the account in Adam, *Vitae Germanorum Medicorum*, 242–246, which is primarily based on Oporinus.

the faculty in Heidelberg, and appointed him his physician. Likewise, on account of his rare prudence and moral integrity, [Frederick] made him one of his councilors. Thomas took on these roles and especially enhanced the Heidelberg academy. Not only has he handled and explicated philosophy and medicine with this erudition, but also theology, in that he was most ready in resolving all questions. Thus, since the Lord's Supper controversy revived in Germany, he has opposed the Lutherans, and [he has maintained,] together with Zwingli, [that] the words of the Lord [in the institution of the Eucharist] should be understood figuratively. This opinion has achieved a dominant position in Heidelberg. Thomas continues in this manner in the same academy, and since he has published several books concerning this topic, he has become well known not only to Germans, but also in foreign lands.

Johannes Oporinus

Since Oporinus also published a book by Erastus in the year he wrote this biographical sketch, it would seem that Oporinus had a pecuniary interest in Erastus's fame. Thus, his piece perhaps falls in the same genre as the biographical blurb that one finds on modern dust jackets. Although it is often vague on details, the account is factually accurate at those points where it can be compared with other sources, though one gets the sense that he wrote it from memory rather than from extensive research.[66] As discussed above, Oporinus's account of Erastus's birth date may be the most reliable estimate we possess.

Beyond his mention that Erastus already possessed a basic Latin education when he arrived in Basel, Oporinus did not illuminate Erastus's early life. From the limited extant sources, we can reconstruct little more than a plausible outline of his childhood and youth. The most basic fact comes from his entry in the Basel University matriculation list, which records that Erastus contributed nothing to the payment of his university fees.[67] With little beyond this fact to go on, scholars have postulated that he came from an artisan or peasant family. Not only was he unable to pay his matriculation fees, but he had to depend on an unnamed patron's

[66] On the surface, Oporinus's account appears to have a factual error in that he leaves out the detail that Erastus was brought to Heidelberg during the reign of Ottheinrich. What I take Oporinus to be saying, however, is that Frederick was already familiar with Erastus's reputation before he ascended to the throne in Heidelberg, and for that reason, he especially prized Erastus among the professors already in residence at the university. There is no surviving correspondence between Erastus and Oporinus, though they must have exchanged some letters in the 1560s. Their relationship is discussed in greater detail in chapter 7.

[67] Wackernagel, *Die Matrikel der Universität Basel*, 30: "Thomas Lüberus Badensis—nihil."

benevolence to finance his studies in Italy. While we can certainly rule out a noble or even a patrician background for Erastus, it is possible that a family that displayed such physical mobility was at least at the level of middling peasants, although well-off peasants—like Luther's parents, for instance—would have been able to pay his university fees. Unlike his Swiss associates Bullinger, Ludwig Lavater, and Johann Jakob Grynaeus, who possessed close social connections with the bourgeois elite of their cities, Erastus clearly was a *novus homo*.[68] Regardless of his origin, an apparent close identification with the interests of the ruling elite was a mentality that he shared with his urban Swiss friends. It is nevertheless noteworthy that he composed many of his early writings, both theological pamphlets and a plague tract, in the vernacular for the benefit of the "common man."

Not surprisingly, Erastus's modest origins made an impact on his adult psychology. He would display a simultaneous humility and arrogance in his later years. Though from humble origins, Erastus appears to have readily taken to the company of magnates. His decade in Italy may have served as something of a finishing school for Erastus; years among the bourgeoisie of Bologna proved a more than adequate preparation for life at a rustic German court. For all his courtliness, his forthrightness in addressing princes suggests that he never lost a peasant's ability to diagnose a situation in a simple manner and express his opinion in straightforward terms. Nevertheless, having risen from a mean estate, Erastus was not quick to question the social and intellectual norms of the establishment.

The exception to his general embrace of conventional social thinking may be found in Erastus's conception of the church, and in particular, his opinion of the role of the clergy. A measure of popular anticlericalism animated Erastus's heated opposition to the imposition of a Calvinist consistory of elders to monitor parishioners. Erastus perceived that the new Calvinist boss was all too similar to the old Roman boss. If the consensus that he was born in Baden in Aargau is correct, one cannot overlook the fact that he likely spent his early years in a Catholic region. This would have provided him with significant experience with the Catholic Church that was later augmented by his extended stay in Italy.

[68] See, for example, Robert Walton, "Heinrich Bullinger, Repräsentant der reichen Bauern und seine Beziehungen zur städischen Oligarchie," in *Reform, Reformation, Revolution*, ed. Siegfried Hoyer (Leipzig: Karl-Marx-Universität, 1980), 132–142.

Another source that complements the Oporinus portrait is a comment that Erastus made in a letter to Bullinger. Here Erastus recounted:

> I hear that somewhere among you dwells a certain Badener, by the name Georg Rockenmann, who once was a monk in a certain monastery in the Black Forest that is named St. Blasien.[69] He together with his brother, who is in the monastery of Müry[70] in your vicinity, were my teachers in order that I began to undertake the study of the Latin language.[71]

This brief remark raises as many questions as it answers. It informs us of the identity of Erastus's early teachers and tends to confirm the suspicion that Erastus likely spent his early days in Catholic circles. It also lends additional evidence to the thesis that he was born in Baden (Aargau), since Erastus mentions "a certain Badener" without having to explain what kind of "Badener" he meant. This makes all the more sense when we remember that Bullinger was from nearby Bremgarten himself. In that light, this aside takes on the dimension of one Badener speaking to another. Unfortunately, the passage does not explicitly state where he attended Latin school, though it may have been St. Blasien or Muri, either of which were relatively accessible to him in geographical terms. The abbey of St. Blasien was an important lord in Grafschaft Baden, holding judicial rights in the districts directly north of the town of Baden.[72] While this is only a thread of evidence, one could speculate that Erastus may have lived in one of these districts associated with St. Blasien.

Education in Zurich and Basel

We are only slightly better informed regarding Erastus's transition to higher education. The limited clues from the surviving evidence suggest that his first experience with higher education may well have been in

[69] The Benedictine abbey of St. Blasien is located a few kilometers north of Waldshut on the Alb, in southern Baden-Württemberg. The Peasants' War began here on May 30, 1524 when St. Blasien's subject peasants refused to fulfill their feudal obligations to the abbey.

[70] He likely means the Benedictine abbey of Muri in Southern Aargau (then the *Freie-Ämter*), roughly between Zurich and Lucerne.

[71] Erastus to Bullinger, Heidelberg, March 11 [1565], StAZ, E II 361, fol. 48: "Audio apud vos alicubi agere quendam Badensem, nomine Gregorium Rockenman/ qui olim monachus fuit in coenobio quodam Silvae Henricinae (Schwartzwald) cui nomen est Sancti Blasii. Is cum fratre, qui est in monasterio vobis vicino Müry/ autores mihi fuerant, ut latinae linguae inciperem dare operam." Benrath, "Die Korrespondenz zwischen Bullinger und Thomas Erastus," 88.

[72] Seiler and Steigmeier, *Geschichte des Aargaus*, 40.

Zurich rather than Basel, as a strict reading of Oporinus would imply. Wesel-Roth suggested that Erastus perhaps studied in Zurich before attending the University of Basel. Robert Walton has supported Wesel-Roth's theory of a sojourn in Zurich, although he has suggested that it may well have occurred some time between 1544–1555, that is, during the timeframe conventionally assigned to Erastus's medical studies in Italy.[73] Alternatively, Gustav Adolf Benrath, who has done the fullest investigation of Erastus's correspondence with Bullinger, apparently assumed that their relationship began only after Erastus arrived in Heidelberg.[74] Like Wesel-Roth and Walton, I find it implausible that the close relationships that Erastus enjoyed with so many Zurich intellectuals and his firm commitment to the Zurich theology did not rest on some more extensive personal experience with the Zurich scene than the surviving sources explicitly confirm.

Putting together what is concretely known about Erastus's whereabouts in the 1540s and 1550s with the pattern of evidence we have in the form of Erastus's surviving correspondence with his early intellectual patrons, it appears likely that Erastus attended the Zurich Academy (*Carolinum*) before moving on to the University of Basel. The Zurich Academy, the ancestor of the modern University of Zurich, was an institute of higher learning that was something between an advanced Latin school and a university specializing in theological education.[75] Leading Zurich ministers such as Zwingli and later Bullinger and Rudolf Gwalther gave exegetical lectures, the *Prophezei*, at the school. With no surviving matriculation list before 1559, any student's attendance at the Carolinum would have to be confirmed on the basis of external evidence.[76] In Erastus's case, his close relations with the Carolinum's faculty appear to connect him to the institution. The Old Testament professor Konrad Pellikan served as Erastus's chief backer in his early academic life, and

[73] Walton, "Der Streit zwischen Thomas Erastus und Caspar Olevian," 211; Wesel-Roth, *Thomas Erastus*, 2–4.

[74] Benrath, "Die Korrespondenz zwischen Bullinger und Thomas Erastus," 89. Benrath includes the rather ambigious comment, "Es wird wohl zutreffend sein, dass sich Bullinger und der zwanzig Jahre jüngere Erast erst aus der Ferne entdeckten, als es um die Förderung der reformierten Konfession in der Pfalz ging."

[75] See J. Wayne Baker, "Zürich Academy," in *OER*, 316–317. Karin Maag, *Seminary or University? The Genevan Academy and Reformed Higher Education, 1560–1620* [St. Andrews Studies in Reformation History] (Aldershot: Scholar Press, 1995).

[76] Maag, *Seminary or University*, 136. While Oporinus does not specifically mention study at the Zurich *Carolinum*, he does confirm a certain level of academic achievement prior to Erastus's arrival in Basel.

Erastus admired Pellikan as a father. It would be difficult to explain how a young man of humble origins from Baden could have come to develop such a close relationship with Pellikan and his family if he had not studied at the Zurich Academy. Though this is not in itself conclusive proof, positing a time of study at the Carolinum provides the most economical explanation for the depth of Erastus's relationships with the Zurich community. Another factor that makes Erastus's study at the Carolinum appear likely is that not only did Erastus know Pellikan extremely well, he also sent greetings in his letters to Pellikan to other members of the Carolinum faculty, such as Bullinger and Theodor Bibliander, as early as 1546. In one letter he refers to himself as their "child and most honest disciple."[77] While this is not hard proof, Erastus tended to be rather reserved and tactful in approaching the famous personages of his day, and in most cases where he extended greetings through a third party, we know from other sources that he knew the individual in question personally. Likewise, since his letters from Italy contain few personal references, it would seem most implausible to suggest that he was not personally familiar with four out of the five individuals whom he asked Pellikan to greet in his name.[78] The simplest explanation for this pattern of contacts is that Erastus studied at the Zurich Carolinum before moving to Basel.[79]

There is no question that Erastus moved to the University of Basel in the early 1540s. Wesel-Roth has suggested that he likely entered the pre-university *Paedigogium* Basel in 1540 and then stood for exams in early 1541 for enrollment in the arts faculty of the university. Thus, in Wesel-Roth's reconstruction, his entry into the Basel matriculation list

[77] Erastus to Pellikan, June 21 [ca. 1546], Zurich, Zentralbibliothek (Simmlersche Sammlung), MS S 60, no. 93.

[78] Erastus to Pellikan, May 17, 1546, ZBZ (Sim.) 60, no. 92. Erastus asked Pellikan on various occasions to greet Bullinger, Bibliander, Rudolf Gwalther, Samuel Pellikan, and Lelio Sozzini. See the Correspondence Register.

[79] The alternate hypothesis of an extended Zurich sojourn after the University of Basel or Bologna would not conform to a conventional academic trajectory and does not fit the evidence from Erastus's correspondence, which indicates well-developed Zurich connections prior to his move to Italy. Erastus's extensive correspondence with Bullinger apparently does not settle the issue one way or the other. That is, no explicit mention seems to be made of Erastus's putative study in Zurich. However, when the correspondence between Bullinger and Erastus picked up in earnest in 1560, it appears that they already knew each other well. The most plausible resolution to this dilemma is that Erastus did study in Zurich, but that he was a protégé of Pellikan and not Bullinger, and thus his contacts with Bullinger were limited prior to Pellikan's death in 1556. Through his entire adult life Erastus appears to have had one primary correspondent in Zurich: first Pellikan, then Bullinger, followed briefly by Josias Simmler, and finally Rudolf Gwalther.

probably reflected his reception of the A.B. in 1542. However, if the thesis concerning a time of study at the Zurich Academy is correct, one does not have to consider this preliminary study in Basel a necessity.[80] Wesel-Roth also asserted that Erastus likely received the M.A. in 1544 since he had already moved on to Bologna by December of that year. There is no proof that Erastus received an M.A. in Basel, however, and Oporinus's report of his attending philosophy lectures in Italy may suggest that he undertook additional studies in Bologna before beginning his medical program. Perhaps it was his patron's willingness to pay rather than the conclusion of his studies which led Erastus to break off his time at the University of Basel.[81] Oporinus's biographical portrait and his later correspondence with Oswald Myconius, Coelio Secundo Curione, Martin Borrhaus, and the Amerbach family suggest that Erastus made a strong impression on the university community and forged enduring connections in the city.[82]

While Erastus would maintain and enhance his Basel connections throughout his adult life, he did not frequently reminisce about his Basel instructors. One professor he did not remember fondly was Luther's former collaborator, and later despised rival, Andreas Bodenstein von Karlstadt, who taught at the university in the late 1530s until his death in 1541 in the same plague epidemic that nearly felled Erastus.[83] With the exception of Karlstadt, Erastus would have had ample opportunity to renew these relationships with the Basel intellectual community during his time in Heidelberg. Given Erastus's close relationship with Basel, it is fitting that the city would serve as a place of refuge after his departure from the Palatinate during the territory's return to Lutheranism in the late 1570s.

Whether or not one accepts the hypothesis that Erastus studied at the Zurich Carolinum, the academic flagship of the Zwinglian Reformation, there is no doubt that Erastus was moving within distinctly Reformed circles by the early 1540s. Though little is known about Erastus's earliest religious experience, which may well have been in the Catholic tradition,

[80] Although Oporinus suggested that Erastus began his studies in Basel in 1540, Bonnard argued that this should be interpreted as an approximate rather than an exact date. To hold to this date too strictly would seem to go against the grain of the generally imprecise nature of Oporinus's portrait. Bonnard, *Thomas Éraste*, 202.

[81] Wesel-Roth, *Thomas Erastus*, 2–3.

[82] Cf. Correspondence Register.

[83] Erastus to Grynaeus, Aug. 15, (15)76, Basel UB, G II 4, fol. 198. After briefly noting his studies there in the early 1540s, Erastus quipped, "Carolostadii et sociorum eius novi artem et artes. Dominus eos perdat."

by the time he was about sixteen he was a Reformed Protestant. As we will see below, his experience as a foreign adherent of an outlawed faith in Italy further consolidated this identity. Since it is clear that Erastus was in the Reformed camp by his mid teens, even if he moved from Catholicism to Protestantism, it would not have been a full-fledged adult conversion. Being a Reformed Protestant was an integral part of his identity, and, unlike many of his conversion-prone friends, Erastus pursued a singular religious vision his entire adult life.

From Oporinus we also learn the curious fact that Erastus switched from writing with his right hand to his left hand. Erastus evidently experienced lameness in his right arm, though Oporinus does not mention this specific disability, as a result of his encounter with the Bubonic plague. During another outbreak of the plague, which drove the Heidelberg court to Mosbach in the winter of 1564, Erastus reflected in a letter to his countryman Gessner that his experience with the plague had begun as a patient, rather than as a physician, while a student in Basel in 1542.[84] In a postscript from a letter to Pellikan from early 1551, Erastus apologized for any mistakes in his letter, saying that he had written hurriedly and with his left hand.[85]

Erastus's early experience as a patient must have played some role in forming a successful bedside manner, which is evidenced in his lucrative practice in attending princes. Perhaps this bout with debilitating disease influenced our young Lüber, who possessed an obvious flair for theological disputation, to pursue a career in medicine. Not unlike today, the financial benefits of a medical career compared to that of a pastor or arts professor would have provided ample inducement. Once Erastus set his sights on a more ambitious academic career with a probable turn to medicine, the natural path was across the Alps into Italy.

---

[84] Thomas Erastus, *Varia Opuscula Medica*, ed., Giacomo Castelvetro (Frankfurt: J. Wechel, 1590), 88: "Sum in praesentia magis dubius, quam unquam fuerim. In causa est, quod nullam unquam pestem aliam vidi, Medicus. Nam cum anno 1542[,] si non fallit memoria, Basileae me corripuisset, parum mihi tunc ista curae erant, ut qui animum ad haec studia nondum appulissem, imo ne cogitarem quidem hisce operam navare. Proinde quae ante annum me putabam scire, hoc anno me ignorare libenter fateor."

[85] Erastus to Pellikan, [early year, 1551], Zurich, Zentralbibliothek (Simmlersche Sammlung), MS S 75, no. 4. This fact perhaps also offers backhanded support for our thesis that Erastus studied at the Zurich Academy before 1541; if his lameness postdated his time in Zurich, this might explain why he felt obligated to explain to Pellikan that he was now writing with his left hand.

Erastus in Italy

Erastus lived in Italy from 1544 to 1555. Moving to Bologna was the final step in the upward trajectory of his education. Not only was he climbing the academic ladder in terms of acquiring degrees (though we know little about the details of these as well), he was clearly ascending in terms of the prestige of the institutions he attended. If Erastus first studied at the Zurich Academy, it would have been natural for a student like him to progress to the more prestigious University of Basel. In fact, Karin Maag has suggested that the Carolinum served as a "springboard for the most talented to study elsewhere."[86] While Basel was the most distinguished institution in Switzerland—it was the only university there—it did not rank among the top universities of Europe, such as Paris, Oxford, and Cambridge.[87] As for medical schools, Bologna, Padua and Montpellier occupied the upper echelon in terms of contemporary appeal, though modern scholars have recognized Padua as the leading medical innovator, especially regarding the advances in anatomy associated with Andreas Vesalius.[88] In heading south, Erastus turned toward the epicenter of the humanistic study of philosophy and medicine and took the most dramatic step yet in transcending the humble status of his birth.

Erastus's time in Italy was a critical period for his professional and personal development. He enjoyed good relations with the Italians, even bringing an Italian bride back home. However, no in-depth study of Erastus's Italian connections exists, although many continued to flourish after he returned to northern Europe. The first firm sources for Erastus's life are the letters composed during his time as a student in Italy. These reveal little about his specific comings and goings, though we learn a good deal about his Protestant sensibilities and some fascinating morsels concerning his intellectual milieu. While we know conclusively that

[86] Maag, *Seminary or University*, 139.

[87] This was certainly the case at mid-century and was arguably the case even after the rise of the Geneva Academy, which has received more scholarly attention. For the University of Basel in the sixteenth century, see Thommen, *Geschichte der Universität Basel 1532–1632*. For a comparison of the various Reformed institutions, see Maag, *Seminary or University*, passim.

[88] Regarding medical schools in general, see Lawrence Conrad et al., *The Western Medical Tradition 800 BC to AD 1800* (Cambridge: Cambridge UP, 1995). For the special case of Padua, see Jerome J. Bylebyl, "The School of Padua: Humanistic Medicine in the Sixteenth Century," in *Health, Medicine and Mortality in the Sixteenth Century*, ed. Charles Webster (Cambridge: Cambridge UP, 1979), 335–370.

Erastus studied in Bologna, it has also been alleged that he studied in Padua.[89] It would not have been unusual for a student to pick up and attend lectures at another institution for a semester, but there is no firm evidence that connects Erastus to Padua. While the majority of letters that he wrote during this time explicitly give Bologna as his place of residence from 1544 to 1552, no letter is recorded as having been composed in Padua. If Erastus had studied in Padua for an extended period of time (e.g., six years as Bonnard suggested, which seems entirely out of the question), his later works would likely have paid some homage to the masters who taught in Padua, such as Giambattista de Monte (1498–1561). This point cannot be pushed too far, since Erastus seldom referred to his Bolognese professors in his works. Nevertheless, there is sufficient evidence beyond the surviving letters written from Bologna to prove that he studied there. Likewise, if he did study in Padua, no one has yet tracked any personal relationships which he continued to foster later in life.[90] Much as his strong connections to Zurich make study at the Carolinum probable, the dearth of later references to Padua make it seem unlikely that he studied there for an extended period of time, though the possibility of a brief sojourn in Padua cannot be ruled out.

Erastus's Protestant convictions were clearly visible in his Italian correspondence. His first surviving letter recounted a lively exchange between an Italian youth and a Catholic friar in Imola, which landed the youth in the hands of the Inquisition. The youth had attacked the friar's assertion that entrance into the kingdom of heaven depended on human merit.[91] Though the youth's audacity impressed Erastus, one does not get the impression that Erastus desired to enter the fray. He apparently attended church services with some frequency and was even impressed

[89] E.g., Bonnard suggested, but offered no proof, that Erastus studied for six years in Padua. Wesel-Roth was much more cautious and noted that the connection linking Erastus to Padua stemmed from a comment from Johannes Wolf which could just as easily be in error. It is noteworthy, but not conclusive, that neither Oporinus nor Melchior Adam mentioned Padua in their early biographies. However, around the publication of Zedler in the early 1700s, the Padua sojourn appeared in many accounts. Zedler, *Universal-Lexicon*, col. 1471; Bonnard, *Thomas Éraste*, 16; Wesel-Roth, *Thomas Erastus*, 3.

[90] The best example of this is, of course, his wife, Isotta de' Canonici, from Bologna, though Erastus also kept up with Camillius Franchinus. The extent to which his later interactions with the physicians Girolamo Mercuriale, Conte da Monte, Girolamo Capodivacca, and Archangeli Mercenari might have been connected to his time as a student in Italy has not been engaged in prior scholarship.

[91] Erastus to Myconius, Bologna/Imola, Dec. 31, 1544, Zurich, Zentralbibliothek (Simmlersche Sammlung), MS S 56, fols. 166^{r}–166^{v}.

by an Augustinian friar's espousal of the absolute dependence on Christ's grace for salvation.[92] Erastus's other letters from Italy are peppered with jabs at the Catholic authorities. He referred to the Dominicans as "Daemonicanes" and cardinals as "Carnales." Erastus reveled in recounting the sordid details of Julius III's pontificate, including the well known story of his special affection for the youth Innocenzo, whom Julius made a cardinal.[93] As Julius had been the cardinal legate of Bologna, Erastus was well placed to pick up inside information on his court and the machinations surrounding the second session of the Council of Trent. Although Erastus's reports betray a clear Protestant slant, they relayed gossip that would have been equally entertaining or scandalous to a Catholic audience.

The most interesting letter from Italy concerns Erastus's attempt to act as an intermediary between Olaus Magnus (1490–1557) and Konrad Gessner, two of sixteenth-century Europe's great naturalists. Olaus Magnus, a Swedish cleric by profession, a geographer and ethnographer by avocation, was living in exile in Italy due to his loyalty to the Roman Catholic Church. Both he and his brother Johannes Magnus had been favored by Rome, and Olaus became titular archbishop of Uppsala and primate of Sweden in 1544—a rather hollow honor as the state-sponsored Lutheran Reformation was taking hold in Sweden. Olaus Magnus is primarily famous for his pioneering work in Scandinavian geography and ethnography including its depictions of sea monsters and naive illustrations of Lapps on skis.[94] As it was known in Bologna that Gessner was preparing his landmark work in zoology, the *Historiae Animalium*, evidently Olaus Magnus approached Erastus with the offer of additional information regarding the species of Scandinavia that he wanted to contribute to Gessner's work. Erastus noted that Olaus had traveled all over "the island of Scandinavia, which contains Sweden, Gothia, and Norway and other realms" and from his own experience and from others had learned of species unknown to the ancients.[95] Erastus complained that

[92] Erastus to Pellikan, May 17, 1546, ZBZ (Sim.) S 60, no. 92.

[93] Later Cardinal Innocenzo Ciocchi Del Monte (1532–1577).

[94] Sten Lindroth, "Olaus Magnus," in *DSB*, ed. Charles Coulston Gillispie (New York: Scribner, [1970–1980]), 9:197.

[95] Erastus to Pellikan, July 9, 1549, ZBZ (Sim.) S 70, no. 168: "Olaus ille Gothus est et totum scandianam insulam, quae Gothiam, Suediam et Norvegiam eum aliis regnis continet, peragravit, plurima vidit ipse ab aliis plurima accepit, de quibus tamen nemo facilius judicaverit, qualia sint, quam is qui et natus in illi locis est et educatus. Pollicitus est mihi, se multa nomina duium et species nosse querum ex antiquis nemo unquam mentionem fecerit."

he had twice written at great length concerning Olaus's offer to Gessner, but to this point he had received no response. This silence had caused Erastus no end of consternation and embarrassment, and he hoped that Pellikan would rectify the situation with Gessner. Apparently the mediation worked, and Gessner included information from Olaus in his monumental work.[96] Erastus likewise continued to pass along information to Gessner concerning the natural world from various contacts, and Gessner would acknowledge him as a source for his *Historiae Animalium*.[97]

This same letter to Pellikan contains another fascinating piece of information which would have been of great interest to Erastus's later enemies in the Heidelberg controversy over church discipline. At the bottom of the letter, Erastus asked Pellikan to pass his greetings to Lelio Sozzini, the Italian biblical scholar generally regarded as one of the fathers of Unitarianism. At this point in his life, Sozzini was simply a precocious foreign student with a magnetic personality who had befriended Melanchthon, Calvin, and Bullinger on his long student tour of Protestant Europe. Although his orthodoxy was already in question, he did not publicly espouse heretical views and his personal confession remained sufficiently orthodox to satisfy Bullinger of the rectitude of his faith. It is difficult to know what to make of Erastus's greeting, as we do not know when Erastus came into personal contact with Sozzini. When this letter was written, Sozzini had already been in Northern Europe for a couple of years, as he had left Italy in 1547. His early period in Zurich seems to have begun in late 1548, when he lodged and studied with Pellikan, but by the summer of 1549, he was back on the road. Sozzini would not return to Italy or visit Bologna, where his father had recently joined the law faculty, until the spring of 1552. He only resettled in Zurich after his trip to Italy in late 1552.[98] Putting their respective chronologies together, it would seem

[96] See Brian W. Ogilvie, *The Science of Describing: Natural History in Renaissance Europe* (Chicago: University of Chicago Press, 2006), 332–343.

[97] E.g., the "Catalogus" of contributors to the *Historiae animalium liber III qui est de Avium natura* (Zurich: Christoph Froschauer, 1555) lists Erastus along with Girolamo Zanchi, Ulysse Aldrovandi, and others. Gessner also quotes Erastus in *Historiae animalium liber IIII qui est de Piscium et Aquatilium animantium natura* (Zurich: Christoph Froschauer, 1558), 533. A surviving letter from 1557 has Erastus attempting to bring Gessner into contact with Dr. Johannes Pontanus, a physician working in Gotha, who possessed pictures of fish from the Baltic. Erastus to Gessner, April 11 (1557), StAZ, E II 361, fol. 56.

[98] Earl Morse Wilbur, *A History of Unitarianism: Socinianism and its Antecedents* (Cambridge, Mass.: Harvard UP, 1947), 239–245; George Huntston Williams, *The Radical*

most likely that Erastus came to know Sozzini in Bologna prior to the Italian's study tour of Northern Europe. While it is possible that Erastus's friendship with Sozzini may have commenced only after his move to Switzerland, it is more likely that Sozzini came into contact with Pellikan through Erastus's mediation. That these two might have become fast friends is wholly in keeping with Erastus's future pattern of close association with individuals of questionable orthodoxy. Erastus mentions Sozzini three times in his Italian letters and appeared to be well informed of his travel plans.[99] While the evidence does not demonstrate that Erastus and Sozzini were especially close, the combination of this with Erastus's likely association with Ulisse Aldrovandi, suggests that Erastus was in contact with the Bolognese circle of religious radicals that had been influenced by Zwinglian theology.[100] These greetings and Erastus's later interaction with Italian intellectuals call for a more in-depth study of his Italian connections, particularly of his contacts with Italian religious dissenters.

The Italian letters also reveal a young man who had very much taken the path of the humanists, best exemplified by his decision to change his name from Lüber to "Erastus." For a man who had studied in Renaissance Basel, this was hardly a novel step. In the wake of Erasmus, Geisshüsler had become "Myconius," Huszgen "Oecolampadius," Herbster "Oporinus," and Theophrastus von Hohenheim (as if that name were not pretentious enough) had taken to styling himself "Paracelsus." As with his decision to take the road to Italy, Erastus laid claim to a place in the world of letters with this bit of self-fashioning. Thomas Lüber was apparently a poor rustic who could not manage his own matriculation fees; Thomas Erastus would become a humanist scholar, philosopher, lay-theologian, professor, councilor of princes, sought-after physician, and academic patron.

Reformation [*SCE&S* 15] 3rd ed. (Kirksville, Mo., 1992), 880–882, 965–972. On Lelio Sozzini's crucial role in the radical movement, see Antonio Rotondò, *Calvin and the Italian Anti-Trinitarians* [Reformation Essays & Studies 2], trans. John and Anne Tedeschi (St. Louis: Foundation for Reformation Research, 1968), 7 ff.

[99] This awareness is quite clear in two letters from 1552 just as Sozzini was stopping in Zurich before his trip back to Italy. Erastus to Konrad Pellikan, May 4, 1552, Zurich, Zentralbibliothek (Thesaurus Hottingerianus), MS F 47, fol. 224; Erastus to Pellikan, June 12, 1552, ZBZ (Hot.) F 47, fol. 232.

[100] Laelius Socinus, *Opere* [Studi e testi per la storia religiosa del Cinquecento 1], ed. Antonio Rotondò (Florence: L.S. Olschki, 1986), 35–36.

In changing his name, young Thomas began the process of forging a new destiny. In a letter from June 1552, Erastus informed Pellikan of his intention to defend his doctoral theses in two months. In January he hoped to visit the "vestiges of the antiquities" in Rome. The Roman trip was not intended as merely a tourist holiday. His chief purpose was to augment his collection of herbs and medicinal plants before returning north of the Alps. He conceded the possibility that if a suitable position could not be arranged, he would perhaps remain in Italy.[101] The letter proved prophetic, as Erastus remained in Italy for at least another three years.

The additional time in Italy was hardly barren; this experience prepared him to become an immediate success as a physician when he returned north.[102] The surviving evidence suggests he remained in Bologna from 1552 to 1555. He assembled a manuscript for one of his first books while in Bologna, titled *A Most Brief & Easy Method for Forming Syllogisms, Not Teaching the Usage from the Art, but Rather, the Art from the Usage*, though the book would not be printed until 1565.[103] This short work (the actual text was less than seventy pages) revealed both Erastus's logical acumen and his commitment to the Aristotelian philosophy, which would be expressed again in his anti-Paracelsian works. In addition to this philosophical text, a manuscript by Erastus "On the Rudiments of the Greek Language," preserved in the papers of Aldrovandi, suggests that he may well have devoted much of his Italian period to humanistic studies.[104] He had also studied with the prominent botanist Luca Ghini.[105] His most auspicious undertaking in Italy was to marry Isotta de' Canonici, a woman of bourgeois or perhaps patrician background from Bologna. She quite possibly brought a handsome dowry to

[101] Erastus to Pellikan, June 12, 1552, ZBZ (Hot.) F 47, fol. 232: "Circiter Ianuarium proficiscar Romam, visurus antiquitatum vestigia quae extant hodie, et plantas aliquas, quales nullo alio in loco reperiri affirmant, qui simplicium hoc est herbarum et aliorum huiusmodi rerum medicorum cognitionem profitentur ut docent. Inde revertar ad vos, si mihi locum aliquem honestam vel apud vos vel alios esse poterit. Nisi hoc intelligam fortasse Italiam non reliquam tam in cito."

[102] Wesel-Roth, *Thomas Erastus*, 4.

[103] Thomas Erastus, *Ratio Formandorum Syllogismorum brevissima & facilima* (Basel: Johannes Oporinus, 1565). Contra Wesel-Roth, the introduction to the 1565 edition of the text suggests that he was in Bologna until 1555 rather than 1553. Erastus, *Ratio Formandorum Syllogismorum*, 4; Wesel-Roth, *Thomas Erastus*, 24.

[104] "Graecae linguae rudimenta authore Thoma Erasto" (58 folios), Bologna, Biblioteca Universitaria di Bologna, MS 1072 (lat. 579), vol. 2, Fasc. 15. I thank Prof. Dr. Joachim Telle for bringing this manuscript to my attention.

[105] Mentioned in Erastus, *Varia Opuscula Medica*, 93, 100.

the marriage, though in the end the marriage was probably more of a financial burden than a boon for Erastus, since Isotta's mother and young sister Lavinia would eventually join the couple in Heidelberg. Although the couple remained childless, Erastus provided for Isotta's sister as if she were their own child, and Lavinia's marriage to Johann Jakob Grynaeus would eventually supply the vital social bond that secured Erastus an intellectual heir. At any rate, if he took on financial burdens, the marriage no doubt brought Erastus additional social prestige.

Henneberg and the Controversy over Astrology

Erastus's first professional position north of the Alps was in the service of the counts of Henneberg from ca. 1555 to 1557. Upon Erastus's arrival, Henneberg was a county in Thuringia ruled by the last count of Henneberg, Georg Ernst (1511–1583) on behalf of his father Count Wilhelm. Though the ruler of a minor territory, Georg Ernst was officially a "prince" of the empire and was well connected with the leading Protestant nobility of Germany. He had honed his social graces and diplomatic talents at the court of Landgrave Philip the Magnanimous of Hesse and had later joined the imperial forces in the war against the Turks. Georg Ernst did not merely rub shoulders with the great; he actually saved the life of Duke Moritz of Saxony in combat. In his concern for his subjects' religiosity and his desire for Protestant unity, Georg Ernst was more a follower of Philip than the crafty Moritz.[106] It is noteworthy that a pious Zwinglian like Erastus would be well appreciated in the court of a zealous, reform-minded prince in the mold of Philip of Hesse.

How Erastus came into contact with the counts of Henneberg remains unclear, though it is possible that the Henneberg native Ortholph Maroldt, who studied medicine in Bologna from 1552 to 1556 and later became the counts' personal physician himself, was the person who brought Erastus to the attention of Georg Ernst.[107] While many sources illuminate Erastus's departure from the Henneberg court and continued relations with the noble family, very little information exists concerning his activities while in residence in Henneberg from 1556 to 1558.

An interesting question is the degree to which Erastus remained in the closet concerning his Zwinglian opinions while in Henneberg. After

[106] *ADB*, 8:671–673.

[107] Hedwig Pfister, *Bad Kissingen vor vierhundert Jahren* [Mainfränkische Hefte 19] (Würzburg, 1954), 18.

his activity on behalf of the Reformed cause in the early 1560s, Erastus would become notorious in south German princely circles for his Zwinglian beliefs. During the church discipline controversy, when Erastus contemplated seeking sanctuary in Henneberg, the prince's Lutheran theologians protested against allowing such an infamous Zwinglian to settle in their midst. Considering how loath Georg Ernst was for Erastus to leave his service in 1557–1558, one suspects that Erastus kept a low profile in Henneberg and practiced making the Reformed perspective sound fully evangelical to his Lutheran hosts.

Just as living as a Protestant in Italy formed Erastus's self-conception, being a well-liked if somewhat clandestine Zwinglian at a Lutheran court gave him opportunity to develop his gifts of tact and persuasion. His time in Henneberg was a crucial preparation for the role he would later play in the Heidelberg Reformation. Even after his opposition to the Gnesio-Lutheran interpretation of the Eucharist became a public issue, Erastus's professional relationship with the counts of Henneberg never seemed to have suffered. Later while in Heidelberg, Erastus sent Georg Ernst a copy of one of his works detailing the Reformed interpretation of the Lord's Supper and pleaded with him to ponder whether interpretations therein were merely Erastus's or truly the mind of Christ.[108] Georg Ernst developed a great attachment to Erastus and nearly every year implored him to accompany him on his cure at various spas in southeastern and central Germany. Clearly Georg Ernst prized Erastus's medical opinions, but one gets the sense that Georg Ernst's interest in Erastus's companionship went beyond his medical position. For example, on one occasion Georg Ernst invited Erastus's wife to join them on the cure. On the basis of both his medical advice and his agreeable personality, Erastus won a patron and friend for life in Georg Ernst.

[108] Erastus to Georg Ernst, Heidelberg, April 28, n.y. [ca. 1562], Meiningen, Gemeinschaftliches Hennebergisches Archiv (GHA) in the Thüringishes Staatsarchiv Meiningen, MS Sekt. I, 5810: "Weiter gnediger f. und herr/ hab ich e.f.g. ein schrifft hinder mir gelassen sambt einem büchlin, bitt underthenig/ wie ich zuvor gebetten sie wollens mit fleiß lesen/ und bedencken ob es meine wort oder Christi und des heiligen geists seien oder nit. Und da sie [f]ünden das es der heiligen göttlichen schrifft/ iha den Worten Christi selbst ungleich were/ sollen sies nit glauben darumb ichs gesagt hab/ auch darumb nit verachten das es andre hohere leut nit gesehen. Den der herr seine gaben austeilt seins gefallens/ damit sich nihemands für vol komen selbst ansehen oder von anderen angesehen wenden möge. Es werden e.f.g. zum wenigsten mehr von diser sachen verstehen lehrnen/ den vil ander/ das auch wo von nöten helffen besser fordern/ das sie für recht und Christlich werden erkennen."

Erastus published the first work of his academic career during his stay in Henneberg, and unwittingly also stirred up a minor intellectual controversy.[109] Upon his return to the German lands from Italy, Erastus had been shocked by the popularity of astrology. As an antidote to this, Erastus decided to translate a treatise by Giovanni Savonarola which assailed the validity of the sidereal prognostications. The work was a rather curious hybrid publication entitled *Astrology Confuted* (Astrologia Confutata): *A True, Well-Founded, Irrefutable Refutation of False Astrology or Idolatrous Soothsaying from the Course of the Heavens and the Stars, Newly Translated into German from foreign and Latin tongues to Steer Towards the Truth and To Serve as Warning to the Common Man.*[110] The centerpiece of the work was a rather free and at times enhanced translation by Erastus of a treatise by Savonarola which was in turn dependent on the prior work of Giovanni Pico della Mirandola. The bulk of Erastus's publication, however, was not the translated piece of Savonarola, but his own lengthy "Summa of a Disputation in which it is proven in three ways that it is impossible for the Astrologers to proclaim out of the alignment of birth any future fortune or misfortune (etc.) for the one who has been born."[111] Finally the book concluded with a brief essay, apparently also by Erastus, on "The Origin of Astrology," which outlined the historical antecedents of astrology in the ancient world.[112]

This was a rather humble debut in the world of letters, though the Thuringian Wald was hardly the center of the publishing trade. The reception of Erastus's publication would prove that confidence in the utility of astrological prognostications was not merely the provenance of unlettered common folk in Germany. Melanchthon learned of Erastus's attack on astrology and was appalled by it. Melanchthon was easily the most prominent imperial Protestant intellectual, leading a humanist-

[109] What follows is a condensed version of "German Protestantism and Astrology: The Debate between Thomas Erastus and the Melanchthon Circle," in *Religion und Naturwissenschaften im 16. und 17. Jahrhundert, Schriften des Vereins für Reformationsgeschichte*, no. 210, ed. Kaspar von Greyerz, Thomas Kaufmann, Kim Siebenhüner, and Roberto Zaugg, 86–101 (Gütersloh: Gütersloher Verlagshaus, 2010).

[110] Thomas Erastus, *Astrologia Confutata. Ein wahrhafte Gegründte Unwidersprechliche Confutation/ der falschen Astrologei oder abgottischen warsagung aus des himels und der gestirnen lauff/ der warheit zu steuer/ unnd dem gemeinen man zur warnung/ aus welsher und Lateinischer sprach/ wie volgend zu sehen/ von neuem ins deutsch gebracht* (Schleusingen: Hermann Hamsing, 1557).

[111] *Astrologia Confutata*, fols. Gvi^r–Ovii^v.

[112] *Astrologia Confutata*, fols. Oviii^r–Pv^v.

inspired reform moment within the imperial educational institutions that led him to be dubbed the *Praeceptor Germaniae*. While investigations into the natural world largely followed a humanist Aristotelian approach in Melanchthon's Wittenberg, like other Aristotelians Melanchthon placed great value in astrology as a form of natural prophetic knowledge, and the subject was prominently represented in the curriculum.[113] Although the chronology of the controversy is not clear, it appears Melanchthon encouraged one of his acolytes, Christoph Stathmion (1509–1585), the city physician of Coburg, to undertake a refutation of Erastus.[114] Stathmion accepted the task and answered Erastus's *Astrologia Confutata* with his own *Astrologia Asserta*.[115] Stathmion rejected Erastus's out-of-hand repudiation of astrology, and argued that there was a proper distinction between authentic natural astrology and illicit divination. Reflecting the general consensus of the Wittenberg school, Stathmion approved of astrology as a science founded on experience and suggested that it was an indispensable tool for medical practitioners.

113 Sachiko Kusukawa, "Melanchthon and Astrology for Lutheran Medics," in *Medicine and the Reformation*, ed. Ole Peter Grell and Andrew Cunningham (London: Routledge, 1993), 33–55, especially, 34. For Melanchthon's larger scientific project, see Sachiko Kusukawa, *The Transformation of Natural Philosophy: The Case of Philip Melanchthon* (Cambridge: Cambridge UP, 1995).

114 *CR* 7:794 (no. 4904): "Hodie literas accepti ab eo, qui docet initia mathematum in Academia Marpurgensi, in quibus scribitur Principem Hessorum Guihelmum praeclare eruditum esse in doctrina Astronomica, ac arte Planetarum motus computare. Dignior hic laude est, quam Medicus aulae Hennebergicae [i.e., Thomas Erastus], qui astris bellum infert magnis clamoribus. Ego judicio adolescentiam ad optimas artes divinitus monstratas summa cura invitandam eas, ex quibus doctrina motuum extructa est, necesse est. Et haec ipsa est per sese μαντιxη, quia testimonium est de Deo, et de providentia. Quaeso ut nobis aliquid de tuo vicino scribas. Bene vale. Calend Junii." The letter is grouped with Melanchthon's letters from 1551 in the *CR*, though the editors acknowledged that the date of the year was uncertain. Melanchthon's letter is dated June 1, and the preface of Erastus's *Astrologia Confuta* was dated May 5, 1557. Melanchthon's letter is thus probably from 1557 or 1558. See also Klaus Matthäus, "Zur Geschichte des Nürnberger Kalendarwesens: Die Entwicklung der Nürnberg gedruckten Jahreskalendar in Buchform," *Archiv der Geschichte des Buchwesens* 9 (1969): cols. 965–1396; especially cols. 1080–1086; *Melanchthons Briefwechsel: Kritische und kommentierte Gesamtausgabe*, ed Heinz Scheible (Stuttgart: Frommann-Holzboog, 1977–) 7:318.

115 Christoph Stathmion, *Astrologia Asserta. Oder ein kurtze unnd gründliche verlegung/ der langen unnd ungegründten schrifft D. Thome Erasti/ Darinne er sich unterstehet/ die Kunst/ so auß der Sternen lauff natürlich urteylet/ zu vernichten* (Nuremberg: Valentin Neuber, 1558).

The conflict did not end with Stathmion's *Astrologia Asserta*. The parties pursued the controversy through an epistolary exchange ca. 1558–1560. Erastus was prompted to publish additional works on the question to defend himself, since Stathmion had passed their correspondence along to Wittenberg.[116] Sometime around 1558, about the time Erastus moved to Heidelberg, he wrote a larger defense of Savonarola's work on astrology in German. By 1568, he had translated this work into Latin and was seeking a publisher. It is well worth noting that Erastus's views on astrology found a more receptive audience in Geneva than in Wittenberg. Theodore Beza, Calvin's successor in Geneva and Erastus's sometime friend, ushered the Latin translation through press on Erastus's behalf in 1569, during the very period in which Beza and Erastus were in the midst of a bitter row over church discipline.[117] In the later treatise Erastus refined his arguments and focused on the philosophical basis of astrology, arguing that it was inconsistent to suggest that a contingent effect could be produced by a necessary cause, which had been more or less the position of the moderate advocates of astrology who wished to avoid the charge of determinism. The final salvo of the controversy would not be launched until 1580, when Johann Jakob Grynaeus edited and published Erastus's letters on astrology to Stathmion and others.[118] Whereas their early vernacular tracts had been more or less centered on whether astrology could be reconciled with Christianity, this correspondence dealt with more recondite issues such as whether Galen's corpus supported the medical use of astrology.[119]

---

[116] Matthäus, "Zur Geschichte des Nürnberger Kalendarwesens," col. 1082.

[117] Contemporary letters document Beza's role in the publication of the work. See chapter 6 below. Thomas Erastus, *Defensio libelli Hieronymi Savonarolae de astrologia divinatrice, adversus Christophorum Stathmionem, Medicum Coburgensem* ([Geneva]: J. Le Preux & J. Petit, 1569). This work is briefly discussed in Don Cameron Allen, *The Star-Crossed Renaissance: The Quarrel about Astrology and Its Influence in England* (Reprint, London: Cass and Company, 1966), 82–83; Thorndike, *History of Magic and Experimental Science*, 5:653–655. See also Beza's response to Erastus's query regarding astrology. Theodore Beza to Erastus, Geneva, [1568], *CB*, 9:208–214.

[118] Thomas Erastus, *De astrologia divinatrice epistolae D. Thomae Erasti, iam olim ab eodem ad diversos scriptae, & in duos libros digestae, ac nunc demum in gratiam veritatis studiosorum in lucem aeditiae, opera et studio Ioannis Jacobi Grynaei* (Basel: Pietro Perna, 1580).

[119] Andrew Wear treats the specific problem of the relationship of medicine and astrology in Galen as well as Erastus's reaction to this (p. 249) in his article "Galen in the Renaissance," in *Galen: Problems and Prospects*, ed. Vivian Nutton (London: Wellcome Institute, 1981), 229–262.

This discussion of astrology, though a cursory overview, displays themes that played prominent roles in Erastus's later work. Particularly noteworthy was his at first almost unconscious assumption that belief in astrology was necessarily an offense to divine honor. In his battle with Stathmion, Erastus was forced to defend and further explicate his views against a member of Melanchthon's circle who had possessed Melanchthon's explicit support. When one takes into account Beza's later role in assisting Erastus, the debate takes on the look of an intramural Protestant dispute on a question of natural philosophy with the traditions of Zurich (with Erastus as their proxy) and Geneva lining up against Wittenberg. Though this split between the Lutherans and the Reformed on the issue of astrology was not absolute, each group's basic theological assumptions conditioned its potential receptivity toward embracing astrology as a legitimate branch of natural philosophy. The heart of the early Lutheran message was simply justification by faith and freedom from the heavy burdens of the merit-based conception of righteousness of the late medieval church. Although the Reformed also embraced Luther's fundamental insight, from early on the restoration of proper worship of God, with its concomitant declaration of war against any idolatrous practice, became the center of Reformed Protestantism.[120]

We will have further opportunity below to discuss Melanchthon's influence on the natural philosophy of German Protestant universities. It is ironic that perhaps the only time that Erastus was able to draw the attention of the *Praeceptor Germaniae* was on the issue on which they disagreed so strongly. Otherwise, Erastus had much in common with Melanchthon. They shared a deep appreciation for Aristotelian natural philosophy. Their interpretations of the Lord's Supper were converging. Likewise, Erastus later befriended many of Melanchthon's favorite disciples, including Zacharias Ursinus, Johannes Crato von Krafftheim, and Albert Hardenberg. The irony becomes more profound when seen in light of the future Philippist-Reformed cooperation in Heidelberg and Erastus's attempt to employ Melanchthon's reputation on behalf of the Heidelberg Reformation.

Although the motivating force of Erastus's attack on astrology was primarily theological, it was more than that. His theological predisposition supplied the lenses through which he perceived that astrological

[120] Here I follow the insights of Steven Ozment, *The Reformation in the Cities* (New Haven: Yale UP, 1975) and Carlos Eire, *War Against the Idols: The Reformation of Worship from Erasmus to Calvin* (Cambridge: Cambridge UP, 1986).

influences had no basis in experience. Even though Stathmion argued more vociferously from the basis of experience, in the end he did not really have experience in his corner. In the case of astrology, Erastus's Reformed *Weltanschauung* was an active agent of disenchantment. There were no intermediary forces influencing the world, only a providential God who had not been inclined to directly intervene in the natural world since the apostolic era.[121] Erastus's war against any perceived superstitious or magical practice, including many of the occult virtues advocated by the Neoplatonists, would continue as perhaps the most pervasive feature of his career.

[121] This would clearly be the case in Erastus's conception of miracles, which he later explicated in *Disputationum de medicina nova de Philippi Paracelsi Pars Prima* (Basel: Pietro Perna, [1571]).

PART I

THE ARRIVAL OF THE REFORMED FAITH IN THE PALATINATE

CHAPTER TWO

EARLY BATTLES: REFORMED PROTESTANTISM'S ARRIVAL IN THE PALATINATE

> "I was first with Boquin in the change of religion here."
>
> Erastus to Johann Jakob Grynaeus, November 24, 1577

With increased attention now given to the confessionalization of the second half of the sixteenth century and especially the "Second Reformation," a study investigating the critical turn of Palatine history requires little justification. The Palatinate was the archetype for imperial territories adopting a Reformed confession and played a fateful role that finally ran its course in the tragedy of the Thirty Years War.[1] Thus any treatment of imperial politics or the nature of the Second Reformation must take the very important case of Heidelberg into account. Given the Palatinate's importance, the nature of its conversion to a Reformed confession remains a vital question. Political histories have generally focused on the personal religious decision of the monarch, Frederick III, the Pious (1559–1576). While the pioneering research in this field was done by August Kluckhohn more than a hundred years ago, in recent decades the late Volker Press enriched this discussion through his studies of the Palatine court and the influence of councilors like the Counts of Erbach. Press argued that the groundwork for the Reformation under Frederick III had been laid by native, Upper German Protestantism[2] and stressed

[1] Henry J. Cohn, "Territorial Princes in Germany's Second Reformation, 1559–1622," 135–166; Meinrad Schaab, ed. *Territorialstaat und Calvinismus* (Stuttgart: W. Kolhammer, 1993); Johannes Merz, "Calvinismus im Territorialstaat? Zur Begriffs- und Traditionsbildung in der deutschen Historiographie," *Zeitschrift für Bayerische Landesgeschichte* 57 (1994): 45–68. See also Claus Peter Clasen, *The Palatinate in European History 1559–1618* (Oxford: Basil Blackwell, 1963).

[2] The expression "Upper German Protestantism" connotes the distinct Reformation tradition that emerged in cities such as Strasbourg and Augsburg—often at some variance to Luther's own teaching (especially regarding the Lord's Supper). Representatives

continuity of the so-called "Calvinist" Reformation under Frederick III with the earlier reforms of Frederick II and Ottheinrich.[3]

Alternatively, theological studies have obsessively and sometimes rather ahistorically focused on the authorship and theological bent of the Heidelberg Catechism. Although a new consensus is emerging regarding the question of the authorship of the Catechism, the document itself can still bear divergent interpretations as to its theological character.[4] The debate has largely centered on whether the Heidelberg Catechism is generally Melanchthonian or Calvinist in character. While not quarreling with the aforementioned approaches, this chapter seeks to contribute to the understanding of the nature of the Heidelberg Reformed movement by investigating the role of one of the primary instigators of the confessional transformation. Erastus played a critical role as both rector of the university and a member of the church council (*Kirchenrat*), as well as through writing and debating on behalf of the Reformed cause. When this late-Zwinglian's role is fully appreciated, one can perceive how much the Reformation of the Palatinate was a pan-Reformed development, built on an Upper German foundation, and not simply a Calvinist or Melanchthonian achievement.

---

of the Upper German Reformation included the signatories of the *Tetrapolitan Confession* (1530). Martin Bucer (1491–1551) was perhaps the classic Upper German reformer. In Reformation scholarship, the description "Upper German" generally embraces the Zwinglians as well.

[3] August Kluckhohn, "Wie ist Kurfürst Friedrich III. von der Pfalz Calvinist geworden?" *Münchener Historisches Jahrbuch für 1866* (1866): 421–521; Press, "Die 'Zweite Reformation' in der Kurpfalz," 108–109. In this essay, Press argued that the term "second Reformation" was not a fitting description of the Palatine Reformation, since there was a great deal of continuity between Frederick's reform of the 1560s and earlier Upper German trends. However, in an earlier article Press himself used the term "second reformation" to describe the "Calvinist" turn in Palatine history. See Volker Press, "Die Grafen von Erbach und die Anfänge des reformierten Bekenntinisses in Deutschland," in *Aus Geschichte und ihren Hilfswissenschaften*, ed. Hermann Bannasch and Hans-Peter Lachman (Marburg: N.G. Elwert Verlag, 1979), 653–685.

[4] E.g., Fred H. Klooster, "The Priority of Ursinus in the Composition of the Heidelberg Catechism," *Controversy and Conciliation: The Reformation of the Palatinate 1559–1583*, ed. Derk Visser (Allison Park, Penn.: Pickwick, 1986), 73–100; Lyle Bierma, *The Doctrine of the Sacraments in the Heidelberg Catechism: Melanchthonian, Calvinist, or Zwinglian?* [Studies in Reformed Theology and History, New Series 4] (Princeton: Princeton Theological Seminary, 1999). See the discussion of the Heidelberg Catechism in chapter 4.

The Confessional Situation in the Holy Roman Empire

When Martin Luther posted his "Ninety-Five Theses" in 1517, he could not have imagined that his internal critique of Catholic practice would ultimately lead to the creation of even one new church, and he would have been horrified to have thought that his protest would spawn three major magisterial churches and many splinter groups on the radical fringe. Luther's message of justification by faith and acceptance of the scriptures alone as being authoritative found a receptive audience among the cities of the Holy Roman Empire, and soon it was no longer Luther's proprietary teaching. A veritable army of preachers took up the evangelical mantle and remolded Luther's ideas. In many cases these preachers applied his principle of *sola scriptura* in a more radical fashion than Luther himself. One such preacher, Huldrych Zwingli, the father of the Swiss-Reformed, led the evangelical movement in Zurich. The difference between how Luther and Zwingli understood the Lord's Supper would be the root of the separation of the continental Protestant movement into two main bodies, Lutheran and Reformed. Whereas Luther had himself attacked Catholic Eucharistic teaching—rejecting the doctrine of transubstantiation as well as the Mass as a merit-generating sacrifice, and calling for giving both bread and wine to the laity—he still embraced the traditional notion that Christ's body and blood were physically present "in, with, and under" the communion elements. Zwingli broke with medieval tradition and asserted that the Lord's Supper was a memorial of Christ's crucifixion. Christ's body and blood were not present in the elements; rather, Christ remained in heaven, and Christians simply remembered his efficacious death in the memorial celebration. An attempt at the Marburg Colloquy in 1529 to bridge the split in the Protestant movement failed. Because Luther considered Zwingli and his followers to be heretics, deep hostility existed between the two centers of Protestantism.

In the 1550s when Protestantism gained official sanction in the Palatinate, the difference of opinion on the Lord's Supper remained of serious consequence to pan-Protestant unity. Whereas the diversity of opinions on the Lord's Supper among Protestants may have looked like two conflicting poles of truth and falsehood to Luther in 1544 when he issued his final condemnation of Zwingli, Oecolampadius, and Schwenckfeld, in the mid-1550s a non-partisan observer might have perceived a gradual continuum of positions. Wittenberg itself, where the Palatinate's most famous son Phillip Melanchthon held sway after Luther's death, remained the foremost Lutheran intellectual center in the empire. Though long a leading proponent of the evangelical message, Melanchthon was hardly a slavish follower of Luther's theology. He showed a willingness to accommodate the Reformed in making changes to the text of the Augsburg Confession in the article treating the Lord's Supper in 1540 (commonly called the *Variata* or altered version of the Augsburg Confession, as opposed to the original unaltered version of 1530, which is known as the *Invariata*). Melanchthon further modified his position concerning the Lord's Supper after Luther's death. He rejected the Lutheran idea of the ubiquity of Christ's human flesh and, like the Reformed, no longer held that Christ's body and blood were physically consumed in the Lord's Supper, leading Gnesio-Lutherans[5] to derisively label Melanchthon and his followers "Crypto-Calvinists." Recent studies have suggested that his Gnesio-Lutheran foes had finally exasperated Melanchthon beyond the point of reconciliation, and he was about to make a more definitive stance on behalf of his beleaguered "Calvinizing" allies at the time of his death in 1560.[6] His brand of Lutheranism, "Philippism," or "Melanchthonianism," remained a potent force in the empire at mid century.

Strasbourg, a relatively short distance from Heidelberg up the well-traveled Rhine corridor, was a more immediate influence on the Palatinate than distant Wittenberg. There a more moderate form of Protestantism had flourished under the tutelage of Martin Bucer, until his departure after the city's acceptance of the Interim of 1549.[7] Strasbourg and its Upper German allies strove for a middle ground between the extremes of Zwingli's memorial understanding of the Lord's Supper and Luther's insistence on the real presence. In the *Wittenberg Concord* (1536), however, Bucer reached an accommodation with Luther and largely abandoned his own, more Zwinglian position.[8] Johann Marbach,

[5] I.e., Lutherans who adhered more strictly to Luther's own teaching, especially on the issue of the Eucharist.

[6] See Wim Janse, "Wittenberg Calvinizans: The Involvement of Melanchthon, Peucer, and Eber in the Bremen Sacramentarian Controversy, 1560," in *Ordentlich und Fruchtbar: Festschrift für Willem van't Spijker*, ed. Wilhelm Neuser and Herman Selderhuis (Leiden: J.J. Groen en Zoon, 1997), 53–68.

[7] The Interim was proclaimed in 1548. Bucer left Strasbourg in 1549. Marbach actually filled Caspar Hedio's post in 1553. See Thomas A. Brady, Jr., *Protestant Politics: Jacob Sturm (1489–1553) and the German Reformation* (Atlantic Highlands, N.J.: Humanities Press, 1994).

[8] Bucer, however, used the *Tetrapolitan Confession* in his will and in his deathbed confession. Philip Schaff, *The Creeds of Christendom*, 3 vols. (1931; Reprint, Grand Rapids: Baker, 1993), 1:529.

a resolute supporter of Lutheran orthodoxy, now headed the Strasbourg clergy and had a direct role in shaping the emerging Palatine Reformation. The city that had once served as Calvin's refuge had not eradicated all Reformed influences, however, and Johann Sturm and Girolamo Zanchi still held influential positions at the Strasbourg Academy. Moreover, individuals who had imbibed Bucer's early, more Zwinglian position could be found throughout southwestern Germany—even in the service of the Palatine court.[9] It is important to note that the Upper German Protestant movement, epitomized by men like Bucer, never saw the Swiss Reformed as heretics.[10]

The duchy of Württemberg also exercised a strong influence on Palatine religious and political developments, especially through the persuasive leadership of Duke Christoph, the dominant Protestant prince in the region. Under the tutelage of Johannes Brenz (1499–1570) and later Jakob Andreae (1528–1590), Württemberg followed Luther's teachings on the sacrament more faithfully than most other Upper Germans and, as the century progressed, would become the center of the Gnesio-Lutheran movement in southwestern Germany.

Hardly beyond the Heidelberg sphere of influence were the cities of the Swiss confederation. Under the leadership of Simon Sulzer (*antistes*: 1553–1585), Basel played a wildcard role, as it refused confessional agreement with the leading Zwinglian Swiss cantons of Zurich and Bern and sought ties with the Lutheran powers of southwestern Germany.[11] Zurich revered the reputation of its fallen apostle Zwingli under the long ascendancy of his protégé Heinrich Bullinger (*antistes*: 1531–1575), although Bullinger moved away from Zwingli's strict memorialism in his interpretation of the Lord's Supper to the extent that he was able to forge an understanding with Calvin in the Zurich Consensus (*Consensus Tigurinus*) of 1549. Geneva was naturally more oriented toward French than German affairs, but was increasingly becoming an intellectual beacon to many who would assist the Heidelberg reform. There was a continuum of

[9] See Press, *Calvinismus und Territorialstaat*, 201.

[10] Michael Bruening has recently demonstrated how much Bucer's efforts to mediate between Wittenberg and the Swiss had made him *persona non grata* within the Swiss confederation. The Swiss thought that he had conceded far too much to the Lutherans. Michael W. Bruening, *Calvinism's First Battleground: Conflict and Reform in the Pays de Vaud, 1528–1559* (Heidelberg: Springer, 2005), 73–91.

[11] Sulzer himself was an important link between Basel and south German Lutherans in his dual role as *Landessuperintendent* of the Markgrafschaft of Baden and *antistes* of the Basel Church.

opinions on the Lord's Supper available in the 1550s, and only a minority of the likely influences reflected what would eventually become the orthodox Lutheran opinion expressed in the *Formula of Concord*.

Like all princes of the Reich, the elector palatine's legal range of action in religious affairs was delineated by the Peace of Augsburg (1555). For the first time, this agreement by the emperor and the imperial estates gave princes the right to make Protestantism the official confession of their territories. From that point onward, the religion of the territorial sovereign determined the principality's confession: a principle captured in the later expression *cuius regio, eius religio*. Though framed as a provisional measure, the basic principles of the Peace of Augsburg were incorporated into the later Peace of Westphalia (1648) and endured until the end of the empire. The Peace of Augsburg offered religious freedom in a limited fashion. It had two major restrictions. First, only princes possessed freedom of religion; the only option for normal citizens was emigration if they disagreed with the faith of the sovereign. Second, only Catholicism and Lutheranism as defined by the Augsburg Confession were the legal options; neither the Reformed faith (either in its Zwinglian or Calvinist form) nor more radical visions (e.g., Anabaptism, Unitarianism) obtained legal standing. The door appeared to be shut to anything more radical than the Augsburg Confession.

The Situation at the University of Heidelberg

When Erastus arrived in Heidelberg in 1558, the territory was ruled by the resolute Lutheran Elector Ottheinrich, who was a leading proponent of further modification of the imperial constitution on behalf of the Protestant cause. Ottheinrich in no way felt bound to a strict interpretation of the Augsburg Confession when it came to furnishing the University of Heidelberg with the finest faculty possible. The year 1558 proved particularly successful in terms of faculty recruitment as the University attracted not only Erastus but also the promising theological student of Melanchthon, Tilemann Heshusius (Hesshus or Heßhusen, 1527–1588).[12]

[12] Heidelberg, Universitätsarchiv Heidelberg, MS A-160/7, fols. 301^{v}–302^{v}; Eduard Winkelmann, *Urkundenbuch der Universität Heidelberg*, 2 vols. (Heidelberg: Carl Winter's Universitätsbuchhandlung, 1886) 2:116; Wesel-Roth, *Thomas Erastus*, 11.

Erastus quickly found himself a leading player in the fluid confessional atmosphere of Ottheinrich's Heidelberg. How he came to Heidelberg remains something of a mystery, though. Wesel-Roth suggested that the court physician Johannes Lange was the key player in his recruitment. Since Lange, the most noteworthy humanist physician of sixteenth-century Heidelberg after Erastus, was a correspondent of Konrad Gessner, the Zurich connection could have come into play.[13] One wonders what role, if any, the controversy spawned by the *Astrologia Confutata* played in Erastus's appointment. With Melanchthon's close relationship to the elector and the University, one would think that he could have had a say on the issue if he had been interested, and his early impression of Erastus was not favorable. At any rate, the University of Heidelberg found itself in something of a bidding war for Erastus as the counts of Henneberg sought to place him on the faculty of the new University of Jena in Saxe-Weimar to keep him close at hand. Erastus decided on Heidelberg. Confessional issues might have played a role in his choice, as Jena was to become a focal point for militant Gnesio-Lutheranism, though it is likely that the higher pay and the prestige of the University of Heidelberg, in addition to its proximity to Erastus's Swiss homeland, were the decisive factors. Beyond the fringe benefits of housing and grain, Heidelberg's offer of 180 florins (fl.) per annum trumped Jena's offer of 120 fl. Heidelberg likely had sweetened its offer to obtain Erastus, since the posted salary for his position was only 160 fl. and he was inserted in the faculty above the third chair (whose salary was only 140 fl. per annum).[14] After his departure from Henneberg, Erastus maintained cordial relations with Count Georg Ernst. Although he left Henneberg, Erastus never left the count's service.

Though there were already two medical professors in Heidelberg, Erastus was slotted above the more junior of the two into the second chair of medicine.[15] The resident occupant of the third chair, Petrus Lotichius

[13] Vivian Nutton, "John Caius und Johannes Lange: Medizinischer Humanismus zur Zeit Vesals," *NTM* 21 (1984): 81–87; Victor Fossel, "Aus den medizinischen Briefen des pfalzgräflichen Leibarztes Johannes Lang, 1485–1565," *Archiv für die Geschichte der Medizin* 7 (1913/14): 238–252; Ralph H. Major, "Johannes Lange of Heidelberg," *Annals of Medical History* (1935): 133–140.

[14] August Thorbecke, *Statuten und Reformationen der Heidelberg Universität vom 16. bis 18. Jahrhundert* (Leipzig: Dunkler & Humblot, 1891), 81; Stübler, *Geschichte der medizinischen Fakultät der Universität Heidelberg 1386–1925*, 36.

[15] This slotting is puzzling, as this jump over Lotichius was exactly the type of maneuver which might cause a protest by the faculty senate. Since Lotichius already possessed the M.D., it cannot be explained away simply on the grounds of credentials. The chairs

Secundus (1528–1560), has earned a more illustrious place in intellectual history than the occupant of the first chair, Jacob Curio (1497–1572). A noted humanist and correspondent of Melanchthon, Lotichius's fame rests on his Latin poetry rather than on his medical reputation.[16] Erastus's friendship with Lotichius, whose greater appreciation of astrology and Paracelsus might have exercised a moderating influence on Erastus, was cut short by Lotichius's premature death in 1560. After Lotichius, with the exception of Philipp Melanchthon's nephew Sigismund Melanchthon, who also died young, a string of unremarkable physicians occupied the third medical chair over the next twenty years. Though far and away the most influential and productive physician on the faculty, Erastus did not receive the first chair until Curio's death in 1572.

Nearly from the day of his arrival, Erastus became a major force at the university and at court. The first sign of Erastus's favored position was his participation in Ottheinrich's *reformatio* of the University of Heidelberg. When the court physician Lange composed the first draft of the new constitution for the medical faculty, the faculty members themselves took part in revising Lange's draft, and it appears that Erastus took the most active role. The prevailing belief among scholars is that the *reformatio* was a collaborative effort of Erastus and Lange, a view that has reinforced the notion that Erastus was in some sense Lange's protégé.[17]

did have different lecturing topics, but one would think that the lecturers were not so specialized that they would have declined a promotion. Perhaps Lotichius voluntarily agreed to the arrangement (as was apparently the case later in Olevianus's resignation of his chair to accommodate Ursinus). Although Erastus was older than Lotichius and had much more practical experience, it would still be unusual for the conventional sense of seniority, based on length of tenure at the institution, to be overlooked. Perhaps Lotichius had less clout as he had only arrived in the preceding year.

[16] Wilhelm Kühlmann and Joachim Telle, "Humanimus und Medizin an der Universität Heidelberg im 16. Jahrhundert," in *Semper Apertus: Sechshundert Jahre Ruprecht-Karls-Universität Heidelberg 1386–1986*, ed. Wilhelm Doerr et al. (Berlin: Springer, 1985), 1:255–289.

[17] For example, Kühlmann and Telle have labeled Erastus as Lange's "*Schützling*." "Humanimus und Medizin," 256. See also Stübler, *Geschichte der medizinischen Fakultät der Universität Heidelberg 1386–1925*, 33. It has been suggested that Lange was Erastus's chief supporter at court, which would explain the extraordinary favor Erastus enjoyed in his first years in Heidelberg. In the opening of his plague tract, Erastus apologized that he could offer nothing better than that which Lange had previously published. In an early letter to Georg Ernst, Erastus noted that he would consult with the more experienced Lange regarding his condition. Thomas Erastus, *Kurtzer Bericht für den gemeinen Mann* (Heidelberg: Johannes Mayer, 1563), Aii; Erastus to Georg Ernst, July 10, n.y., GHA, Sektion I, 5810.

But if Erastus was Lange's protégé, the two nevertheless took differing stands on the Islamic-Arabic medical tradition. Writers like Avicenna and Rhazes had been standard fare in medieval curricula. Lange included those standard Islamic authorities in his early draft of the faculty curriculum. The revised draft banished the Arabic authors from the curriculum, leaving an all-Greek syllabus larded with Galen and Hippocrates, with a sampling of the lesser authors Alexander of Tralles and Paul of Aegina.[18] Erastus made other suggestions that sought to remake the Heidelberg program in the image of the great Italian faculties. Provisions were made for bedside instruction, the collection and study of medicinal plants, instruction in anatomy, and holding more frequent disputations on the model of the theological faculty.[19] The first chair was held responsible for giving instruction in therapeutics; the second, pathology; and the third, physiology. The actual institution of anatomical lectures with a human cadaver seems to have been in place by the late 1560s, which apparently followed the Italian norm of having a surgeon perform the dissection with a learned physician offering commentary, and Erastus apparently filled the latter function at times.[20] Though Erastus did not engage anatomical questions at length in his medical works, he clearly kept abreast of developments in this arena and corresponded with the renowned anatomist Volcher Coiter. With the *reformatio*, the medical faculty became a cutting edge institution which was completely in step with the Hellenism of the "medical Renaissance" of the sixteenth century. It also shared the limitations of this movement in privileging the academic disputation as the primary mode of critical inquiry in the

[18] Thorbecke, *Statuten und Reformationen*, 78–79. According to Thorbecke, many of the significant changes to the document were actually in Erastus's hand (See especially pp. 78, 81).

[19] Thorbecke, *Statuten und Reformationen*, 76–91. See also Stübler, *Geschichte der medizinischen Fakultät der Universität Heidelberg 1386–1925*, 32–39; Kühlmann and Telle, "Humanimus und Medizin," 257: Wolgast, *Die Universität Heidelberg*, 36.

[20] For example, in a letter to Bullinger from Feb. 2, 1569, Erastus recounts his efforts to procure a cadaver (StAZ, E II 346a, fols. 549–550). He later gave an account of Simon Grynaeus's involvement in anatomical instruction: "Simon noster nunc est in Anatome corporis occupatus: quod Italus Chirurgus [Pigafetta] secat. Discimus ex eo multum." Erastus to Grynaeus, Jan. 24, [1570]. Basel UB, G II 4, fol. 278. Erastus's protégé Christoph Schilling reflected on his anatomical instruction in Heidelberg in a letter to Andreas Dudith from Padua on Jan. 22, 1579: "Memini cum Heidelbergae Pigofetta primum ostenderet, & Erastus postea assumeret...." Lorenz Scholz, ed. *Epistolarum philosophicarum, medicinalium, ac chymicarum a summis nostrae aetatis philosophis ac medicis exaraturum, volumen* (Frankfurt: Wechel, 1598) cols. 111–112 (no. 77).

scientific arena. Erastus's imprint on Ottheinrich's *reformatio* serves as a testament both to his medical Hellenism and to his influence within the University.[21]

Although Erastus had only arrived in the city in April of 1558, he was chosen as rector of the university in December 1558 to serve through the 1559 academic year.[22] His elevation reflected perhaps not so much his immediate popularity among the other faculty as it did the patronage of Ottheinrich. In a later reflection on his first year in Heidelberg, Erastus sheepishly recounted: "I was created Rector the same year on 19 December against practices, customs and laws [of the university]. Concerning my ignorance, and the fact that I had not even established a home or any such thing but had recently come from school, I won't add any more."[23] In elevating him to the position of rector, Ottheinrich had unwittingly given the neophyte Erastus a trump card to play in the confessional conflicts which would erupt in the coming months.

Erastus was not the only ambitious young academic who had recently unpacked his bags in Heidelberg; Tilemann Heshusius, the energetic young student of Melanchthon, joined the theological faculty in 1558.[24] Johann Marbach's nomination, paired with a recommendation from Melanchthon, had secured Heshusius the general superintendent position that Marbach himself had twice declined. As general superintendent of the church, occupant of the first chair of theology, and member of the church council, the orthodox Lutheran Heshusius was in a position to wield wide influence over Palatine religious developments. The conventional historical narrative of the Palatinate, primarily dependent on sources stemming from his Reformed opponents, has not been kind to the volatile Heshusius. One scholar even quipped, "He had all the qualities of a dog, except the loyalty."[25]

---

[21] These developments in the history of medicine are discussed in more detail in chapter 8.

[22] UAH, A-160/7, fols. 320^{r}–322^{r}.

[23] "Heidelbergam veni Anno .58. die 25. April. sub Ottone Henrico Principe. Creatus Rector eodem anno contra mores et consuetudinem ac leges (De mea imperitia, qui ne domu quidem aut rem familiarem unquam institueram aut curaram, sed ex Scholis nuper veneram, nihil hunc dicam)...." Erastus to Abraham Musculus, Nov. 23, (15)77, Zofingen, Staatsbibliothek und Stadtarchiv, MS no. 1.53. http://www.heidelberg-frueheneuzeit.uni-hd.de/themen/uni/quellen/erastus_quelle01-01.html.

[24] Alternatively referred to as Tilemann Heßhus/Hesshus, Heshusen or Heshusius in early modern sources and modern secondary literature.

[25] Wolfgang Menzel, *Geschichte der Deutschen bis auf die neuesten Tage* (Stuttgart, 1855) 3:153.

While the conventional portrait of Heshusius has been unflattering, Peter Barton sought to rehabilitate Heshusius and was partially successful in arguing that "Gnesio-Lutheran" was an ill-suited label for this erstwhile student of Melanchthon.[26] Heshusius was a fine theologian who actually held to a rather moderate Lutheran position between the Philippists and some Gnesio-Lutherans. For example, he rejected the doctrine of ubiquity of Christ's flesh as outlined by the Württemberg theologians.[27] Likewise, Heshusius was on good terms with Melanchthon until their falling out in 1559. To portray Heshusius as a genuinely sympathetic figure, however, remains an unlikely prospect. Particularly in his absolute refusal to countenance any compromise with the Reformed on the Lord's Supper, Heshusius displayed a Gnesio-Lutheran spirit, if not a full Gnesio-Lutheran theology. Erastus described Heshusius to his friend Bullinger in less than charitable terms: "The man is approximately 34 years old, tedious, lean, full of gall, of a boiling and an irascible temperament; uncommonly ambitious, audacious, brash, confident; more obstinate and tenacious of his own opinions, than I can express."[28] This quotation reveals Erastus's talent for summing up an individual's character with a couple lines, and we encounter his uncharitable pen directed against friend and foe alike on many other occasions. When we recall Erastus's later reminiscence about his own audacious naïveté at this juncture, it is clear that Erastus and Heshusius had much in common in the way of youthful overconfidence. Heshusius's intemperate zeal and aversion to compromise had already cost him positions in Goslar and Rostock, and he would experience further abbreviated tenures and frequently quarrel with his orthodox Lutheran brethren before his death.

Heshusius's most obvious theological rival was the French-born Pierre Boquin, who held the chair of dogmatic theology at the university. The

[26] Peter F. Barton, *Um Luthers Erbe: Studien und Texte zur Spätreformation Tilemann Heshusius (1527–1559)* (Witten: Luther Verlag, 1972); Thilo Krüger, *Empfangene Allmacht: die Christologie Tilemann Heshusens (1527–1588)* [Forschungen zur Kirchen- und Dogmengeschichte 87] (Göttingen: Vandenhoeck & Ruprecht, 2004).

[27] David Steinmetz examined Heshusius's controversy with Calvin in "Calvin and his Lutheran Critics," in *Calvin in Context* (Oxford: Oxford UP, 1995) 172–186.

[28] Erastus to Bullinger, Oct. 8, (1560), StAZ, E 361, fol. 83a^{r}: "Homo est 34 plus minus annorum, longus, gracilis, biliosus, praefervidi et iracundi ingenii, mire ambitiosus, audax, temerarius, confidens, Supra quam dici potest obstinatus, et suae sententiae tenax." He gives a similar description of Heshusius in a letter to Albert Hardenberg. Erastus to Hardenberg, Heidelberg, Feb. 4, 1560, Bremen, Staats- und Universitätsbibliothek, MS 10, no. 41, fols. 74^{r}–76^{v}. See Wim Janse, *Albert Hardenberg als Theologe: Profil eines Bucers-Schülers* (Leiden: Brill, 1994), 401.

former prior of the Carmelite monastery of Bourges, Boquin quit the monastery in 1541 and studied both in Basel and Wittenberg.[29] Earlier in his career, he was considered too much of a partisan Lutheran to head the French exile congregation in Strasbourg, with its large Reformed contingent. In time, Boquin came increasingly under the influence of Philippism and Calvinism and eventually assumed a Reformed interpretation of the Lord's Supper. Boquin's difficulty with the German tongue and his reluctance to become too deeply engaged in politics kept him from becoming the popular leader of the Reformed party in Heidelberg. Yet Boquin played a critical role in the theological transition of the early 1560s, as Erastus himself acknowledged, and his role in Palatine church history has undoubtedly been underappreciated by modern historians.[30]

Beyond Erastus and Boquin, the emerging Reformed faction did not lack men of political savvy within the university. The jurist and future privy councilor Christoph Ehem was an avid proponent of the Genevan variety of Protestantism.[31] The majority of faculty members at the university, however, apparently favored a moderate form of Lutheranism à la Melanchthon or Bucer.[32] It would not be strength of numbers, but tact and cunning that would decide the outcome in the brewing conflict over the Lord's Supper.

---

[29] Boquin's time in Basel seems to have overlapped with that of Erastus, though I have yet to find any suggestion that they befriended one another at that time. Wackernagel, *Die Matrikel der Universität Basel*, 2:26, 30. Regarding Boquin's call to Heidelberg, see Winkelmann, *Urkundenbuch der Universität Heidelberg*, 2:112.

[30] See Press, *Calvinismus und Territorialstaat*, 240; Wesel-Roth, *Thomas Erastus*, 20; G.P. Hartvelt, "Petrus Boquinus," *Gereformeerd theologisch tijdschrift* 62 (1962): 49–77; idem, "De Avondmaalsleer van de Heidelbergse Catechismus en haar Toepassing in de Prediking," *Homiletica en Biblica* 20 (1964): 121–140.

[31] See Press, *Calvinismus und Territorialstaat*, 213–215, passim.

[32] Among the faculty members, the only individuals of a manifest Reformed orientation were Erastus, Boquin and Ehem. It is perhaps wise not to seek to categorize conversion-prone jurist François Baudouin, who was to depart Heidelberg in the spring of 1561. See discussion in Donald Kelley, *François Hotman* (Princeton: Princeton UP, 1973), 135–138. With no recognizable Gnesio-Lutherans other than Heshusius, the Philippist label would appear an adequate description for the remainder of the university, though admittedly this is more of a designation by default than a positive characterization. Against the prevailing historiographic trend, Barton preferred to label the majority of the university faculty "Kryptocalvinisten" since they migrated so easily to the Reformed position.

The Heidelberg Lord's Supper Controversy

Act 1: Stephan Sylvius's Promotion

If the confessional composition of the university was itself potentially volatile, the actual spark that ignited the controversy arrived in the promotion of the Frisian theology student Stephan Sylvius.[33] Heshusius had intended Sylvius to defend theses which he himself had written containing virulent attacks on Zwinglianism and Catholicism. Sylvius objected to this proposal and desired to defend his own theses. Sylvius argued that he did not wish to offend his Catholic lords in the Netherlands, and that he could not take such a strong position against Zwingli since he did not know the Swiss reformer's works.

Boquin, the *prodekan* of the theology faculty, supported Sylvius's cause. Nevertheless, Heshusius attempted to obstruct Sylvius's promotion on the grounds that he could not sanction the unbiblical and Zwinglian views that he found in the opinions of Sylvius. Thus, the promotion of Sylvius became an internal university squabble that happened to fall into the lap of Erastus in his position as university rector. Although we can fairly assume that Erastus favored Sylvius's theological position, he was careful not to make this dispute a transparent test of confessional rivalries.

The issue before the university senate concerned whether or not Sylvius had the right to choose his own doctoral theses. The corollary question regarded whether Heshusius had unfairly blocked Sylvius's promotion. The faculty senate saw Heshusius as attempting to overstep his authority within the university. It decided against him and barred him from attending future senate meetings. Thus, on the eve of Frederick III's ascension, the Lutheran Heshusius had already succeeded in making himself *persona non grata* within the university. The Reformed had won the first battle of the so-called "Heidelberg Lord's Supper Controversy" (*Heidelberger Abendmahlsstreit*), though the Philippists within the university could hardly have thought that Lutheranism itself was under siege. The first round of the battle had been about academic freedom and the

[33] Although Erastus calls him "Petrus" rather than "Stephanus" in the letter to Musculus cited below, he is called "Stephanus" in the university records in Erastus's own hand and in Erastus's correspondence with Hardenberg. He later became minister in Leeuwarden, Friesland. See J. de Wal, *Nederlanders, Studenten te Heidelberg* (Leiden, 1886), 42–43.

university's privileges. In the midst of this controversy, Elector Ottheinrich died on February 12, 1559, leaving a talent-filled, if strife-laden, university as his primary bequest to his successor Frederick III.[34]

Act 2: Frederick III and the Heshusius/Klebitz Affair

Elector Frederick III, the Pious (1559–1576), had already assumed the position of presumed heir to the Palatine crown as governor (*Statthalter*) of the Upper Palatinate early in the reign of Ottheinrich. Frederick had converted to Protestantism through the influence of his wife Maria of Brandenburg-Kulmbach and demonstrated this conviction through his resistance to the Interim in 1548. While Frederick was hostile toward the emperor and his Catholic associates, the duplicitous treatment of his brother-in-law Albert Alcibiades (*Albrecht Alkibiades*) at the hands of Lutherans, according to Owen Chadwick, "led him to eye the chief Lutheran princes critically."[35] Nevertheless, Frederick remained in the Lutheran fold and, as governor, implemented Ottheinrich's Reformation in the Upper Palatinate. Upon the death in 1557 of his father, Johannes II of Pfalz-Simmern, who had remained loyal to the old church, Frederick introduced the Palatine church order into his patrimonial lands. From all public manifestations, Frederick remained a moderate Lutheran when he moved to Heidelberg to take the reins of the Palatine government.[36]

The controversy over the Lord's Supper was far from settled when Frederick arrived in Heidelberg in February of 1559. The second flashpoint of this dispute likewise originated in the university. While Heshu-

[34] UAH A-160/7, fols. 324–336; Winkelmann, *Urkundenbuch der Universität Heidelberg*, 2:119; Erastus to Abraham Musculus, Nov. 23, (15)77, Zofingen, no. 1.53; Wesel-Roth, *Thomas Erastus*, 18–21; Barton, *Um Luthers Erbe*, 200–201; Press, *Calvinismus und Territorialstaat*, 219.

[35] Owen Chadwick, "The Making of a Reforming Prince: Frederick III, Elector Palatine," in *Reformation, Conformity and Dissent*, ed. R. Buick Knox (London: Epworth, 1977), 56.

[36] Barton argues that the Counts of Erbach had already begun to exercise a Reformed influence on Frederick before he began his reign as elector. On that account, he terms Frederick a "latenter Kryptocalvinist" on the date of his accession, based on a suggestion from Frederick's wife Maria's correspondence from 1559. Barton, *Um Luthers Erbe*, 197. Goeters, however, contends that, "Friedrich III. war bei seinem Regierungsantritt unzweifelhaft lutherisch gesonnen...." *EKO*, 14:37. Goeter's opinion reflects the preponderance of evidence and represents the scholarly consensus. See also Benrath, "Die Eigenart der pfälzischen Reformation und die Vorgeschichte des Heidelberger Katechismus," in *Heidelberger Jahrbücher* 7 (1963): 20; Chadwick, "Making of a Reforming Prince," 56–61; Press, *Calvinismus und Territorialstaat*, 222–223, 226.

sius was out of town attending his mother's funeral that winter, Boquin used the opportunity to confer a bachelor's degree upon Wilhelm Klebitz, a deacon of Heshusius at the *Heiliggeistkirche*. Klebitz defended distinctly Reformed theses on the nature of the Eucharist.[37]

Upon his return, Heshusius, incensed by the developments, sent copies of Klebitz's theses to Lutheran associates for their assessment. The controversy escalated with both Heshusius and Klebitz using the pulpit to condemn the other's position. At this juncture, Elector Frederick was away at the Augsburg Reichstag, leaving Count Georg von Erbach as governor in his stead. Georg admonished both parties to refrain from making the controversy public. Georg also arranged for a dialogue between the two disputants, but this only served to cement Heshusius's conviction that his opponent was an unrepentant Sacramentarian.[38]

Heshusius attempted to settle the controversy by removing Klebitz from his post and later excommunicating him. Since the elector would not sanction Klebitz's removal from his office, however, Heshusius's actions had no practical effect. After both parties were ordered to offer a written account of their positions to the elector, Klebitz again assaulted Heshusius from the pulpit, which led to another excommunication by Heshusius. Elector Frederick intervened in the controversy after Klebitz's excommunication and ordered him reinstated to communion. He also forbade usage of the explicit Lutheran formulae "in the bread" and "under the bread" that Frederick found divisive. That pronouncement proved to be more than the proud Heshusius could bear, and he sealed his own downfall when he denounced the elector's decree. Frederick sought to restore the peace by dismissing both Heshusius and Klebitz on September 16, 1559. In this act, Frederick eliminated both the leading Lutheran authority as well as the most conspicuous Reformed agitator from the Palatine scene.[39]

---

[37] Regarding Klebitz, see Wim Janse, "Non-conformist Eucharistic Theology: The Case of the alleged 'Zwinglian Polemicist' Wilhelm Klebitz (c. 1533–1568)," *Nederlands Archief voor Kerkgeschiedenis/Dutch Review of Church History* 81 (2001), 5–25; idem, "Die Melanchthonrezeption des Nonkonformisten Wilhelm Klebitz (ca. 1533–1568)," in *Melanchthon und der Calvinismus*, ed. Günter Frank and Hermann Selderhuis [Melanchthon-Schriften der Stadt Bretten 9] (Stuttgart-Bad Cannstatt: Frommann-Holzboog, 2005), 257–290.

[38] Barton, *Um Luthers Erbe*, 204. Heshusius also had the temerity to warn Georg of the nobleman's own error.

[39] Barton, *Um Luthers Erbe*, 200–217; Chadwick, "Making of a Reforming Prince," 62; Press, *Calvinismus und Territorialstaat*, 227–228; Wesel-Roth, *Thomas Erastus*, 18–24; Benrath, "Die Korrespondenz zwischen Bullinger und Thomas Erastus," 90.

With the chief troublemakers out of the picture, Frederick sought Melanchthon's advice in bringing peace to the Palatine church.[40] As Luther's successor and a Palatine native, Melanchthon possessed unrivaled influence, a position strengthened by his associates and relatives in Palatine service. By nature a peace-loving and tolerant man, Melanchthon had no sympathy for the agitators of the Heidelberg disturbance, and he issued a strong rebuke to those involved that conveyed the sense of a man already exasperated by the Gnesio-Lutheran party. Although he had actually recommended him for the Heidelberg position, Melanchthon had little sympathy for Heshusius's role in the controversy. Melanchthon responded to Frederick with a personal letter commending the elector's action to silence both of the disputing parties.[41] Melanchthon also composed a *Judgment* on the controversy to accompany the letter. This brief work not only condemned Heshusius's actions, but also went out of its way to denounce the positions of the Gnesio-Lutherans Joachim Mörlin and Erasmus Sarcerius. He condemned speculation concerning the mode of Christ's presence in the Eucharist and the recent formulations that suggested that the bread was the "true body of Christ" or "the substantial body of Christ." Melanchthon, rather, recommended dropping contentious formulae and emphasizing the Pauline formulation, that the bread was the *koinonia* (κοινωνια, fellowship) of the body of Christ.[42] Moreover, he pointedly rejected the Lutheran doctrine of ubiquity and suggested that it was merely a "novel dogma" brought forward by modern scholars.[43] The irenic reformer was hardly temperate when he asked, "What is the great authority of Heshusius, that we should agree with him rather than with so many approved ancient writers...."[44] The old

[40] *CR*, 9:960–963. For an English translation of Melanchthon's letter, see Lowell C. Green, *Melanchthon in English* (St. Louis: Center for Reformation Research: 1982), 23–28. Frederick's private secretary, Stephan Cirler, who was something of a Reformed partisan, hand delivered the request.

[41] Melanchthon to Frederick, Nov. 1, 1559: "I therefore approve the plan of the Most Illustrious Elector because he commanded silence on the part of those quarreling on both sides in order that there not be a distraction in the young church and its neighbors." Translation, Green, *Melanchthon in English*, 25; *CR*, 9:961.

[42] *CR*, 9:962: "Et in hac controversia optimum esset retinere verba Pauli: Panis quem frangimus, κοινωνια εστι του σωματος."

[43] *CR*, 9:963: "Postea fingunt, quomodo includant pani: alii conversionem, alii transubstantiationem, alii ubiquitatem excogitarunt. Haec portentosa omnia ignota sunt eruditae vetustati."

[44] *CR*, 9:963: "Quae est igitur tanta auctoritas Heshusii, ut ipsi potius assentiamur, quam tot probatis veteribus scriptoribus...." Translation from Green, *Melanchthon in English*, 27.

Melanchthon's weariness with the theologians' fury was clearly manifest in his aside concerning the "men whose savagery I also know from experience."[45] Although Melanchthon recommended that both of the quarreling sides be silenced, it was abundantly clear that the Gnesio-Lutherans were the prime object of his wrath.

The letter was generally well received in Heidelberg. Naturally, it had to have been reassuring to the elector that Melanchthon had sanctioned his decision to fire both Heshusius and Klebitz. The Reformed had every reason to rejoice; their loss of Klebitz, a minor clergyman, was hardly comparable to the loss of the superintendent and professor Heshusius. Ironically, the Philippists in the university expressed the least enthusiasm for Melanchthon's *Judgment*; when Frederick sought to have the letter printed, the university, utilizing its right to censor publications, refused to grant its consent. This refusal suggests that the majority of the faculty were not enthusiastic supporters of the emerging Reformed party and that these Philippists were all too aware that Melanchthon's letter could be misused. The elector sought the letter's publication anyway. Erastus sent copies to Bullinger and tried to have him publish them in Zurich. Erastus also arranged for the publication of the letters in Basel by Johannes Oporinus. Many editions of Melanchthon's *Judgment* flowed from the presses of Germany and Switzerland in the ensuing months.[46] Erastus was interested in collecting more of Melanchthon's later letters to demonstrate that he had abandoned Luther's position on the Lord's Supper.[47] The Reformed eagerly capitalized on Melanchthon's apparent rejection of Lutheran orthodoxy.

[45] *CR*, 9:963: "quorum saevitiam et ego experior." Translation from Green, *Melanchthon in English*, 27.

[46] Erastus to Bullinger, Oct. 8, [1560], StAZ, E 361, fol. 83[a] and Oct. 30, [1560], StAZ, E II 361, fols. 85a[r]–85b[v]. Erastus corresponded with Johannes Oporinus over the publication of Melanchthon's *Judgment* and sent copies of Melanchthon's letters to him. (See the letters from Oporinus to Bullinger, printed in *CO*, 18 (nos. 3275 and 3281.)) Melanchthon's *Judgment* was printed at least twelve times in 1560 and 1561 (eight Latin and four German editions; see VD 16, 13:418–420). From the discussion in the letters of Erastus and Oporinus, it is clear that Erastus had a hand in Oporinus's two editions. For a discussion of the controversy regarding the publication of Melanchthon's letter in Heidelberg, see Erdmann K. Sturm, *Der junge Zacharias Ursin: Sein Weg vom Philippismus zum Calvinismus* [*BGLRK* 33] (Neuenkirchen-Vluyn: Neukirchener Verlag, 1972), 229–230, Wesel-Roth, *Thomas Erastus*, 29.

[47] Erastus also sought a copy of the letter from Melanchthon to Johannes Crato von Krafftheim, which contained a metaphorical explanation of the words of institution. Erastus's correspondence with Hardenberg also concerned Melanchthon's opinions. Janse,

In retrospect, the arrival of Melanchthon's *Judgment* marked the zenith of Philippist Lutheranism in the Palatinate. Melanchthon died less than six months after writing the letter. Had he lived a few years longer, the confessional history of the Palatinate would probably have evolved much differently. Given the apparent Philippist majority, with the right combination of advice and appointments, Melanchthon might have turned Heidelberg into another Wittenberg. In the vacuum that had been left by Philipp's death, the Heidelbergers looked to Zurich and Geneva for advice. Thus Melanchthon's efforts proved to be a catalyst which ultimately served to facilitate the Palatinate's entry into the Reformed camp.[48]

With the exception of Frederick, and perhaps Melanchthon, none of the principle players in this conflict distinguished themselves in their display of Christian charity. Heshusius's overbearing style and stubbornness created more difficulty for him than his theological position. His position had once been nearly unassailable. He had possessed supporters at court, influential friends abroad, and a broad Lutheran majority in the university. Ehem, Boquin, and Erastus were the only manifestly Reformed faculty members. As general superintendent and holder of the first chair of theology, Heshusius led both the church and university; the confessional evolution of the Palatinate should have been clay in his hands. It is tempting to see Heshusius's confessional zeal as his chief fault and thus cast him as a prime example of an era increasingly characterized by confessional strife. Although Heshusius was obviously eager to maintain the integrity of the Lutheran Reformation, it was only when his zeal was paired with an equally acute lack of political savvy that it undermined all that he held dear.

While past historiography has sometimes portrayed Erastus as the wily puppet master behind the scenes, it is doubtful that either Erastus or Boquin would appear so cunning if Heshusius had not been so inept.[49] Attempting to force Sylvius to defend inflammatory theses against his

Hardenberg, 401–403. For the letter from March 21, 1559, see *CR*, 9:784–786 (no. 6714). Erastus would later come into personal contact with Crato and exchange letters of mostly medical content. See chapter 8.

[48] Melanchthon died April 19, 1560. See Press, *Calvinismus und Territorialstaat*, 228–229.

[49] For example, Barton relates, "Erastus hat während des Heidelberger Abendmahlsstreites eine Schlüsselposition bessesen, er hat freilich darbei stark vom Hintergrund aus operiert." Barton, *Um Luthers Erbe*, 198–199. See also Press, *Calvinismus und Territorialstaat*, 227; *EKO*, 14:38.

will was not a plot hatched by Erastus or Boquin. Certainly, they displayed a measure of sleight of hand in holding Klebitz's baccalaureate disputation while Heshusius was away burying his mother, but the confessional fate of a principality does not normally turn on a B.A. examination. Again, it was Heshusius's conduct that escalated this episode into a confessional shibboleth and state crisis.[50] The fact that Heshusius alienated both the Philippist-dominated university and his former patron Melanchthon demonstrates his propensity to fail despite having the deck stacked in his favor. In the final analysis, Heshusius's ineptitude was a more important factor than the Reformed faction's cunning in the transition of the Palatinate from Lutheranism to Reformed Protestantism.[51]

The behind-the-scenes machinations of the controversy have also sullied the reputations of Erastus and Boquin. The men have been faulted for allowing Klebitz to go down with Heshusius, a complaint made vociferously by Klebitz after his departure—with much of his animus directed at Erastus.[52] The issue here is the extent to which Klebitz was an independent player rather than merely a "tool" of the Reformed leaders, as he has traditionally been seen.[53] Beyond Klebitz's promotion at the university, however, no one has produced evidence to suggest that Boquin or Erastus fomented his every move. In fact, Klebitz's public feud with Heshusius—especially his assault from the pulpit—differed from Erastus's more tactful approach. Klebitz does not appear to have been his protégé, and Erastus later communicated a certain disdain for him, alleging that he was

---

[50] Barton, *Um Luthers Erbe*, 223. My reading of the events directly opposes the interpretation advanced by Barton that "Heshusius had neither induced or hardly provoked the confessional conflict of the Palatinate, rather he only made it manifest and public."

[51] I take this to be the import of Cirler's comment: "Wen geleich Doctor Tileman nicht wer in die Pfaltz gekommen, so were daerumb die Pfaltz nicht undergegangen." Quoted in Wilhelm Klebitz, *Victoria Veritatis, Ac Ruina Papatus Saxonici* ... (Freiburg: Daniel Delenus, 1561), F1^{v}.

[52] From Klebitz's account, one receives the impression that Erastus was a central player in the controversy, alongside the clerics Michael Diller and Pantaleon Blasius. Klebitz's hard feelings toward Erastus were apparently more focused on the aftermath of the controversy rather than any putative role Erastus might have had in instigating the conflict. That said, Klebitz did heap scorn on Erastus for abandoning him and blamed his inability to find a pastoral post in Germany on Erastus. Klebitz, *Victoria Veritatis*, F[4]^{v}–G2^{v}.

[53] E.g., Press, *Calvinismus und Territorialstaat*, 228: "Ihr Werkzeug Klebitz ließen sie nach Heshusens Sturz fallen, ohne zu zörgern." Barton, *Um Luthers Erbe*, 202: "Clebitius war in dem ganzen Handel kein Akteur, mochte er sich selbst auch dafür halten, sondern Werkzeug."

as contentious and ambitious as Heshusius.[54] In contrast, when another Reformed colleague was dismissed in 1567, Erastus revealed much more compassion and expended a considerable amount of energy to find him a new position.[55] Clearly, Erastus felt no such obligation to the belligerent Klebitz. Rather than reading too much significance into the theological positions of the lead players, one can assert that this controversy was actually a much less complicated affair. It was not quite the "Heidelberg Lord's Supper Controversy" that historians have made it, but more of an overblown row between two irascible clerics; an assessment also expressed by Frederick and Melanchthon. Regardless of how significant these events seemed in 1559, the removal of Heshusius and the begging of the question of the meaning of the Lord's Supper were to have significant impact upon the Palatine church in the following years.

The Heidelberg Lord's Supper Disputation (1560) and its Aftermath

A distinct Reformed tendency surfaced in the Palatine Reformation during the Heidelberg Disputation of June 1560. While the majority continued to favor a moderate form of Lutheranism, the Reformed were growing more influential both in the university and at court. To this point, the only marked Reformed accomplishment had been the removal of Heshusius, which at the time must have seemed much more of a victory for Philippism than for Zwinglianism or Calvinism. German Lutherans noticed the Palatine developments, and after his expulsion, Heshusius became a vocal critic of confessional changes in the Palatinate. These concerns found an influential champion in the person of the elector's wife Maria. Fearing that her husband was falling under the influence of

[54] Erastus to Bullinger, Oct. 8, (1560), StAZ, E 361, fol. 83av: "Clebitzium hic habuit adv[er]sarium, hominem non minus contentiosum simul et ambitios[um] ut nihil praeterea dicam, cum quo si litiget parum sibi gl[o]riae fore putat." Benrath suggested that the candor of Erastus's comments to Bullinger regarding Klebitz shows that he was not fully aware of all the Zurichers' plans. Bullinger still supported Klebitz and entreated Frederick to have Klebitz reinstated, but to no avail. Benrath, "Die Korrespondenz zwischen Bullinger und Thomas Erastus," 90; Hollweg, *Heinrich Bullingers Hausbuch*, 242–243. See also Erastus's comments to Albert Hardenberg: "Ad omnes alios accessit Klebitius, de quo nemo melius est meritus me, quem acerbissimè tamen et improbissime prosequitur. Ingratiorem hominem per omnem anteactam vitam non vidi." Erastus to Hardenberg, Heidelberg, Nov. 11, 1560, SUB Bremen, 10, no. 49, fols. 87^{r}–87^{v}.

[55] The person in question here was Johannes Brunner. See the discussion in chapter 5.

Zwinglian heretics, Maria expressed alarm to members of the Saxon Wettin court.[56] Later, the marriage of the Palatine princess Dorothea Susanne to Johann Wilhelm of Saxe-Weimar became the occasion to stage a disputation over the mode of Christ's presence in the Eucharist between the Saxon court theologians and representatives of the Palatinate.

A most colorful report of this disputation from the Reformed side is found in a letter from Caspar Olevianus to John Calvin. According to Olevianus, the Saxons hoped to use the perceived leadership vacuum in Heidelberg to place one of their own clerics in the church superintendent office recently vacated by Heshusius. The duke desired to lead the lost Palatine sheep back into the fold, and even before the debate the Saxon court preacher Johann Stössel insinuated in a sermon that Frederick had been seduced by his councilors.[57] External pressure was mounting for Frederick to eliminate the heretical forces at work in the Palatinate, which ironically served as a catalyst for his definitive move to the Reformed camp.

The ground rules of the disputation stipulated a one-on-one debate between a Saxon theologian and a Palatine theologian. Stössel and Boquin were the chief participants, though other theologians sat in on different days. Olevianus's account implies that the Lutherans placed no small hope of victory in the fact that Boquin was ill-suited for the task, and Olevianus even suggested that Frederick was tricked into agreeing to the terms of debate. Once the event was proposed, however, Boquin could hardly back out. Both sides were to have a moderator who sat at the same table with the disputants as well as a scribe to record the debate. The event, which was held June 3–7, 1560, was open to the general public, and the princes were seated on a balcony above the disputants. Boquin began the disputation by defending theses that set forth the Reformed interpretation of the Lord's Supper. These theses were very similar to the ones Klebitz had defended in his bachelor's exam.[58] Boquin's presentation pleased the elector but failed to win the sympathy of the audience.

[56] Maria's concerns were initially addressed to her son-in-law Duke Johann Friedrich II of Saxe-Gotha (son of Johann Friedrich the Magnanimous and grand nephew of Frederick the Wise) who had married Elizabeth of the Palatinate. Wesel-Roth, *Thomas Erastus*, 22. Press, *Calvinismus und Territorialstaat*, 226.

[57] *CO*, 18:191–196 (no. 3250). See Sturm, *Der junge Zacharias Ursin*, 223.

[58] D. Seisen, *Geschichte der Reformation zu Heidelberg von ihren ersten Anfängen bis zur Abfassung des Heidelberger Catechismus* (Heidelberg, 1846), 99. Although they are often described as Klebitz's theses, I consider it just as likely that they were actually theses written by Boquin which he supplied for Klebitz's promotion. Sources for the disputation are printed in Seisen, *Geschichte der Reformation zu Heidelberg*, 99–106 and Carl

According to Olevianus, Boquin lacked the debating skill to ward off Stössel's heavy-handed tactics. More critically, most of the audience could not understand him because of his thick French accent. Consequently, the boisterous Stössel easily bettered Boquin.

In the midst of the debate, Frederick proposed a change that was to fundamentally alter the psychological impact of the disputation. He summoned Erastus and ordered him to sit with Boquin in order to clarify his arguments. Olevianus suggests that Duke Johann Friedrich did not originally resist this suggestion, which must have sounded more like an innovation for the sake of linguistic clarity rather than a tactical move. According to the account that a Swiss student sent to Bullinger, Frederick first publicly addressed Erastus before he took part in the debate:

> We have already often heard that you have been accused of error in the Sacrament. We desire today that you defend your theses, in order that your opinion in this controversy will be clearly understood. My son-in-law has consented and desires to hear your opinion with me.[59]

The Saxons, however, quickly lamented their decision to allow Erastus to enter the debate. Erastus both expressed the Reformed case eloquently and deftly eluded Stössel's rhetorical ploys. Olevianus relates, "When [Erastus] had attended Boquin for about half an hour, and had summarized and elucidated some [of the Reformed] arguments, it was amazing how the empty confidence of the adversary was lowered."[60] Erastus's theological preparation in Switzerland apparently served him well. Olevianus marveled at the speed with which Erastus reeled off his arguments. Stössel protested that according to the original conditions of debate he was only supposed to be facing Boquin. He refused to continue the debate if Erastus actively participated. Stössel supposedly pledged that he

---

Büttinghausen, *Ergözlichkeiten aus der Pfälzischen und Schweizerichen Geschichte und Literatur* (Zürich bey Drell, 1766–1768), 31–36. Accounts of the disputation are included in Kluckhohn, "Wie ist Kurfürst Friedrich III," 40–44; idem, *Friedrich der Fromme, Kurfürst von der Pfalz, der Schützer der reformirten Kirche, 1559–1576* (Nördlingen, 1879), 69–73 (which largely repeats Kluckhohn's earlier work verbatim); Wesel-Roth, *Thomas Erastus*, 23–24; and Sturm, *Der junge Zacharias Ursin*, 222–229.

[59] Letter of Thuring Ruost (Turingus Rustius) to Bullinger. "Audivimus iam saepe te accusari erroris Sacramentarii, cupimus igitur, ut tu publice hodie theses illas vestras defendas, ut quae tua sit hac de controversia sententia perspicue intelligatur. Assensit filius meus, idemque mecum audire cupit." Quoted in Sturm, *Der junge Zacharias Ursin*, 227.

[60] *CO*, 18:192–193: "Is quum hora fere dimidia assedisset D. Boquino, atque argumenta aliquot collegisset et explicasset, mirum quam deiiceretur adversarii inanis confidentia, adeo perspicue apte et graviter negotium velut in transcursu explicabat."

would first debate Boquin and later have a second debate with Erastus. When it came time for Stössel to debate Erastus individually, however, he declined, saying that the duke did not desire a second debate. Moreover, he added the weak objection that he did not wish to debate with a physician but with a theologian.[61]

Even from Olevianus's rather one-sided account, one receives a clear impression that it was exactly the sort of debate in which either side could claim unequivocal victory. No doubt Stössel had gotten the better of Boquin, but Erastus had embarrassed Stössel, as Erastus himself reminisced years after the debate.[62] From the perspective of the Heidelberg Reformed, the debate proved to be an unparalleled success. Frederick was impressed by the simplicity of the Reformed arguments to such an extent that it apparently confirmed his doubts concerning the Lutheran doctrine of Christ's physical presence in the sacrament. Whether or not they had actually won the debate, Boquin and Erastus had expressed the heart of the Reformed argument in a manner that the elector found persuasive. From this point forward, the elector could no longer be considered an orthodox Lutheran in terms of his view of the Lord's Supper.[63] Erastus remarked that prior to the disputation "the prince still wavered" with regard to the Lord's Supper, but at the disputation "he learned more correctly. Thus little by little the Reformation had begun."[64] Frederick would convincingly display this new commitment by his decisive actions over the coming months.

Before continuing with Erastus's role in the confessional developments, it is fitting to reflect on the nature of Frederick's conversion. Even if one accepts Press's conclusion that the elector's move to the Reformed camp can be dated from the Heidelberg disputation, we might still ask to what the prince had actually been converted.[65] Though Frederick is

[61] Ibid, 193.

[62] Erastus to Abraham Musculus, Nov. 23, (15)77, Zofingen, no. 1.53: "Venit res ad disputationem, ubi Stoesselium obiter pudefacio."

[63] Chadwick, "The Making of a Reforming Prince," 65–66.

[64] Erastus to Abraham Musculus, Nov. 23, (15)77, Zofingen, no. 1.53: "Princeps tunc nutans adhuc rem, discit rectius. Ita paulatim coepta est reformatio."

[65] Press, *Calvinismus und Territorialstaat*, 229. August Kluckhohn actually marked the elector's conversion with the appearance of Erastus's *Grundtlicher Bericht* and asserted, "Es war eine weitläufige Darstellung der calvinischen Abendmahlslehre, so daß mit Recht gesagt worden ist, mit dem Erscheinen jener Schrift sei der Uebertritt Friedrichs zum Calvinismus im Grunde schon entschieden gewesen." Kluckhohn, *Friedrich der Fromme*, 131. See also Derk Visser, *Zacharias Ursinus: The Reluctant Reformer* (New York: United Church Press, 1983), 107.

frequently labeled a "Calvinist" from this point, there was little that was per se Calvinistic about the early Reformed developments in the Palatinate; the early Palatine Reformed movement lacked a specifically Calvinist understanding of the Lord's Supper or church discipline. In fact, the elector always eschewed the term "Calvinist." Rather, he was converted to a more amorphous understanding of the Reformed faith, which included the elimination of images and the acceptance of the tenet that Christ was not physically present in the Lord's Supper—the two issues Bullinger defined as essential to a Reformed perspective.[66] The first Reformed marker, iconoclasm, had already largely been accomplished by Ottheinrich, highlighting the continuity of the Reformed movement with the earlier Palatine religious developments. The second Reformed distinctive, a memorial understanding of the Eucharist, grew stronger after the Heidelberg disputation.

Reflecting on the prince's conversion does not answer the question of what was attractive to him about the Reformed standpoint. In one of the few English-language attempts to grapple with this issue, Chadwick offered a psychological interpretation of Frederick's conversion in which Frederick's disenchantment with his fellow Lutheran princes, due to their abandonment of his relative Albert Alcibiades, opened the door for his departure from the Lutheran fold.[67] Frederick was an avid Bible reader, and the Reformed vision of a more thorough Reformation appealed to him. One cannot overlook the fact that laymen like Erastus, Christoph Ehem, and the Counts of Erbach played a critical role in his conversion. While it may have seemed that Erastus was at a tremendous disadvantage in having to match swords with men of superior theological pedigrees in the Heidelberg disputation, Erastus was able to seize the advantage through his ability to speak directly to the commonsense concerns of the elector.

To fully understand the nature of Frederick's conversion, we must depart from the finer theological points and assess how the theological transformation may have reflected larger issues in his *Weltanschauung*. For the Gnesio-Lutheran perspective to have remained cogent, Frederick had to accept the proposition that as "Sacramentarians" the Reformed were heretics. The notion that the Reformed were anything less than

[66] See Jaroslav Pelikan, *The Christian Tradition: A History of the Development of Doctrine, vol. 4, Reformation of Church and Dogma (1300–1700)* (Chicago: University of Chicago, 1984).

[67] Chadwick, "The Making of a Reforming Prince," 56.

committed brethren became exceedingly difficult to maintain in light of the spread of the Reformed teaching in Western Europe. Many people in France, Spain, and the Netherlands, in Melanchthon's words, "who share our faith, but yet have the opinion that Christ is not physically eaten with the mouth and teeth in the Lord's Supper," were being martyred by the Catholic authorities.[68] If a theologian like Melanchthon could not maintain the intellectual distinction that the Reformed were false brethren inspired by the devil, how much harder must it have been for Frederick, who had been deeply disenchanted by the duplicity that the Lutheran princes had displayed in the Schmalkaldic Wars. In the end, all three factors—the Lutheran princes' placement of politics above piety, the Reformed self-representation as a more thorough, Biblical form of Reformation, and the manifest devotion and courage of the Reformed Christians in France and the Netherlands—likely played a role in bringing the elector to the Reformed faith. Likewise, once the momentum had shifted in the direction of a Reformed understanding of the Eucharist in the Palatinate, well-meaning attempts by Lutheran princes and theologians to retard these developments came to be seen as unfriendly meddling in internal Palatine affairs.[69]

The period between the Heidelberg disputation (June, 1560) and the publication of the Heidelberg Catechism (January, 1563) marked the era of Erastus's greatest influence on the Palatine church. Erastus was made a member of the church council that undertook the further reform of the church. Unfortunately, the early history of this commission is shrouded in obscurity. According to Press's reconstruction, the council consisted of Erastus, Ehem, Boquin, the court preacher Michael Diller, and Frederick's private secretary Stephan Cirler.[70] Soon afterwards, Olevianus and Wenzel Zuleger, both of whom had studied in Geneva, joined the council. The decisively Reformed orientation of the church council was unmistakable, offering further proof of Frederick's new resolve to move the

[68] *CR*, 9:759 (no. 6704): "... die unsers Glaubens sind, doch die Opinion haben, daß Christus wesentlich nicht also im Nachtmahl mit dem Munde und Zähnen gegessen werde." Melanchthon offered these reflections in a letter to Philip of Hesse and Johann Friedrich of Saxony on March 7, 1559.

[69] See, for example, Elector Frederick's annoyance at the Strasbourg theologians' support for Heshusius after his dismissal. C. Schmidt, *Der Antheil der Strassburger an der Reformation in Churpfalz*, 47–53.

[70] Regarding Stephan Cirler, see Press, *Calvinismus und Territorialstaat*, 240. Cirler was early on assailed as a Zwinglian and can fairly be considered a partisan of Erastus.

Palatine church in a Reformed direction.[71] Frederick also began to lay the basis for the successful defense of his new religious outlook. At the Naumburg *Fürstentag* (princes' assembly), the leading Lutheran princes recognized the *Invariata* of the Augsburg Confession as the official evangelical confession of the empire. However, Frederick won the concession of the acceptance of the *Variata*, with its more open language on the Lord's Supper, as an acceptable interpretation of the *Invariata*.[72] This would give Frederick the opportunity to claim that he had not broken the religious peace after the publication of the Heidelberg Catechism (1563). On his return journey from Naumburg, Frederick read Luther's "Short Confession on the Holy Sacrament" and was unimpressed with Luther's intemperate anti-Zwinglian polemic. Ironically, Frederick's conversion to the Reformed faith seems to have been confirmed by his displeasure in reading Luther.[73]

Among this church council, two figures began to rise to a position of dominance: Erastus and Olevianus. The measure of leadership they displayed led Erdmann Sturm to conclude that "the driving forces of

---

[71] Press, *Calvinismus und Territorialstaat*, 239–240. Erastus joined the body either in late 1559 or early 1560—most likely before the disputation. Barton offers a list with Cirler, Erastus, Ehem, Diller, Boquin, and Pantaleon Blasius, although he notes that Pantaleon Blasius was soon removed. Heinrich Alting suggested that Erastus had been on the first constituted church council during the reign of Ottheinrich, though Wesel-Roth and Press have rejected this notion. Alting, *Historia de ecclesiis Palatinis*, 49 (ch. 27); Barton, *Um Luthers Erbe*, 224; Wesel-Roth, *Thomas Erastus*, 17; Press, *Calvinismus und Territorialstaat*, 218 (in note). For the general role of the church council, see Press, *Calvinismus und Territorialstaat*, 114–129.

[72] The Naumburg *Fürstentag* of 1561 revealed the confusion regarding the document. The princes were unable to find the original Latin version of 1530. The *Variata* (1540) had such a wide currency that it was actually the document used at the Peace of Augsburg in 1555. The exact language of the Naumburg agreement recognized the *Variata* as an "etwas stattlichere und ausführlichere Wiederholung" of the *Invariata*. Quoted in J.F. Gerhard Goeters, "Die Rolle der Confessio Helvetica Posterior in Deutschland," in *Glauben und Bekennen: Vierhundert Jahre Confessio Helvetica Posterior*, ed. Joachim Staedtke (Zürich: Zwingli Verlag, 1966), 81. See Robert Calinich, *Der Naumburger Fürstentag 1561* (Gotha, 1870); Chadwick, "The Making of a Reforming Prince," 66–67; Gunnoe, "The Reformation of the Palatinate and the Origins of the Heidelberg Catechism," 42–44; Karl Schornbaum, "Zum Tage von Naumburg," *ARG* (1911): 181–214; Walter Henss, *Der Heidelberger Katechismus im konfessionspolitischen Kräftespiel seiner Frühzeit* (Zürich: Theolgischer Verlag, 1983), 46; Cf. Bard Thompson, "An Historical Reconstruction of Melanchthonianism in the German Reformed Church based on Liturgical Evidence" (Ph.D. diss., Columbia University, 1953), 340–345; Wesel-Roth, *Thomas Erastus*, 27. Erastus regarded the outcome of the colloquy as tolerable. Erastus to Hardenberg, Heidelberg, Sept. 11, 1561, SUB Bremen, 10, no. 54, fol. 95.

[73] Chadwick, "The Making of a Reforming Prince," 66–68.

the reconfiguration of the Palatine church were not the elector and the church council as a whole, but Olevianus and Erastus."[74] A native of Trier, Olevianus was to become the leading administrator of the Palatine church. Though originally trained in law, Olevianus became an avid student of Reformed theology, learning at the feet of Calvin, Beza, Martyr, and Bullinger.[75] Olevianus demonstrated the strength of his convictions in his courageous if foolhardy attempt, at the encouragement of Guillaume Farel, to introduce the Reformed faith to his hometown. For his audacity in holding Protestant sermons in Trier—one of the leading ecclesiastical territories of the empire—he was rewarded with a sojourn in the city hall jail. The advocacy of Frederick III and other Protestant powers won Olevianus's release after two months of incarceration.[76] Olevianus then followed Frederick's envoys back to Heidelberg and quickly joined in the work of reforming the Palatine church, though mostly behind the scenes at first. Although at first favored more by the elector than respected as a theologian, in time Olevianus would become the chief organizing force behind the Palatine church. Initially Olevianus and Erastus worked closely to establish the Reformed faith in Heidelberg. After 1564, they became increasingly alienated from one another until eventually they were arch-enemies in the conflict over church discipline. Olevianus became the primary advocate of instituting a Genevan style consistory of elders in the Palatinate and rightly saw Erastus as his primary obstacle. After winning the controversy over church discipline, Olevianus hounded Erastus's partisans mercilessly and was the driving force behind Erastus's exclusion from church life in the mid-1570s. His feud with Erastus aside, Olevianus was the most significant proponent

[74] Sturm, *Der junge Zacharias Ursin*, 233: "Aus den gennanten Briefen gewinnt man den Eindruck, daß die treibenden Kräfte bei der Umgestaltung der Pfälzer Kirche nicht der Kurfürst und der Kirchenrat als ganzer, sondern Erast und Olevianus waren."

[75] He does not seem to have made much of an impression on Bullinger, however, as Bullinger referred to him as "Olivetanus" after he had been in Zürich some months. Goeters has nevertheless argued that Olevianus did not travel to Zürich so much to study with Bullinger as with Peter Martyr Vermigli. J.F. Gerhard Goeters, "Caspar Olevianus als Theologe," *Monatshefte für Evangelische Kirchengeshichte des Rheinlandes*, 37–38 (1988–1989): 293–294.

[76] See Günther Franz, "Piscators Kurzer Bericht vom Leben und Sterben Herrn D. Gasparis Oleviani," in Caspar Olevianus, *Der Gnadenbund Gottes 1590: Faksimile-Edition mit einem Kommentar*, ed. Gunther Franz, J.F. Gerhard Goeters, and Wilhelm Holtmann (Cologne: Rheinland-Verlag, 1994), 450–466. Piscator's *Kurzer Bericht* itself is printed on pp. 19–36. See also Lyle Bierma, *German Calvinism in the Confessional Age: The Covenant Theology of Caspar Olevianus* (Grand Rapids: Baker, 1997).

of genuine Calvinism in Germany and one of the first covenant theologians. Both he and Erastus played crucial roles in the foundation of the Reformed Church in Germany.

Although Olevianus's influence was growing, Erastus remained the leader of the reform effort. Even Ursinus's biographer Sturm has concluded: "Without a doubt Erastus had the greatest influence, due to his good relations with the Zurichers, and due to his theological education and his skilled argumentation."[77] Not only did the powers of persuasion that he demonstrated in the disputation of 1560 endear Erastus to Frederick, he also enjoyed the elector's respect as a physician. Though he would later boast that he had always rendered medical service to the princely family free of charge, he was not forgotten in the university's allocation of "extraordinary" income. His medical service no doubt increased his opportunity to advise the elector personally.[78] Erastus's relationship with Frederick grew quite intimate, as evidenced in a comment that Erastus related to the Zurich theologian Rudolf Gwalther regarding his lord:

> You know how much princes fear and how slowly they ponder these things. I estimate that I have said things to the prince, which he has never heard from any preacher or councilor, and that in council and not just once. The most pious prince is in no way offended by my liberty but declares [that] my eagerness is welcome to him. If only he were not so cautious, everything would progress better.[79]

Erastus had the elector's ear, and through his position at the university, his seat on the church council, and his international connections, he played a leading role in reorganizing the Palatine church in a Swiss-Reformed manner.

---

[77] Sturm, *Der junge Zacharias Ursin*, 233: "Den größten Einfluß hatte wegen seiner guten Beziehungen zu den Zürchern, wegen seiner theologischen Bildung und seiner geschickten Argumentation zweifellos Thomas Erast." Note the similar assessment of Curt Horn: "So trat der Führer der reformierten Partei ins Vordertreffen, der Arzt Thomas Erast." Curt Horn, "Johann Sylvan und die Anfänge des Heidelberger Antitrinitarismus," *NHJ* 17 (1913): 238. See also J.G. Hautz, *Geschichte der Universität Heidelberg* (Mannheim, 1864), 2:73.

[78] See also Press, *Calvinismus und Territorialstaat*, 240; Wesel-Roth, *Thomas Erastus*, 24.

[79] Erastus to Gwalther, Oct. 31, [1560], Zurich, Zentralbibliothek (Thesaurus Hottingerianus), MS F 38, fol. 271. "Nosti quam principes multa metuant, quamque tarde de hisce rebus cogitent. Ego me ea dixisse principi puto, quae à nullo unquam puto concionatore aut consiliario audivit, idque in consilio et non semel. Nihil est mea libertate piisimus princeps offensus sed gratum sibi meum esse studium ostendit. Nisi esset paulo tardior, melius omnia procederent." For a German translation of this passage, see Sturm, *Der junge Zacharias Ursin*, 233–234.

Of course, Erastus was not alone in pushing the Heidelberg church in the Reformed direction. Although the decision of the elector was decisive, Press has clearly demonstrated that the high council, some of whose members had served since the reign of Frederick II and represented the earlier school of Upper German Protestantism, supported the territory's transition from Philippism to the Reformed standpoint.[80] In the wake of the Lord's Supper controversy, Gnesio-Lutheran councilors and theologians were released. The reconstituted church council faced the task of filling the parishes with qualified preachers. Erastus lamented the poor state of the church and at one point reckoned that it only possessed four qualified pastors.[81] That at least some of the Palatine clergy were receptive to the Reformed faith can be observed in a comment that Erastus made to Bullinger: "How God marvelously helps us. The Lord has completely provided our church with the best men, who had lain hidden like Nicodemus .... Who would have believed before, that such men lie hidden among us?"[82] This comment provides anecdotal evidence to support the notion that vestiges of the former tradition of Upper German Protestantism lived on in the Palatinate and cooperated in the transition to Reformed worship.

From being an obscure physician whose only notable contacts had been with other Swiss intellectuals like Konrad Pellikan and Oswald Myconius, Erastus became an important contact for the German-speaking Reformed movement. Erastus's correspondence blossomed at that time, most notably with Bullinger, with whom Erastus stayed in close communication until the latter's death in 1575.[83] Erastus turned to Bullinger for all manner of assistance in the Heidelberg reform, much as Olevianus did with Calvin. In time, Erastus acted as a de facto agent of Zurich in Heidelberg. Swiss students and pastors came to Heidelberg to study and labor, and Erastus was normally the chief contact for these individuals, especially at the university.

[80] Press, *Calvinismus und Territorialstaat*, 225–227, 233.

[81] Just who made the grade is unknown, though Erastus must have included Johannes Willing. Erastus to Wolf, Heidelberg, Sept. 29, (15)61, ZBZ (Hot.) F 38, fol. 272.

[82] Erastus to Bullinger, Heidelberg, Jan. 1, [1561], StAZ, E II 361, fols. 63–63[a]. "Deus mirabiliter nos iuvat. Ecclesiae nostrae penè optimis viris prospexit dominus, qui latebant quasi Nicodemi. Adversarii nostri fatentur, nunquam fuisse melioribus viris exornatam, aut melius institutam, et ad huc non est, ut speramus nos facere posse, constituta tamen. Quis credidisset, tales apud nos viros latere ante?"

[83] See the Correspondence Register.

Although no longer rector after 1559, Erastus took an active part in reconstituting the university after the departure of the Lutheran theologians Heshusius and Paul Einhorn.[84] Even before the Lord's Supper debates, Erastus had invited the prominent Reformed theologian Wolfgang Musculus to assume the top spot at the Heidelberg church and academy in the name of the church council. Erastus's letter gushes with praise for Musculus, whom the committee saw as the most qualified person to take the post. It would have been a fitting end to Musculus's career if this dynamic former leader of the Augsburg Reformation, and later steady hand in the state-dominated Bernese church, had been able to foster the growth of the native tradition of Upper German Protestantism in the Palatinate after the Schmalkaldic Wars had nearly eliminated it from the empire. However, Musculus cited a number of reasons, chief among them his age, for declining the offer.[85]

As Boquin was the lone remaining theologian, he was given the first chair as professor of New Testament. Needing at least two more qualified theologians, the University of Heidelberg attempted to win the services of Peter Martyr Vermigli, but, even with the prodding of Calvin, the much-traveled Vermigli, as Musculus, declined on account of his age.[86] As an alternative, Vermigli recommended John Immanuel Tremellius (Giovanni Emanuele Tremellio), an Italian of Jewish origin who converted to Christianity through the encouragement of Reginald Pole. A renowned Hebraist, Tremellius had been the king's reader of Hebrew at Cambridge before the accession of Mary Tudor. Tremellius accepted the

[84] The noted humanist Wilhelm Xylander (Holtzman) was also recruited in 1558 at Erastus's suggestion. Daniel Ludwig Wundt, *Magazin für die Kirchen- und Gelehrten-Geschichte des Kurfürstenthums Pfalz* (Heidelberg, 1789) 1:171; Sturm, *Der junge Zacharias Ursin*, 237.

[85] UAH, A-160/7, fol. 398ᵛ. See the letters to and from Musculus from March of 1560 printed in Reinhard Bodenmann, *Wolfgang Musculus (1497–1563): Destin d'un autodidacte lorrain au siècle des réformes* [*THR* 343] (Geneva: Droz, 2000), 444–449. See the Correspondence Register.

[86] Erastus to Bullinger, Oct. 8, [1560]. StAZ, E II 361, fol. 8: [from the postscript] "Caremus adhuc professore in Schola, et in ecclesia concionatore. Unicornum princeps arbitror dimittet. Iam cum Emanuele Tremelio, qui D. Martyri notus est, agitur. Spero eum nobiscum futurum, quofacto .2. habebimus. Deest tertius, si nos iuvare poteris, rogo te plurimum, ut iuvare velis. Boquino dabimus primum locum. Emanueli secundum, et Tertium ei, quem nobis Deus offeret. Concionatore bono et pio valde indigemus. Cupimus in hac quoque parte à te consilium et auxilium. D. Martyrem plurimum cupio, meis verbis salutari. Voluimus Zanchium nuper ad nos vocare, sed nimium bene aiunt ei cum Marpachio convenire iam, De doctrina coenae non puto eos consentire." Regarding the various machinations, see Sturm, *Der junge Zacharias Ursin*, 232–233.

university's offer and was given the second chair in theology.[87] The university still lacked a third theologian. Its leaders considered calling Girolamo Zanchi from Strasbourg—who eventually would succeed Ursinus in the third chair in 1568—but at this point it was rumored that he held an excessively Lutheran conception of the Lord's Supper.

Given his later fame as a Reformed theologian, it appears curious in hindsight that Olevianus was not immediately appointed to fill the third chair, as he had already been in Heidelberg for some months. However, it took some time for Olevianus to emerge as a theologian and preacher.[88] Initially, either he was unwilling to join the faculty or the university considered him an unacceptable candidate. Later, the university senate debated calling either Olevianus or Adam Neuser (c. 1530–1576) to the third chair of theology. Neuser was a south German native of the territory of Brandenburg-Ansbach who had apparently studied with Musculus in Bern. Later a cleric at the *Peterskirche* and the *Heiliggeistkirche*, Neuser would cause no end of scandal with his Antitrinitarian opinions in the early 1570s.[89] Though the faculty favored Neuser, Olevianus was awarded the position at the behest of the elector.[90]

Not long after Olevianus's appointment was arranged, however, the Protestant diplomat Hubert Languet recommended the Silesian theologian Zacharias Ursinus to the Palatine representatives at the princes' colloquy at Naumburg.[91] Ursinus was a student of Melanchthon who increasingly moved in Reformed circles after Melanchthon's death. When he received the call to Heidelberg, Ursinus was studying with Bullinger and Vermigli in Zurich. Erastus wrote Bullinger and sought his counsel regarding the suitability of Ursinus. From the sources that survive, one gets the impression that Erastus took the leading role in

[87] John Tedeschi, "The Cultural Contributions of Italian Protestant Reformers in the Late Renaissance," in *Schifanoia: notizie dell'Istituto di studi rinascimentali de Ferrara* (Modena: Panini, 1986), 127–151.

[88] For instance, Erastus remarked to Bullinger that Olevianus was reluctant to preach. Erastus to Bullinger, Oct. 30, [1560], StAZ, E II 361, fol. 85ᵃ: "Oleviani opera uti nequeamus in concionibus in causa qui concionari non vult."

[89] Christopher J. Burchill, *The Heidelberg Antitrinitarians* [Bibliotheca Dissidentium 11], ed. André Séguenny (Baden-Baden: Editions Valentin Koerner, 1989), 107–111.

[90] Burchill, *The Heidelberg Antitrinitarians*, 113. Erastus to Bullinger, Heidelberg, Jan. 1, [1561], StAZ, E II 361, fols. 63–63ᵃ: "Dominus Olevianus uxorem Argentinae duxit, et hic tertium in Schola inter theologos locum est habiturus." UAH, A-160/8, fol. 32. See Goeters, "Caspar Olevianus als Theologe," 295.

[91] On Jan. 25, 1561, Lanquet mentioned in a letter to Caspar Peucer that he had recommended that Ursinus be called to Heidelberg. Sturm, *Der junge Zacharias Ursin*, 237.

recruiting Ursinus for Heidelberg and that Bullinger's advice on the decision was considered critical.[92] By July of 1561, Ursinus had accepted the call to Heidelberg.[93] This strategic recruitment had an enduring impact on the development of the Heidelberg theology and served to forge a closer link between Reformed Protestantism and Philippist Lutheranism. After the university secured Ursinus, Olevianus transferred to a post at the *Heiliggeistkirche* to make room for Ursinus on the university faculty.[94] Olevianus's transfer had a large impact on future confessional struggles. When Olevianus later emerged as the leading cleric of the Palatinate, he did not possess a direct role in the university. No future cleric ever wielded the combined powers of Heshusius, who had been both the general superintendent of the church and the holder of the first chair of theology. In the later struggle over church discipline, Olevianus's authority was limited to the ecclesiastical realm. The clergy had a tough time implementing their will in the university, and the university thus remained a haven of intellectual dissent.

Also at the university, Erastus acted to secure a position on the faculty for his Swiss countryman Johannes Brunner. With Brunner it seems that the Swiss influence had reached such a high level that it had engendered something of a backlash. Erastus and his associates found it prudent to send Brunner to a nearby parish for a few months to help soften his Swiss accent. He was eventually recalled to the university, but even then his posting was opposed by some members of the arts faculty.[95]

---

[92] Erastus to Bullinger, May 19, [1561], Zurich, Staatsarchiv des Kantons Zürich, MS E II 345, fol. 736. "Audivimus etiam apud vos istic esse virum bonum et doctum Zachariam Ursinum a Huberto Lanqueto nobis commendatum; eum valde cuperemus, si minister ecclesiae esse vellet ac nobiscum esse, de conditione ei non mala prospiceremus. Si putaveris eum usui nobis esse posse, vehementer te oramus, ut cum eo colloquaris et, quid animi habeat, nobis, quamprimum poteris, significes; erit id nobis omnibus quam gratissimum."

[93] Sturm, *Der junge Zacharias Ursin*, 237.

[94] While most pro-Olevianus historiography has not seen his resignation from the theological faculty as a slight, it is possible that this change, as well as the earlier reluctance to appoint Olevianus to the faculty, offers a clue regarding Olevianus's reputation as a theologian among his contemporaries. See also Press, *Calvinismus und Territorialstaat*, 242.

[95] Brunner, like Zwingli himself, was from the lordship of Toggenburg in eastern Switzerland. Brunner matriculated in Heidelberg as Professor of Ethics on Oct. 3, 1561 (Toepke, *Die Matrikel der Universität Heidelberg*, 2:26). Brunner's arrival and various postings (pastor in Weinheim, *Collegium Sapientiae*, university arts faculty) can be tracked in Erastus's letters to the leaders of the Zurich church. Erastus to Gwalther,

Investigation of Erastus's correspondence leaves little doubt that he played a significant role in acquiring these future leaders of the Heidelberg church. Beyond Erastus's personal influence, one should not overlook the fact that both of the new theologians (Tremellius and Ursinus) were recruited with the assistance of Zurich.

Erastus's influence on Palatine religious developments mirrored the unrivaled status that Bullinger and the Zurich church possessed as outside theological authorities in the early days of the Palatine Reformed movement. The emerging Palatine church was nourished by Bucerian, Melanchthonian, Calvinist, and Zwinglian streams. While the Zwinglian party was perhaps the most influential group in the early days of the "Second Reformation," the Calvinist faction enjoyed immense influence at court, which would increase with the flood of French and Dutch refugees into the Palatinate in the mid-1560s.

Heidelberg, Dec. 5, [1560], ZBZ (Hot.) F 38, fol. 269; Erastus to Bullinger, Heidelberg, Jan. 1, [1561], StAZ, E II 361, fols. 63–63[a]; Erastus to Bullinger, Sept. 18, (15)61, StAZ, E II 345, fol. 491; Erastus to Bullinger, Heidelberg, Nov. 21, [1561], StAZ, E II 361, fol. 29. See also Benrath, "Die Korrespondenz zwischen Bullinger und Thomas Erastus," 93–94.

CHAPTER THREE

THE LORD'S SUPPER IN THEORY AND PRACTICE

> And further my gracious prince and lord, I have left your grace a text together with a booklet, and I humbly beseech you, as I have asked before, that if you will, you might read it with diligence, and consider whether it be my word or if it be that of Christ and the Holy Spirit.
>
> Erastus to Count Georg Ernst, April 28, [ca. 1562]

The Gründtlicher Bericht

In the early 1560s, Erastus headed the cadre of academics, preachers, and court officials who prodded Elector Frederick III, the Pious, towards the Reformed camp. While Erastus had previously worked behind the scenes, the Heidelberg Lord's Supper disputation of 1560 pushed him into the spotlight. Now recognized for his theological expertise, he endeavored to write theological works for a popular audience. His first work was a Reformed interpretation of Eucharistic proof texts entitled *Thorough Account, Regarding How the Words of Christ, 'This is my body, etc.,' Should be Understood* (Gründtlicher Bericht).[1] After writing the tract in 1561 and circulating it among friends, he published it anonymously in 1562. He intended the work to serve as an apology for the Reformed interpretation of the Lord's Supper. Erastus sought to win over the vernacular

[1] Thomas Erastus, *Gründtlicher bericht/ wie die wort Christi/ Das ist mein leib/ etc. zuverstehen seien* (Heidelberg: Ludwig Lück, 1562). Though the work was published anonymously, there is no doubt regarding Erastus's authorship of the tract. Not only is the authorship attested in Erastus's letters (referenced below), but the French translations of the tract bore his name. He also defended the work in a response to Johann Marbach. See Henss, *Der Heidelberger Katechismus*, 18. Note that another anonymous work (this time by Ursinus) was published under a similar title: *Gründtlicher bericht Vom heiligen Abendmal unsers Herren Jesu Christi/ aus einhelliger Lere/ der heiligen Schrifft/ der alten rechtglaubigen Christlichen kirchen/ und auch der Augspurgischen Confession. Gestellt Durch der Universitet Heydelberg Theologen* (Heidelberg: Johann Meyer, 1564).

reading public and to defuse Lutheran criticism by stressing both the Scriptural authenticity and soteriological heart of the Reformed understanding of the Eucharist.[2] As an apologetic text, the treatise possessed both educational and ecumenical purposes. His primary audience was the pastors of the Palatinate, as he commented in a letter to Bullinger:

> I have written crudely for unlearned ones, but in such a manner that [Caspar] Olevianus, Petrus Colonius, [Wilhelm] Xylander, our council, and others have asserted that they have never read anything more clear or equally frank on the topic. I have written for certain of our quite uneducated preachers; but they are also pious and think rightly, [and] since having received a certain foundation they desire to relate to the people the same thing more successfully, having set aside all [their] questions.[3]

Beyond discerning the tract's intended audience from this quote, one can see that Erastus was quite pleased with his tract and with the reception that it had received from his theological associates. Erastus likely also had men like Frederick and his own former lord Georg Ernst von Henneberg in mind in composing his tract and, in fact, he apparently sent Georg Ernst a copy of the treatise.[4] Such literate laymen had likely only heard of the doctrine of Zwingli from the mouths of his enemies. One cannot overvalue how Erastus's experience as a Zwinglian serving in a Lutheran court in Henneberg affected both his personality and his work. Having lived with Lutherans, he was surely well-informed of the misrepresentations of Zwinglian theology as well as of popular prejudice against Zwinglians. A poignant example of this prejudice can be seen in the need for Bullinger's son Christoph's need to pass under an assumed name at the Lutheran Henneberg court lest he reveal his close connections to the leaders of the Zurich Reformation.[5]

---

[2] *Gründtlicher Bericht*, 3. Wesel-Roth, *Thomas Erastus*, 32–33.

[3] Erastus to Bullinger, March 18 and 25, (1561), ZBZ (Hot.) F 38, fol. 264. "Meum de coena domini Scriptum ei legendum tradidi, cuius exemplum ad te mittam, ubi Heidelb[ergam] rediero. Scripsi rudibus ruditer, sed ita ut Olevianus, Petrus Colonius, Xylander, noster Senatus, atque alii nihil se unquam legisse asseverent magis explicatè aut aequè apertè hac de re scriptum. Propter concionatores nostros quosdam rudes admodum, sed pios tamen et rectè sentientes, scripsi, ut accepto certo fundamento felicius populo proponere quirent ipsam rem quaestionibus omnibus omissis."

[4] Erastus to Georg Ernst, Heidelberg, April 28, [ca. 1562], GHA, Sekt. I, 5810. See chapter 1.

[5] Erastus had secured Christoph a place at the Henneberg court and suggested he call himself "Christoph Adlisweiler" rather than be known as "Christoph Bullinger." After explaining the hostility to those called Zwingilians, Erastus explained to Bullinger: "Sed et illic arte opus fuit, et nomen mutandum. Itaque pro Bullingero sese appellat Adlisweiler." Erastus to Bullinger, Oct. 8, (1560), StAZ, E II 361, fols. 7 and 83. "Adlischwyler" was the

His time at the Henneberg court had also made Erastus something of an apologist, if a clandestine one, for the Reformed cause. He avoided waving flags that might alert his Lutheran associates of a Zwinglian message. Rather than directly confronting the Lutherans, Erastus proceeded with a strategy that made the rejection of Christ's physical presence in the Lord's Supper appear only natural corollary to justification by faith; he attempted to sound a tone that was more evangelical than that of the Lutherans themselves.

He sent the tract to Bullinger to learn his opinion of the work and to seek a printer for it in Zurich. Erastus made the curious suggestion that if the tract pleased Bullinger, and if he could improve the text, Erastus would be happy for it to be published under Bullinger's name; Erastus claimed that he had no desire to see it published as his own work.[6] Although on the surface Erastus appeared to lack confidence in his own work, this suggestion may also betray a touch of hubris. Erastus may have felt that he had communicated the Reformed understanding of the Lord's Supper so successfully that it was likely to find wide appeal. In this light, it would be fitting that the work should bear the official stamp of the Zurich church, so that all could see that this was the actual teaching of the Swiss. Whether one interprets his comments to Bullinger as a mark of humility or pride, it is clear that Erastus did not doubt that the work conformed to the Zurich conception of the Lord's Supper.

As the title suggests, the work focused on Christ's words of institution of the Lord's Supper: "This is my body." This simple phrase had been the stumbling block to pan-Protestant confessional unity since the 1529 Marburg colloquy. According to reports of the colloquy, Luther dramatically demonstrated his reliance on the words *Hoc est corpus meum* by writing them in chalk on a tabletop in the Marburg castle. Thus, Erastus was not avoiding controversy but addressing the problem directly with his tract. According to Erastus, the key question to the meaning of "This is my body" focused solely on the meaning of the word "this." Erastus conceded that many believe that it means what it literally expressed; i.e., that the bread that Christ offered the disciples was literally Christ's

maiden name of Heinrich Bullinger's wife Anna. See also Benrath, "Die Korrespondenz zwischen Bullinger und Thomas Erastus," 89.

[6] Erastus to Bullinger, March 18 and 25, (1561), ZBZ (Hot.) F 38, fol. 264: "Non iudicium modo, sed si edendum putes, id quod omnes hucusque à me improbè flagitarunt, tuo nomine edas, ubi pro arbitrio tuo cuncta in eo mutaveris. Nomen meum hac ratione legi neque volo neque velle debeo."

body. Erastus contended, however, that this literal reading was indefensible when one interpreted the passage in the light of other scriptural texts, and, thus, that the passage could not be understood "according to the letter."[7]

Erastus organized his argument in three sections to prove his point. First, he endeavored to show that Paul's words in 1 Corinthians excluded a literal interpretation. He then argued that other statements by Christ in the Gospels suggested a symbolic rather than literal understanding of "This is my body." Finally, Erastus assembled a brief list of Patristic witnesses to bolster the orthodox heritage of the Reformed Eucharistic theology.

In the treatise's first section, Erastus began his discussion of the Eucharistic teaching of Paul by taking up 1 Corinthians 10:16: "The cup of blessing which we bless, is it not the communion of the blood of Christ? The bread which we break, is it not the communion with the body of Christ?"[8] Although this was a common proof text for Eucharistic theology which had also been referred to by Zwingli, it is likely that the prominent place Melanchthon had given the passage in his *Judgment* alerted Erastus to its rhetorical potential.[9] Here was a text that offered an amplification of that ever-troublesome phrase "This is my body." Erastus argued that Christ's words of institution recorded in the Gospel accounts needed to be reinterpreted in light of Paul's text. Erastus confidently asserted that Paul had the same understanding of the Lord's Supper as Christ and the apostles. The Holy Spirit, however, had inspired Paul to communicate a more complete explanation of the Lord's Supper than was present in the Gospel accounts. Thus, in this passage, Paul fleshed out the truth that had been latent in the Gospels; namely, that "is my body" actually meant "is the communion of the body of Christ."[10] Erastus asserted that Christ's words should be taken to mean: "This bread which I break with thanksgiving and give or offer you is the communion of my body which is given for you."[11]

---

[7] *Gründtlicher Bericht*, 4. "Wie der büchstab lautet."

[8] KJV.

[9] Goeters has also noted Erastus's dependence on Melanchthon in the piece. [Goeters] in *EKO*, 14:39.

[10] *Gründtlicher Bericht*, 6.

[11] Ibid.: "Das brot das ich mit dancksagung gebrochen/ eüch zuessen übergebe oder darbiete/ ist die Gemeinschafft meines leibs/ der für eüch geben wird."

From this Pauline perspective, Erastus suggested that anyone who knew the meaning of the German word *Gemeinschaft*[12] could easily understand what the Lord's Supper was originally intended to symbolize. The "communion" that Christians have with the body of Christ was analogous to a citizen's enjoyment of full right of citizenship in a village or town community.[13] Zwingli had made a very similar point, though he had used slightly different vocabulary. Regarding the meaning of "communion" in 1 Corinthians 10:16, Zwingli related: "Once we see this point it is easy to understand the word communion [*gemeinsame*], for we have simply to give it the sense of community [*gemeind*]."[14] Erastus used *Gemeinschaft* instead of Zwingli's *Gemainsame* but developed a similar analogy of comparing communion with Christ to the civic community. In the case of a village, *Gemeinschaft* meant two or more people having power or right to possess and use the same water or field with others. These individuals were thus fellow members in the *Gemeinschaft* of the same resource. Erastus argued that *Bürgerrecht* (citizenship) was also a fitting analogy to a Christian's communion with Christ. When individuals acquired the right of citizenship, they became joint members of the city and enjoyed the freedom and privileges of citizenship.[15] Likewise, Erastus argued, to have communion with Christ meant to have authority and right with all believers to receive the merits and benefits of Christ's death.[16] It simply meant that Christians were joint heirs and fellow partakers of all heavenly benefits in Christ. Here Erastus could almost be writing at the cue of twentieth-century historians who emphasized the appeal of the Reformation to the late medieval *Gemeinde* in that he takes the metaphor of membership in the civic community to be functionally identical to a Christian's communion with Christ.[17] Erastus's equation of civic communion and spiritual communion was reminiscent of

[12] Ibid. Spelled *Gemainschafft* in Erastus's text.

[13] The Greek range of *κοινωνια* would not exclude this interpretation, though it more commonly denoted association or partnership among individuals. Walter Bauer et al., *A Greek-English Lexicon of the New Testament and Other Early Christian Literature*, 2nd ed. (Chicago: University of Chicago, 1979), 438–439.

[14] Z, 4:860. "Demnach verstat sich das wort 'gemeinsame' wol, doch das du es für 'die Gemeind' verstandist." Translation from G.W. Bromiley, ed., *Zwingli and Bullinger* (Philadelphia: Westminster Press, 1953), 236.

[15] *Gründtlicher Bericht*, 7.

[16] Ibid., 8, "Vollmacht und Gerectigkeit."

[17] E.g., Bernd Moeller, *Imperial Cities and the Reformation*, trans. H.C.E. Midelfort and M.U. Edwards (Philadelphia: Fortress, 1972) and Peter Blickle, *Gemeindereformation: die Menschen des 16. Jahrhunderts auf dem Weg zum Heil* (Munich: Oldenbourg, 1985).

the "miniature *corpus christianum*" which Bernd Moeller has suggested characterized late medieval south German and Swiss towns.[18] In Erastus's thought, however, the communal themes have a different effect. Rather than encouraging the town council to usurp formerly ecclesiastical functions for the community's salvation, which had been the case in the communal Reformation, in his discussion of the sacrament, communal relations had become normative for Christian experience. Worldly communion defined a Christian's communion with Christ, and this communion was as much a shared quality with other Christians as it was a participation in Christ's sacrifice.[19]

Communal metaphors were an important resource for Erastus in his effort to explain the symbolic nature of the Lord's Supper. He maintained the traditional distinction between the symbol and the reality symbolized, which characterized early Swiss Reformed theology. The strength of Erastus's presentation was that in emphasizing the *Gemeinschaft* metaphor, he employed an analogy that could not bear a literal interpretation. Erastus argued that a Christian's *Gemeinschaft* with Christ was analogous to a burgher's citizenship rights. Therefore, the Lord's Supper was a tangible sign of that *Gemeinschaft* in the same way that a letter of citizenship or (legal) seal was a tangible sign of citizenship. One protected this letter of citizenship assiduously, since it guaranteed one's civic rights. However, the letter could never be identified with citizenship itself; it was only a legal witness of citizenship. Likewise, the Lord's Supper was a sign of a Christian's *Gemeinschaft* with Christ. It was a tangible symbol that guaranteed the underlying spiritual reality. The bread and the wine were authentic signs, *Wahrzeichen*, of a Christian's communion with Christ. Christians called the communal elements Christ's "body" and "blood." Nevertheless, as in the case of citizenship, this *Gemeinschaft* with Christ that the communal elements symbolize remained invisible and intangible.[20] The direct analogy that Erastus made between *Gemeinschaft* with Christ and *Gemeinschaft* with a civic community gave a powerful example of how the Lord's Supper could be conceived as a symbol

---

[18] Moeller, *Imperial Cities and the Reformation*, 49.

[19] Unlike Zwingli, Erastus does not emphasize the communion of the body of Christ as the "transubstantiation" of the congregation into Christ's body, as some scholars have characterized Zwingli's Eucharistic thought. Erastus's focus is on a Christian's communal right to enjoy Christ's benefits. See W.P. Stephens, *The Theology of Huldrych Zwingli* (Oxford: Oxford UP, 1986) 230.

[20] *Gründtlicher Bericht*, 10: "unsichtbar und ungreifflich."

of a spiritual or forensic reality rather than a physical reality.[21] Erastus put forward a theology of the Lord's Supper in which participation in the rite objectively conveyed Christ's benefits to the believer. Any notion of Christ's physical presence in the elements, however, would seem quite beside the point in Erastus's theory. The Heidelberg Catechism later employed the identical theme of objective participation in Christ's benefits in the Lord's Supper without affirmation of Christ's physical presence in the Eucharistic elements.

In the second and longest section of the *Gründtlicher Bericht*, Erastus sought to prove the Reformed understanding of the Eucharist from the Gospel accounts. He first focused on Christ's words: "Take, eat; this is my body which is given for you." Erastus suggested that, even in the words of Christ, the focus was not on the direct physical correlation between bread and body. Rather, in Christ's presentation, the Eucharistic elements inherently point to the crucifixion. That is to say, the object of Christ's teaching was not his body and blood in the elements, but rather his sacrifice on the cross. Thus, when Christ said, "This is my body," Erastus suggested he was clearly alluding to the sacrifice of his human flesh on the cross.[22] Like Zwingli, Erastus here made the concluding phrase "which was given for you" the key to understanding the passage. Humans do not partake in Christ's body in a physical eating and drinking of his flesh and blood, but partake of Christ's body only "in so far as" he has died and shed his blood to save them. The bread and the wine were symbols of Christ's sacrificial death; the true object of the Lord's Supper remains the crucifixion.

Next Erastus considered Christ's commendation to "Do this in my remembrance." He argued that the Holy Spirit also clarified this command in the writings of Paul by adding, "You shall proclaim the death of the Lord until he returns."[23] The Lord's Supper was therefore a symbolic proclamation of the crucifixion. Erastus deduced from this that Christians partake in the body and blood of Christ only "in so far as" Christ surrendered himself on the cross. The phrase "in so far as" was a continual refrain in the work, and he used it to forge a symbolic parallelism between the reception of the elements and Christ's death on the cross. Erastus suggested that, properly understood, the passage might read, "You ought to eat and drink this bread and wine, so that you remember and are assured,

---

[21] Ibid., 9–10.

[22] Ibid., 16–18. See Stephens, *The Theology of Huldrych Zwingli*, 247.

[23] 1 Cor. 11:25.

that the surrender of my body and the shedding of my blood are food and drink for you for eternal life."[24] Thus, Christians only eat and drink the body and blood of Christ to the extent that he has died for them. The Lord's Supper can only be understood from the perspective of the cross. The point of eating and drinking was to assure Christians that the crucifixion of Christ secured their entrance to heaven.

Erastus expanded his list of texts of Christ's teaching on the Lord's Supper by including the sixth chapter of John in which Jesus said, "Very truly I tell you, unless you eat the flesh of the Son of Man and drink his blood, you have no life in you."[25] The early leaders of the Reformed movement such as Zwingli and Oecolampadius had argued that John 6 pertained to the Eucharist, whereas Luther rejected the notion that Christ was here speaking of the Lord's Supper.[26] Erastus naturally joined his Swiss spiritual forebears and argued that since John 6 is the only place in the scriptures where Christ speaks of eating and drinking his flesh and blood, our understanding of the words of institution must conform to the teaching of this passage. He bolstered that assertion by citing the application of this text to the Eucharist teaching by Augustine and Chrysostom and contended that from the early church to his day there had been no debate on whether John 6 pertained to the Eucharist.[27] He also noted the similarity between the texts of the Synoptic accounts of Christ's institution of the Lord's Supper and John 6 to stress that Eucharistic theology must take the passage into account.

In Erastus's vision, the clear absurdity of Christ's words in John 6, if interpreted literally, proved that the Lord's Supper must be understood spiritually. Here Christ explicitly taught that "I am the living bread that came down from heaven. Whoever eats this bread will live forever; and the bread that I will give for the life of the world is my flesh."[28] Indeed, the gospel writer recorded that the disciples themselves murmured over this difficult saying. Erastus maintained that the point of Christ's difficult saying, however, was to direct them away from "fleshly eating." Christ taught

[24] *Gründtlicher Bericht*, 19–20: "Ir sollet diß brot und wein essen und trincken/ auff daß ir erinnert und versichert werden/ daß eüch die hinngebung meines leibs und vergeissung meines bluts speise und trencke zum ewigen leben."

[25] John 6: 53, New Revised Standard Version (NRSV).

[26] Pelikan, *The Christian Tradition*, 4:195–196; David Steinmetz, "Scripture and the Lord's Supper in Luther's Theology," in *Luther in Context* (Bloomington, Indiana: Indiana UP, 1986), 76.

[27] *Gründtlicher Bericht*, 21–26.

[28] John 6:51, NRSV.

"that he did not desire that they should eat and drink the substance or being of his body and blood in a fleshly manner," but rather that his words should be understood spiritually.[29] Furthermore, the favorite Zwinglian proof text John 6:63, "the flesh is of no use to life," clearly implied that the fleshly eating could provide no benefit.[30] Erastus concluded that only spiritual consumption can deliver the fruit of life and that John 6 ruled out a literal interpretation of "This is my body."

In his last section on Christ's teaching on the Eucharist, Erastus addressed the passage from the book of Luke: "This drinking vessel or cup is the new testament in my blood, which is shed for you."[31] The significance of this passage for Erastus lay in the fact that Christ did not say that the wine "*is* my blood." A literal reading of Luke did not suggest that the wine is actually transformed into Christ's blood, and thus Erastus argued that the other Gospel accounts should be understood in the light of Luke. To explicate the passage, Erastus first engaged the meaning of a testament. A testament could be either one's final wishes or the document that recorded these last wishes. Erastus suggested that Christ used the latter sense and spoke of "testament" in the sense of a document or a sign, but that this naturally referred back to his last wishes. Since Christ's final wishes were that Christians should receive forgiveness of sins through his death, the "new testament" which the symbol of the Lord's Supper was designed to communicate was nothing other than the forgiveness of sins. The passage could just as well read, "this wine is the new testament or the forgiveness of sins in my blood."[32] To explain the meaning of "testament," Erastus turned to its equivalent in the Greek N.T. text, διαϑηκη (*diatheke*). Although διαϑηκη was translated *Testament* in Luther's translation, Erastus suggested that the word was more commonly understood to mean a *Bund* or covenant in Scripture. This covenant is nothing other than the divine promise "that for the sake of

[29] *Gründtlicher Bericht*, 27.

[30] Ibid., 27: "Das flaisch sei kain nutz zuom Leben."

[31] Ibid., 28–29: "Diß trinkgeschir oder kelch ist das neüwe Testament in meinem blut/ das für euch vergossen wird." Luke 22:20. There is some ambiguity in the Greek text as to whether the phrase "which is shed [or: poured out] for you" modifies "cup" or "blood." The vulgate translated: "hic est calicem novum testamentum in sanguine meo quod pro vocis funditur." In this rendering, "which is shed for you" actually refers to "testament" rather than "blood" or "cup." The translators of the NRSV render the passage: "This cup that is poured out for you is the new covenant in my blood." Erastus's reading of the text is consistent with the wording of the modern *Luther Bibel* (Stuttgart: 1984) and the KJV and can be considered the traditional reading.

[32] *Gründtlicher Bericht*, 38.

Christ he will account us righteous."[33] Erastus's explication of the Lord's Supper as new testament or covenant supported his contention that the words of institution must be understood symbolically.

In the last section of the tract, Erastus cursorily dealt with the Patristic support for a symbolic interpretation of "This is my body." Since the early days of the controversy over the Lord's Supper, the Reformed had claimed that the early church Fathers were on their side. Erastus did not display an extensive knowledge of the Fathers, and his citations of Augustine and Chrysostom could have been culled from Zwingli or Oecolampadius.[34] Such Patristic knowledge would have been common in Erastus's humanist intellectual circle at the University of Basel. Erastus emphasized that the opinion of the early church was not decisive in itself, since Christians were obliged to follow the scriptures rather than the opinions of men. Nevertheless, the testimony of the Fathers was useful to Erastus since he found it to be in total agreement with his interpretation of scripture on this point. He also argued that their opinion was important since they wrote in a time when there was no controversy on the issue.[35] Erastus emphasized the Patristic notion of what a sign or sacrament was intended to communicate. He suggested that the Fathers possessed a clear understanding that signs were meant to represent something beyond themselves.[36] Likewise, to Erastus's mind, they understood figures of speech, and so that even if the communion elements were referred to as the "body" and "blood" of Christ, the Fathers realized that the elements were holy signs or sacraments rather than Christ's actual flesh and blood.

Erastus did all that he could, from his basically Zwinglian position regarding the mode of Christ's presence in the Eucharist, to construct a theology that highlighted the efficacy of the sacraments. For instance, he described the sacraments as *Wahrzeichen*, literally "real signs," a term that had been used by Johann Brenz and which would be later employed in the Heidelberg Catechism.[37] Nevertheless, he maintained the fundamental distinction, so often stressed by the Reformed, between symbols and

---

[33] Ibid., 44.

[34] In the five-page section, Erastus cites Augustine and Chrysostom repeatedly, Cyprian once, and includes [Pseudo-]Dionysius and Theodoret in a list. Augustine was clearly Erastus's favorite, and he calls him the "fürnemsten Vatter und Lehrer."

[35] *Gründtlicher Bericht*, 54.

[36] Ibid., 54–58.

[37] Cf. Bard Thompson, "An Historical Reconstruction of Melanchthonianism," 273. The term had already been used in the First Helvetic Confession. Schaff, *The Creeds of Christendom*, 3:225.

the spiritual reality they represented. The Lord's Supper was a tangible symbol of forgiveness of sins through Christ, since actual forgiveness "cannot be grasped, seen, or taken with the human mouth."[38] In fact, even Christ's body and blood were not actually the forgiveness of sins, rather they were the treasures by which forgiveness of sins was acquired. Since the body and blood were not themselves the forgiveness of sins, Erastus suggested that it was clear that the words of institution must not be understood literally. Like all symbols, whether Biblical ones like circumcision or baptism, or worldly examples like an IOU or a diplomat's credentials, there remained a distinction between the symbol itself and the reality it represented.[39]

In line with the Reformed interpretation of baptism as being analogous to circumcision as a symbol that marks entrance into the faith community, Erastus saw the Lord's Supper as the New Testament analogy of the Passover. Like the Old Testament practices, these New Testament sacraments were nothing more or less than signs of God's covenant with his people, his promise to deal with them under certain terms.[40] Although this may seem like a further argument for a low memorial understanding of the sacrament, Erastus turned it around to argue for the efficacy of the Lord's Supper. As eating food offered to idols made one a partaker in the idol, participation in the Lord's Supper made one a member of the body of Christ.[41] Erastus used the analogy of Old Testament symbols to suggest that the Lord's Supper was a sacrament that had the effect of constituting the Christian community. The Lord's Supper was a sacrament, true sign, deposit, seal, and undoubted witness, in which communion with Christ is "promised, assured, empowered, and sealed."[42]

Erastus's understanding of the Lord's Supper was inherently tied to his conception of faith and, in turn, to his notion that the Eucharistic elements only had meaning to the extent that they referred to the cross. As with Zwingli, the believer's faith was a prerequisite for communion in Erastus's scheme. Individuals who commune truly were the ones "who do not doubt that he was nailed to the cross for their sins."[43] Another

[38] *Gründtlicher Bericht*, 41.

[39] Ibid., 41–47.

[40] Ibid., 45.

[41] Ibid., 12–14. Erastus obviously does not push this motif to its logical conclusion, which would tend to suggest the reality of *manducatio infidelium*.

[42] Ibid., 10. "Sacrament," "wahrzeichen," "sigel," "pfand," "ungezweifelt zeügnuß," pp. 42–43.

[43] Ibid., 18.

motif that Erastus takes from Zwingli was his insistence that the object of the communicant's faith must be in Christ's sacrificial death on the cross and not in the communion elements themselves. At one point, Erastus approached Augustine's dictum, "Believe and you have already eaten," when he suggested that to eat and drink means "to believe firmly in one's heart without doubt."[44] Concomitantly, Erastus clearly rejected the notion of *manducatio infidelium*, that is, an actual consumption of the flesh of Christ by an unbeliever. Erastus came close to espousing the doctrine of limited atonement when he contended that "Christ has neither promised nor given this food and drink for anyone other than those for whom he gave his life and shed his blood."[45]

For all his debt to Zwingli, Erastus did make thematic as well as theological choices that distinguished his theology of the Eucharist from the father of the Swiss Reformation. Unlike Zwingli's classic *A Clear Instruction on the Lord's Supper*,[46] which throughout was focused on scriptural arguments bearing on the meaning of "This is my body," the force of Erastus's presentation was more soteriological than hermeneutical. For instance, Erastus did not belabor the meaning of the "is" in "This is my body" and never suggested that it would be better understood as meaning "this 'signifies' my body." Perhaps Erastus sought to avoid commonplaces that would identify him as a blatant Zwinglian. He simply said that the text cannot be understood "according to the letter" and denied "fleshly eating." Rather than relying on hermeneutical necessity, Erastus argued that the idea of the physical presence of Christ in the Eucharist was erroneous, since it reflected a misreading of Christ's passion and a lack of appreciation for his central purpose. That soteriological theme was also present in Zwingli, but since many of his Eucharistic works were controversial pieces designed to undermine his opponents' hermeneutical arguments, that cross-centered mandate for a symbolic interpretation was more plainly visible in Erastus's tract than in Zwingli's work.

The difference between Erastus's and Zwingli's theology of the Lord's Supper went beyond a mere difference in emphasis. Erastus offered an alternative opinion of how the sacrament influenced faith. As previously

[44] *Gründtlicher Bericht*, 20: "essen ... und trincken haisse: naemmlich in seinem herzten vestiglich on alles zweiflen glauben...."

[45] Ibid., 18: "daß Christus dise speis und tranck niemand verhaissen hab und gebe/ denn den jenigen/ fur die sein leib gegeben/ und sein blüt vergossen ist."

[46] Zwingli, *Eine klare Unterrichtung von Nachtmal Christi*, in *Z* [*CR* 91], 4:773–862.

mentioned, both agreed that faith remained an absolute precondition for participation in the Lord's Supper. In Zwingli's thought, faith was a rather static quality that was not enhanced or strengthened by taking part in the Eucharist.[47] The Lord's Supper imparted no grace nor inherently strengthened faith; it was simply a memorial. Erastus broke with Zwingli on this point in that he conceived of the sacrament as a faith builder. The purpose of the sacrament was that all believers may be "powerfully convinced that they are in the communion and society of the body of Christ."[48] The Lord's Supper offered great assurance to the Christian in order that "we should no longer doubt that we are children of God, and fellow heirs with Christ in eternal life."[49] This faith-enhancing aspect of the Lord's Supper possessed an objective quality in that communicants were as assured of their acceptance into Christ's kingdom "*as certainly as* we receive the bread and the wine."[50] This was an internal, spiritual process which required faith to participate. Nevertheless, the agent in this strengthening of faith was the Holy Spirit, not the individual's will or intellect. Erastus asserted that it was wrong to say that the bread and the wine were "empty signs which have no effect,"[51] because through the agency of the Holy Spirit, the sacraments brought a real transformation in the heart of the believer.

In the *Gründtlicher Bericht*, Erastus explicated a late Zwinglian[52] understanding of Christ's presence in the Lord's Supper; Christ was not physically present in the sacrament nor did communicants consume the flesh of Christ. Erastus suggested that the sacrament of the Lord's Supper could have meaning only in Christ's sacrifice of his body and blood on the cross. Only that sacrifice obtained the Christian's salvation. However, the Lord's Supper was no empty symbol. Although the Lord's Supper required faith for participation, it also inspired faith. Understood as a parallel of the Old Testament practices of circumcision and the Passover, the Lord's Supper

47 Stephens, *Theology of Huldrych Zwingli*, 249.
48 *Gründtlicher Bericht*, 11.
49 Ibid., 44–45.
50 Ibid., 49. The emphasis is mine.
51 Ibid., 50.
52 "Late Zwinglian" is an expression that has been coined to describe the Eucharistic theology of Swiss German theologians after Zwingli. Late Zwinglians moved beyond Zwingli's strict memorial understanding of the Lord's Supper. Heinrich Bullinger is the classic example of a "late Zwinglian" and his *Second Helvetic Confession* perhaps the finest expression of late Zwinglianism. Erastus should also be considered a prime example of late Zwinglianism. Discussed more fully in chapter 4.

established and sealed the faith community; it was a holy "true-sign" of Christ's sacrifice. Though Erastus had a rather "high" view of the sacrament's efficacy for a Zwinglian, one should also note what he did not say in the work. Erastus never addressed the issue of whether grace was tangibly received as a result of participation in the sacrament. At minimum, however, his characterizations of the Lord's Supper assumed a distinct parallelism between the participation in the sacrament and the reception of grace.

Befitting the work's apologetic purpose, it was quite non-polemical for its time, with the exception of a few barbs tossed in the direction of Roman Catholicism. Erastus did not use party labels in the tract and never mentioned Zwingli by name. He appeared to be attempting a measure of accommodation with Lutherans by maintaining the "realist" language of eating and drinking the body and blood of Christ, even though he explained that this did not occur in a fleshly manner.

The work proved a moderate success in Reformed circles. It was well received by Erastus's Reformed friends—both of the Calvinist and Zwinglian persuasion—and printed at least six times in German. Petrus Colonius (Pieter van Keulen, Pierre de Cologne), a Netherlandish theologian ministering in Heidelberg, translated it into French, and this translation was also reprinted at least twice.[53] There is also evidence that the treatise was translated and printed in English, though there are no known surviving copies.[54]

Not surprisingly, the tract was less successful in convincing Lutheran theologians of the authenticity of Reformed Eucharistic theology. Any attempt at accommodation would be difficult in an age when theologians had become experts in accentuating their differences and misrepresenting the opinions of their opponents. Even though Erastus had expressed his thoughts in as inoffensive a language as possible, many elements in the work rightfully alarmed orthodox Lutherans; for example, his rejection of the ubiquity of Christ's human nature and *manducatio infidelium*. Johann Marbach refuted Erastus's tract in a polemical work published in 1565, which led Erastus to write his *Resolute Rejection of the Unfounded Accusation, in which Dr. Johann Marbach has Attempted to Impugn the*

[53] *Vraye & droite intelligence de ces paroles de la Saincte Cene de Iesus Christ, CECY EST MON CORPS, &c.* (Metz, 1564). Henss, *Der Heidelberger Katechismus*, 45. See the bibliography.

[54] See the bibliography. [Thomas Erastus, *The true Understanding of those Words: This is my Bodie* (London, 1578).]

Booklet of the Physician Thomas Erastus, concerning the Understanding of the Words of Christ 'This Is My Body, etc.'[55] Martin Chemnitz also contemplated refuting Erastus but was apparently satisfied with Marbach's retort.[56] Naturally, the book was not appreciated in Catholic circles and may have been the work that landed Erastus on the *Index of Prohibited Books* as early as 1569.[57]

The *Gründtlicher Bericht* illuminates the character of the emerging Heidelberg theology from the perspective of its most important early activist. Though Erastus maintained Zwingli's chief insights, he modified the Zwinglian legacy to include a faith strengthening vision of the Lord's Supper and a notion of assurance that was not dependant on the mood of the participant. He reinterpreted the sacrament of Christ's body and blood not as a simple memorial meal but as a powerful event in which the divine promise was spoken. He conceptualized the Lord's Supper as a dynamic, transforming event. His emphasis on the transforming purpose of the Lord's Supper remained a consistent theme in his Eucharistic writings as well as in his later works on church discipline. As Erastus would later conclude, to debar someone from participation in the Lord's Supper was fundamentally wrongheaded, since the prohibition subverted the chief purpose of these "provocations and allurements to religion and piety."[58] Struggling Christians in particular needed this medicine. The impression that one receives of the purpose of the sacrament was quite unlike Zwingli's straightforward memorial approach in which the primary communion that the believers entered into was a fellowship or

[55] Thomas Erastus, *Bestendige Ableinung der ungegründten beschuldigung/ damit D. Johann Marbach/ das büchlein Thomae Erasti Medici, vom verstand der wort CHRisti/ Das ist mein Leib/ etc. unterstehet verdechtig zu machen* (Heidelberg: Johann Mayer, 1565).

[56] Martin Chemitz to unknown [Johann Marbach ?], Braunschweig, Aug. 5, 1565, printed in Johannes Fecht, ed., *Historiae Ecclesiasticae a.n.c. XVI. Supplementum* (Frankfurt and Speyer, Christoph Olffen, 1684), 203: "Illud, quod omninò necessarium fuit, valde probo, quod Heidelbergensis Sacramentarios nominatim taxas & refutas. Nam ego rei dignitate permotus aliquoties mihi proposueram, Erasti Medici scripto responsionem aliquam opponere, sed existimavi, per alios in vicinia rectius hoc fieri posse. Et illud iam à te factum esse gaudeo."

[57] Franz Heinrich Reusch, *Die Indices librorum prohibitorum des sechzehnten Jahrhunderts* (Stuttgart, 1886), 284, etc.

[58] Thomas Erastus, *Explicatio Gravissimae Quaestionis utrùm Excommunicatio, quatenùs Religionem intelligentes & amplexantes, à Sacramentorum usu, propter admissum facinus arcet; mandato nitatur Divino, an excogitata sit ab hominibus* ([London: John Wolfe], 1589), thesis 19. Discussed more fully below in chapter 6.

communion with one another. Put another way, Erastus maintained the central insight of his great countryman (the lack of physical presence in the sacrament), but reinterpreted Zwingli's theology of the Lord's Supper by infusing it with a certain Lutheran quality. Erastus was not original in this inclination to add evangelical cogency to Reformed Eucharistic doctrine. This "Lutheranizing" trend had been evident in the *First Helvetic Confession* of 1536.[59] Reformed theologians like Peter Martyr Vermigli and John Calvin had likewise sought to enrich the Reformed doctrine of the sacrament, understanding it as a faith-inspiring event in which the sacrament represented the "visible words of Christ." Scholars are generally aware of Calvin's own attempt to move the Reformed understanding of the Lord's Supper away from Zwingli "memorialism" and towards Luther, even if many Lutherans were likewise loath to recognize the Reformed as their brethren.[60] It is easy to lose sight of the degree to which "late Zwinglians" like Bullinger and Erastus were pursuing a similar path of accommodation.[61] As discussed below, Erastus's teaching would resurface in the Heidelberg Catechism's sacramental doctrine. The irony here is that after scholars have argued for decades whether the Palatine Reformation was essentially Calvinist or Melanchthonian, one is surprised to discover that a late Zwinglian is perhaps the best example of what many historical theologians have considered the movement's most appealing qualities. Indeed, the chief characteristics that have often been hailed as the Melanchthonian spirit of the Heidelberg Catechism—the clear message of assurance and consolation, use of accommodating language, and judicious silence on divisive doctrines—were visible in the work of the Palatinate's most conspicuous Zwinglian representative.

[59] See Alfred C. Cochrane, ed., *Reformed Confessions of the 16th Century* (Philadelphia: Westminster, 1966), article 22, pp. 108–109.

[60] Regarding the evolution of Calvin's thought, see Wim Janse, "Calvin's Eucharistic Theology: Three Dogma-Historical Observations," in *Calvinus sacrarum literarum interpres: Papers of the International Congress on Calvin Research* [Reformed Historical Theology 5] ed. Herman J. Selderhuis (Göttingen: Vandenhoeck & Ruprecht, 2008) 37–69.

[61] The modifications of the Zwinglian heritage are clearly appreciated in the work of David Steinmetz, Paul Rorem, and B.A. Gerrish. See the bibliography. Bruening has argued that the most promising path for mediation on the question of the Eucharist had not been Bucer's efforts but rather direct contact between Bullinger and Melanchthon. Bruening, *Calvinism's First Battleground*, 86.

Das Büchlein von Brotbrechen

Erastus's second theological work was a short treatise on the *fractio panis* (breaking of bread, or simply "fraction") entitled *Account of Some of the Reasons, why the Precious Sacrament of the Last Supper of Our Lord and Savior Jesus Christ, Should Not Be Held without the Breaking of Bread.*[62] It was of vital importance for the liturgical development of the Palatinate. Though this work, commonly known as *Das Büchlein von Brotbrechen*,[63] was not published until early 1563, Wesel-Roth uncovered evidence which suggested that the rite of breaking bread had been introduced in the Palatine church as early as 1561.[64] Other evidence suggests that it took some time for the rite to be uniformly instituted throughout the territory, and thus Erastus's tract addressed a current concern.[65] The introduction of bread breaking gave yet another evidence of the firm commitment of the elector to the Reformed faith. The significance of this change in cultic practice cannot be underestimated. As Bodo Nischan has argued, such clear changes in ritual practice "came to symbolize basic theological disagreements that otherwise were not readily apparent."[66] The *fractio panis* appealed to the Reformed both as a restoration of proper worship as outlined in the Scriptures and as a manifest rejection of any notion of the real presence of Christ's body in the communion bread. It was an action

---

[62] [Thomas Erastus], *Erzelung Etlicher ursachen/ warumb das hochwirdig Sacrament des Nachtmals unsers Herrn/ und Heylandts Jhesu Christi/ nicht solle ohne das brodbrechen gehalten werden* (Heidelberg: Johann Mayer, 1563; reprint, Heidelberg: Johann Mayer, 1565).

[63] Erastus's Lutheran adversaries dubbed the tract "Das Büchlein von Brotbrechen." This fact made it difficult for the first generation of modern Reformation scholarship to concretely identify the work. Albrecht Wolters and J.I. Doedes rediscovered the tract in the second half of the nineteenth century.

[64] Stephan Cirler to Bullinger, Heidelberg, Dec. 11, 1561, StAZ, E II 363, fol. 79, printed in Wesel-Roth, *Thomas Erastus*, 131: "Introducimus his diebus fractionem panis explosis rotundis particulis. Deus nobis suam gratiam concedat, ut reliqua quoque emendare liceat. Principis pietatem ac constantiam nolo encomiis elevare. Er sitzt fürwar im Sattel und soll noch einem großen theologo, der sich etwas zu sein dünkt, zu schaffen geben. Ipsemet legit perpendit examinat ... nec ab aliorum iudicio more reliquorum principum pendet." Klebitz's description of the events leading to his dismissal in the fall of 1559 makes it clear that the breaking of bread was already an issue of contention and was being introduced by some ministers. Klebitz, *Victoria Veritatis*, D3^{v}.

[65] Ursinus expressed the populace's reluctance to accept the new practice in a letter to Crato from August 1563, printed in August Kluckhohn, ed., *Briefe Friedrich des Frommen Kurfürsten von der Pfalz mit verwandten Schriftstücken*, 2 vols. (Brunswick, 1868–1872) 1:443–448, see especially, 447.

[66] Bodo Nischan, "The 'Fractio Panis': A Reformed Communion Practice in Late Reformation Germany," *CH* 53 (1984), 18.

loaded with symbolic importance, and as such, became something of a shibboleth in the confessional age. The Reformed insisted on breaking the Eucharistic bread while the Lutherans rejected the practice and began to suspect anyone who advocated the breaking of bread as being a Crypto-Calvinist.

Over the last one hundred years there has been a fair amount of interest in Erastus's short pamphlet on the breaking of bread. Jakob Isaac Doedes reprinted it in 1891 but did not know the identity of the author. M.A. Gooszen made a tentative case for Erastus's authorship by comparing the text of the *Büchlein von Brotbrechen* with the *Gründtlicher Bericht* and a manuscript defense of the *Büchlein* found in the Saxon state archive in Dresden. Auguste Bonnard likewise theorized that Erastus was the author of the *Büchlein* on the basis of comments made in Erastus's correspondence.[67] It was not until Wesel-Roth undertook a more careful study of Erastus's correspondence in the Zurich state archive that Erastus was definitively identified as the author. The key piece of evidence comes from a letter to Bullinger, in which Erastus related:

> The catechism is now published, as you see it here sent to you. I have added a pamphlet, which I have published for the unlearned concerning the breaking of bread—without my name by will of the prince—because they judged [it] thus better.[68]

This letter also yields a clue regarding the semi-official status of Erastus's early publications. Erastus's decision to publish the *Büchlein* was not an individual action but a matter of state religious policy. Though its primary purpose was to give a Biblical rationale for the *fractio panis* to the Palatine clergy, it seems to have played a secondary role in justifying the transformation of ritual practice to the outside world. Pierre Boquin also published a Latin tract defending fraction the same year.[69] This pattern of

---

[67] J.I. Doedes, *Das Büchlein vom Brotbrechen* (Utrecht: Kemink & Zoon, 1891), xii–xiii; M.A. Gooszen, *De Heidelbergsche Catechismus en Het Boekje van de Breking des Broods, in het jaar 1563–1564 bestreden en verdedigd* (Leiden: Brill, 1892), 238–242; Bonnard, *Thomas Éraste*, 204–205.

[68] Erastus to Bullinger, Feb. 26, [1563], StAZ, E II 345, fol. 735; Wesel-Roth, *Thomas Erastus*, 133: "Catechismus editus est, ut vides, hic tibi missus. Addidi libellum, quem de fractione panis propter rudiores ex principis voluntate omisso nomine edidi quod melius ita iudicarent."

[69] Pierre Boquin, *Canones quibus defenditur ΔΙΑΝΟΙΑ in verbis Christi, hoc est corpus meum: et controversiae de coena domini atque similium dijudicandae certissima ratio demonstratur. Item assertio ritus frangendi, in manusque sumendi panis in celebratione coenae Domini* (Heidelberg: Michael Schirat, 1563). See Henss, *Der Heidelberger Catechismus*, 18–19.

simultaneous action by Erastus and Boquin suggests an intentional collaboration of the two which is not readily discernible in other surviving sources from the era. The fact that the *Büchlein* was published simultaneously with the Catechism and is often found bound together with it has led to the scholarly consensus that the *Büchlein*'s publication possessed official sanction.[70] This conclusion would seem to be more than justified, especially considering the fact that the earliest opponents of the Heidelberg Catechism also attacked the *Büchlein* and noted its appearance with the Catechism.[71]

Das Büchlein von Brotbrechen was a primitivist work, harking back to the early Zwinglian scripture principle that all church ceremonies had to be expressly commended in scripture. It argued that because Christ himself had broken bread in the last supper and because he had enjoined his disciples to do the same, there could be no imaginable grounds for contemporary Christians to depart from Christ's own practice.[72] Erastus asserted that the disciples themselves maintained the custom of breaking bread (they had to, since Christ had commanded it). The practice continued into the early church "until Satan had twisted the holy Lord's Supper of Christ into the idolatrous Mass."[73] Erastus contended that the contemporary Catholic misuse of fraction revealed that even Satan realized that it would have been inconceivable to totally remove the practice. Erastus

[70] Doedes, *Das Büchlein vom Brotbrechen*, xii–xiii; Wilhelm Port, "Johann Mayer, Ein Reformierter Drucker des 16. Jahrhunderts," *Zentralblatt für Bibliothekswesen* 59 (1942): 143–144; Walter Hollweg, *Neue Untersuchungen zur Geschichte und Lehre des Heidelberger Katechismus* [*DGLRK* 13 & 28] 2 vols. (Neukirchen-Vluyn: Neukirchener Verlag des Erziehungsvereins, 1961–1968), 1:183–184; J.F. Gerhard Goeters, "Genesis, Formen und Hauptthemen des reformierten Bekenntnisses in Deutschland. Eine Übersicht," in *Die reformierte Konfessionalisierung in Deutschland* [*SVRG* 195], ed. Heinz Schilling, 44–59 (Gütersloh: Gerd Mohn, 1986), 52. Even more closely related to the Catechism was the tract *Christliche Gebet/ die man daheim in heusern/ und in der Kirchen brauchen mag*, which is often found bound with the Catechism and is sometimes listed on the Catechism's title page. Ironically, the Württembergische Landesbibliothek's copies of the *Christliche Gebet* and *Erzelung Etlicher ursachen* are not bound with the Catechism but with each other.

[71] For example, Duke Christoph, Margrave Karl, and Count Palatine Wolfgang sent a joint letter of protest to Elector Frederick that included a refutation of the *Büchlein von Brotbrechen* in addition to the "Verzeichnis der Mangel," which was the Württemberg theologians' refutation of the Heidelberg Catechism. Printed in Albrecht Wolters, *Der Heidelberger Katechismus in seiner ursprünglichen Gestalt* (Bonn, 1864), 184–192 ("Verzeichnis der Mangel," pp. 164–184).

[72] [Erastus], *Erzelung Etlicher ursachen*, 3.

[73] Ibid., 7.

argued for fraction based on the phrase "Do this in my remembrance" by asserting that the breaking of bread engendered greater remembrance of Christ's death than either eating or drinking.[74] Erastus appreciated fraction as a ritual memorial of Christ's sufferings. In fact, any holding of the Eucharist without the breaking of bread was something less than an authentic Lord's Supper.[75] Erastus also asserted that Christians must use one loaf of bread for true communion, rather than individual communion wafers.[76] Without the one loaf, the church lost the image that they were all members of one body. He concluded the work with the challenge that all who considered themselves "evangelical" ought to conform to the practice and asserted that he knew of no famous pious theologian who had taken a position against the breaking of bread.[77]

Erastus's treatise offered a persuasive and biblically grounded, if often circular, justification for the necessity of breaking bread in the Lord's Supper. That his rationale for this definitive Reformed rite arrived precisely at the historical juncture when the practice was taking root on German soil has caused historians like J.F. Gerhard Goeters to recognize his significant contribution to the liturgical development of the German Reformed church.[78] That this Zwinglian's work has been labeled the "classic Calvinist statement on the fraction"[79] offers yet another example of how the term "Calvinism" is a rather arbitrary designation for the religious tradition that emerged in the sixteenth-century Palatinate.

[74] Ibid., 10–11.

[75] Ibid., 6.

[76] Ibid., 16–17.

[77] Ibid., 22.

[78] Goeters, "Genesis, Formen und Hauptthemen," 48, 52–53. The 1568 Synod of Wesel declared fraction "absolutely necessary because it was obviously instituted by Christ." Nischan, "The 'Fractio Panis,'" 20.

[79] Oliver Olsen as quoted in Nischan, "The 'Fractio Panis,'" 20.

CHAPTER FOUR

THE EPIPHANY: THE HEIDELBERG CATECHISM

> We have composed a catechism, in which all the heads of doctrine as well as the Sacraments are explained clearly and in great detail ... For some time now I have been totally absorbed in it. For I was always eager to make our doctrine public.
>
> Erastus to Bullinger, January 30, [1563]

The Heidelberg Catechism, composed in late 1562 and published in January 1563, arguably became the most important confessional document in the history of Reformed Christianity. It was the first manifestly Reformed confession adopted by a principality of the Holy Roman Empire and, as such, stood as a direct challenge to the Religious Peace of Augsburg. Its adoption signaled the beginning of the so-called "second Reformation," in which many principalities and cities of the Holy Roman Empire moved from Lutheranism to the Reformed faith.[1] For no reason other than this, the Heidelberg Catechism occupies a prominent place in the history of the Reformation. Beyond its political importance, the catechism became one of the most popular confessional documents of the Reformation era. It has been translated into more than twenty languages and retains confessional status in many Reformed denominations around the globe. It played a formative role in the histories of German and Dutch immigrant communities in North America. It has also been considered one of the most theologically cogent and appealing confessions of the Reformation era. Since the catechism did not directly affirm the most controversial tenets of Calvinism, it has also been considered one of the most irenic documents of the era. Theologians from Heinrich Bullinger to Karl Barth have lauded its presentation of the

[1] Henry J. Cohn, "Territorial Princes in Germany's Second Reformation, 1559–1622," in *International Calvinism 1541–1715*, ed. Menna Preswich (Oxford: Oxford UP, 1985), 135–166; Press, "Die 'Zweite Reformation' in der Kurpfalz," 104–129; Goeters, "Genesis, Formen und Hauptthemen," 44–59.

Christian faith in a manner which is simultaneously theological and devotional. Members of the Reformed communion have also hailed its literary quality—a fondness no doubt enhanced by familiarity—and the devotion shown it is akin to an Anglican's love for the *Book of Common Prayer*.[2]

Thus, when probing the origins of the Heidelberg Catechism, historians must be aware that they are standing on holy ground. Like other celebrated texts, the story of its composition has become obscured over the centuries in the haze of legend and hagiography. One could cite many accounts of the Heidelberg Reformation which would be better suited for a Sunday school room than the history seminar. The paean of the leading Mercersberg theologian John Nevin captures the pious enthusiasm regarding the catechism's origins:

> It is something wonderful in the first place, that the catechism should be in fact the production of two authors; for it appears to be certain, that the double authorship was of the most real and positive character, involving throughout not simply an outward, but a true inward coöperation also, which it is curious to note, and by no means easy to understand. The catechism was not the work of Ursinus, approved by Olevianus, nor on the other hand the work of Olevianus, approved by Ursinus; it was the joint production of both; and it was this, not in the way of any mechanical putting together of their different contributions to the work, but in the way of an organic fusion, which refers the whole work to both authors, and makes it impossible to know or say, what in it belongs to one and what to the other.[3]

Were this account true, the composition of the catechism truly would have been a sublime affair that would have been the exception rather than the rule in this era of confessional strife. Research published around the four hundredth anniversary of the publication of the catechism, however, has demonstrated conclusively that this hagiographic depiction of the writing of the catechism must be severely revised.

Since the traditional conception of the dual authorship of Caspar Olevianus and Zacharias Ursinus has been set aside (more below), the opportunity is ripe to investigate the roles of other likely members of the authorship circle, such as Thomas Erastus. To orient this study, it is

---

[2] See Lyle D. Bierma et al., *An Introduction to the Heidelberg Catechism: Sources, History, and Theology* (Grand Rapids: Baker, 2005).

[3] [John W. Nevin] in *The Heidelberg Catechism, in German, Latin and English: with an Historical Introduction* (New York, 1863), 33.

necessary to review the question of the authorship of the catechism both in the historiographic tradition as well as what can be proven on the basis of sixteenth-century sources. To investigate Erastus's role, special attention will be paid to the catechism's Eucharistic theology and Erastus's probable influence upon it. Many sources link Erastus quite closely to the composition of the catechism. Ultimately, I will argue that Erastus played a much larger role in the composition of the catechism than is commonly acknowledged and that he should be considered a co-author.

The Composition of the Heidelberg Catechism

The traditional image of Ursinus and Olevianus as the joint authors of the catechism was based on the account found in *Historia de Ecclesiis Palatinis* by the Emden theologian Heinrich Alting (1583–1644) that was published in 1644.[4] According to Alting, Elector Frederick specifically assigned the work of composing a new catechism to Olevianus and Ursinus. Both theologians proceeded to write their own rough drafts: Ursinus, two catechisms, and Olevianus, a treatise on the covenant. Afterwards, both writers worked together to produce a single text based on each man's preliminary efforts.[5] Nevin's rhapsody on this harmonious cooperation, quoted above, was merely an elaboration of Alting's account.

This portrayal of the Heidelberg Catechism, with some modifications, basically held the field until the four hundredth anniversary of the catechism's publication.[6] The only substantial change in the story dealt with Olevianus's draft, which Alting had described as a "popular declaration of the convent of grace." Since no document was found that could be

[4] Alting's account was written more than fifty years after the event. His first mention of the joint authorship of Olevianus and Ursinus was written ca. 1619–1620—after he had left the Palatinate following the invasion of the Bavarian Army in the Thirty Years' War. His classic version of the catechism's composition was written even later, while he was in the Netherlands, and not published until 1644. (See chapter 1, note 1.)

[5] Alting, *Historia de ecclesiis Palatinis*, 81–82 (ch. 43): "Id negotii datum duobus Theologis Doctoribus, Oleviano & D. Ursino 1562 tanquam Germanis & Germanice scribere doctis. Et uterque in chartam conjecit ejus specimen. Olevianus populari declaratione *foederis gratiae*: Ursinus scripto duplici Catechisimo; majore pro provectoribus, minore pro junioribus. Ex utroque contracta est *Catechesis Palatina*, quae a loco natali *Heidelbergensis* appellari solet" (italics in the original).

[6] There were some, such as Arnout van Schelven, who doubted the large role ascribed to Olevianus. Goeters, "Caspar Olevianus als Theologe," 301.

identified with that described by Alting, historians modified Olevianus's role in the composition and subsequently credited him as the redactor of Ursinus's preliminary efforts, the *Catechesis minor* and *Catechesis maior*— works which manifestly served as sources for much of the Heidelberg Catechism.[7] In that role, Olevianus still received praise for turning the solid preliminary efforts of Ursinus into a stylistic and devotional masterpiece. As August Lang, one of the leading scholars of the catechism wrote, "The final German edition, with its popular, robust, faith-kindling speech, should in all likelihood be credited to Olevianus, the author of the church order."[8]

In 1961, Walter Hollweg shattered this image with his groundbreaking essay "Did Caspar Olevianus revise the German text of the Heidelberg Catechism?"[9] Hollweg demonstrated that contemporaneous evidence was wanting for ascribing a large role to Olevianus in the composition of the catechism. First, he argued that the famous reputation as a preacher that Olevianus had garnered over the centuries, whether or not it was well deserved, did not prove that he was qualified to transform Ursinus's rough drafts into a work of literary excellence. In any

---

[7] Both Ursinus's *Catechesis Maior* (also known as *Summa theologiae*) and the *Catechesis Minor* are reprinted in August Lang, *Der Heidelberger Katechismus und vier verwandte Katechismen* (1907). English translations are available in Bierma, *An Introduction to the Heidelberg Catechism*, 141–223. The *Catechesis Maior* has 323 questions and is written in Latin. The *Catechesis Minor*, a German catechism with 109 questions, is clearly the document upon which the Heidelberg Catechism has the most textual dependence. "Im Aufbau und weithin sogar in der Formulierung," concluded Goeters, "steht dieser Ursinische Katechismusentwurf dem später publizierten, unserem Heidelberger Katechsimus, am nächsten." J.F. Gerhard Goeters, "Entstehung und Frühgeschichte des Katechismus," in *Handbuch zum Heidelberger Katechismus*, ed. Lothar Coenen (Neukirch: Neukirchener Verlag, 1963), 13. There is actually some debate whether or not this Catechism was solely the work of Ursinus, although it has long been ascribed to him, since a manuscript of it was found which was written in his own hand. See Wilhem Neuser, "Die Väter des Heidelberger Katechismus," *Theologische Zeitschrift* 35 (1979): 178–179.

[8] "Die deutsche Endredaktion mit ihrer volkstümlichen, kernigen, glaubenswarmen Sprache ist aller Wahrscheinlichkeit nach Olevian, dem Verfasser der Kirchenordnung, zu verdanken...." Lang, *Der Heidelberger Katechismus*, 77.

[9] Walter Hollweg, "Bearbeitete Caspar Olevianus den deutschen Text zum Heidelberger Katechismus," in *Neue Untersuchungen zur Geschichte und Lehre des Heidelberger Katechismus* (Neukirchen-Vluyn: Neukirchener Verlag, 1961), 1:124–152. Hollweg does acknowledge the dissenters from the mainstream opinion that preceded him, especially Johannes Brauer, who had maintained that there was no evidence for the role traditionally ascribed to Olevianus (p. 126). Hollweg was later to issue a second volume of essays on the Heidelberg Catechism: *Neue Untersuchungen zur Geschichte und Lehre des Heidelberger Katechismus. Zweite Folge* (Neukirchen-Vluyn: Neukirchener Verlag, 1968; hereafter these works will be cited as *Neue Untersuchungen* 1 [i.e., 1961] and 2, respectively).

event, it was Ursinus, and *not* Olevianus, who that same year had translated Calvin's *Geneva Catechism* into German, suggesting that Ursinus felt himself more than competent to translate a Latin theological work into German.[10] Thus, if Ursinus translated the catechetical works of others into German at this time, it would seem extremely unlikely that the unpublished Olevianus would have been charged with the task of perfecting the German text of Ursinus's own work.[11] The older historiography had also frequently asserted the great similarity between the Heidelberg Catechism and Olevianus's other works as proof for his role in the redaction of the catechism—though no one had demonstrated this similarity conclusively.[12] Regardless of whether or not such a similarity existed, Hollweg maintained that this assumed affinity offered no proof for Olevianus's role. Since Olevianus published his entire theological corpus after the Heidelberg Catechism, any likeness may have as easily reflected

[10] Hollweg, "Zur Quellenfrage des Heidelberger Katechismus," in *Neue Untersuchungen*, 2:38–47. This point is especially telling in view of the fact that Olevianus had previously attempted to translate Calvin's Geneva Catechism before abandoning the task. Hollweg documents Olevianus's lack of self-confidence as a translator, based on a letter of Olevianus to Beza from 1561 (pp. 40–42).

[11] Hollweg, *Neue Untersuchungen*, 1:142. Hollweg here makes much of a comment that Olevianus made to Calvin regarding Ursinus, "who supersedes me in the faculty of language" ("qui me facultate linquae superat"). Hollweg suggests that Olevianus was chiefly making a concession about his own literary abilities in this comment, rather than his translating skills, since his knowledge of Latin had to be excellent and he was in all likelihood far superior to Ursinus in his facility in French. Bierma is right to challenge how much can be drawn from such a self-deprecating comment in which Olevianus's chief goal was to assure Calvin that the translation of his work has been handled with care (Lyle Bierma, "Olevianus and the Authorship of The Heidelberg Catechism: Another Look," *SCJ* 13 (1982): 23). Bierma then argues that Olevianus was only speaking of his translating skills and not his ability, as Hollweg had suggested, "gedanklich schwer geladenen Schriften kongenial in einer anderen Sprache neue Gestalt und Form zu geben" (Hollweg, *Neue Untersuchungen*, 1:145). I would argue that both Hollweg and Bierma force the dichotomy between the technical proficiency in languages and stylistic capacity. However, Bierma (himself an able translator) would likely concede that excellence in translating goes far beyond knowledge of the language out of which one is translating, and thus, even though Hollweg perhaps makes too much out of Olevianus's comment to Calvin, the simple fact that Ursinus had such recognized linguistic abilities undercuts the traditional rationale for why Olevianus could putatively have been called upon to rework Ursinus's Latin drafts. However, Olevianus's letter offers more of a positive endorsement of Ursinus than it says anything per se negative about Olevianus's verbal skills. Nevertheless, Hollweg's basic point holds, although Bierma is correct to add that "the possibility that Olevianus had a hand in the final redaction has not at all been ruled out" (p. 23).

[12] Bierma's translation of Olevianus's *Vester Grundt* documents this case more fully. Caspar Olevianus, *A Firm Foundation*, ed. and trans. Lyle D. Bierma (Grand Rapids, Baker: 1995).

the catechism's influence on Olevianus rather than any influence he might have exerted on the catechism.[13] Another fact that argued against ascribing much credit to Olevianus for the catechism was his dissatisfaction with question thirty-six concerning the benefit of the "holy conception and birth of Christ," which was revealed in a later controversy in Heidelberg. If Olevianus had theological reservations with part of the catechism, this would at least beg the question of how influential he had been in its composition.[14] Finally, Hollweg also revealed some of the dark side of Olevianus's personality, and questioned whether he were the man from whom such a warm and inspiring catechism might have been conceived. Although one might argue that Hollweg's critique of Olevianus's personality went beyond what was strictly relevant to the question of authorship of the catechism,[15] his basic arguments proved decisive and a new scholarly consensus has emerged in the wake of Hollweg's essay. Though Ursinus's contribution remains unquestioned, most scholars now maintain that there is little contemporaneous evidence to suggest that Olevianus played a large part in the composition of the catechism.[16] J.F. Gerhard Goeters, the leading modern authority on Palatine church history, sum-

[13] Hollweg, *Neue Untersuchungen*, 1:141. The late Fred Klooster should be added to this list of skeptics regarding the supposed similarity between the works of Olevianus and the Heidelberg Catechism. See Klooster, "Priority of Ursinus," 87.

[14] Hollweg, *Neue Untersuchungen*, 1:146–150. The row was basically between Olevianus and his erstwhile ally in the church discipline controversy, Petrus Dathenus. Goeters has furthered the discussion with Olevianus's relative discontent with the original form of the Heidelberg Catechism by noting his "enhancement" of the catechism by the insertion of the infamous eightieth question, which condemned the idolatry of the papal Mass. Of course, all of his colleagues would have no doubt agreed that the Mass was idolatrous, but it was nevertheless a noteworthy departure from the irenic tone of the catechism. Likewise, Olevianus also intimated some discontent with some passages of the catechism that could not really be successfully translated from German into Latin. Goeters has concluded that, "Dem Olevianus ist der Katechismus zu deutsch, das heißt zu melanchthonisch." Goeters, "Caspar Olevianus als Theologe," 304–305.

[15] Hollweg is rather uncharitable toward Olevianus in the article. Beyond attacking his character, he questioned whether Olevianus was particularly talented in composing catechisms. Bierma has censured what he termed the "unhelpful" comments of Hollweg, particularly in view of the fact that Hollweg took some of the most damning evidence from the lips of Olevianus's enemies (namely Erastus). Bierma, "Olevianus and the Authorship of The Heidelberg Catechism: Another Look," 22.

[16] E.g., Goeters, "Entstehung und Frühgeschichte des Katechismus," 15: "Diese Ansicht ist von Hollweg mit zumeist schlüssigen Argumenten, die sich noch vermehren ließen, wiederlegt worden." Neuser, "Die Väter des Heidelberger Katechismus," 177: "Ein hervorragender Beitrag Olevians ist auszuschliessen." See also Klooster, "Priority of Ursinus," 87 and 99; Press, *Calvinismus und Territorialstaat*, 230; Visser, *Zacharias Ursinus*, 118–119; Ulrich Hutter, "Zacharias Ursinus und der Heidelberg Katechismus,"

marized: "Olevianus was a member of the commission like the others. He was personally not content with the final version of the catechism. He had wanted it to be more Calvinist. As a senior church leader, however, he took an active role in the ecclesiastical introduction of the catechism."[17]

In an essay in which he sought to counter Hollweg's arguments and reinvigorate Olevianus's claim to authorship of the Heidelberg Catechism, Lyle Bierma argued that "modern historians have too quickly dismissed the 1644 Alting account as erroneous."[18] Indeed, it is disheartening to undermine the authority of one of the chief narrative accounts of Palatine history, especially since so many of the sources that he may have consulted are no longer extant. To Reformed theologians this rejection might seem a double blow, since it might be perceived equally as a knock on Alting, a respected theologian who served as a delegate to the Synod of Dort. It is not, however, that Alting's account is blatantly false; his portrait of events reflects a telescoping of the facts surrounding the composition of the catechism and displays a measure of understandable confusion regarding some of the catechism's potential sources.[19] Given that Olevianus and Ursinus were to become the most well known Palatine theologians, the memory of whom was no doubt especially honored in Alting's circles, it is not unnatural that Alting would magnify the roles they played in the composition of the catechism.[20] One could submit that what Alting's account supremely expresses is a reading of affairs backward in time,

in *Martin Luther und die Reformation in Ostdeutschland und Südosteuropa*, ed. Ulrich Hutter (Sigmaringen: Jan Thorbecke, 1991), 79–105, especially 82–87. See discussion of Bierma below.

[17] J.F. Gerhard Goeters, "Zur Geschichte des Katechismus," in *Heidelberger Katechismus: Revidierte Ausgabe 1997*, 3rd ed. (Neukirchen-Vluyn: Neukirchener Verlag, 2006), 89.

[18] Bierma, "Olevianus and the Authorship of the Heidelberg Catechism: Another Look," 17–27.

[19] I am referring here especially to his comment regarding the "populari declaratione *foederis gratiae*," a work which he credited to Olevianus. Neuser commented regarding this text: "die letztgenannt ist unbekannt und gehört wohl 'ins Reich des Mythos.'" Neuser, "Die Väter des Heidelberger Katechismus," 177. Olevianus's most important works have been reprinted in Caspar Olevianus, *Der Gnadenbund Gottes 1590: Faksimilie-Edition mit einem Kommentar*, ed. Gunther Franz, J.F. Gerhard Goeters and Wilhelm Holtmann (Cologne: Rheinland-Verlag, 1994). For the *Vester Grundt*, see pp. 37–203. See especially J.F. Gerhard Goeter's article "Olevians Fester Grundt: Entstehung, Geschichte, Inhalt" (467–490) in the same. Note that this volume, which celebrates the work of Olevianus, does not advance the argument that Olevianus had a major role in the composition of the catechism.

[20] I omit Girolamo Zanchi, who did not arrive in Heidelberg until 1567, from this comparison.

giving the men who were later recognized as the chief heroes of the tradition the greatest role in the authorship of the catechism. Since this view has been agreeable both to those who would stress the Calvinist (here Olevianus) or the Melanchthonian (there Ursinus) dimensions of the catechism, we need not wonder that Alting's depiction would have enjoyed such a long life. Its longevity was perhaps also sustained by the hope that it reflected a basis in long-missing source materials of the church council in Heidelberg. Alting's account of Palatine church history is indispensable, but it must be used with caution. Since Alting did not write the account when he was in the Palatinate or before the probable destruction of source materials due to the Thirty Years' War, and likewise since the account is not reliable on other details, historians can no longer give his narrative the benefit of the doubt, much less assume that it is always based on better sources than we now have at hand.[21] In summation, given its late date and the difficulty of reconciling its depiction with that of sources contemporaneous to the catechism's composition, Alting's account must be set aside in order that our conception of the catechism's composition can be anchored on more reliable sources.[22]

While there is no contemporary evidence to argue for an especially large role for Olevianus, the links between Ursinus and the catechism are so strong that a consensus has emerged in which he is considered the primary author of the Heidelberg Catechism. Ursinus is recognized as the author of two catechisms, the *Catechesis minor* and the *Catechesis major*, which demonstrably influenced the Heidelberg Catechism. Beyond the textual dependence of the Heidelberg Catechism on his earlier works,

[21] For example, Alting has been demonstrated to be incorrect regarding his depiction of the date of the composition of the church order of 1556 (Goeters, "Caspar Olevianus als Theologe," 299–300; *EKO*, 14:23). He also places Erastus on the church council prematurely (Press, *Calvinismus und Territorialstaat*, 218). He gives the wrong year for Erastus's reconciliation with the church (Alting, *Historia de ecclesiis Palatinis*, 108; also see chapter 7 below). His account of the treatment of Johann Sylvan and the Heidelberg Antitrinitarians is biased (Burchill, *The Heidelberg Antitrinitarians*, 55, 66, passim). Similarly, his narrative of the church discipline conflict is one-sided and murky on the details. These reservations aside, it must be noted that Alting was not a blind devotee of Olevianus; he implicitly criticizes him at points. See, for example, Olevianus's attempt to convert an elderly Lutheran minister to a Reformed view of the Lord's Supper (Alting, *Historia de ecclesiis Palatinis*, 112–113 (ch. 60)). Here Olevianus's assertiveness compares rather poorly to Elector Frederick's moderation and sagacity.

[22] More recently Bierma conceded, "There is indeed no solid evidence for the longstanding claims that Olevianus was one of two main authors of the HC or that he was responsible for the final German redaction." Bierma, "The Purpose and Authorship of the Heidelberg Catechism," in *An Introduction to the Heidelberg Catechism*, 67.

which absolutely assures his consideration as an author, is the fact that after the catechism's publication he became its chief defender and expositor; he took up the pen on many occasions to defend the teachings of the catechism against its Lutheran assailants.[23] Furthermore, his copious lectures on the catechism were transformed by his students into a comprehensive commentary on the catechism, which is still a standard reference work in the Reformed community.[24] No one begrudges Ursinus primary credit for the catechism. Nevertheless, Ursinus never claimed sole responsibility for the work. Likewise, the collector of his works, Quirinius Reuter, while stressing the Heidelberg Catechism's dependence on Ursinus's preliminary drafts, did not deny that the composition had been the work of a committee.[25] Since it has long been acknowledged that the catechism was a group project, the search remains open regarding other possible contributors.

In seeking to make a list of likely contributors, the quest must begin with Elector Frederick's own introduction to the first printed edition of the catechism. On January 19, 1563, he explained the rationale behind the decision to commission a new catechism with these words:

> And accordingly we have composed and authorized, with the counsel and assistance of our entire theological faculty here, also with all the superintendents and prominent servants of the church, a summary instruction or catechism of our Christian religion from the word of God, in both Latin and German, that henceforth not only should the youth be blessedly instructed and therewith unanimously maintained in the churches and schools in such Christian doctrine but also [that] the preachers and the schoolmasters themselves may have a certain and constant custom and standard, how they ought to conduct the instruction of youth and not undertake daily changes or introduce offensive teachings at their whim.[26]

[23] See Klooster, "Priority of Ursinus," 88.

[24] The first edition was published posthumously without the permission of Ursinus's family. The work was refined and reprinted numerous times in the late sixteenth and early seventeenth centuries and translated into English and Dutch. Zacharias Ursinus, *Doctrinae Christianae compendium; seu Commentarii catechetici* ... (Geneva: Eustache Vignon, 1584); *The Commentary of Dr. Zacharias Ursinus on the Heidelberg Catechism*, trans. G.W. Willard (Columbus, 1852). See Christopher Burchill, "On the Consolation of a Christian Scholar: Zacharias Ursinus (1534–1583) and the Reformation in Heidelberg," *Journal of Ecclesiastical History* 37 (1986): 578.

[25] Goeters, "Caspar Olevianus als Theologe," 301–302.

[26] Reprinted in *EKO*, 14:343: "Und demnach mit rhat und zuthun unserer gantzen theologischen facultet allhie, auch allen superintendenten und fürnemsten kirchendienern einen summarischen underricht oder catechismum unserer christlichen religion auß dem wort Gottes beides, in deutscher und lateinisher sprach, verfassen und stellen lassen, damit fürbaß nicht allein die jugendt in kirchen und schulen in solcher christlicher

That the catechism was actually a team project, and not the work of one or two men alone, has long been an insight available to those who would take the elector's preface seriously.[27] Two factors, however, have encouraged historians to overlook Frederick's testimony of team authorship. First, it is difficult to imagine how such an acknowledged masterpiece of catechetical literature could have been composed by committee. The theological antecedents to the catechism have not been so elusive, but its stylistic excellence seems to beg the question of the identity of the literary genius that lay behind it. Second, in many works published anonymously or with claimed joint authorship in Heidelberg, scholars have since been able to establish the author. Not surprisingly, given the Lutheran hostility toward works thought to have a Calvinist or Zwinglian flavor, Heidelberg authors often omitted their names from publications in an attempt to garner an audience instead of being summarily dismissed as "Sacramentarians." Indeed, even Calvin's *Geneva Catechism* was published in a German translation in Heidelberg in 1563 without mentioning the reformer's name on the title page.[28] Likewise, as previously discussed, Erastus anonymously published his booklet on the breaking of bread and the *Gründtlicher Bericht*, as well as later works. Sometimes the Palatine theologians simply wanted to put forth a common front, as in the case of the defense of the Heidelberg Catechism published in 1564, which, although composed by Ursinus, was published in the name of the theological faculty.[29] Considering this proclivity to hide behind anonymity or group authorship, it is not strange that historians would have ignored the preface's claims and searched for the true author or authors. While this tendency was perhaps understandable, none of these reasons is compelling enough to force modern historians to discard the elector's account—or worse yet give it secondary billing to Alting's nar-

---

lehre gottseliglichen underwiesen und darzu einhelliglichen angehalten, sonder auch die prediger und schulmeister selbs ein gewisse und bestendige form und maß haben mögen, wie sie sich in underweisung der jugendt verhalten sollen und nicht ires gefallens tegliche enderungen fürnemen oder widerwertige lehre einfüren."

[27] Although reprints of the first edition of the catechism have been widely available the last hundred years, few allowed Frederick's words to take a preeminent place over the account of Alting. M.A. Gooszen gave Frederick's testimony credence but was also an enthusiastic supporter of the idea that Olevianus was the primary redactor of the German text of the Heidelberg Catechism. M.A. Gooszen, *De Heidelbergsche Catechismus: Textus Receptus met Toelichtende Teksten* (Leiden: Brill, 1890).

[28] Hollweg, *Neue Untersuchungen*, 1:143.

[29] [Zacharias Ursinus], *Verantwortung Wider die ungegründten aufflagen* … (Heidelberg: J. Meyer, 1564).

rative, which was written more than fifty years later. A more prudent approach is to take Frederick's account at face value and then determine if other sixteenth-century evidence complements or undermines it.

Frederick's preface even offers an explicit list of those involved: the theological faculty, the superintendents, and the prominent servants of the church. Along with Ursinus, Immanuel Tremellius and Pierre Boquin were members of the theological faculty. Since neither Tremellius nor Boquin was a native German speaker, they have not generally been considered serious candidates for a large role in composing the catechism—especially not in influencing its German text.[30] Little is presently known about the nine district superintendents, which is a reflection of the relative dearth of Palatine archival records from the period. The office of general superintendent was abandoned after the dismissal of Heshusius. Since Olevianus was both a superintendent and a member of the church council, he most certainly took an active part in the deliberations. The other clerical members of the church council included Boquin and the court preacher Michael Diller, who had already played a significant role in the history of Protestantism as the first evangelical preacher in Speyer and was probably a more important player in the conversion of the Palatinate to the Reformed faith than is currently recognized.[31] The lay members of this body were Wenzel Zuleger and Stephan Cirler, along with Erastus himself. Since even the bureaucrats Cirler and Zuleger were quite theologically engaged, it would be premature to exclude any of these church council members from the authorship circle without just cause.[32] The court preacher Johannes Willing, from whom a number of printed sermons survive, may well have played a role in the catechism's production. Erastus reckoned Willing to be among the Palatinate's most able preachers.[33] Likewise, Petrus Dathenus, leader of the Dutch refugee community at Frankenthal and future court preacher to Frederick, also

[30] Regarding Boquin's role, see G.P. Hartvelt, "Petrus Boquinus," 76–77.

[31] *NDB*, 3: 719.

[32] Regarding the composition of the church council, see Goeters, "Entstehung," 15; Goeters, "Caspar Olevianus als Theologe," 298; Klooster, "Priority of Ursinus," 79–80; Press, *Calvinismus und Territorialstaat und Territorialstaat*, 238–243. We have already had a glimpse of Cirler's Reformed zeal in his role as messenger to Melanchthon in the Heshusius affair.

[33] Erastus to Wolf, Heidelberg, Sept. 29, (15)61. ZBZ (Hot.) F 38, fol. 272. From Erastus's correspondence it is clear that Willing was in the Palatinate as early as 1561, though curiously he is generally left out of discussions of the composition of the catechism's editorial committee. For his biography, see Werner Seeling, *Johannes Willing (1525–1572), ein*

likely took part in the sessions and is thought to have introduced Jan Łaski's Emden Catechism of 1554 into the source milieu of the catechism.[34] Other figures who possibly should be added to the authorship circle include the ethics professor Johannes Brunner, who would later convert to Catholicism, and Adam Neuser, the future Antitrinitarian and alleged Muslim, both of whom were regarded at that point as theologians of roughly similar standing as Olevianus.[35] It appears doubtful that the other future Antitrinitarian, Johann Sylvan, took part in the composition of the catechism, as he apparently did not take up his position of superintendent in Kaiserslautern until later in 1563—though it is not clear when he arrived in the Palatinate.[36] Beyond these individuals, Goeters suggests local ministers Petrus Macheropoeus and Tilemann Mumius may have taken part in the proceedings, as well as Konrad Marius, the leader of the *Collegium Sapientiae*.[37] Likewise, one cannot exclude the jurist, councilor, and Reformed partisan Christoph Ehem, whom Volker Press has characterized as the lead agitator for Calvinism in the territory.[38] Finally, it was after all Elector Frederick's catechism, and he personally claimed to have enhanced it on a number of points.[39] While Ursinus may well have been the theological leader of this brain trust, a

Schicksal zwischen Luthertum und Calvinismus: Versuch einer Biographie [Veröffentlichtungen des Vereins für pfälzische Kirchengeschichte 11] (Otterbach: Argobast, 1972).

[34] Goeters, "Enstehung und Frühgeschichte des Katechismus," 14. Thompson argued the catechism's famed comfort motif was in fact taken over from Jan Łaski. Thompson, "An Historical Reconstruction of Melanchthonianism," 263–265.

[35] As discussed earlier, Neuser had actually competed with Olevianus for the theological chair at the University of Heidelberg. In fact, the faculty senate actually favored Neuser, but Olevianus prevailed with the assistance of the elector. Burchill, *The Heidelberg Antitrinitarians*, 113. The Switzer Brunner was clearly Erastus's protégé as discussed in chapter 2 (note 95). He was first given a pastoral position in nearby Weinheim, then moved to a post at the *Collegium Sapientiae*, and finally joined the university arts faculty as professor of ethics in 1561.

[36] Both Seeling and Burchill can only affirm his presence in Kaiserslautern by midyear (certainly by March) 1563. Alternatively, Goeter's discussion suggests that he was already in place in Kaiserslautern by January 1563. Werner Seeling, "Johannes Sylvan, Neue Erkenntnisse über die Hinrichtung eines kurpfälzischen Theologen im Jahr 1572," *Blätter für pfälzische Kirchengeschichte und religiöse Volkskunde* 40 (1973): 91; Burchill, *The Heidelberg Antitrinitarians*, 24 and 31; Goeters, "Enstehung und Frühgeschichte des Katechismus," 16.

[37] Goeters, "Caspar Olevianus als Theologe," 303.

[38] Press, *Calvinismus und Territorialstaat*, 213, passim.

[39] Henss, *Der Heidelberger Katechismus*, 26.

long list of potential collaborators for the project existed, any number of whom may well have had a substantial impact on either the theological content of the catechism or its literary style.

Before considering the actual evidence that points toward a large role for Erastus in the composition of the catechism, it is fitting to reflect on how relatively influential the likely contributors were at the time of the composition. This exercise should correct the description of the catechism's composition offered by Alting, who apparently let the later reputations of the participants color his account. Although Ursinus never became a court insider during his long stay in the Palatinate, he was considered a rare theological talent from the moment Erastus and others began to recruit him for the university. They sought qualities in Ursinus that were apparently lacking in Boquin and Olevianus—specifically, they sought a true systematic theologian who could also defend the emerging Palatine theology with the pen and in public debate. Although Olevianus's dedication and organizational skills may have been apparent, in late 1562 there was little evidence to suggest that his colleagues regarded him as a budding theological talent. Furthermore, Olevianus displayed a tendency to decline certain preaching assignments—especially those closely associated with the work of catechization.[40] Alternatively, Erastus was at his pinnacle of influence in church affairs. He had just written two tracts that appear to have possessed the official sanction of the elector. He was personally close to the elector and apparently in a strong position on the church council. He had also been empowered to recruit a theologian for the university—a task apparently not entrusted to Boquin or Olevianus. Erastus possessed a certain *auctoritas* in Heidelberg intellectual life; he was ten years older than either Ursinus or Olevianus and was manifestly confident of his own opinions. It is no exaggeration to assert that Erastus's theological works are the best witnesses of the nascent Palatine theology before the Heidelberg Catechism. From his relative influence alone, we have every reason to expect that Erastus

[40] See above in chapter 2 (note 88) for Erastus's comment to Bullinger regarding Olevianus's reluctance to preach. In August 1563, Ursinus disclosed that he had to take over the Sunday afternoon catechetical lectures for Olevianus, despite his own heavy work load, as the position "required a man who was a teacher and skilled, and who might also succeed in connecting with the less educated people and the youth in accommodating his speech" ("requirens hominem διδακτικον et exercitatum quique ad captum rudioris populi et iuventutis accomodata dictione valeat"). Ursinus to Johannes Crato von Krafftheim, August 1563, in Hans Rott, ed., "Briefe des Heidelberger Theologen Zacharias Ursinus aus Heidelberg und Neustadt a.H," *NHJ* 14 (1906): 59.

would have played a prominent part in the composition of the catechism. The question that remains is whether we can find corroborating sources to support his role.

Although many records from the sixteenth-century Palatinate are no longer extant—in particular, the actual minutes from the sessions in which the catechism was approved—a modest quantity of letters from Erastus, Olevianus, and Ursinus, has survived. These sources fail to identify any particular person as the author of the catechism; indeed, neither Olevianus nor Ursinus—the two favorites of Reformed historians since Alting—claimed an especially prominent role in the catechism's composition.[41] What follows is an investigation of the extant correspondence, focusing particularly on sources that shed light on Erastus's role in the composition of the catechism.

While a good number of Ursinus's letters survive, there are not many surviving letters by Ursinus from the period of the catechism's composition. One letter from 1562 to Konrad Gessner in Zurich documents his involvement in the project but otherwise sheds little light on the composition itself. In discussing his role in reforming the Palatine church, Ursinus related, "In this we are currently occupied that a type of catechism may be written of our own making suitable for the populace and youth."[42] Here we learn, in line with the elector's introduction, that the catechism was a collective composition (thus the first person plural) and, not surprisingly, that Ursinus was part of this group. What is equally noteworthy here is what is not said; for example, no explicit mention about any close collaboration with Olevianus, Erastus, or anyone else, is included.[43]

The extant letters from Olevianus from this period also tend to support the group authorship thesis, and ironically turn our focus to Olevianus's future rival Erastus. A source which is particularly suggestive regarding Erastus's role in the catechism's creation is a letter from Olevianus to Bullinger. In it he praised the Swiss Germans, declaring, "If

[41] Hollweg, *Neue Untersuchungen*, 1:135.

[42] Gustav Adolf Benrath, ed., "Briefe des Heidelberger Theologen Zacharias Ursinus (1534–1583)," *NHJ* 8 (1964): 100. Ursinus to Gessner, Frankfurt, March 22: "In eo iam sumus, ut forma catechismi populo et iuventuti nostrae instituendae idonea conscribatur, ministerii et disciplinae ratio constituatur."

[43] It can also be noted that while earlier scholarship nearly made Olevianus and Ursinus to be the Lennon and McCartney of the sixteenth century, it does not seem they were particularly close, and Olevianus's name only appears infrequently in Ursinus's correspondence.

there is any clarity in these [the Latin and German versions of the catechism] we owe a good measure to you and the lucid abilities of the Swiss." He continued with a remark that sheds insight on the group authorship of the catechism: "the pious thoughts have not been gathered from one but from many."[44] The interpretation of this passage hangs on the word *cogitationes*, which I have translated as "thoughts." Though one could perhaps make the case that Olevianus was speaking here of the *cogitationes* in terms of the various sources reviewed in preparation of the catechism, it is more likely that Olevianus meant to suggest the actual input of the members of the catechism committee. This interpretation is buttressed by Olevianus's comment to Calvin concerning the composition of the catechism: "Such is the difficulty of reconciling from many heads and reducing them to one."[45] It bears noting that Olevianus's own words are much more in line with the account given in the elector's preface rather than Alting's later rendition of events. Another sentence in the letter to Bullinger has proved even more difficult for modern historians to interpret. Here Olevianus lamented,

> Surely it was a careless mistake, that [the catechism] was not sent to you sooner, but I was unwilling in haste and too quick in my liberality, to take away praise from my most dear colleagues, *chiefly Erastus*. But, be that as it may, I send these books to you in all of our names.[46]

Olevianus apologized for his delay in sending the catechism. This fact seems strange on the surface, since Erastus had already sent Bullinger a

[44] Olevianus to Bullinger, April 14, 1563, printed in Sudhoff, *C. Olevianus und Z. Ursinus*, 482–483: "Gratiam ac pacem. Gratias tibi ago, Venerande pater ac frater in Christo pro libro ad me misso: et remitto Catechismos nostros latinos et Germanicos. Certe si qua in iis est perspicuitas, eius bonam partem tibi et candidis ingeniis Helvetiorum debemus. Gloria redeat ad solum Deum. Non unius sed multorum sunt collatae piae cogitationes. Certe factum est negligenter, quod citius ad te non est missus, sed ego nolui festinatione et praepropera liberalitate mea laudibus praeripere carissimis Collegis meis, Erasto praecipue. Sed utut sit, communi nostro nomine hosce libellos ad te mitto. Iudicium tuum valde desidero." Wesel-Roth, *Thomas Erastus* also prints most of this selection with some variations (chiefly: "laudem praecipere" instead of "laudibus praeripere" and "Sed ut id" instead of "sed utut"). Wesel-Roth, *Thomas Erastus*, 133. See also Hollweg, *Heinrich Bullingers Hausbuch*, 238–239; Fred Klooster, "Calvin's Attitude toward the Heidelberg Catechism," in *Later Calvinism* [*SCE&S* 22], ed. W. Fred Graham (Kirksville, Mo., 1992), 315; Visser, *Zacharias Ursinus*, 118–119; Neuser, "Die Väter des Heidelberger Katechismus," 181; and Bierma, "The Purpose and Authorship of the Heidelberg Catechism," 54.

[45] *CO*, 19:685: "Tanta est difficultas in conciliandis multis capitibus et redigendis in unum."

[46] The emphasis is mine. See the Latin text above in note 44.

copy of the catechism nearly two months earlier.[47] However, rather than interpreting this as a misunderstanding between Erastus and Olevianus, it is perhaps best to understand this letter as Olevianus's official communiqué to Bullinger as the leading clerical member of the church council. Olevianus sent both the German and Latin texts of the catechism, including the infamous question eighty which declared the papal Mass "accursed idolatry."[48] It is also worth noting that Calvin received a copy of the catechism a month after Bullinger. More germane to the question of authorship of the catechism is Olevianus's mention of Erastus. The text appears to credit Erastus for the quality of the catechism.[49] While he did not directly name Erastus as an author, his comment implies Erastus's participation; otherwise, it would be difficult to understand how Olevianus could steal praise from Erastus for the catechism if in fact Erastus had had little to do with its composition. An alternative interpretation would be that Olevianus and Erastus were already on bad terms in early 1563, and the letter's reference to Erastus combined with Olevianus's ignorance of Erastus's activities reflected a measure of hostility between the two. Indeed, this estrangement would come, although we are fairly well informed that it did not take place before 1564. In fact, in a later letter from 1563, Olevianus calls Erastus his "brother and most dear friend."[50] Given that Erastus and Olevianus were on good terms in 1563, it is more likely that the letter implies that Erastus merited praise as one of the individuals whose "pious thoughts" had contributed to the catechism.

Another source suggests in an even more definitive fashion that Erastus played a role in the catechism's composition. Erastus sent a letter to Bullinger on January 30, 1563 announcing the completion of the catechism, in which he declared:

[47] Erastus reports sending Bullinger the catechism in a letter from Feb. 26, 1563. Cf. Wesel-Roth, *Thomas Erastus*, 83, note, 84; Hollweg, *Neue Untersuchungen*, 1:135.

[48] *CO*, 19:633–635 (no. 3925). See Goeters, "Caspar Olevianus als Theologe," 304. "Teufelswerk" was later added for good measure. This question would again become a source of mischief in the early eighteenth century when the electors of the Palatinate were again Catholic. See Schaab, *Geschichte der Kurpfalz*, 2:173–174.

[49] Hollweg and Benrath have disagreed over the interpretation of the letter. Hollweg found the letter quite clear and asserted that "Olevianus ... ausdrucklich die Mitarbeit des Erast erwähnt." Hollweg, *Neue Untersuchungen*, 1:135. Benrath, alternatively, remarked that he did not discern such an explicit confirmation of Erastus's role in the catechism in Olevianus's letter. Benrath, "Die Eigenart der pfälzischen Reformation," 25, note 37.

[50] Olevianus to Bullinger, Oct. 25, 1563. Sudhoff, *C. Olevianus und Z. Ursinus*, 483–485. Of course, we should take these formulaic niceties with a grain of salt. Nevertheless, after they had fallen out, their estrangement is readily apparent in Erastus's correspondence.

> *We have composed a catechism*, in which all the heads of doctrine as well as the Sacraments are explained clearly and in great detail according to the work's intent, which the most illustrious prince desires to be taught in schools and churches in general. It is now in press and should be complete within a couple of days. I will send it to you soon. I suppose that no one at all will say regarding us [that we] are hiding. *For some time now I have been totally absorbed in it.* For I was always eager to make [our] doctrine public.[51]

On the surface, the first line, "We have composed a catechism," yields an even more explicit testimonial to taking part in the composition of the catechism than the above mentioned quotation from Ursinus. The obvious question that arises is how to interpret Erastus's use of "we." Does he mean this literally (i.e., that he was one of the composers of the catechism) or is he only using "we" in an impersonal collective sense, much like when a person remarks of her favorite sports team, "We won." The latter interpretation is certainly plausible; after all, the catechism was not only the personal confession of a few theologians, but the guiding rule of faith for the entire principality. This non-literal reading of Erastus's quotation seems so obvious that it probably explains why prior historians have not used this text to argue for Erastus's authorship.[52] A close reading of the remainder of this passage, however, suggests that Erastus meant the literal sense, i.e., that he was intimately involved in writing the catechism. This interpretation turns on Erastus's statement, "For some time now I have been totally absorbed in it." The context around this passage leaves no doubt that the "it" he was talking about was the catechism. Perhaps it could be argued that he was merely speaking of tasks not directly related to the composition of the catechism such as monitoring the committee, influencing opinion at court, and writing letters on behalf of the Palatine cause. While Erastus may well have been involved in

[51] Erastus to Bullinger, Jan. 30, [1563], StAZ, II 361 fol. 86: "Catechismum composuimus, in quo cum alia Doctrinae capita, tum Sacramenta aperte et (fus)è pro ratione propositi operis explicantur, quem illlustrissim[us] Princeps in Scholis et Ecclesiis vult omnino doceri. Sub pressu est et intra biduum perficietur. Proxime ad te mittam. Nemo arbitror, dicet aliquid à nobis dissimulari. Iam diu in eo totus fui. Cupivi enim semper doctrinam publicam fieri."

[52] For instance, Wesel-Roth reproduced this quotation in her text without pausing to reflect upon the implications it might have regarding Erastus's role in the composition of the catechism (*Thomas Erastus*, 35). Wesel-Roth does not seem to have been especially interested in the question of the composition of the catechism. More significantly, she wrote in a time when the orthodoxy of the dual authorship of the catechism by Ursinus and Olevianus had not been seriously questioned. Certainly Hollweg, among others, was familiar with the quote, but again his purpose was to discredit the theory of Olevianus's authorship, not to prove that Erastus was an author.

various campaigns on behalf of the catechism, it would be sidestepping the most straightforward interpretation of the meaning of these passages if we read them not to suggest that Erastus was an active participant in the catechism's composition. Especially considering Erastus's reputation at this juncture as a theological authority and his fervent desire to bring the Palatinate to an explicitly Reformed stance, we are forced to accept that Erastus is saying exactly what he appears to be saying, namely, that he and others have composed a catechism and that his involvement was so extensive that it had in fact absorbed much of his time.

The evidence from these sixteenth-century letters suggests that Erastus had a significant role in the composition of the catechism. To engage this possibility more thoroughly, it is fitting to take a closer look at the text of the catechism to discern areas where Erastus's influence might have been felt. Since Erastus's contemporaneous writings concern the Lord's Supper, the best place to test this hypothesis regarding Erastus's role in the catechism's composition is the Eucharistic teaching of the Heidelberg Catechism.

The Heidelberg Catechism's Doctrine of the Lord's Supper

The theologians of the Palatinate explicated their doctrine of the Eucharist in questions 75 through 79 of the Heidelberg Catechism. The catechism's primary motif was to direct the believer toward receiving the benefits of Christ's crucifixion and away from contemplation of the elements themselves. The catechism asserted with the precision of a mathematical equation that those who truly received the elements in faith would receive the benefit of forgiveness and eternal life, while rejecting the notion that the benefit was achieved through a transformation of the elements themselves. In this line, participation in the symbol of communion guaranteed the partakers that Christ's body and blood were sacrificed for them and that Christ's crucified body "nourishes my soul to eternal life." "Eating" was defined as embracing Christ's sufferings and being united to his "sacred body by the Holy Spirit." The same passage that Melanchthon had emphasized in his *Judgment* was brought forward for special notice in the catechism's proof texts for the doctrine. The authors rejected any notion of the elements actually becoming the body and blood of Christ as in the doctrine of transubstantiation; however, the catechism did not explicitly refute the notion that the elements might contain the body of Christ as in the doctrine of Consubstantiation. There was simply no explicit discussion of Christ's presence in the Eucharist, affirmative or negative, in the catechism. It maintained that according to traditional usage the elements are called the body and blood of Christ, but explained that this was an analogy to the spiritual truth that Christ's body and blood are believers' "food and drink" for eternal life. Even more importantly, the reception of the "true-signs" assures believers that Christ's sacrifice benefits them personally. Like the rest of the catechism, the emphasis of its Eucharistic teaching was centered on the assurance and consolation of the believer.

The Eucharistic teaching of the Heidelberg Catechism was explicitly anti-Catholic but only implicitly anti-Lutheran. There was no discussion about Christ's presence in the Eucharist. However, in its direct statement that Christ's body is in heaven, the catechism took a posture against the Gnesio-Lutheran idea of the ubiquity of Christ's human flesh, and by implication undermined the notion that Christ's human flesh could be present "in, with, and under" the elements, as most Lutherans held. The Palatine theologians certainly could and did make the argument that the Eucharistic teaching of their catechism was not at variance with the Augsburg Confession (at least the *Variata*) and could therefore claim that they had not broken the stipulations of the Religious Peace of Augsburg. In sum, it was clearly not classic Lutheran theology, but it was not per se anti-Lutheran. Although this assessment might appear strange, given that the Palatinate is often held up as the prototype of "Calvinism" in the Holy Roman Empire, the catechism's teaching on this touchstone doctrine was by no means distinctively Calvinist either. For example, it lacked the specific Calvinist vocabulary of *sursum corda*, the notion that believers' hearts were lifted up to commune directly with the ascended Christ.[53] Even more strikingly, the catechism did not affirm that communicants take part in Christ's body "substantially." Both Lutherans and Calvinists included the term "substantially" in their confessions, whereas Zwinglians adamantly rejected the use of the term. The lack of specific Calvinist teaching in this section of the catechism led Wilhelm Neuser to

[53] *Sursum corda* comes from the part of the Mass that many English prayer books translate as, "lift up your hearts." Calvin's notion was that Christ did not physically come down from heaven to be present in the elements, but that by the agency of the Holy Spirit, believers were tangibly joined with him in heaven. My contention here is in opposition to the interpretation of Fred Klooster, who suggests the idea of *sursum corda* is expressed in question 76 of the catechism. Though question 76 clearly emphasizes the Holy Spirit's agency in facilitating this communion with the ascended Christ, I do not discern an explicit dependence on Calvin's idea of *sursum corda* in the catechism. Klooster, "Calvin's Attitude toward the Heidelberg Catechism," 328.

describe its theology of the Lord's Supper as "late-Zwinglian."[54] While it might be prudent to simply regard the catechism's teaching as representing Heidelberg, as opposed to trying to force an association with Geneva, Zurich, or Wittenberg, Neuser's characterization has perhaps a modicum of validity regarding the modesty of the doctrine that the catechism confirms. Looking at the glass "half empty," as it were, one might characterize the catechism as a late Zwinglian document in its failure to explicitly teach real participation in Christ's body and blood in the sacrament or concretely affirm that grace is bestowed in the sacrament. Nevertheless, seeing the glass "half full," in the sense that it strove to inspire faith in an objective manner, regardless of the emotional state of the participant, one could say that it still retained a Lutheran feel, if devoid of Lutheran substance. Similarly, questions such as no. 76 seem to echo Calvin's theology of the Lord's Supper without explicitly endorsing aspects of this theology which would not be palatable—that is, no explicit affirmation of communion with Christ's substance—to those who held to a more straight-forward memorial interpretation of the Eucharist. It surely was not anti-Calvinist; the catechism was enthusiastically embraced by most Calvinists other than Calvin himself, whose feelings toward it seem to have been rather lukewarm (see below). The Heidelberg teaching on the Eucharist was in essence a union of the late Zwinglian/Calvinist position of the Zurich Consensus with a now fully "Sacramentarian" Philippist understanding of the Lord's Supper. It was analogous to the attempt to move a Zwinglian understanding closer to a Melanchthonian Lutheran interpretation, which was seen in the Eucharistic teaching of the *First Helvetic Confession*. The catechism was thus more than a mere compromise, but perhaps even had something of the quality of a magical mirror in that a reasonably broad spectrum of Zwinglians, Calvinists, and moderate Lutherans could see their own interpretations of the Lord's Supper reflected in the document.[55] Unqualified confessional labels do not help

[54] Neuser, "Die Väter des Heidelberger Katechismus," 185. Neuser is not alone in this view that the Eucharistic theology of the Heidelberg Catechism is closer to Bullinger's thought than Calvin's. For example, B.A. Gerrish has written: "Despite the contrary judgments of Schaff and Müller, it does not seem to me that the catechism teaches a full Calvinistic doctrine of the sacraments." Later he states, "And yet it is not so much anti-Calvinistic as timidly Calvinistic." B.A. Gerrish, *The Old Protestantism and the New: Essays on the Reformation Heritage* (Chicago: University of Chicago Press, 1982), 125 and 129. See also Burchill, "On the Consolation of a Christian Scholar," 570.

[55] Bierma thoroughly reviews this ground in *The Doctrine of the Sacraments in the Heidelberg Catechism: Melanchthonian, Calvinist, or Zwinglian?* [Studies in Reformed Theology and History, New Series, 4] (Princeton: Princeton Theological Seminary, 1999).

us much here, as the catechism's teachings are quite removed from the impasse of Zwingli or Luther from 1529, and while its Eucharistic theology is closer to Calvin than to Luther or Zwingli, it equally reflects the efforts of Beza, Bucer, Bullinger, and Vermigli to find a workable middle ground in the wake of Marburg.

It is instructive to review the opinions of Bullinger and Calvin on the catechism, even if this task does not directly address the authorship question. The degree to which the catechism's view of the Lord's Supper was in complete agreement with Bullinger's theology can be drawn from his comment to Ambrosius Blarer on the Heidelberg Catechism: "You will have never seen a more felicitous presentation of the entire matter of the faith; likewise, as far as it concerns the Lord's Supper; in everything we agree wholeheartedly."[56] As late as 1566, Frederick still found the need to refute the rumor that Bullinger had written the catechism himself: "The report that I have had my *Catechism* and *Kirchenordnung* prepared in Zurich by Bullinger and his associates is an open and barefaced lie."[57] Whereas Bullinger's assessment of the catechism was unequivocal, Calvin's never gave his direct blessing to the catechism—despite having been explicitly asked for an assessment by Olevianus.[58] Fred Klooster argued that Calvin possessed a favorable opinion of the Heidelberg Catechism, which he indirectly communicated by dedicating his Jeremiah commentary to Elector Frederick. In this he hails Frederick for authorizing "sound doctrine" about the Lord's Supper—but still withholds any direct praise of the catechism. Reading between the lines, one gets the sense that Calvin must have found the catechism palatable, perhaps no more or less so than the preceding *Consensus Tigurinus* to which he was a party, but that he was not enthusiastic about its sacramental theology, which probably did not go far enough in his eyes. From my perspective, rather than displaying manifest approval or disapproval

[56] Quoted in Walter Hollweg, *Der Augsburger Reichstag von 1566 und seine Bedeutung für die Entstehung der reformierten Kirche und ihres Bekenntnisses* [BGLRK 17] (Neukirchen-Vluyn: Neukirchener Verlag, 1964), 168. See also idem, *Heinrich Bullingers Hausbuch*, 238. Of course, the Palatines were alternatively derided as "Calvinists," "Zwinglians," and "Sacramentarians" by their Lutheran critics.

[57] Letter from Nov. 1, 1566, quoted in Thompson, "The Palatinate Church Order of 1563," 350.

[58] Klooster, "Calvin's Attitude toward the Heidelberg Catechism," 311–331 (especially 318–320). It is also interesting to note that Calvin's letter to Olevianus from October 1562, apparently the very time the catechism was being composed, says nothing about the catechism but a great deal about church discipline. See below. *CO*, 19:563–565 (3869); Sudhoff, *C. Olevianus und Z. Ursinus*, 482.

of the catechism, Calvin used the opportunity of the introduction to the Jeremiah commentary as a teachable moment both to praise the Palatines for their accomplishment and to offer the elector and his theologians an elevated view of sacramental efficacy and participation with the substance of Christ's body and blood. In short, Calvin makes explicit in his dedication what had only been implicit in the catechism, and in doing so paved the way for succeeding Calvinists to read his theology into the document. While Bullinger was more enthusiastic about the catechism's sacramental doctrine in the short run, perhaps Calvin's views won out in the long run, in that he provided the lenses through which succeeding generations have most commonly read the catechism.[59]

However if we focus on the Heidelberg context in 1562–1563 rather than looking abroad, the document that shared the greatest affinity with the Lord's Supper teaching of the Heidelberg Catechism was Erastus's *Gründtlicher Bericht*, which was published in 1562. Goeters and Neuser previously suggested that the catechism's doctrine of the Lord's Supper could likely be attributed to Erastus, and Irena Dingel called it the "cornerstone" of confessional transformation leading to the Heidelberg Catechism.[60] Even the Calvinist scholar Karl Sudhoff, the biographer of Olevianus and Ursinus and a chief proponent of Olevianus's authorship, declared of the *Gründtlicher Bericht*: "We will encounter entirely the same teaching in the Heidelberg Catechism."[61] In both works the driving motif was to suggest that the sacrament of the Lord's Supper can have meaning only with reference to Christ's passion. In both, the Lord's Supper was viewed as a faith-inspiring event. Indeed, this faith-enhancing aspect of the Lord's Supper has a certain objective quality in that communicants are as assured of their acceptance into Christ's kingdom "as certainly as we receive the bread and the wine."[62] In all of this there was no discus-

[59] Klooster, "Calvin's Attitude toward the Heidelberg Catechism," 326–328. For the dedication of the Jeremiah commentary, see *CO*, 20:72–79. Partial translation in John Calvin, *Commentaries on the Book of the Prophet Jeremiah and the Lamentations*, trans. by John Owen, 5 vols. (Grand Rapids: Eerdmans, 1950), 1:xvi–xxiv. See also Bierma, *The Doctrine of the Sacraments in the Heidelberg Catechism*, 39.

[60] Neuser, "Die Väter des Heidelberger Katechismus," 185: "Thomas Erastus … hat sich aller Wahrscheinlichkeit nach in den Abendmahlsfragen 75 bis 79 durchgesetzt." Goeters, "Entstehung und Frühgeschichte des Katechismus," 3–23. Irene Dingel states, "wird bereits hier der Grundstein für die spätere Bekenntnisbildung im Heidelberger Katechismus gelegt." *Bibliotheca Palatina* [Textband] ed. Elmar Mittler (Heidelberg: Editions Braus, 1986), 169.

[61] Sudhoff, *C. Olevianus und Z. Ursinus*, 87.

[62] *Gründtlicher Bericht*, 49.

sion of the presence of Christ in the Lord's Supper in the Heidelberg Catechism—whereas Erastus's unwillingness to admit this in principle was more explicit in the *Gründtlicher Bericht*. All in all, there is a fundamental harmony between the Eucharistic teaching of Heidelberg Catechism and Erastus's *Gründtlicher Bericht*, which adds further weight to the presumption that Erastus was extensively involved in the catechism's preparation.

Complementing the theological agreement of the *Gründtlicher Bericht* with the Heidelberg Catechism is a linguistic similarity between the catechism and Erastus's works. Both the Heidelberg Catechism and the *Gründtlicher Bericht* speak of sacraments as *Warzeichen* (true-signs) and as a *Pfand* (deposit). Another case of terminological similarity seems to go right to the heart of the catechism's faith-kindling quality. Ernst Bizer found the use of "so certainly" and "as certainly as" language to be the quintessential formulation of the catechism.[63] An example of this comes in question 75: "and further, that with his crucified body and shed blood he himself feeds and nourishes my soul to everlasting life, as certainly as I receive from the hand of the minister and taste with my mouth, the bread and cup of the Lord, which are given to me as true-signs of the body and blood of Christ." This phrasing is likewise to be found in Erastus's *Gründtlicher Bericht*, which sounded a similar chord: "That we do not doubt that he feeds and refreshes us, *so certainly* with the communion of his crucified body and shed blood for eternal life, *as certainly as* we receive the bread and the wine."[64] While this vocabulary was not unprecedented in Reformation theology prior to the catechism[65] and some of the terminology simply reflects the biblical proof texts favored by the catechism's authors, if we are going to postulate how this language found its way into the catechism, we would have every right to assume the influence of the person who was employing this language in Heidelberg immediately prior to the catechism's composition and for whom we have firm evidence that puts him in the circle of its composition. It would nevertheless be overstating the case to say the

[63] Ernst Bizer, *Studien zur Geschichte des Abendmahlsstreits im 16. Jahrhundert*, 2nd ed. (Darmstadt: Wissenschaftlicher Buchgesellschaft, 1962), 303. Bizer was quite taken by this terminology and commented: "Diese Formulierung erscheint nun überaus glücklich."

[64] *Gründltlicher Bericht*, 49: "daß wir nit zweiflen er speise und tränke uns so gewiß mit der gemainschafft seines gekreutzigten leibs und vergoßnen blüts zum ewigen leben/als gewiß wir brot und wein empfahen."

[65] Bierma, "The Purpose and Authorship of the Heidelberg Catechism," 56.

Eucharistic teaching of the Heidelberg Catechism belongs exclusively to Erastus.[66] The catechism's Eucharistic doctrine had many fathers, and there is a line of evolution that began with the debates of 1559–1560, developed further in the printed works of Boquin and Erastus, and which found definitive expression in the catechism. Erastus had been the most effective exponent of this tradition in German both in debate and in treatises prior to the catechism's publication. The harmony of the catechism's language and teaching corresponds to what we would expect to find, were Erastus to have had a prominent role in the catechism's composition, and it corroborates the circumstantial evidence that closely associates Erastus with the catechism's composition.

Conclusion: Erastus's Role in the Catechism's Creation

On balance, the evidence for ascribing a leading role to Erastus in the composition of the catechism, or at bare minimum, of the portion of the catechism dealing with the Lord's Supper, is quite strong. To summarize the arguments in Erastus's behalf: first, Erastus was a person of unparalleled influence with the elector, at the university, and within the church itself at the time of the catechism's composition. Without any additional evidence one would assume that he would have taken part in the committee's activities. Second, statements from contemporary letters link Erastus more closely to the catechism than either Ursinus or Olevianus and give the distinct impression that he was deeply involved in the work of constructing the catechism. Third, the catechism's Eucharistic doctrine was in close agreement with Erastus's *Gründtlicher Bericht*, a fact that has long been recognized, and the catechism even deployed some of the characteristic expressions and vocabulary also present in Erastus's work.

Taken together, these points shed new light on the work of the committee that assembled the catechism. It is not my goal to refute the Ursinus-Olevianus dual authorship thesis to replace it with an Ursinus-Erastus thesis. The chief import of this analysis, rather than placing Erastus in the role of the primary author of the catechism, is to suggest that the elector's preface must be taken seriously and to assert once again that the

[66] In fact, Erastus would later directly oppose the catechism's firm authorization of excommunication. However, as Erastus reported, at this point he supported the basic notion of excommunication, so this section of the catechism (Q & A 81–85) apparently matched Erastus's opinions in 1562. See chapter 6.

catechism was actually composed by a larger group than the dual authorship hypothesis allowed. While not refuting the notion that the dogmatic clarity of the work should be credited to Ursinus, here we have a case where the fingerprints of another agent can be seen on the work. Erastus stands out as the one member of the committee besides Ursinus whose participation is most explicitly confirmed by the sources.

If the dual authorship thesis is rejected (though it remains ubiquitous and no doubt will enjoy "virtual" immortality as Internet reference works cannibalize one another ad infinitum) and we accept Ursinus's priority, how should we weigh the relative influence of the other participants in the process? Perhaps we might think of the catechism's authorship team as a three-stage pyramid, with Ursinus at the top as the leading spirit of the catechism. Ursinus gave the catechism its structure, harmonized theological motifs drawn from different sources—which he knew better than anyone else in the circle—and likely influenced the German text of the catechism, given his recognized linguistic talents. In the middle we might place individuals like Erastus and Olevianus, who we know stood out among the organizers of the Palatine church and regarding whom we also possess corroborating evidence to associate with at least some stage of the catechism's production. While the current consensus is that Olevianus does not deserve recognition as a full co-author of the catechism, he was apparently the most prominent of the superintendents and the late addition of question eighty has been ascribed to him. Both Olevianus and Erastus certainly had the authority at this juncture to influence the text of the catechism, if they had the inclination. Given the tenacity that both of these men showed in later ecclesiastical developments in the Palatinate, it is hard to imagine either taking an overly passive role when such an important document was drafted. On the bottom tier of the pyramid we would place the larger pool of individuals named in the elector's preface whose roles were probably limited to discussing the lead authors' work in committee. It is unlikely that the actual composition of the body of the catechism was effected by the entire ten-to-fifteen person group. Above the pyramid we naturally have the elector himself, who undoubtedly had a free hand to steer the catechism according to his wishes, and below, the Palatine clerics who accepted the catechism at the January "synod." The pyramid model accommodates the available evidence for the catechism's composition and takes into consideration the practical constraints of composing a document that evidences an impressive consistency of style and theological vision. Future research will likely continue to debate the relative contributions of Ursinus as opposed to the rest of the committee and probe whether individuals such as Boquin might move up a level in the authorship pyramid.

Placing Erastus in a prominent role in this authorship circle has not been invented out of whole cloth, but follows up the leads suggested by the last century of scholarship. One might call it a latent thesis; it was rather obvious for anyone who would consider the possibility of a larger role of Erastus as an author and compare the prior conclusions of Hollweg, Goeters, Neuser, Sudhoff, and Auguste Bonnard. That it has not been advanced earlier is due largely to the dominance of the old thesis in the historiography. Since much of the prior debate has been over the Calvinist vs. Philippist Lutheran quality of the catechism, it was easy to overlook the contributions of someone conventionally labeled a "Zwinglian" in their midst.

Perhaps it is most fitting to allow Erastus's future rival Olevianus, the man who has at times received too much credit for the catechism's composition, to write our conclusion. Olevianus reveled in Erastus's theological gifts and exclaimed to Calvin that "Erastus is nearly unsurpassed in Germany as a theologian." The irony of this story was that although Olevianus was unwilling to rob Erastus for the credit of the catechism, for three hundred years his own promoters have done exactly that. If Olevianus himself was unwilling to defraud Erastus of the honor due him for his role in the composition of the catechism, I submit we must also recognize Erastus as a prominent member of the committee which composed the catechism.

Viewing the events in Heidelberg as they unfolded alters our view of the significance of the shapers of the Heidelberg Reformation. The old hagiography of "Three Men Came to Heidelberg"[67] must be severely revised. Boquin and Erastus, with the political cover of Christoph Ehem and the counts of Erbach, were the theological leaders who first swung Heidelberg into the Reformed camp. Alternatively, Olevianus and Ursinus consolidated, and, in the case of Olevianus, further transformed the movement begun by Boquin and Erastus. The Heidelberg Catechism represented the genuine cooperation of all these men, and it was not merely the work of Ursinus and Olevianus. However, the epiphany of 1562–1563, when Philippists, Zwinglians, and Calvinists all worked together, proved to be the exception for the Heidelberg Reformation. The cooper-

[67] I.e., Frederick III, Olevianus, and Ursinus.

ation of 1562–1563 represented the eye of the hurricane. The Reformed had vanquished their Gnesio-Lutheran rivals but had not yet discovered the issues that divided them from each other. The harmony would not be long lived.

PART II

CHURCH DISCIPLINE AND THE DESTRUCTION OF THE REFORMED CONSENSUS IN HEIDELBERG

CHAPTER FIVE

THE REFORMED CONFESSION IN STORM AND STRESS

> New Presbyter is but Old Priest writ large.
> John Milton

The period of cooperation that went into winning the elector to the Reformed faith and constructing a pluralistic Reformed confessional accord came to an end in the mid-1560s. At that point dissension over the proper form of church discipline split the Palatine church into hostile camps. The leading cleric Caspar Olevianus, with the backing of John Calvin and Theodore Beza in Geneva, steadfastly worked to erect a consistory on a Genevan model that would have independent power to excommunicate wayward believers. While the Palatine church had made great strides in establishing clear Reformed teaching, this group, which has been dubbed the "disciplinists,"[1] thought the fulfillment of the Reformation awaited the creation of a consistory with effective oversight over moral infractions. Many influential figures of the Palatine government, church, and intellectual community resisted this effort, and thus became an opposing "anti-disciplinist" party. Erastus would emerge as the champion of the anti-disciplinist, and thus anti-Calvinist, party and give his name to an alternative conception of church-state relations know as "Erastianism."

Erastus largely owes his enduring fame in the English-speaking world to the terms "Erastian" and "Erastianism." Although dictionaries often attempt to define the terms with reference to Erastus, it has been frequently observed that their popular usage has little connection to Erastus himself. While the *Oxford English Dictionary* recognizes two senses of the adjective "Erastian," I have discerned three uses of the term which naturally possess some overlap in meaning.[2] The most common sense of

[1] I.e., those who desired to establish a consistory of elders with independent authority to excommunicate recalcitrant sinners on roughly a Genevan model.

[2] *Oxford English Dictionary*, 2nd ed. s.v. "Erastian." The origin and early use of the term "Erastian" will also be engaged in the epilogue.

"Erastianism" connotes a general "ascendancy of the state over church in ecclesiastical matters,"[3] whose most common reference point is the Anglican Church in the era of Henry VIII. A second usage of the term connects directly to Erastus's program and emphasizes the notion that ecclesiastical authorities have no independent disciplinary role in a Christian commonwealth.[4] This connotation of "Erastian Erastianism" should be regarded as the most authentic use of the term, and while its usage was fairly common from the seventeenth into the nineteenth centuries, it might be considered somewhat archaic at present. The third usage of "Erastian" asserts the absolute right of the state to determine religious policy, regardless of the theological orthodoxy of the magistrate. This "Hobbesian" or "Statist Erastianism" goes well beyond Erastus's own thought. As we will see in the epilogue, this tendency likewise sprung from the context of Erastian debates of seventeenth century Europe.[5]

The focus of this section is not the history of Caesaropapism or an investigation of the contribution of Erastus's ideas to seventeenth-century English debates—though the later point will be engaged in the epilogue. This section aims to tell the story of the Heidelberg conflict regarding church discipline and reveal how Erastus's ideas crystallized during that conflict. The Heidelberg conflict focused on the question of who should police the moral lives of the faithful in a Christian state. Erastus sought to give a theoretical basis for a Reformed state church in which power over church discipline lay in the hands of the magistrate. While Erastus's arguments sought to do little more than justify the status quo, his Calvinist rivals saw his ideas as having radical and potentially "atheist" tendencies that would undermine all Christian discipline. The Heidelberg conflict, rather than being an isolated controversy, was only one of many clashes—though it may well have been the defining battle—within the Reformed communion on the question of proper church discipline and what role, if any, the Christian magistrate should have in its exercise.

---

[3] F.L. Cross, ed., *The Oxford Dictionary of the Christian Church*, 3rd ed. (Oxford: Oxford UP, 1997), 558.

[4] E.g., "The essence of Erastianism, or what had come to be called Erastianism, was that all power of discipline, ecclesiastical as well as civil, belongs ultimately to the State." David Masson, *The Life of John Milton* (London: 1871) 2:606.

[5] E.g., "Modern Erastianism develops an idea of Hobbes that political representatives even though they are non professing, may legislate upon religious matters." William B. Hunter, "Erastianism," in *A Milton Encyclopedia*, ed. idem, et al. (Lewisburg: Bucknell UP, 1978), 3:68.

The Palatine church discipline controversy was a bitter conflict among former allies who waged a cold war against one another until the advocates of the Genevan style of church discipline gained the upper hand. Nearly every move in the university, at court, or in the church became a proxy skirmish in the larger war over church discipline.

Further Consolidation of the Palatine Reformed Church

The process of establishing Reformed belief in the Palatinate continued with the acceptance of the Heidelberg Catechism at a territorial synod in January of 1563. Further work was to be done in shaping the Palatinate's ecclesiastical structures and liturgical practices. The revised formulary (*Agende*) for celebrating the Eucharist was first employed on October 24, 1563 while the Palatine court had fled to Mosbach to avoid the plague. The proclamation of a new church order (*Kirchenordnung*) on November 15, 1563 further consolidated the Reformed orientation of the Palatinate. Like the catechism, the church order of 1563 drew on multiple sources for its inspiration and, thus, is difficult to characterize as Lutheran, Calvinist, or Zwinglian.[6] Also like the catechism, the liturgical models it contained would have an enduring impact on the larger Reformed community.

Following the church order, the publication of the "Church Council Order" (*Kirchenratsordnung*) in July of 1564 regulated the administrative structure of the Palatine church and its disciplinary competence. This order addressed church discipline and mandated excommunication, though the manner of its administration—under the hands of the superintendents in a system of visitations under the authority of the church council (*Kirchenrat*)—was more in keeping with a territorial state church

[6] Printed in *EKO*, 14:333–408. Goeters discusses the background and sources of the church order in the same (pp. 43–47), emphasizing the free borrowing from Zurich and Genevan antecedents, with some influence of Upper German and Dutch refugee church models. Alternatively, Ernst Walter Zeeden had stressed the Calvinist elements of the document, though in the wake of Goeter's analysis his emphasis appears overstated. Zeeden, "Calvinistische Elemente in der Kurpfälzischen Kirchenordnung von 1563," in *Existenz und Ordnung* (Frankfurt: Klosterman, 1962), 183–214. See also Thompson, "The Palatinate Church Order of 1563," 339–354; Bruno Bürki, "The Reformed Tradition in Continental Europe: Switzerland, France and Germany," in *The Oxford History of Christian Worship*, ed. Geoffrey Wainwright and Karen B. Westerfield Tucker (Oxford: Oxford UP, 2006), 448–450.

than the Genevan consistory.[7] While the Heidelberg theologians and church councilors did a masterful job synthesizing theological motifs and creating works that genuinely represented Heidelberg, as opposed to being merely slavish imitations of foreign precedents, it was not possible to sweep all of the theological and structural differences away or even produce documents that were thoroughly consistent with one another. J.F. Gerhard Goeters noted the marked dissonance between the church council order on the one hand, which left the final say on the issue of excommunication to a fundamentally state-controlled body, and the catechism and church order on the other, with their mandates that discipline should be exercised by ecclesiastical authorities.[8] Furthermore, this legislation did not establish the consistorial-presbyterial structure of discipline desired by Calvinist members of the church council such as Christoph Ehem and Wenzel Zuleger—who apparently composed the directive themselves.[9]

Before proceeding, it is fitting to ponder why the Palatinate did not become fully Calvinist in 1563–1564 in terms of its ecclesiastical organization. First is the rather obvious point that erecting a system which would empower a largely clerically controlled body vis-à-vis the state was going against the grain of post-Reformation church-state relations in the setting of a territorial church, even if such an organization might offer some benefit to the state in acquiring another tool for social control. Second, the experience of the highhanded tactics of Tilemann Heshusius, including excommunicating his subordinates under his own authority as church superintendent, no doubt made it difficult for many to see unfettered consistorial discipline whose primary sanction was excommunication as an effective panacea for reform. In fact, Frederick's creation of the

[7] *EKO*, 14:48–50 (commentary); 409–424 (text). It should be noted that the terms "consistory" (*consistorium*) and "church council" (*Kirchenrat*) were by no means synonymous in the Palatine context as they sometimes were in other Reformed settings.

[8] *EKO*, 14:47. See the Heidelberg Catechism, questions 82–85. The German version of the Catechism was not definitive on this point, as it mandated that sinners were to be reported "der kirchen oder denen, so von der kirche darzu verordnet seind" (Q&A 85). Nevertheless, the clear expectation of the catechism is that excommunication is biblical and a matter pertaining to the church. Schaab also noted this contrast between the church order and the catechism and characterized the 1564 order as "more Erastian." Meinrad Schaab, "Obrigkeitlicher Calvinismus und Genfer Gemeindemodell: Die Kurpfalz als frühestes reformiertes Territorium im Reich und ihre Einwirkung auf Pfalz-Zweibrücken," in *Territorialstaat und Calvinismus* (Stuttgart: W. Kolhammer, 1993), 45. See also Paul Münch, *Zucht und Ordnung* (Stuttgart: Klett-Cotta, 1978), 102–104.

[9] *EKO*, 14:48–49.

church council, which was fundamentally an appendage of the elector's high council, can be seen in part as a move to bring potentially arbitrary clerical power under state control. Finally, Erastus remained influential in church affairs and was satisfied with the status quo, which inclined more to the Zurich model of church-state relations.

The enactments of 1563–1564 marked the consolidation of a moderate Reformed confession in the Palatinate. Here the more inclusive term "Reformed" is used intentionally to signify that the religious policy that prevailed was a combined Melanchthonian, Zwinglian, and Calvinist achievement, built upon a native, Upper German base. There were legitimately Calvinist elements in the Palatine Reformation; however, it is fair to label the Palatinate as "Calvinist" in 1563–1564 only if one intends it as a general synonym for "Reformed." This does not suggest that the Palatine Reformation did not possess Calvinist themes and that the leaders of the Palatine Reformation were not looking to Geneva, as well as Zurich, for inspiration. As we shall see in the following, it was only through the controversy over church discipline that the Palatine church took a distinctively "Calvinist" turn, and even those developments were subject to revision.

The Palatine Confession under Attack: The Maulbronn Colloquy

Opinions were sharply divided in the mid-1560s as to whether the Heidelberg Catechism deviated from the Augsburg Confession and thus violated the Peace of Augsburg (1555). Walter Hollweg has argued that most Reformed theologians could, and many did, subscribe to the Augsburg Confession. Reformed theologians from Jan Łaski to Calvin embraced the modified 1540 version of the confession, known as the *Variata*, with its much more open-ended language concerning the Lord's Supper.[10] The Heidelberg theologians argued that their new catechism stood in harmony with the Augsburg Confession. Ursinus used this argument in his defense of the Heidelberg Catechism, and the Augsburg Confession itself would be printed in the Palatinate as part of their self-representation that they had not broken the religious peace.[11] Thus, it was a legitimate

[10] Hollweg, *Der Augsburger Reichstag von 1566*, 83.

[11] [Zacharias Ursinus], *Gründtlicher bericht Vom heiligen Abendmal unsers Herren Jesu Christi/ aus einhelliger Lere/ der heiligen Schrifft/ der alten rechtglaubigen Christlichen kirchen/ und auch der Augspurgischen Confession.*

question of interpretation as to whether the Palatinate had manifestly transgressed the religious peace or whether they had merely pushed the envelope of the acceptable with their new catechism.

The leading Lutheran princes of southwestern Germany and their theologians understood the matter differently. Even before the publication of the catechism, Duke Christoph of Württemberg had warned Frederick in clear terms of the danger of his deviation to "Calvinism." With the publication of the catechism, Christoph's worst fears were realized. Although many sections of the catechism offended the southwestern German princes, they especially complained of its "Zwinglian and Calvinist" teaching of the Lord's Supper.[12] After the publication of the catechism, Christoph led a coalition against Frederick which included Margrave Karl II of Baden-Durlach and Count Palatine Wolfgang of Pfalz-Zweibrücken. They sought to exclude the Palatinate from the provisions of the Peace of Augsburg. If they were successful, Frederick could have come under the imperial ban and forfeited his territories, and the Palatinate would have been restored to Lutheranism or Catholicism. This was a serious and painful development, as these princes not only were the traditional allies of the Palatinate, but Frederick had family connections with each of them. Friends and family aside, however, they were also individuals who had much to gain if Frederick's territories should be liquidated. For example, Wolfgang had a personal score to settle related to his displeasure with the disposition of Ottheinrich's testament.[13] The princes' motivations were not merely egocentric, however, and there was something of a parallel religious zeal in Christoph's abhorrence of Zwinglianism and Frederick's politically inconvenient attraction to the Reformed faith. Not only were the Lutheran princes lining up against Frederick, but Maximilian II, who as King of the Romans was in line to succeed his father Ferdinand as emperor, agreed with the Lutherans that the new catechism violated the religious peace. Though Maximilian was a Catholic who was often rumored to possess evangelical tendencies—he thought the church should concede the cup to the laity and clerical marriage—he possessed little sympathy for "Sacramentarians" who denied that Christ was physically present in the Lord's Supper. In Maximilian's assessment, the catechism was Zwinglian in its sacramental teachings and thus in

[12] Count Palatine Wolfgang, Duke Christoph, and Margrave Karl to Elector Frederick, May 4, 1563, printed in Wolters, *Der heidelberger Katechismus in seiner ursprünglichen Gestalt*, 155–164.

[13] Press, *Calvinismus und Territorialstaat*, 236.

violation of the religious peace.[14] With the Lutheran princes conspiring against him and having no support at the imperial court, the situation looked bleak for Frederick and the Palatine Reformed movement.[15]

There was one major attempt at accommodation between the Palatinate and its chief theological opponents in Württemberg. During the reign of Duke Christoph (1550–1568), Württemberg had generally enjoyed a close relationship with the Palatinate. The new confession of the Palatinate undercut this traditional alliance. In an attempt to stem the regional tension between the Palatinate and its neighbors, Frederick and Christoph met in Hilsbach in February of 1564. There they agreed to stage a colloquy between their theologians on the grounds of the former Cistercian monastery of Maulbronn in northern Württemberg territory adjacent to Melanchthon's hometown of Bretten. As always, the chief issue of contention was the Lord's Supper. Unlike the Marburg Colloquy of 1529, however, which had chiefly centered on hermeneutical questions, at Maulbronn Christological questions touching on Christ's presence in the Eucharist took center stage.[16]

The princes and their representatives met in Maulbronn from April 10 to 15, 1564. According to the published accounts, two primary theologians represented each side. On the Palatine side, the protocol listed the court preacher Michael Diller and the superintendent Olevianus as the primary disputants; Johann Brenz and Jakob Andreae faced them. Both sides possessed a person who acted as the chair of the proceedings as well as a notary. Wilhelm Xylander (1532–1576), a former Tübingen student, served as the Palatine notary; Lucas Osiander for Württemberg.[17] In addition to those listed as the primary disputants, three additional

[14] Maximilian II to Frederick, April 25, 1563, printed in A. Wolters, *Der heidelberger Katechismus in seiner ursprünglichen Gestalt*, 153–155. Synopsis in Kluckhohn, *Briefe Friedrich des Frommen*, 1:398–399.

[15] Hollweg, *Der Augsburger Reichstag von 1566*, 41–45; Andreas Edel, *Der Kaiser und Kurpfalz: Eine Studie zu den Grundelementen politischen Handelns bei Maximilian II. (1564–1576)* [Schriftenreihe der Historischen Kommission bei der Bayerischen Akademie der Wissenschaften 58] (Göttingen: Vandenhoek & Ruprecht, 1995).

[16] *Protocoll Des Gesprächs zwischen den Pfältzischen und Würtenbergischen Theologen/ im Aprill des 1564. Jars zü Maulbrunn gehalten* (Tübingen, 1565); *Protocoll Das ist/ Acta oder Handlungen des Gesprechs zwischen den Pfältzischen und Wirtembergischen Theologen/ von der Ubiquitet oder Allenthalbenheit des Leibs Christi* ... (Heidelberg: Johann Mayer, 1565); Robert Kolb, "Maulbronn Colloquy," OER, 3:34–35; Visser, *Zacharias Ursinus*, 135–139; Bizer, *Studien zur Geschichte des Abendmahls Streits*, 335–351; Henss, *Der Heidelberger Katechismus*, 48–50; Goeters, "Olevianus als Theologe," 311–312.

[17] *Protocoll Des Gesprächs zwischen den Pfältzischen und Würtenbergischen Theologen*, [305].

Palatine theologians took part, including court preacher Petrus Dathenus and theology professors Boquin and Ursinus.[18] Erastus was present at the debate, though the published protocols do not mention his participation.[19] Perhaps Erastus's doubts as to the wisdom of holding such a debate might have been a factor in his non-participation.[20] It seems more likely, however, that some sense of disciplinary competencies had been restored in Heidelberg. Unlike the Heidelberg Disputation on the Lord's Supper in 1560, at this point the Palatinate possessed enough theological talent to hold their most conspicuous lay-theologian in reserve.

The Württemberg side brought along reinforcements as well, including Balthasar Bidenbach (Bidembach), Dietrich Schnepf and Valentin Vannius (Wannenmacher); however, their participation was negligible. Though Brenz took part in the discussions, Andreae dominated the debate for the Württemberg side. Historians judge both Brenz and Andreae among the most influential Lutheran theologians of the sixteenth century, though by this point Brenz, who had attended Luther's famous disputation at Heidelberg in 1518 and had taken part in the Marburg Colloquy, was clearly reaching the twilight of his career. Erastus was singularly unkind in his assessment of the elderly statesman of south German Lutheranism: "The man Brenz is backward and stupid and is seen to be led around by the advice of Andreae in all things."[21] The fact that Brenz had been a harsh critic of Bullinger perhaps explains why Erastus felt free to unleash such an intemperate remark against this hero of the south German Reformation. Alternatively, Andreae was at the peak of his powers. Andreae, who would be remembered primarily as one of the co-drafters of the *Formula of Concord*, was in many senses Brenz's spiritual successor. Although he had been conciliatory toward Calvin and the Genevan theologians as a younger man, by the time of the Maulbronn Colloquy, Andreae had absorbed Brenz's strict Lutheran teaching on the Lord's Supper that basically precluded any rapprochement with the Reformed.

[18] Kolb's fine article is mistaken in its description of the Heidelberg participants. Neither Dathenus nor Olevianus were members of the university faculty in 1564. Olevianus had briefly held the third chair of theology in 1561–1562. Kolb, "Maulbronn Colloquy," *OER*, 3:34–35.

[19] Erastus is listed along with Ehem among the "Politici" in attendance. [Johannes Brenz], *Warhafftiger, vnd Gründtlicher Bericht, Von dem Gesprech zwischen deß Churfürsten Pfaltzgraffen, vnd deß Hertzogen zu Wirtemberg Theologe, von deß Herrn Nachtmal zu Maulbronn gehalten* (Frankfurt: Peter Brubach, 1564).

[20] Wesel-Roth, *Thomas Erastus*, 36.

[21] Erastus to Bullinger, April 20, [1564], StAZ, E II 345, fol. 731: "Brentius homo est rusticus, stupidus, et qui videatur Iac. Andreae consilio omnia agere."

Erastus's assessment of their relationship was somewhat off target, since Andreae had imbibed far more from Brenz than vice versa. As much as the Palatine side resented Andreae's attacks on their theology, one has the sense that they would have liked to have possessed a theologian with his ferocious tenacity in their camp. Although Ursinus may have been more than his equal with the pen, he did not relish the disputation as did Andreae.

For five days the two sides engaged in an instructive if ultimately fruitless exchange of views. From the start, they debated the doctrine of the ubiquity of Christ's human nature.[22] Brenz had been one of the chief proponents of this doctrine, which held that wherever Christ's divine nature was present his human nature must also be present, because of the eternal quality of the union of Christ's two natures in one person. This formulation was needed to explain how the resurrected Christ, seated at the right hand of God, could be physically present in the Eucharist. Although this doctrine was to become standard Lutheran orthodoxy as enshrined in the *Formula of Concord*, at mid-century many Philippist Lutherans rejected it. The Reformed likewise unanimously rejected what they considered an unbiblical and overly sophistic doctrine. Alternatively, the Reformed held to the notion that the resurrected Christ was seated literally at the right hand of God; i.e., the resurrected body of Christ was located in a specific place in heaven. Since Christ's human nature was genuinely human, like other humans it was finite, thereby excluding the possibility of Christ's physical presence in the elements. The Palatine theologians also maintained that Christians received all the benefits of the Lord's Supper through faith and rejected the notion of *manducatio infidelium*, the eating by those without faith, against the Württemberg theologians who maintained that Christ's presence in the Eucharist did not depend on the faith of the participant. Most of the arguments put forward at the colloquy were battle-tested by this point. Perhaps the greatest novelty of the colloquy were some of the unusual syllogisms employed by the participants. Since both sides had already staked out their opinions on this topic, the chances of confessional reconciliation were slim.

The colloquy resulted in the further entrenchment of the two antagonistic camps. The debate broke little new ground but defined the impasse that existed between the Gnesio-Lutherans and the Reformed in the Holy

[22] It should be noted that the Lutherans did not favor the term "ubiquity." They preferred to speak of a full and real understanding of the communication of attributes (*communicatio idiomatum*) between Christ's divine and human natures.

Roman Empire and, in focusing on the question of ubiquity, set the stage for the coming decades of confessional conflict. Although the princes had agreed that reports from the colloquy would not be printed, rumors of victory or defeat as well as epistolary reports of the debate circulated, which supplied the impetus for the Württemberg camp to break the non-publication pledge first.[23] The Palatine theologians, who had been preparing their version of events before the Württemberg account was in print, soon responded. Erastus opposed the colloquy, and its failure to reach a positive understanding with the Lutherans did not surprise him. Yet the colloquy had a positive impact on Palatine morale that he had not anticipated. In his analysis of the colloquy, the Palatine side and Ursinus in particular had acquitted themselves well. Erastus was also quite impressed by the fortitude that the elector displayed in the colloquy and thought that the colloquy had buoyed his Reformed convictions. Perhaps the most dramatic moment of the colloquy had come when the Elector Frederick interrupted Andreae's long, Luther-dependent monologue with the assertion "Luther was no apostle; [he] too could err."[24] The colloquy also represented something of a coming of age for Olevianus. Some quirky syllogisms aside, he held his own under difficult circumstances in the debates.[25] The fact that Erastus could not spare a kind word for Olevianus's performance might suggest that some friction had developed between the two. Erastus's correspondence from the summer and fall of 1564 reveals that he was involved in assembling a compendium of the colloquy himself, though no one has yet identified which of the published accounts of the colloquy should be credited to him or even if his compendium was ever published.[26]

[23] Wesel-Roth, *Thomas Erastus*, 37. Brenz's *Warhafftiger, vnd Gründtlicher Bericht* from 1564 (above note 19) was the first published account of the colloquy.

[24] *Protocoll Das ist/ Acta oder Handlungen des Gesprechs* (Heidelberg, 1565), 101: "Luther ist kein Apostel gewesen/ hat auch irren können." See also Benrath, "Die Korrespondenz zwischen Bullinger und Thomas Erastus," 100.

[25] Here Olevianus employed the syllogism "The Ocean circles the globe. Antwerp lies on the ocean, thus Antwerp circles the world" as a characterization of Andreae's position. It is not surprising that the superior dialectician Erastus would have frowned on Olevianus's performance. Visser, *Zacharias Ursinus*, 138.

[26] Erastus to Bullinger, August 25, [1564], StAZ, E II 361, fol. 81: "Disputationis Maulbrun. compendium heri, excepta praefationem, quae ad te dirigetur (Statui enim, si per principem licebit excudi curare, ita tamen, ac si me inscio factum fuisset, de qua re aliàs) perfeci benè tarde. Totam hanc septimanam in id operis consumpsi, rebus ordinariis perfectis. Ubi descriptum fuerit exemplum, ad te statim mittam. Puto te inventurum esse, quae sint placitura, habita circumstantiarum r[ation]e. Ursinus noster omni

In late 1564 Erastus resigned his position on the church council to devote more time to his medical profession and his academic career. Judging his work in the Palatine Reformation to be complete, he nevertheless volunteered to advise the council on important decisions. In fact, he does not seem to have left the council until late 1565 and continued to advise the prince on religious affairs at least into 1567.[27] Perhaps equally important to the later religious developments of the Palatinate, Frederick promoted Erastus's friend Stephan Cirler from his position as secretary of the church council to private secretary (*Kammersekretär*). Erastus expressed great pleasure with the development, as it placed his supporter in close proximity to the elector.[28] With Cirler's promotion, however, Erastus also lost an ally on the church council. This restructuring of the Palatine bureaucracy signaled a changing of the guard in terms of influence on religious affairs. Most of the senior officials who had

meruit laudem." Erastus to Bullinger, Oct. 13, [1564], StAZ, E II 361, fol. 68: "Nunquam ab initio huius causae peiore loco res nostrae fuerunt quam sunt hodie propter aeditum scriptum Wirtenberg[icorum] Theolog[orum]. Numquam etiam meliore fuerunt. Dementarunt quidem mendaciss[imo] scripto o[mn]i[u]m a[n]i[m]os. At rem ad summum pertraxerunt, unde necesse sit vel nos vel illos cadere. Non iam de causa loquor, quam scire nobis D[omi]n[u]s defendet pro suo sancta voluntate. Sed aut nos aut illi pro Nebulonibus porrò habebimur. Spero imò certo scio, si d[omi]n[u]s nostris concesserit vitam et facultatem perficiendi quod coeperunt, mundum cogniturum esse et nostram innocentiam, et adversariorum effusam et incredibilem impudentiam. Tibi dico soli haec. Edetur protocollum diligenter. Attexetur eorum extractum ut vocant, cum nostrarum ad singulas partes [r]esponsione uberiore, et ubique tamen remittetur lector ad protocolli lectionem citato semper folio [verso] et loco, ut petulantiss[ima] eorum mendacia cunctimet ipsi videant imò palpent. Res acta germanicè est. Ego compendium feci latinum, et verba utriusque partis servavi. Videbis interea vel ex hoc compendio hominum illorum probitatem."

If Erastus's labors went into any of the published versions, the following would seem to be the most likely candidate: *Protocollum, hoc est, Acta colloquii inter Palatinos et Vvirtebergicos theologos, de Ubiquitate sive Omnipraesenta corporis Christi, Et de sensu verborum Christi, Hoc est corpus meum, &c. Anno M.D.LXVIII. Mulbrunnae habiti. Item Vvirtembergicorum Theologorum de hoc ipso Colloquio eodem anno edita Epitome. Cui addita est Palatinorum Theologorum vera et constans Responsio, … a quodam Theologiae studiose Latinè reddita* (Heidelberg, 1566). Cf. the VD 16 entries B 7854 and B 7855.

[27] Wesel-Roth, *Thomas Erastus*, 48; Press, *Calvinismus und Territorialstaat*, 243; Erastus to Bullinger, July 29, [1564], StAZ, E II 361, fol. 66: "Princeps Senatum Ecclesiasticum redintegravit, et D. Willingum et duos alios cooptavit. Mihi dimissionem propter infinita negocia, ita dedit, ut non nisi in gravioribus[us] causis vocer." A letter to Bullinger from Jan. 1, 1566 names Johannes Junius as Erastus's successor, but does not give precise information regarding when Erastus actually left the council. StAZ, E II 361, fol. 10.

[28] Benrath, "Die Korrespondenz zwischen Bullinger und Thomas Erastus," 102; Press, *Calvinismus und Territorialstaat*, 240.

connections with the earlier tradition of Upper German Protestantism died in the early 1560s.[29] Olevianus and Zuleger—two ardent advocates of the Genevan theology and church discipline—ascended to new heights of influence in religious affairs.[30] The influx of Dutch and Walloon refugees also began to add weight to a thoroughgoing Calvinist vision of church reform in the Palatinate.

Iconoclasm in the Palatinate

Another factor which signaled a change in the religious policy of the Palatinate was the state-mandated iconoclasm, which began in the late summer 1564 and continued into 1565. Iconoclasm was not in itself new to the Palatinate. While Lutherans are conventionally viewed as being more tolerant of images than the iconoclastic Reformed, many of the neighboring Lutheran territories such as Württemberg, Baden-Durlach, and Pfalz-Zweibrücken—Frederick's current persecutors regarding the catechism—had taken steps similar to Ottheinrich's efforts to eliminate images. Thus, Frederick's iconoclasm hardly signaled the arrival of "Calvinism" in itself. What was problematic about the iconoclasm of 1565 was that Frederick embarked on this new campaign in territories where his legal right to do so was at best contested.[31] Frederick's religious enthusiasm, and that of his advisors, emboldened him to act in an impolitic fashion. Frederick felt obliged to act in every location where he possessed patronage rights and in every common lordship. He personally took part in the iconoclasm, not merely by attending, but by destroying images with his own hands. The advisors who seem to have been the chief supporters of the iconoclasm were Olevianus, Zuleger, and Diller.

In early May 1565, Frederick and seventy knights arrived at the abbey of Neuhausen near Worms. Upon Frederick's arrival, the abbey's *scholasticus* Johann Deubinger implored the elector to respect their traditional rights and liberties. Frederick answered that as their "patron and protector" (*Schirm und Schutzherr*), he had come to put an end to the idolatry. He justified the action against the monastery not only on the basis of end-

[29] Press, *Calvinismus und Territorialstaat*, 233–234.

[30] Press, *Calvinismus und Territorialstaat*, 242. Both Olevianus and Zuleger, who had been on the church council since 1562, had studied in Geneva.

[31] Rott, "Kirchen- und Bildersturm," 243. Most of Frederick's actions were in areas of joint jurisdiction with the bishops of Speyer, Worms, or the Margrave of Baden.

ing the transgression of the second commandment,[32] but also because of the dissolute lives of the monks who lived in concubinage and mismanaged the affairs of their foundation. Before removing the images, Frederick forced the monks to join him and his partisans for a meal, which degenerated into a row over the meaning of the Lord's Supper. Olevianus reportedly took a piece of consecrated communion wafer and asked the monks if Christ's body was to be found inside of it. When they answered his question in the affirmative, he took the host and crushed it before their eyes, declaring that "it was only a bread-god, or rather an enchanted anti-God."[33] The meal served as the prelude to the main event. First Frederick and his men entered the church and broke open the tabernacle and confiscated the hosts. Next he brought in eighty peasants with their tools to break up the idolatrous images in the church. The following day they destroyed the altar, crucifix, and organ. The entire affair concluded with a great bonfire, in which Olevianus and Zuleger allegedly took part.[34]

Still attached to the church council, Erastus was certainly informed of these actions. As a committed Reformed Christian who abhorred "idolatry" and anything smacking of "superstition," Erastus's sympathies likely were with the iconoclasts. Erastus informed Bullinger of the iconoclasm, however, in a fashion that suggested that he approved of the elector's goals but questioned his tactics. He noted that Frederick destroyed the images in a church in Ladenburg that was under the joint lordship of the elector and the bishop of Worms. He also mentioned that rumors were afoot regarding the monasteries on Frederick's list that housed imperial knights. After listing these dubious actions without much commentary, Erastus summed up his narrative: "I hear indeed that [Frederick] does a noble thing but not in a noble fashion due to certain men who neither want nor have learned how to pursue a good cause well. *These you have known well enough*."[35] Here Erastus's censure was subtle and more implicit than explicit. Olevianus and Zuleger would seem to be the obvious targets of his critique. This was one of the first signs that Erastus had begun to question his Calvinist colleagues.

---

[32] I.e., the Second Commandment according to the numeration of the Heidelberg Catechism.

[33] Rott, "Kirchen- und Bildersturm," 249: "Es sei nur ein brodtgott, ja ein bezauberter nichtiger gott."

[34] Rott, "Kirchen- und Bildersturm," 248–252.

[35] Erastus to Bullinger, April 25, [1565], StAZ, E II 361, fol. 40: "Audio quidem fieri rem optimam non optimè, propter certos homines, qui causam bonam benè agere neque volunt neque didicerunt. Eos tu satis novisti."

The Diet of Augsburg (1566) and Its Aftermath

That Frederick would dare to make such legally questionable moves at a time when the very legal standing of his confession in the empire was in doubt offers an additional testimony to the passion of his convictions. Since the iconoclasm would lead to protracted legal claims against Frederick in the imperial court, it certainly did not help his image in the empire. Not all of Frederick's actions prior to the Diet of Augsburg in 1566 were so heedless of public opinion. To gain recognition of the catholicity and orthodoxy of the Reformed position, Frederick's advisors launched a plan to solicit confessions from Reformed churches from around Europe. This was part of the larger Palatine desire to have Protestantism defined on an international, as opposed to an imperial, level. The long-term goal of this policy was to hold an international evangelical council that would have accented the strength of the Reformed throughout western and central Europe, unlike their isolated position in the Holy Roman Empire. A preliminary step in this direction was the request for confessions from the principal Reformed churches. The personal confession that Bullinger modified to satisfy the Palatine request took on a much more important life of its own, as it was recognized by the majority of the Protestant Swiss cantons and became known as the *Second Helvetic Confession*. Although Frederick's request had spurred this Zurich-led effort to promote confessional accord, the *Second Helvetic Confession* was not officially endorsed by the Palatinate, though the elector expressed warm personal gratitude to Bullinger for his efforts. In the event, the *Second Helvetic Confession* did not play a large role at the Diet of Augsburg.[36]

The imperial diet of 1566, which was the first since the publication of the Heidelberg Catechism and church order in 1563, proved to be a turning point in the history of Reformed Protestantism in the Empire. Maximilian II, now Holy Roman Emperor (r. 1564–1576), conspired with the leading southwestern German princes to exclude Frederick III from the religious peace. Not only were the evangelical estates alarmed by the perceived deviation from the faith of Luther, the resurgent Catholic Church, represented by shrewd and resolute figures such as the Jesuit Peter Canisius, also viewed the advance of "Calvinism" into the empire as a threat.[37]

---

[36] Hollweg, *Der Augsburger Reichstag von 1566*, 163–176; Benrath, "Die Korrespondenz zwischen Bullinger und Thomas Erastus," 108–109; Goeters, "Die Rolle der Confessio Helvetica Posterior in Deutschland," 80–98.

[37] Hollweg, *Der Augsburger Reichstag von 1566*, 2–3.

That the Palatinate's Reformed confession survived the imperial diet was largely due to the political matrix that existed in the 1560s. The plans of the emperor failed because of the resistance of the most powerful Lutheran prince, Elector August of Saxony. August was motivated not by sympathy but by a desire to avoid chaos and protect his own interests since he felt insecure in his hold on the electoral dignity, stolen not that long ago by his brother Moritz from the Ernestine branch of the Wettin dynasty. Like his more famous brother, he refused to subordinate political decisions to confessional interests. The fact that a Melanchthonian brand of Lutheranism was still ascendant in Saxony also aided the Palatine cause. Philip of Hesse likewise was more interested in confessional unity than in persecuting Frederick, whose personal piety he genuinely appreciated. A decade later the situation would look quite different. By then Philip of Hesse was dead, and August had sacked his Melanchthonian advisers.[38] The Palatine success in surviving the diet was in part dependent on the timing of the confessional change. Credit must also be given to elector himself, however, for his courageous stand at the diet and his insistence on maintaining the Augsburg agreement in good conscience. His cunning also contributed to the Palatine success; for example, he claimed his opinions were merely biblical and maintained that he had not read a single word of Calvin.[39]

After surviving the imperial diet of 1566, the Reformed movement possessed a free hand to continue its work of renewing the Palatine church. Their position, immensely strengthened since the failure of the estates to bring a judgment against the Palatinate, meant, as Press argued, an implicit recognition of the legality of their actions.[40] The agreement between the leading south German Protestant princes in May of 1567 to refrain from further polemics regarding the Lord's Supper also enhanced the position of the Palatinate.[41] Thus, some eighty years before the Peace of Westphalia made it explicit, the Palatinate succeeded in wedging the door open for the Reformed faith in the empire.

[38] Press, *Calvinismus und Territorialstaat*, 236–238.

[39] Alting, *Historia de ecclesiis Palatinis*, 93–99 (chs. 51–53); Press, *Calvinismus und Territorialstaat*, 229.

[40] Press, *Calvinismus und Territorialstaat*, 237.

[41] Kluckhohn, *Briefe Friedrich des Frommen*, 2(1):49–50, 94. The participants were Baden, Hesse, Württemberg, and the Palatinate.

The International Scene

The decade of the 1560s would prove to be something of a hinge in the history of Reformed Christianity. There had been some very encouraging developments prior to 1566. Not only had a de facto recognition been achieved in the empire, but England was back under a Protestant sovereign who welcomed home exiles from Geneva and Zurich, whose return gave birth to the Puritan movement during Elizabeth's reign. Affairs were even more promising in France and the Netherlands. The 1560s were the high water mark for the wild growth of Huguenot congregations in France. Likewise, the Reformed faith found many adherents in the Netherlands, especially in southern provinces like Flanders. The fate of the Reformation in France and, in particular, the Netherlands exercised a decisive influence on the developments in the Palatinate. The fact that these "churches under the cross" much more naturally inclined to the Genevan model of church organization would put pressure on the Palatine church leaders to organize their church along the lines of what was coming to be seen as the "universal" and "biblical" form from the vantage of La Rochelle, Nîmes, or Emden. What would ultimately prove crucial to tying religious developments in France and the Netherlands closely to the Palatinate was the presence of large exile communities in the Palatinate. These communities exercised an enormous influence on the ecclesiastical and cultural life of the Palatinate and in turn served as avenues for the dissemination of lessons learned in the Palatinate back to their home communities.

As the decade advanced, however, the situation for Reformed Protestantism worsened considerably. The French Wars of Religion commenced in 1562, and forces from the Palatinate would intervene militarily on behalf of the Huguenots in 1568 and again in 1576 under the leadership of the gallant Count Palatine Johann Casimir, a younger son of Elector Frederick. Religious tensions increased in the Netherlands following the iconoclasm of the Wonderyear (spring 1566 to spring 1567) and the subsequent installation of the Alba regime to quash the rabble rousers. Civil war would follow, lasting for decades. From this juncture German mercenaries would be as influential as Genevan missionaries in insuring the viability of the Reformed faith in western Europe. Ironically, it would be precisely in these years, when the survival of Reformed Christianity was under threat, that the Heidelberg Reformed community would fall out so bitterly with one another over the question of church discipline.

Not surprisingly, as a chief contact for the Swiss churches in the empire, Erastus's letters are full of news and rumors of the latest events in the Netherlands and France. Erastus celebrates the victories and laments the defeats of the Protestant forces in these countries as if each tide of battle were advancing or undermining God's kingdom on earth. In time, however, Erastus soured on the adventurism and hawkishness of his coreligionists, and began to ascribe more worldly motivations to the political champions of Protestantism. His friend Ursinus more vociferously decried the foolhardiness of those political agents in Heidelberg who supported intervention in France and the Netherlands.[42] After Erastus had become embittered against Palatine court preachers of French and Dutch origin, he also became suspicious of the motivations of their military champions. Later, Erastus began to question whether there could really be any scriptural justification for subjects to take up arms against their divinely sanctioned princes.[43]

Amberg and Erastus's Alienation from Olevianus

After having successfully weathered the imperial diet and the machinations of the Lutheran princes, the Palatinate's immediate diplomatic difficulties were relieved. In the fall of 1566, Frederick renewed his campaign to implement the new Palatine religious policy on the Upper Palatinate. Though constitutionally part of the elector's inalienable territory, the Upper Palatinate was geographically separate from the Lower Palatinate and enjoyed a tradition of autonomous administration. Lutheranism had put down firmer roots in the Upper Palatinate, and the fact that the validity of the Heidelberg Catechism in imperial law was still contested no doubt emboldened the populace to cling to their Lutheran convictions. Since the governor of the province, Frederick's eldest son, the future Ludwig VI, remained a Lutheran, Frederick faced an awkward problem in implementing his religious policy in the Upper Palatinate. Because he feared that the emperor would back his Upper Palatine subjects in the event of an all-out confessional struggle, Frederick was forced to use more subtle methods to accomplish his will. In

[42] Visser, *Zacharias Ursinus*, 147–170. See below.

[43] Letters of Erastus to Bullinger from Sept. 24, [1572], StAZ, E II 361, fols. 32–32[a] and Sept. 7, [1572], StAZ, E II 361, fol. 80. See Benrath, "Die Korrespondenz zwischen Bullinger und Thomas Erastus," 128–129.

an effort to bring the leading pastors into the Reformed camp, Frederick personally visited the territory with his leading councilors in late 1566.[44]

It was a sign of Erastus's continuing engagement in religious affairs that he traveled with the prince, councilors, and theologians to Amberg and remained there from late October into December, 1566.[45] Against the advice of Erastus and other councilors, it was decided to hold a disputation. Olevianus represented the Reformed party in the debate, and from the beginning, he fared poorly. Erastus ventured that Olevianus's Lutheran opponent was a good measure cleverer. Erastus would have intervened in the debate, but he knew that in doing so he would necessarily attack Olevianus's position as well. Since he did not want to strengthen the Lutherans' cause by creating the appearance of strife within the Heidelberg camp, he refrained. The Upper Palatine Lutherans apparently took heart from the exchange and later asked Frederick if the disputation could be continued. When they rejoined the disputation, which Erastus again thought a bad idea, Frederick asked Ursinus to take Olevianus's place. Erastus noted, "The prince had seen that Olevianus was losing the struggle, and in the meantime he had called Ursinus. But he did not want to join the colloquy since he anticipated that it would bear little fruit, having resolved that it would not be possible to correct what the other [Olevianus] had already spoiled."[46] While the episode is doubtless an indication of Ursinus's reserve and his weariness of unproductive confrontations, his refusal to come to Olevianus's aid also suggests that he was not as personally close to Olevianus as the traditional hagiography, which has generally cast them as enthusiastic collaborators, has assumed.[47]

After Ursinus declined the invitation, Olevianus returned to the debate. He eventually arranged an agreement with the preachers of the Upper Palatinate on the basis of these three statements:

> Every promise of grace is received through grace alone.
> All that is promised to us in the Lord's Supper, with the exception of external signs, is and belongs to the promise or the word of grace.

[44] Press, "Die Grundlagen der kurpfälzischen Herrschaft in der Oberpfalz," 43–47; Kluckhohn, *Friedrich der Fromme*, 261–285; Goeters, "Olevianus als Theologe," 313.

[45] Benrath, "Die Korrespondenz zwischen Bullinger und Thomas Erastus," 110.

[46] Erastus to Bullinger, March 28, [1567], StAZ, E II 361, fols. 67–67[a]: "Viderat Princeps Olevianum causam perdere, atque interea vocaverat Ursinum. At is congredi noluit, quod sine fructa futurum videret, neque corrigere se posse cerneret quae alter corrupisset."

[47] Visser, *Zacharias Ursinus*, 145–146.

> Therefore, what is received in the Lord's Supper, without and beyond the external signs, can only be consumed and received through faith.[48]

Erastus was in no sense satisfied with these results, as his comments revealed: "These [propositions] are seen to be consistent with oral eating and corporeal presence."[49] In other words, the Upper Palatine pastors could freely hold a Lutheran view of the Lord's Supper. For all intents and purposes the elector's attempt to introduce the Reformed confession in the Upper Palatinate had gone shipwreck. The only additional moves he dared to make were to replace a handful of the most militant pastors and to found a new Latin school in the hope of winning the next generation. Lutheranism would survive for decades in the Upper Palatinate.[50]

Beyond the failure of the elector's religious policy, the episode revealed the developing strains among the Palatine Reformed. Erastus offered a bitter assessment of Olevianus, labeling him "a weak-hearted youth" who possessed no facility in the art of disputation.[51] From this point forward, it becomes hard to assess whether the rift between Erastus and Olevianus centered more on personality or theology. The beginning of the fissure was likely theological. From early in his stay in Heidelberg, Olevianus had not hidden his desire to implement the Genevan program of church discipline.[52] Olevianus's formative Protestant experience had been in the underground Huguenot congregation in Bourges, and he desired to put into practice the self-regulating form of church discipline that he experienced there. Early in his tenure at Heidelberg he had been given explicit instructions from the master himself on implementing discipline in the Palatinate. Calvin had recommended that the prince "nominate two of his councilors, two from the university, and four from the city council, who will meet together with the pastors of the church, and they are to be the censors of morals." Calvin's words proved prophetic in a dual sense. First, his suggestions had some impact on the form of the consistory as it took shape nearly a decade later. Second, Calvin had frankly

[48] Erastus to Bullinger, March 28, [1567], StAZ, E II 361, fols. 67–67ª: "Alle verheissung der Gnaden wird allein durch den glauben empfangen. Alles so uns in Nachtmal verheissen wird, ausgenommen die eusserlichen Zeichen/ ist und gehört zur verheissung oder zum wort der gnaden Ergo. Was ihm nachtmal ohne und uber die eusserlichen zeichen empgangen wird/ kan allein durch glauben genossen und empfangen werden."

[49] Erastus to Bullinger, March 28, [1567], StAZ, E II 361, fols. 67–67ª: "Videbant hinc cadere oralem manducationem, corporalem praesentiam."

[50] Press, "Die Grundlagen der kurpfälzischen Herrschaft in der Oberpfalz," 46–47.

[51] Erastus to Bullinger, March 28, [1567], StAZ, E II 361, fols. 67–67ª.

[52] Wesel-Roth, *Thomas Erastus*, 45.

acknowledged that erecting such a system was difficult, perhaps even odious, in a state ruled by a prince.[53] Alternatively, Erastus favored the Swiss-German model of discipline, which left the oversight of morals in the hands of the state. In the eyes of the Swiss-Germans, the intervention of the state in ecclesiastical affairs had been the salvation rather than the perversion of true religion. Thus, Olevianus and Erastus had different conceptions of church discipline that not only were rooted in the theological matrices of their respective traditions, but whose authenticity had been confirmed in their own life histories. Erastus had come of age in the Swiss-German Reformed church, which left control of morals in the hands of the magistrate, and the tolerant humanist atmosphere of Basel. He compared this experience most favorably against his Italian sojourn, where the oppressive specter of the Holy Office menaced. Alternatively, having grown up in Catholic Trier, Olevianus's formative experience in dynamic Protestantism had been in an underground, self-disciplining Reformed congregation in France, and his attempt to institute the Genevan model of church discipline was in part an attempt to reproduce that experience in a German state church that seemed only partially reformed in his eyes.[54] Inevitably such divergent visions of the future course of the Palatine church led to conflict. Erastus's acerbic and condescending attitude, coupled with Olevianus's obsessive zeal (and that is how even his friends saw it) made a volatile mix.[55] As much of an intractable foe as Olevianus would later prove himself to be, Erastus may well have provoked the antagonism. Over time Erastus squandered the good will that he once possessed with Olevianus. Even during their years

[53] Calvin to Olevianus, Oct. 27, 1562, *CO*, 19: 563–565 (no. 3869): "Quod de constituendae disciplinae ratione consilium meum postulas, vix occurrit quod respondeam, nisi optandum esse ut duos Princeps de consilii sui sententia nominet, duos universitas, quatuor autem commune urbis, qui una cum Pastoribus Ecclesiae praesint, ac sint morum censores. Hoc enim modo partes quae alioqui suis ordinibus distinctae sunt, coalescerent in unum corpus, Ecclesia jus suum retineret; nullus autem gravaretur. Modis quidem omnibus instandum est, ut est mediocrem saltem disciplinam obtineat.

Difficilis labor et molestus, fateor, addo etiam odiosus, sed ubi Christum habes ducem, non est quod unquam fatigeris. Si tibi cum Juris consultis certandum est, scias hoc hominum genus ubique fere esse Christi servis adversum: quia non existimant se gradum suum posse tueri, si quae vigeat Ecclesiae authoritas. Constanter tamen pergendum, quod eo facilius erit, quia adiutores nactus es non fidos modo, sed etiam animosos et strenuos."

[54] Goeters, "Olevianus als Theologe," 293.

[55] See Friedrich Rudolf, "Die Kirche in Heidelberg nach den letzen Briefen Bullinger-Beza," *Zwingliana* 8 (1944), 95–107, especially p. 103. For his detractors' less charitable assessments, see Hollweg, *Heinrich Bullingers Hausbuch*, 276–277, idem, *Neue Untersuchungen*, 1;140–141, 151–152. See also chapter 6.

of the close cooperation, ca. 1560–1564, Erastus never singled out Olevianus for praise. In fact, Erastus later took some of the blame for the breakdown of the relationship on himself, stating, "The hatred that Olevianus has for me stems from this, that first at Maulbronn and later at Amberg, I reproached him sharply in the midst of the debate."[56] Events would prove that Erastus should not have underestimated Olevianus's ability or his resolve in pursuing his vision of a true church.

Erastus's Dialogue with Jakob Schegk

In the years following the Maulbronn colloquy, Erastus engaged in a curious if little studied exchange with the Tübingen philosopher and medical professor Jakob Schegk (1511–1587). Erastus may well have first met Schegk behind the scenes of the colloquy itself. Another avenue of contact for Erastus with Schegk was Erastus's close friendship with Schegk's former pupil Xylander. The literary exchange began when the duke of Württemberg asked Schegk to offer a response to a philosophically-based assault on the Württemberg Eucharistic theology by Theodore Beza.[57] Erastus perceived that Schegk's analysis of the philosophical concepts underlying the Christological controversy opened a door for a possible rapprochement between the Reformed and Lutherans. Erastus had his anonymous approach to Schegk printed with Beza's assistance in Geneva, with a preface by the philosopher Simone Simoni.[58] Erastus's basic thrust was to argue that if one could clarify the terms of the debate between the Heidelberg and Württemberg theologians, they really disagreed very little about the central meaning of the Eucharist. While Wesel-Roth has argued that Erastus's claims were so dramatic here that she even questioned whether Erastus himself thought these ideas might be constructively engaged in Württemberg, a contemporaneous letter to Albert Hardenberg suggests that Erastus genuinely felt that the long running impasse over the Lord's Supper might be resolved through this

[56] Erastus to Grynaeus, Jan. 27, (15)76, Basel UB, G II 4, fol. 195: "Odium Oleviani erga me originem inde habuit, quod eum Maulbrunnae primum, deinde Ambergae res turbantem acriter reprehendi."

[57] Jakob Schegk, *De una persona, & duabus Naturis Christi, Sententia Iacobi Schegkij* ... (Frankfurt: Peter Braubach, 1565).

[58] [Thomas Erastus], *Declaratio eorum, quae in libello D.D. Iacobi Scheckij, summi & clarissimi Philosophi, De una Persona & duabus Naturis Christi nunnullis obscuriora, et Ubiquitati corporis Christi patrocinari sunt visa* (Geneva: Jean Crespin, 1566).

interchange with Schegk.[59] After a further clarification by Schegk, Erastus continued the dialogue with a book whose subtitle reveals its object: *In which Next It is Demonstrated from the Beginning, that the Heidelberg and Württemberg Theologians Do Not Disagree Greatly in the Disputation concerning the Presence of the Body of Christ in All Places* [i.e., ubiquity], *and Also in the Same Lord's Supper*.[60] In this text Erastus promoted a high view of sacramental efficacy while also maintaining his aversion to corporeal presence in the Eucharist. Though Schegk pursued the dispute further with Simoni, he only offered a brief response to Erastus to ensure his readers that he did not really agree with the Heidelberg theologians as much as one might think by reading Erastus alone. Nevertheless, Schegk wrote in an irenic tone and only made clarifications in emphasis or noted where Erastus had not engaged his full views.[61] It was by no means a polemical rebuke.

While only a preliminary assessment of the encounter can be offered at this juncture, these points seem fairly clear. Erastus was quite satis-

---

[59] Wesel-Roth, *Thomas Erastus*, 38–39; Erastus to Hardenberg, Dec. 10, [1565 ?], SUB Bremen, 10, no. 56, fol. 100: "D. Jacob[us] Scheckius summus philosophus aetate nostra Tubengensis professor, iussu Ducis scriptum edidit, ut dicitur, quo [necessitatem] concordiae sternere conatur. Hoc est à Theologis approbatum, ut an principio et fine libri desertè scribit. Imo, aiunt tertio eum corrigere coactum fuisse iubentibus Theologis. Scribit valde obscurè, atque hic natura habet, in omnibus suis scriptis [etc.] Sed summa libelli (quem ego declaravi fuisse admodum. Nunc describ[itur] meus alias misissem exemplum) est haec, humanitas Christi Substantiam sive essentiam non nisi uno in loco esse, Ubique dicere esse, absurditatem omn(ium) vincere. At ubique dici personaliter atque id etiam impropriè et per accidens. Haec summa est, sed obscurè admodum proposita. Spero nos finem controversiae mox visuros, aut certe magnam mutationem expecturos."

[60] *Responsio Thomae Erasti, ad Libellum D. Iacobi Schegkii, quo nuper Anonymo libro sui, de una persona & duabus in Christo naturis interpreti respondit: in qua mox ab initio demonstratur, Theologos Heydelbergenses et Vvirtebergicos in disputatione de praesentia carnis Christi in omnibus locis, ac in ipsa quoque coena Dominica, non dissentire amplius* (Geneva: Jean Crespin, 1567). Schegk's rejoinder had been the *Responsio Iacobi Schegkii Schorndorffensis, ad libellum Anonymi interpretis libri sui de una persona & duabus naturis in Christo* (Tübingen: Ulrich Morhart, 1566).

[61] Schegk's "Breve Responsum ad Scriptum D. Thomae Erasti, quo explicatur hactenus non consentire Schegkium cum Erasto" is an addendum to *Responsum Iacobi Schegkii Schorndorffensis, ad Simonis Simonii libellum* ... (Tübingen: Ulrich Morhart, 1568), 169–171. Simoni had continued the controversy with *Interpretatio eorum quae continentur in praefatione S. Simone ... cuidam libello affixa ... In qua omnia fere, quae ex physicis D.J. Scheckius ad ubiquitatem carnis Christi, eiusdemque in coena Domini praesentiam corporalem astruendam sumpsit, confutantur* ... [Geneva, 1567] and *Antischegkianorum liber unus* (Basel, 1570). Christoph Sigwart, "Jacob Schegk, Professor der Philosophie und Medizin," in *Kleine Schriften* (Freiburg, 1889), 1:274–277; Wesel-Roth, *Thomas Erastus*, 38–39.

fied with the outcome of the exchange and reported to Bullinger that he had learned via Xylander that Schegk had also approved of Erastus's text.[62] Ironically, Beza, who helped Erastus see the books through press, thought that Erastus had conceded too much to the Lutherans.[63] Erastus emphasized the positives of the exchange to Beza and exalted in the fact that he had been able to get Tübingen's leading philosophical authority to author a book which "omitted a defense of ubiquity" and did not take a firm position on *manducatio impiorum* in the Eucharist.[64] It seems clear that the gesture did not meet with great resonance among Württemberg Lutherans such as Andreae. Likely, the long run impact of the exchange was to marginalize Schegk's position with the Württemberg theologians.

Thus, rather than in any way painting Erastus and Schegk as rivals, they must be seen as fellow travelers; in fact, they were nearly philosophical doppelgangers.[65] The relatively small gap between Schegk's Melanchthonian and Erastus's late-Zwinglian Eucharistic theologies and their common Aristotelian philosophical background enabled them to discuss the Lord's Supper in such a way that emphasized their commonality without demonizing the other's position. Likewise, Schegk's own tepid embrace of ubiquity made it difficult for him to cogently distance himself from Erastus's overtures, which makes for strange reading and had to be problematic for Schegk in the Württemberg context. Erastus and Schegk would find much to agree about in the future debates as well. Erastus would fully endorse Schegk's repudiation of the philosophical novelties of Petrus Ramus, and Schegk in turn would praise Erastus's rejection of the medical world view of Paracelsus.[66] Erastus was quite deferential to the elder Schegk, whom he acknowledged as the leading philosophical

[62] Erastus to Bullinger, July 13, 1567, StAZ, E II 361, fol. 11: "Fuit apud D. Schegkium Xylander noster ante paucos dies, itemque alii boni viri. Hi mihi narrant eum meo scripto contentum esse."

[63] Beza to Bullinger, Feb. 20, 1567, *CB*, 8:72 (no. 538). Bullinger, alternatively, was pleased. Bullinger to Beza, March 31, 1567, *CB*, 8:97 (no. 547).

[64] Erastus to Beza, April 17, [1568], *CB*, 11:344–345 (no. 601bis): "Schegkium videbis omissa defensione Ubiquitatis, tantum nescio quid obscure de impiorum participatione scribere, ne putent homines suos theologos prorsus succubuisse."

[65] Unfortunately, the probable correspondence that passed between Erastus and Schegk has not been preserved. A more thorough analysis of Schegk's correspondence network would likely shed further light on his relationship with Erastus.

[66] See the discussion of the Ramus affair in chapter 7. On Schegk and Paracelsus, see J. Schegk, "De occultis seu abiditis et manefestis medicamentorum facultatibus viribusque ...," in *Disputationum Physicarum et Medicarum Libri VIII* (Frankfurt: Johannes Wechel, 1590), 9.

authority of the age. Erastus's approval of Schegk was confirmed by dubbing him "our Schegk" in his later correspondence. As the situation in Württemberg became increasingly inhospitable for Schegk during the run up to the *Formula of Concord*, Erastus and Simon Grynaeus attempted to get a book by Schegk published in Zurich, only to have the initiative quashed by the resistance of Andreae and the University of Tübingen.[67] In short, Erastus and Schegk appear to have become close intellectual admirers, and Schegk was still around after Erastus's death to remember him fondly in a letter to their common friend and sometime nemesis Beza.[68]

The Dismissal of Johannes Brunner

Seen from the perspective of hindsight, the first skirmish in the struggle to establish the Genevan system of church discipline in the Palatinate was won by the Calvinist "disciplinists" with little anti-disciplinist opposition. In the summer of 1567, before the public outbreak of the controversy, the Swiss-German theologian Johannes Brunner was dismissed from his university post. Brunner had come to Heidelberg through the recommendations of Bullinger, Rudolf Gwalther, and Johannes Wolf and held the chair of ethics on the arts faculty at the university. Though at one time regarded as a theologian with a bright future and still judged by Erastus to be an able scholar, the fact that he published nothing during his years in Heidelberg suggests that he had never quite lived up to expectations. His lack of production alone would likely have been tolerated had he not also possessed a difficult personality. In any event, a controversy over the Lord's Supper paved the way for his dismissal.

In the controversy, largely of Brunner's own making, he revealed himself to be a fairly crude Sacramentarian. He argued that the sacrament did not act as an agent of strengthening faith "in itself and properly" (*per se et proprie*) but only "incidentally" (*per accidens*).[69] This was a return

[67] Erastus to Gwalther, Dec. 11, (15)76, StAZ, E II 345, fols. 724–725: "Addem hoc etiam caeteris nihil laetius. Reformator ille Schmidl[in]us a nescio quo Cacodaemone edoctus, Schegkium per me libr[um] suum curare Tiguri excudi, Ducem Wirtemb. monuit." See the discussion of the letter from Simon Grynaeus to Rudolf Gwalther from Nov. 23 [likely 1576] in *CB* 25:241 (no. 1706; see note 5).

[68] Schegk to Beza, Sept. 9, 1584, *CB* 25:240–242 (no. 1706).

[69] Erastus to Haller, Heidelberg, Sept. 12, 1567, printed Hermann Hagen, *Briefe von Heidelberger Professoren und Studenten* (Bern, 1886), 31–32: "Rei summa haec est: non

to Zwingli's own assertion that the sacrament possessed no power "*per se et proprie*" to strengthen faith.[70] It is important to make clear that this return to such an early Zwinglian position was clearly against the trend of late-Zwinglianism or "Bullingerism" at mid-century, which Erastus himself espoused. The late-Zwinglian interpretation of the Lord's Supper accepted what B.A. Gerrish has termed a "symbolic parallelism" between participation in the Lord's Supper and the reception of grace.[71] In such a framework, late-Zwinglians like Erastus played up the Eucharist's faith-enhancing quality, using the "as certainly as" language discussed in chapter three to describe the relationship between participation in the sacrament and reception of Christ's benefits. Though Erastus did not explicitly say that the sacrament strengthens faith *per se* or concretely bestows grace, these conclusions would seem to be the obvious implications of his thought. Given that Erastus's conception of the Eucharist differed from Brunner's, it is not difficult to understand why Erastus did not come to his aid at an early stage of the controversy.[72]

Curt Horn, in an interpretation which was later followed by Wesel-Roth, detected a change in Erastus's opinion of the Brunner affair after he began to realize that the proponents of church discipline on the Genevan model had been behind Brunner's dismissal. The evidence for this putative change was the contrast between a rather harsh letter that Erastus wrote to Bullinger that placed the blame squarely on Brunner for his discharge and a later, more sympathetic version of events that he sent to Johannes Haller in Bern. Ironically, this plausible hypothesis was wholly based on a typographical error found in Karl Sudhoff's *C. Olevianus und Z. Ursinus* in which the author attributed a letter to Erastus that

---

concedit, Sacramentis per se et propiè fidem nostram accendi vel augeri aut etiam per se obsignari, sed in usu eorum nos confirmari et roborari per accidens, ut in omni pietatis exercito."

[70] Horn, "Johann Sylvan und die Anfänge des Heidelberger Antitrintitarismus," 248.

[71] Gerrish, *The Old Protestantism and the New*, 124, 128.

[72] I dissent from Wesel Roth's assessment that Erastus shared Brunner's conception of the Eucharist. Wesel-Roth suggested that the statements Erastus used to sum up Brunner's position in his letter to Haller more or less agreed with his own understanding of the Lord's Supper. I disagree with Wesel-Roth because of the dissimilarity of Brunner's position with Erastus's published works. Erastus clearly described Brunner's opinions without necessarily advocating them in the letter. Note that Benrath has also seen Brunner as something of an outlier, labeling his conception "eine extrem zwinglische Abendmahlslehre." Benrath, "Briefe des Heidelberger Theologen Zacharias Ursinus," 96; Wesel-Roth, *Thomas Erastus*, 50–51; Erastus to Haller, Heidelberg, Sept. 12, 1567, Zofingen, Staatsbibliothek und Stadtarchiv, MS no. 2.34 (printed in Hagen, *Briefe von Heidelberger Professoren und Studenten*, 31–32).

was actually composed by Ursinus.[73] When this piece of misinformation is removed from the picture, it becomes clear that Erastus's opinion of Brunner did not change as the earlier scholarship suggested. In both Erastus's actual letter to Bullinger and in the letter to Haller, Erastus took a charitable stance toward Brunner, though he did not absolve him of responsibility for his dismissal.[74] The letter to Haller was not a ringing endorsement of Brunner, but rather a carefully worded and kind gesture on behalf of a fallen colleague. Brunner's conception of the Eucharist was not beyond the pale in what Erastus likely saw as a continuum of acceptable Zwinglian to Philippist teachings. His misreading of the evidence aside, Horn correctly saw this episode as a harbinger of the coming of the church discipline controversy. In the letter to Haller, Erastus explicitly noted that behind Brunner's dismissal were those who desired to introduce a form of discipline that Erastus said should be labeled tyranny rather than discipline.[75]

Before moving ahead to the public controversy on church discipline, it is fitting to note Brunner's later exploits. His dismissal from Heidelberg must have engendered something of a crisis of faith for Brunner. From Erastus's descriptions, one gets the sense that Brunner was deeply pious and perhaps inclined to push theological propositions to the breaking point. Ironically, this one-time, hard-line Zwinglian later crossed the Rubicon and sided with Rome. He later authored a public profession of the Catholic faith that he published after joining the faculty of the University of Ingolstadt and moved on to the Catholic academy at Freiburg im Breisgau.[76] The coming church discipline struggle would shake the faith of many more.

[73] Sudhoff, *C. Olevianus und Z. Ursinus*, 372–373. A corrected version of the letter is printed in Benrath, "Briefe des Heidelberger Theologen Zacharias Ursinus," 105–106.

[74] Erastus to Bullinger, July 31, [1567], StAZ, E II 361, fol. 46; Erastus to Haller, Heidelberg, Sept. 12, 1567, printed in Hagen, *Briefe von Heidelberger Professoren und Studenten* 31–32: "Nec ob aliam causam est dimissus, quam quod causam non prudentius egit."

[75] Erastus to Haller, Heidelberg, Sept. 12, 1567, printed in Hagen, *Briefe von Heidelberger Professoren und Studenten*, 31–32: "Inprimis autem cupiunt nescio quam disciplinam, utinamne rectius appellem tyrannidem, cuius forma nec in sacrs literis nec in antiquorum historia traditur, introducere." Erastus's friendly if tepid recommendation did not secure Brunner the post he sought.

[76] Johannes Brunner, *Professio Catholica* (Ingolstadt: Wolfgang Eder, 1582). Brunner's life receives a full overview in Erich Wenneker's entry in Traugott Bautz, *Biographisch-Bibliographisches Kirchenlexikon* (Nordhausen, 2003) 21:155–158. http://www.bautz.de/bbkl/b/brunner_jo.shtml.

Clouds were gathering on the horizon, and Erastus was only beginning to fathom the intensity of his Calvinist colleagues' desire to impress their vision of authentic discipline on the Palatinate or the lengths they would go to achieve their goal. At the same time as Brunner's dismissal, the university senate contemplated extending a call to the able Italian theologian Girolamo Zanchi to join the university. Zanchi later played an important role on the Calvinist side in the church disciplinary controversy by composing a rebuttal of Erastus's theses and by modeling the presbyterial system of church governance in the Heidelberg foreigners' church. He would also serve as the primary theological expert responsible for ferreting out the orthodoxy of Erastus's one-time anti-disciplinist allies in the later Antitrinitarian affair. In retrospect, it is quite ironic that Erastus avidly supported the effort to bring Zanchi to Heidelberg. Erastus had earlier corresponded with Zanchi and must have been enthusiastic about his erudition as well as his Aristotelian philosophical standpoint. Given Ursinus's increasing reluctance to engage in theological controversies, adding a qualified controversialist of Zanchi's stature was an obvious move. In an odd sense, it was due in part to Erastus's dissatisfaction with Olevianus's performance at Maulbronn and especially at Amberg that he wanted to call Zanchi; but calling Zanchi only strengthened Olevianus's hand. As Benrath has noted, Bullinger's opposition to calling Zanchi to Heidelberg might suggest that Bullinger was already aware of the threat posed by the desire to advance the Genevan brand of church discipline and that he must have numbered Zanchi a proponent of the same.[77] Zanchi proved to be a contentious colleague at the University of Heidelberg, while maintaining something of an independent voice on theological questions.[78] Heading into the conflict, Erastus apparently misjudged both his own influence and the intensity of the Calvinist desire to establish their particular vision of biblical discipline.

---

[77] Benrath, "Korrespondenz zwischen Bullinger und Thomas Erastus," 111–112. Bullinger also viewed Zanchi as something of a traitor to Reformed Eucharistic teaching for signing on to the Strasbourg Consensus. See Amy Nelson Burnett, "Simon Sulzer and the Consequences of the 1563 Strasbourg Consensus in Switzerland." *ARG* 83 (1992): 158–159; Visser, *Zacharias Ursinus*, 157–158. Zanchi arrived in Heidelberg in September of 1567. Toepke, *Die Matrikel der Universität Heidelberg*, 2:44.

[78] Zanchi's repeated requests to have his salary raised above the normal pay for his position and various other quarrels are on display throughout the records of the UAH from the late 1560s into the 1570s. See Christopher Burchill, "Die Universität zu Heidelberg und der 'Fromme' Kurfürst," in *Semper Apertus*, 1:238–239.

CHAPTER SIX

THE HEIDELBERG CHURCH DISCIPLINE CONTROVERSY

> To one of those churches which lived in most peaceable sort, and abounded as well with men for their learning in other professions singular, as also with divines whose equals were not elsewhere to be found, a Church ordered by Gualther's discipline, and not by that which Geneva adoreth: unto this church, the Church of Heidelberg, there cometh one who craving leave to dispute publicly defendeth with open disdain of their government, that *To a minister with his Eldership power is given by the law of God to excommunicate whomsoever, yea even kings and princes themselves*. Here were the seeds sown of that controversy which sprang up between Beza and Erastus about the matter of excommunication....
>
> Richard Hooker, *Of the Laws of Ecclesiastical Polity*.

Richard Hooker, no sympathizer of Theodore Beza and the Genevan mode of discipline, correctly identified the Palatinate as the scene of one of the most bitter intramural confrontations in the history of Reformed Protestantism. The controversy had perhaps been looming since 1562, and with a strong disciplinist party dominating the church council with ready access to the prince, naturally Olevianus and his allies desired to implement what they considered to be a more complete form of church discipline. Olevianus wanted to create an independent consistory which would place control over the discipline of moral offenses in the hands of a joint lay/clerical body. The key notion here was to renew authentic Christian discipline independent of state control on a New Testament model. Fundamentally it was an effort to change who controlled discipline, but the Calvinist church leaders also envisioned a more proactive disciplinary regime than that which was currently in effect in Heidelberg. As theologically justified from the Calvinist perspective as their attempt was, their impulse would have fateful consequences for the Palatine church. Unlike the working consensus that existed among the Reformed on the issue of the Lord's Supper, there was no united Reformed opinion on the issue of church discipline.[1] Thus, seeking to implement a more stringent

[1] On the Zurich Consensus, see Paul Rorem, "Calvin and Bullinger on the Lord's Supper," *Lutheran Quarterly* 2 (1988): 153–178, 359–384.

form of discipline inevitably brought the competing traditions of church discipline of the mother Reformed churches of Zurich and Geneva into conflict.

Reformed Theories of Church Discipline

The coming of the Reformation and the attack on the hierarchical structure of authority of the Western Catholic Church led by the papacy naturally opened wide the question of church-state relations. Many factors coalesced in the early years of the Reformation to greatly favor the authority of the state vis-à-vis the church: pervasive anticlericalism, a sense of historical exploitation by the papacy which was particularly acute in the Holy Roman Empire, and the relatively easy opportunity for the enhancement of political power and fiscal resources offered to both princes and town councils by usurping ecclesiastical jurisdictions. Luther famously challenged political leaders to cross over traditional boundaries of church and state in his *Address to the Christian Nobility of the German Nation*. Luther then developed his doctrine of the two swords, redefining the areas of competence of church and state. The "Humpty Dumpty" of independent ecclesiastical authority, which could stand toe-to-toe with political leaders and whose roots lay in the high medieval Gregorian reform movement, had been definitively shattered, never to be reassembled in such a menacing fashion within a Protestant German state church. While the new order gave explicit recognition to a certain autonomy of the church, by necessity the Lutheran state Reformation was "Erastian" in common parlance, and if ecclesiastical authorities at times were given putative authority to determine proper doctrine, they did so with the sufferance of the magistrate. The 1555 Peace of Augsburg's *cuius regio, eius religio* had been the de facto rule since the 1520s. Thus, the magisterial Reformation by its very nature had a strong Erastian tendency, though there were many questions left open for future development or elaboration. These questions largely break into three interlocking areas: church-state relations, the structural organization of the church, and church discipline. The early continental Reformation might be described as both adiaphoristic and opportunistic on these fronts; that is, not being too concerned whether the church was effectively controlled by the town council, an oligarchic church council with a general superintendent, or in some cases even retaining bishops, as long as a break from Catholic ecclesiastical authorities took place.

The perceived need in some quarters for more effective church discipline to facilitate true reform among the unwashed masses further begged the question of larger church structure, which concomitantly brought up the issue of how this structure would relate to the state. Urban reformers from Upper Germany and Switzerland quickly pushed beyond Luther on these crucial issues, as they had done before on the question of the Lord's Supper. Broadly speaking, two competing solutions to these questions arose within the Upper German-Swiss Reformation.

The first Reformed theory of church discipline grew out of the Zwinglian Reformation. Since the Reformation in Zurich was enacted by decision of the town council, from the earliest juncture the civil authorities assumed ecclesiastical jurisdiction. Robert Walton has suggested that this pattern was a natural expression of the church-state relations that had developed before the Reformation. According to Walton, the control over church affairs that the state established during the Reformation "marks the end rather the beginning of the progress."[2] In line with the general pattern of state dominance of the church, the state usurped control over the traditional competence of ecclesiastical courts to police moral infractions after the establishment of the Reformation. While there was some internal debate among the Swiss reformers as to the validity of such overweening state influence, Huldrych Zwingli quite early argued for the scriptural legitimacy of what J. Wayne Baker has labeled the Zurich-Bern "single sphere" model.[3] This view held that there was no scriptural justification to erect a separate ecclesiastical institution to supervise morals distinct from that of the magistrate in a Christian commonwealth. Indeed Ryan Reeves now argues that Erastus's early supporter Konrad Pellikan weighed in with a reading of Psalm 82 which acknowledged the divine nature of earthly rulers and which had a decisive impact on emerging Protestant political theory in both Zurich and England.[4] The key figure in

[2] Robert C. Walton, "The Institutionalization of the Reformation at Zurich," *Zwingliana* 13 (Heft 8, 1972): 497. The classic English language study is Robert C. Walton's *Zwingli's Theocracy* (Toronto: University of Toronto Press, 1967).

[3] J. Wayne Baker, "Zwinglianism" in *OER*, 4:323–327. Baker has written many articles on this topic (See the bibliography), of which the most important for our purposes is "Church Discipline or Civil Punishment: On the Origins of the Reformed Schism, 1528–1531," *Andrews University Studies* 23 (1985): 3–18.

[4] Ryan M. Reeves, "'Ye Gods': The Magistrate and Political Obedience in Humanism, Zürich and English Protestantism, c. 1525–1540," Sixteenth Century Studies Conference, Geneva, May 2009.

the articulation of this theory was Zwingli's successor Heinrich Bullinger, who not only upheld the state's right to oversee morals and punish sinners in a Christian society, but also even questioned whether excommunication, in the strict sense of barring sinners from taking communion, was a valid ecclesiastical censure.[5] Bullinger's *Decades* or *Hausbuch*, which was one of the more popular theological compendia of the century, disseminated the basic Zurich concept, if in a somewhat muted fashion.[6] The third major advocate of the "single sphere" conception of state relations and church discipline was the reformer Wolfgang Musculus, who worked in Augsburg prior to the Interim and ended his distinguished career as the leading minister in Bern, the most powerful Swiss canton. Musculus offered ideas that complemented the Zurich position; for example, that the precedent of the Israelite state in the era of the Davidic monarchy was a fitting analogy for contemporary church-state relations. He had a rather extreme view of the superiority of the divinely sanctioned "magistrate" over the humble "minister" of the church and drew his arguments both from Scripture and nature.[7] He also delineated part of Erastus's future line of argumentation in the later Heidelberg debate by asserting that excommunication was a power possessed by the church only "if it lacke a Christian Magistrate."[8] The last major figure from the Swiss Reformation to emerge as a vigorous advocate of the Zurich-Bern "single sphere" model was Bullinger's protégé and eventual successor Rudolf Gwalther, whose ideas evolved in dialogue with those of Erastus himself.[9]

---

[5] See Bullinger's noteworthy letter to Berchtold Haller from July 1531 in *Heinrich Bullinger Werke, 2. Abteilung Briefwechsel*, ed. Fritz Büsser, et al. (Zurich: Theologischer Verlag, 1972), 1:205–216.

[6] See most recently Torrance Kirby, "The Civil Magistrate and the 'cura religionis': Heinrich Bullinger's prophetical office and the English Reformation," in *Heinrich Bullinger (1504–1575): Leben, Denken, Wirkung. Internationaler Bullingerkongress 2004*, ed. Emidio Campi and Peter Opitz (Zurich: Theologische Verlag, 2006), 935–950. Bullinger is quite deferential, though not perhaps to the degree as Musculus, to magisterial authority throughout the *Decades*. Discipline remains under its purview. He does not challenge the concept of excommunication per se, but employs the concept in two primary contexts: one a very negative association of the excessive claims to spiritual authority of the papacy within the Catholic Church and the other as an exclusion from the community, but not explicitly a debarment from the sacraments. Heinrich Bullinger, *The Decades of Henry Bullinger*, ed. Thomas Harding (Cambridge, 1849).

[7] Wolfgang Musculus, *Common Places of Christian Religion* … (London, 1563), 1283–1340. See James Thomas Ford, "Wolfgang Musculus on the Office of the Christian Magistrate," *ARG* 91 (2000): 149–167.

[8] Musculus, *Commonplaces*, 636.

[9] Wesel-Roth, *Thomas Erastus*, 102–107.

The Zurich Reformation also created two institutions to deal with issues of discipline and regulation of clerical affairs, which had a broad impact on the Upper German-Swiss Reformation. The "synod" was a biannual gathering of clergy more analogous perhaps to the Venerable Company of Pastors of Geneva than what is conventionally termed a "synod" in much of the Reformed world. Policing *the clergy* per se was the chief object of this body.[10] The institution which had broader jurisdiction over the morals of the community at large was the "marriage court" (*Ehegericht*), which had been established in 1525. This institution was the successor of the court of the bishop of Constance, who had been the ecclesiastical overlord of the Zurich commune. Though this institution was a marriage court by name, it soon expanded its jurisdiction so that it became in effect a wide ranging morals court. Clerics played an active role in its proceedings, but it was essentially a civil institution dominated by the magistrate. While the Genevan Consistory has received much more attention from historians, and likewise, more negative press, the Zurich marriage court could also be petty and vindictive.[11] Ministerial influence was so strong in the marriage court and on state policy in general in the late 1520s that many observers have marked the "theocratic" tendencies of the Zurich Reformation. The relative influence of clerics lessened after the death of Zwingli, and the state directly controlled the marriage court and oversaw the operation of the synods. The clergy had an advisory or "prophetic" role, which of course could be substantial considering the deep penetration of spiritual concerns in sixteenth-century social life and politics. Analogous institutions were created in cities such as Bern, Basel, and Schaffhausen.[12]

[10] See Pamela Biel, *Doorkeepers at the House of Righteousness. Heinrich Bullinger and the Zürich Clergy 1535–1575* [ZBRG 15] (Bern: Peter Lang, 1991), 207–203 (with a translation of the 1532 synod mandate) and Bruce Gordon, *Clerical Discipline and the Rural Reformation: The Synod in Zürich, 1532–1580* [ZBRG 16] (Bern: Peter Lang, 1992), passim.

[11] For example, Norman Birnbaum almost makes the marriage court look like a forerunner of a revolutionary tribunal: "Zwingli used it to terrorise the political opposition (espionage and denunciation were some of its techniques), as well as to punish sinners and encourage, if that is the word, the morally weak." "The Zwinglian Reformation in Zürich," *Past and Present* 15 (1959): 35.

[12] Walther Köhler, *Zürcher Ehegericht und Genfer Konsistorium, vol. 1, Das Zürcher Ehegericht und seine Auswirkung in der deutschen Schweiz zur Zeit Zwinglis* [Quellen und Abhandlungen zur schweizerischen Reformationsgeschichte 7] (Leipzig: N. Heinsius Nachfolger, 1932); Walton, *Zwingli's Theocracy*; J. Wayne Baker, "Calvin's Discipline and the Early Reformed Tradition: Bullinger and Calvin," in *Calviniana: Ideas and Influence of Jean Calvin* [SCE&S 10], ed. Robert V. Schnucker (Kirksville, Mo., 1988),

This model had much to recommend itself to the leading Swiss cantons. It apparently had strong biblical sanction by analogy with the respective roles of church and state in the Hebrew Scriptures. Perhaps more critically, however, this state-dominated model was threatened by an alternative sectarian vision of the church as a gathered community drawn out of society that should administer its own discipline. Thus, in their encounter with the Anabaptists, the Swiss Reformed had a very early negative exposure to a "precisianist" group that deployed excommunication or the ban to purify itself. Since the Swiss Reformed viewed the Anabaptists' gathered church as a malevolent and seditious threat to the conventional notion of the city as a Christian community, the constructive features of their program, however strong their biblical rationale, tended to have a negative association. Finally, from the state perspective it seemed clerics had exercised too much influence over society and politics at large in the tumultuous decade which culminated in the Second Kappel War (1531). With Zwingli's passing on the battlefield, his able successor Bullinger had a difficult task even reasserting a prophetic advisory role for the clergy in Swiss politics. State dominance over the church and exclusive jurisdiction over moral infractions became the rule in the German-speaking Reformed Swiss Cantons.

The Calvinist-Reformed tradition, however, had initiated a program of church discipline along different lines. The central concept of this system was to give authority over church discipline to an assembly of elders and ministers working in concert—the consistory. Johannes Oecolampadius, the reformer of Basel and Zwingli's close collaborator, first propounded this theory in the late 1520s. Martin Bucer was the most important early advocate of more effectual church discipline—even regarding it as a mark of the true church—though he was never given full sanction to implement a more rigorous model with independent church control over excommunication in Strasbourg. Bucer was nevertheless a critical influence on John Calvin, who became the chief advocate of consistorial discipline to the larger Reformed world.[13] Calvin viewed exercising power over excommunication as critical to the church's mandate to purify itself.

107–119; Hans Ulrich Bächtold, *Heinrich Bullinger vor dem Rat: Zur Gestaltung und Verwaltung des Zurcher Staatswesens in den Jahren 1531–1575* [ZBRG 12] (Bern: Peter Lang, 1982).

[13] See Amy Nelson Burnett, *The Yoke of Christ: Martin Bucer and Christian Discipline* [SCE&S 26] (Kirksville, Mo., 1994).

In fact, his insistence on an independent sphere of ecclesiastical authority was one of the major factors that led to his expulsion from Geneva in 1538.[14] Such a "presbyterial" order mandated a clear separation of the spheres of competence of church and the civil authority, but Calvin and his followers hoped that the two spheres would work in collaboration rather than conflict. Calvin had to struggle for much of his time in Geneva to make his vision a reality, and it was only after the Servetus trial and the exile of prominent members of the Libertine faction in 1555 that Calvin's allies were able to fully implement their program. Without this autonomous, self-regulating feature, Calvinists considered the church's integrity threatened.[15]

What did this consistorial-presbyterial model look like on the ground? First, a word about vocabulary. The word "consistory" traditionally referred to a church court whereas "presbytery" denoted a gathering of elders—though "presbyter," of course, was also the etymological root for "priest." Although the words "consistory" and "presbytery" might be used interchangeably, they eventually came to denote different levels of governance within Reformed church polity. Ironically, Calvin and Beza became prime exponents of "presbyterian" or "presbyterial" church polity in a community that did not formally have a body bearing that title.[16] What was essential in their views was that a body of elders, in Geneva the consistory, exercise proper authority over matters which pertained to the church—especially oversight of matters of morals and belief. In the case of Geneva, the consistory was a city-wide institution, rather than being based on an individual parish, which also had jurisdiction over the outlying rural districts. The consistory in Geneva was a joint lay-ecclesiastical body, and all members of the Venerable Company of Pastors were ex officio members of the consistory, though they did not always attend.

---

[14] William G. Naphy, *Calvin and the Consolidation of the Genevan Reformation* (1994, repr. Lexington: Westminster John Knox Press, 2003) 28–33; Bruening, *Calvinism's First Battleground*, 163–165.

[15] Pelikan, *The Christian Tradition*, 4:215–216; Baker, "Calvin's Discipline and the Early Reformed Tradition," 108–111. For Calvinist discipline in general, see Philip Benedict, *Christ's Churches Purely Reformed: A Social History of Calvinism* (New Haven: Yale UP, 2002), 460–489.

[16] I intentionally employ "presbyterial" instead of "Presbyterian" in this chapter to emphasize the role of elders in church polity rather than a direct identification with a modern denomination. In the French-Dutch Calvinist tradition, the term for the local oversight body is "consistory," the regional body a "classis," and the national or international gathering a "synod." For Presbyterians the structure would run "session," "presbytery," and regional "synod," with a "general assembly" at the highest level.

While the lay members were appointed by the town council, the pastors influenced the selection of suitable elders during the institution's heyday in the second half of the sixteenth century. A layman, one of the leading syndics or magistrates of the city, presided over the Genevan consistory. Individuals who were cited to appear before the consistory after a brief inquest and counseling session might endure sanctions including admonishment, required attendance at sermons, humiliating acts of public penance, and finally excommunication. The most common form of excommunication was more of a short-term suspension from taking part in the Lord's Supper. Individuals who were unrepentant or unwilling to submit to the authority of the consistory might suffer the major ban (formal excommunication), and thus be cut off from church life. While in theory the Geneva Consistory was a non-coercive institution to which people voluntarily submitted themselves, the social stigma of excommunication was great and bore with it great civil liabilities, such as the exclusion from participation in baptism and the prohibition from entering a Christian marriage.

While the Genevan consistory in combination with the preaching and catechetical ministry of the pastors seems to have done a superb job over a few decades in inculcating a Reformed vision of the Christian faith in Geneva, this success came at a price, the chief burden of which was a high degree of prying into areas of life that modern Westerners would consider private. E. William Monter has calculated that one in fifteen Genevans were called before the consistory annually in the period of the 1560s and 1570s and that at its highpoint the consistory excommunicated nearly three hundred people per year.[17] Robert Kingdon, the leading modern authority on Calvin and the Genevan Reformation, has bluntly concluded that the consistory was a "remarkably intrusive institution."[18] However, for many sixteenth-century observers the consistory's value in effecting a genuine reformation of morals served as a tremendous confirmation of the theology behind it. While the system had its detractors (some of whom we will soon meet), the success of consistorial discipline in turning Geneva into a Godly community was one of its chief attractions to sixteenth-century Protestants.

[17] E. William Monter, "The Consistory of Geneva, 1559–1569," *Bibliothèque d'humanisme et de la renaissance* 38 (1976), 84.

[18] Robert Kingdon, "The Genevan Consistory in the Time of Calvin," in *Calvinism in Europe, 1540–1620*, ed. Andrew Pettegree et al. (Cambridge: Cambridge UP, 1994), 22 and 34. See Robert Kingdon, et al. eds., *Registers of the Consistory of Geneva in the Time of Calvin*, vol. 1, 1542–1544 (Grand Rapids, Eerdmans, 2000).

While Geneva became *the* example of a successfully reformed community, it was easier to export the consistorial model than it was to fully replicate the Genevan experience. Geneva represented a unique political and sociological laboratory with its unusual position as a quasi-independent city-state allied to the Swiss confederacy. Geneva's singular religious climate turned it into a Mecca for Protestant refugees at mid-century, and the flood of refugees in turn further transformed the Genevan Reformation and empowered the Calvinist church leaders. Geneva's peculiar model of ecclesial organization with *auctoritas* in church matters lying with the Venerable Company of Pastors could not easily be reproduced: Geneva was distinct in the size of the community, the quality of the ministerial staff, but even more importantly in possessing Calvin's charismatic leadership. A system of discipline developed along parallel lines in the French church "under the cross," due in part to the direct involvement of the Venerable Company. Of course, the practical functioning of the system varied from community to community, and, not surprisingly, Huguenot lords were not nearly as eager to erect such a system of consistorial discipline as were bourgeois town councils. The Genevan Company of Pastors remained a resource of theological authority and a clearinghouse of ministerial candidates for the French churches—in effect, an ersatz papal curia. In general these local consistories were dominated by influential lay bourgeoisie and tended to be more moderate in their exercise of discipline than the Genevan consistory in the 1560s and 1570s.[19]

The church's ability to administer discipline was seen by most later Calvinists as a distinctive mark of a true church (*notae ecclesiae*), alongside preaching the gospel and the correct administration of the sacraments.[20] While Calvin was likely the century's most forceful advocate of effective church discipline, he did not include it among the *notae ecclesiae*. Some scholars have attempted to distinguish between Calvin, who at these junctures is seen to have retained a measure of his Erasmian humanist ethos, and his more hard-line followers who pushed

[19] Raymond Mentzer, "Marking the Taboo: Excommunication in French Reformed Churches," Raymond Mentzer, ed., *Sin and the Calvinists: Morals Control and the Consistory in the Reformed Tradition* [*SCE&S* 32] (Kirksville, Mo., 1994), 97–128; Glenn S. Sunshine, *Reforming French Protestantism: The Development of Huguenot Ecclesiastical Institutions, 1557–1572* [*SCE&S* 66] (Kirksville, Mo.: Truman State UP, 2003), 121–142.

[20] E.g., article 29 of the Belgic Confession of 1561.

his formulations to uncomfortable extremes, whether on predestination or church discipline, without Calvin's pastoral heart. The theological gulf between Calvin and his rigorist followers, whether they be labeled "Gnesio-Calvinists," "disciplinists," or "precisianists," is not that great.[21] On the one hand, if Calvin did not recognize the proper exercise of church discipline as a fully fledged mark of an authentic church, he did see it as a mandatory adjunct of the proper administration of the sacraments. Therefore, the tendency of later theologians and creeds to add church discipline to the marks of the church would appear to be a natural extension of Calvin's thought. On the other hand, going beyond Calvin and turning this discipline into a *nota ecclesiae*, was a stone of offense to other Protestants who did not practice as rigorous a discipline as the Genevans or the Calvinist church "under the cross." Thus, the expression "Gnesio-Calvinist" has some explanatory utility in marking a group whose rigorous devotion to a particular vision of authentic Calvinism alienated others within the Reformed movement. This fissure is analogous in part to the division within the Lutheran community between "Gnesio-Lutherans" and their moderate or Philippist antagonists. In both cases the "Gnesio" faction largely succeeded in assuming control over the tradition and redefining its boundaries.

There had been earlier skirmishes within the Reformed communion on the issue of church discipline. One of the early flash-points was in the Pays de Vaud, a French-speaking territory under Bernese control, where Calvin advocated the Genevan position from abroad and his ally Pierre Viret vigorously worked from within to establish consistorial discipline. The Bernese authorities who ultimately controlled the religious policy of the Vaud would tolerate consistories, but steadfastly refused to grant the nascent Calvinist church organization independent authority over excommunication. They were fortified in their rejection of a Genevan model of discipline by the arrival in Bern of Musculus, who advocated the classic Swiss-German position that Erastus would later espouse. The Zurich church naturally weighed in on this controversy as well, and

[21] I borrow the expression "Gnesio-Calvinist" from Heiko A. Oberman, *The Two Reformations: The Journey from the Last Days to the New World*, ed. Donald Weinstein (New Haven: Yale UP, 2003), 135. Theodore Dwight Bozeman has recently illuminated this tendency in Anglo-American Reformed Protestantism in *The Precisianist Strain: Disciplinary Religion and Antinomian Backlash in Puritanism to 1638* (Chapel Hill: University of North Carolina Press, 2004).

while it by no means supported Viret's drive to establish consistorial discipline, the most recent analysis of the conflict has depicted Bullinger's primary role in the conflict as that of a peacemaker. The final result of this conflict was the mass exodus of Viret and the other Calvinist personnel in 1559 after they failed to establish consistorial discipline.[22] Before the Heidelberg controversy, the French Reformed church had also been racked by strife on this question of church discipline and its concomitant structural issues. Though he did not attack church discipline per se, Jean Morély argued that the final source of authority should be the local church—though perhaps conceived more on a diocesan rather than strictly a congregational model—and implied that the conventional Calvinist disciplinary model placed too much authority in the hands of the clerically dominated consistory. He also faulted the Calvinist system for withholding a role for the magistrate in discipline. In a predictable twist, Morély's opponents in Geneva arranged his excommunication for his opposition to the Calvinist vision of discipline. Petrus Ramus championed Morély's vision of ecclesiastical organization at the synod of La Rochelle in 1571, though their views were again repudiated.[23] The issue of church discipline would later be the source of strife in both the Netherlands and Britain. The Heidelberg controversy was thus not an isolated event but one episode in a series of controversies over church discipline.

George Withers and the Outbreak of the Controversy

The rivalry between disciplinist and anti-disciplinist factions in the Palatinate intensified until open conflict erupted in June of 1568. Like the earlier controversy over the Lord's Supper, the promotion of a foreign doctoral student opened the dispute. The English cleric George With-

[22] Bruening, *Calvinism's First Battleground*, 253–255.

[23] On Jean Morély see Philippe Denis and Jean Rott, *Jean Morély (ca. 1524 – ca. 1594) et l'utopie d'une démocratie dans l'Eglise* [THR 278] (Geneva: Droz, 1993); Robert M. Kingdon, *Geneva and the Consolidation of the French Protestant Movement 1564–1572* [THR 92] (Geneva: Droz, 1967); Michael Graham, *The Uses of Reform: "Godly Discipline" and Popular Behavior in Scotland and Beyond, 1560–1610* [SMRT 58] (Leiden: Brill, 1996), 320–322; Sunshine, *Reforming French Protestantism*. On Ramus's role in these developments, see James Veazie Skalnik, *Ramus and Reform: University and Church at the End of the Renaissance* [SCE&S 60] (Kirksville, Mo.: Truman State UP, 2002).

ers (1540–1604) advocated a more thorough Reformation than that espoused by the church hierarchy under Elizabeth I. Like his Puritan brethren, he resented such "Romish" vestiges as clerical vestments and stained glass, but also desired the erection of a genuinely Reformed system of church discipline. During the Vestiarian Controversy of 1564–1566, Withers had refused to wear the "square cap" prescribed by the 1559 Prayer Book. Withers was one of the representatives of the emerging Puritan party who traveled abroad in an effort to influence church leaders in Zurich, Geneva, and beyond on its behalf.[24] While the party received a sympathetic hearing in Geneva, Bullinger and Gwalther eventually came to see Withers and his ilk as unwelcome troublemakers.[25] A long, undated petition from Withers to Elector Frederick III has survived in which he outlined the evolution of the religious scene in England from King Henry to the present. He asserted that Satan was now undermining the cause of true Reformation through the machinations of careerist clergy who were bowing to the whims of the queen and her lackey bishops. Withers was not only dismayed by the persistence of traditional worship forms, he also lamented that a more biblical version of church discipline had not been installed in England. In line with other Gnesio-Calvinists, Withers asserted in his petition: "For there being three chief parts of the church, wholesome doctrine, the pure administration of the sacraments, and a rightly constituted ministry, which part also includes a vigorous discipline." In England, alternatively, "The ministry is in fact nothing at all, nor is there any discipline."[26] As part of this larger campaign on behalf of the Puritan party, Withers had arrived in Heidelberg by the spring of 1568 and apparently sought both to advance his scholarly pedigree and to create a little controversy.[27] While he was not able to influence the elector to champion the cause of further reformation with the queen directly, Withers secured a long, impassioned plea on the English Puritans' behalf from

[24] Brett Usher and John Craig, "Withers, George (bap. 1540, d. 1605)," in *Oxford Dictionary of National Biography* (Oxford: Oxford UP, 2004); Laquita M. Higgs, *Godliness and Governance in Tudor Colchester* (Ann Arbor: University of Michigan Press, 1998), 204.

[25] For Zurich's and particularly Gwalther's uncomfortable position between the English factions during the Vestiarian controversy, see Patrick Collinson, *The Elizabethan Puritan Movement* (Berkeley: University of California Press, 1967), 79–83.

[26] "George Withers to the Prince Elector Palatine," in Hastings Robinson, trans., *The Zurich Letters* (Second Series) (Cambridge, 1845), 156–164 (no. 62).

[27] Withers was inscribed on the Heidelberg matriculation list on March 22, 1568. Toepke, *Die Matrikel der Universität Heidelberg*, 2:45.

the pen of the university theologian Girolamo Zanchi which decried the Satanic temptations of Popish vestments.[28]

Along these lines, Withers's original intention seems to have been to defend theses on clerical vestments, which the Heidelberg theology faculty wisely disallowed, as it did not want to be seen as fomenting discord within the English church. The alternative plan to defend theses on church discipline was equally incendiary, as events in Heidelberg would later prove. Unfortunately, the extant sources for the early stages of this controversy are rather thin. It does not seem possible to answer the most fundamental question about Withers's theses, viz., who was the driving force behind them. Unlike modern doctoral dissertations and theses, the actual defense of the theses was the crucial step in earning the degree rather than the original composition of the text. Frequently the theses proposed for attaining academic degrees would have been composed by the sponsoring professor rather than the person pursuing the degree. In this case, no background information has been uncovered which shows whether Withers himself or the sponsoring professor Pierre Boquin actually composed the theses. A third option would be that Withers was encouraged by leading figures within the Palatine church such as Olevianus, Dathenus, or Zuleger to defend these theses as a test balloon. Since there is no conflict in seeing all three entities as playing some role in arranging Withers's promotion, it is not necessary to single one party out: all were evidently on board.

The defense of the theses commenced on June 10 and continued for some days, though the extant sources do not fully illuminate this stage of the controversy. The theses contained a couple of provocative assertions which may have seemed rather commonplace among French or Dutch Protestants, but which were quite inflammatory in context of a German state church. Withers upheld the divine right of presbyterial rule, and, granting a clerically led presbytery power over excommunication, even maintained that the presbytery ought to have power to excommunicate the prince. Furthermore, he implied that presbyterial discipline was a mark of the true church, alongside preaching the word and administering the sacraments.[29] Erastus does not appear to have been directly involved

[28] "Hierome Zanchius to Queen Elizabeth," Heidelberg, Sept. 10, 1571, *The Zurich Letters* (Second Series), appendix 1, 339–353.

[29] Theses 12 and 13 are printed in Ursinus, *Opera Theologica*, ed. Quirinus Reuter (Heidelberg: Johann Lancellot, 1612), 3:801; reprinted in Alting, *Historia de ecclesiis Palatinis*, 101 (ch. 54). "Thesis XII: Ad sinceram verbi Divini praedicationem & legitimam Sacramentorum administrationem, oportet in Ecclesia gubernationis vigere officium.

at this juncture. When reminiscing about the controversy many years later, Erastus would recount that he had been preoccupied with treating the sick and wounded from Johann Casimir's recent military campaign in France when the controversy erupted and thus had been unable to take part in the debate. Alting reports that Adam Neuser, a popular preacher of the *Peterskirche*, represented the nascent "anti-disciplinist" side in opposing Withers in the theses defense. Despite the opposition, Withers was subsequently awarded his degree on June 20. Neither his sponsor Boquin nor Erastus himself regarded the fact that Withers had defended controversial theological theses as being out of order.[30] Unfortunately for the Palatinate, Withers's theses became the impetus in which the passionate disagreement regarding church discipline became a matter of public discussion, among both university students and the Palatine clergy.

The summer and fall of 1568 would prove to be the most heated public phase of the Heidelberg church discipline controversy. Erastus's first letter to Bullinger after the start of the controversy in June did not even mention the quarrel but did ominously report that it was not currently possible to print Bullinger's work in Heidelberg.[31] Erastus did not inform Bullinger about how a "certain Englishman" had stirred up a tempest in Heidelberg until August, and he commented that he saw "neophytes and adolescents" behind it.[32] Sensing the disciplinary fervor in the air,

Thes. XIII. Officium autem hoc voco, ut Ministri cum Presbyterio quovis peccantes (etiam Principes) arguendi, increpandi, excommunicandi, reliquaque ad disciplinam Ecclesiasticam pertinentia peragendi facultatem habeant & exerceant." See also Sudhoff, *C. Olevianus und Z. Ursinus*, 343; Bonnard, *Thomas Éraste*, 45–48.

[30] Heidelberg, Universitätsarchiv Heidelberg, MS A-160/9, fols. 75r–75v; Erastus, *Explicatio gravissimae quaestionis*, [A6r]; Alting, *Historia de ecclesiis Palatinis*, 102 (ch. 54); Wesel-Roth, *Thomas Erastus*, 53–54. Alternatively, Alting has Erastus protesting along with Neuser that not enough time had been given for the opposing views. Erastus fairly explicitly says that he did not take part in the disputation ("Itaque ne ego aliquid movere aliquid, nec propter negotia, interesse potui.") Neuser's participation is not mentioned in Boquin's account in the university protocols but is perhaps likely.

[31] Erastus to Bullinger, July 18, [1568], StAZ, E II 361, fol. 35: "Librum tuum hic imprimi impossibile est. Valde cupiunt, qui eum viderunt, etiam Ursinus, excudi. Ipse quoque te oro, ut operam des, quo vel à nundinis statim vel etiam ante imprimatur Basilienses iuuare te poterunt, puto."

[32] Erastus to Bullinger, August 21, [1568], Zurich, Staatsarchiv des Kantons Zürich, MS E I 25, 8, fol. 52. "Venit ad nos huc nuper (tibi soli dico) Anglus quidam, ut Doct[or] crearetur, et proposuit Theses ad disputandum, in quibus oportere scribit Disciplinam in omni vera Ecclesia vigere, qua ministri cum presbyterio quosvis peccantes, etiam Principes excommunicent. Peperit ea res turbas et dissensiones, ac verendum est, ne gliscat odium conceptum, serpatque longius. Quocirca commentarium ipse mihi ea

Erastus responded in the summer of 1568 with 103 theses on the topic of church discipline that circulated freely among the Heidelberg students. Rather naturally, a conflict between the Zurich and Geneva visions of church discipline drew in the interests of the respective home churches, and both parties would attempt to influence the outcome of events in the Palatinate. The conflict would severely strain relations between the Zurich and Genevan Reformers, though ultimately the restraint of Bullinger and Beza mollified the impact of this bitter disagreement. The following section will offer a brief analysis of Erastus's critique of the Calvinist vision of church discipline before returning to a narrative of the events in Heidelberg.

The Explicatio gravissimae quaestionis

The most famous document to come out of the Heidelberg controversy over church discipline was Erastus's treatise on excommunication, the *Explicatio gravissimae quaestionis*. This work had a rather twisted redaction history. The actual *Explicatio* consisted of Erastus's 75 theses on excommunication, distilled from his original 103 theses written sometime in 1569. The theses made up the first quarter of the book, which was published posthumously (discussed below in the epilogue). The published edition also contained Erastus's lengthy rebuttal of Beza entitled *Confirmatio thesium*. Besides these materials, the book also printed assorted letters of Bullinger and others relating to the controversy. Further complicating the redaction history is the existence of an unpublished 1568 manuscript by Bullinger bearing the title *Tractatus de Excommunicatione* which shares some material with Erastus's *Explicatio gravissimae quaestionis*. I follow Baker in assuming that the last parts of Bullinger's *Tractatus de Excommunicatione* were probably culled from Erastus's work.[33]

de re conscripsi ferè; in quo, quid de hac re sentiendum, sit; perspicuè et ex verbo dei validissime ostendere, me puto. Cum perfecero exemplum tibi mittam. Una verbo dicam, quicquid de ea dicatur, non poterit ea forma in nostras Ecclesias sine certa ruina induci, quam Neophyti quicquid et Adolescentuli urgent, suaeque amibitionis causa cum perniciae Ecclesiae stabilire exoptant. Sed D[omi]n[u]s ista curabit."

[33] J. Wayne Baker, "In Defense of Magisterial Discipline: Bullinger's 'Tractatus de Excommunicatione' of 1568," in *Heinrich Bullinger 1504–1575: Gesammelte Aufsätze sum 400. Todestag* [*ZBRG* 7], 1:141–144. It is likely that Baker's supposition "Indeed the last

The title of Erastus's treatise focused on the question, "whether excommunication ... is based upon Divine Mandate or is contrived by men."[34] That Erastus had narrowed his topic to precisely excommunication as removal from the sacrament was significant. His Swiss predecessors had used the word excommunication as a synonym for discipline. This usage produced the novelty of a church that practiced "excommunication" (i.e., discipline) without formal excommunication (exclusion from the sacrament).[35] While Erastus used the question of excommunication as a vehicle to address church discipline in general, the heart of the work was focused specifically on whether there was biblical precedent for using access to the sacraments as means of discipline. Erastus did not reject discipline in general or the private responsibility of pastors and laymen to admonish wayward brethren. He even suggested that something like the practice of shunning may be suggested by the Bible.[36] He could find no justification, however, for the notion that the admission to or refusal of the sacrament had been intended as a disciplinary tool.

Erastus not only rejected the sacraments' putative connection to discipline, he also questioned the church's theoretical power over the disposition of human souls. In the early sections of his treatise, Erastus issued a frontal assault against a millennium of church teaching when he implicitly rejected the power of the keys (*potestas clavium*). A critical component of the rationale for excommunication was that the visible church possessed the power to "bind and loose" things in heaven. The church's absolution was the word of divine forgiveness; the church's anathema condemned a person for eternity. Erastus rejected this notion by denying any necessary relationship between the invisible and visible churches. Erastus asserted that faith alone was the quality that makes a

nine folios may well be a copy of the entire lost 'Tractatio' of Erastus" (p. 144) is correct. See also Wesel-Roth, *Thomas Erastus*, 148.

[34] Thomas Erastus, *Explicatio Gravissimae Quaestionis utrùm Excommunicatio, quatenùs Religionem intelligentes & amplexantes, à Sacramentorum usu, propter admissum facinus arcet; mandato nitatur Divino, an excogitata sit ab hominibus* ([London: John Wolfe], 1589). Since the Latin version of the work is separated into 75 numbered theses, as are the later English translations, thesis numbers are included in addition to the page numbers. Latin quotations will be given in the notes and the documents (English and Latin) shall be collectively referred to as the *Explicatio gravissimae quaestionis*. The circumstances surrounding the publication of the treatise are discussed in the epilogue.

[35] Baker, "Church Discipline or Civil Punishment," 13.

[36] *Explicatio gravissimae quaestionis*, 14–15, 23–24, 61 (theses 31, 37, & 75).

person a Christian: "And indeed we are made members of Christ, that is, are joined to the internal and spiritual fellowship of Christ, and the faithful, by that faith alone which works by charity."[37] Because of this spiritual link to Christ through faith, Erastus maintained that association with the visible church and participation in its sacraments did not possess a necessary relationship to salvation. Since a person might belong to the visible church and not achieve salvation, being rejected from the visible church or cut off from its sacraments did not in itself damn a person because it was impossible for any human being to separate a true believer from Christ.[38] This was a sentiment shared by both Zwingli and Bullinger that had been earlier espoused by Marsilius of Padua, the great critic of the exalted powers of the medieval papacy.[39]

If participation in the visible church and her sacraments had no necessary relationship to a person's ultimate salvation, one could legitimately ask what role sacraments played. Though Erastus did not repudiate his late Zwinglian understanding of the sacraments as outlined in his earlier Eucharistic works, he placed stress in the *Explicatio gravissimae quaestionis* on the simple Zwinglian notion that the Lord's Supper served primarily as a commemoration of the death of Christ and thanksgiving for the redemption it achieved.[40] Erastus argued that personal faith alone remained far more important than participation in the sacrament. One of the reasons Erastus thought the concept of excommunication was wrongheaded was that it seemed to carry the reverse implication that salvation itself was limited to the sacraments.[41] Erastus thought it sent the wrong signal to forbid someone from participating while at the same time allowing them to attend sermons, since this would seem to suggest that sacraments were superior to preaching of the word.[42]

[37] Ibid., 2 (thesis 4). "Ac membra quidem Christi efficimur, id est, internae spiritualiq; Christi, & fidelium societati coniungimur, per solam fidem, quae charitatem est efficax."

[38] Ibid., 2–3 (theses 2–4). Zwingli had likewise argued that excommunication did not damn someone per se; rather, it was only a sign of damnation. See Stephens, *The Theology of Huldrych Zwingli*, 270–274. For a comparative look at the later Eucharistic theologies of Zurich and Geneva, see Rorem, "Calvin and Bullinger on the Lord's Supper."

[39] Walton, "Der Streit zwischen Thomas Erastus und Caspar Olevian," 234; Marsilius of Padua, *The Defender of the Peace*, trans. Alan Gerwirth (New York: Columbia UP, 1965) see vol. 2, ch. 6.

[40] *Explicatio gravissimae quaestionis*, 23–24 (thesis 37).

[41] Ibid., 58–60 (thesis 72).

[42] Ibid., 24–25 (thesis 38).

Sacraments played only a positive role in Erastus's thought as "incitements and allurements to religion and piety." Unlike his fellow partisans Sylvan and Brunner, who seemed to retreat to a strict memorial interpretation of the sacrament during the controversy over church discipline, Erastus still maintained the efficacy of the sacrament by arguing that "by the frequent use of these ordinances, rather than being deprived of them, people are made better;" whereas, "if men are deprived of this invitation they will never grow better but always worse."[43] Erastus also maintained that a person can commune to his or her "damnation" if he or she lacks faith.[44] While solemnity is needed in approaching sacraments to avoid the pitfall of "unworthy" eating, Erastus insisted that Christ taught believers to examine *themselves*—not one another.[45] Thus, Erastus would not limit access to the sacraments to Christians though naturally the unbaptized—"Mohammedans and unconverted pagans"—should not be allowed to commune.[46] Erastus conceived his opposition to the Calvinist disciplinary model as a battle to preserve the liberty of the individual Christian and to defend the exclusively positive function of the sacrament. This particular argument would have a long life among American and English Protestants, both in Stoddardeanism and Latitudinarianism.[47]

Since the sacraments functioned to nurture faith, Erastus argued that it was a cold irony that those who needed them most, manifest sinners, should be deprived of them. Erastus was convinced that the evangelical faith was only beginning to penetrate the hearts of the people in the Palatinate when the controversy over excommunication broke out. Erastus wryly mocked the enthusiasm of the disciplinists for excommunication, "when we neither had men to excommunicate or fit excommunicators; for scarcely a thirtieth part of the people did understand and approve of the reformed religion."[48] Rather than serving the good

[43] Ibid., 13 (thesis 19). "Sacramenta, incitamenta seu invitamenta esse ad pietatem: Et horum frequenti usu potius, quam privatione homines reddi meliores...."

[44] Ibid., 23–24 (thesis 37).

[45] Ibid., 22–23 (thesis 35).

[46] Ibid., 24–25 (thesis 38).

[47] See, for example, E. Brooks Holifield, "The Intellectual Sources of Stoddardeanism," *The New England Quarterly* 45 (1972): 372–392.

[48] *Explicatio gravissimae quaestionis*, introduction (A4^r): "Mirabar eos tum haec agitare consilia, cum neque excommunicandos, neque excommunicatores idoneos haberemus. Etenim vix trigesima populi pars doctrinam intelligebat, & approbabat." Translation from Erastus, *Theses of Erastus Touching Excommunication*, trans. Robert Lee (Edinburgh, 1844), 2.

of the people, Erastus asserted that the pro-consistory party was more concerned with strengthening ecclesiastical power by gaining the authority to take these "allurements to piety" away. In his opinion, the ministers should emphasize preaching the gospel and the proper use of sacraments in the attempt to nourish the Reformed faith among the populace. Both Erastus and disciplinists perceived the need for further Reformation of the Palatine church. Erastus offered the carrot; the disciplinists the stick.

Erastus likewise maintained that the entire idea of excommunication had become obsolete since it was tied to the Roman Church's sacramentalism. Excommunication had been used to heighten the role of the sacrament, which in turn had resulted in an increase of the church's power. Through this development, "excommunication made men look for salvation in the sacrament."[49] In the era of the Reformation, however, Protestants had rejected the sacramental system of medieval Catholicism. Erastus suggested that the natural corollary to this rejection was the repudiation of the practice of excommunication. Excommunication was an historical aberration, which Christians must now set aside like the many other "catholic errors."[50] Erastus had conducted preliminary historical researches to determine the origin of the custom. He believed that the practice began around 200 AD. Erastus did not impugn any ill-intent on the Christians who initiated the practice, although he did contend that excommunication should have ended with the conversion of the Roman Empire. He argued that the practice lived on, since bishops in Late Antiquity were reluctant to yield this power which enabled them to control kings. Whereas many theologians approved of the famous example of Ambrose's excommunication of Theodosius, Erastus condemned the action of this great Latin father and asserted that in excommunicating the emperor, Ambrose had erred more gravely than Theodosius himself.[51]

The church discipline controversy forced Erastus to rethink his conception of the relationship between church and state. In doing so he returned to the Scriptures and particularly the Old Testament (O.T.). Erastus's contemplation of the relationship between priest and ruler

---

[49] *Explicatio gravissimae quaestionis*, 58 (thesis 72): "ut Sacramentis salutem homines adscribere coeperint."

[50] Ibid., 56 (thesis 69): "errores catholicos."

[51] Ibid., 46–49, 57–58 (theses 59, 70). See also Walton, "Der Streit zwischen Thomas Erastus und Caspar Olevian," 239.

among the ancient Israelites made a definitive impact on his concept of church-state relations. The examples of the Hebrew kings of the O.T. seemed normative to Erastus since these rulers were analogous to the godly princes he served in Reformation Germany. In the O.T. he found no examples of dual governmental competencies. Therefore, he argued that there should be only one government in a Christian nation and asserted that the state should possess the exclusive right to punish wrong-doers.

In his vision of the relations between church and state, Erastus followed the well-marked line of his Swiss predecessors. The Zurich tradition had made little effort to differentiate the spheres of church and state and, as Walton has commented, "the basic institution that Zwingli thought of when he spoke of the church congregation was the political assembly of the city."[52] Erastus, likewise, did not distinguish between religious and civil authority. For example, he suggested that in the New Testament "synagogue," which generally denoted a place of assembly, and "Sanhedrin," the Jewish council, both referred to the same thing: a Jewish assembly of magistrates. Thus, to be "cast out" of the synagogue as described in John 9:22 was to suffer a civil rather than a religious penalty.[53] When he considered 1 Corinthians 5:5 and its admonition to "hand over this man to the devil," he likewise interpreted this "handing over" as turning the offending party over to the civil authorities.[54] He also argued that it transgressed the plain sense of the text to think that this "handing over to the devil" could have meant banishment from the sacrament. In this blurring of any possible distinction between a civil and a religious jurisdiction, all religious offenses became public offenses.[55]

This same association of the church body and the civil magistrate was made in Erastus's interpretation of the classic proof text for excommunication, Matthew 18:15–18.[56] This passage states that unrepented sins

[52] Walton, *Zwingli's Theocracy*, 129. Cf. Moeller, *Imperial Cities and the Reformation*, 46; Blickle *Gemeindereformation*, 98.

[53] *Explicatio gravissimae quaestionis*, 15–17 (thesis 22). Whereas "συναγωγη" generally means "gathering place," "συνεδριον" means council and specifically the Jewish high council in most N.T. usages. Cf. Bauer, *A Greek-English Lexicon*, 782 and 786.

[54] *Explicatio gravissimae quaestionis*, 46–49 (thesis 59). "παραδιδωμι."

[55] Cf. Heinz Schilling, "'History of Crime' or 'History of Sin?'—Some Reflections on the Social History of Early Modern Church Discipline," in *Politics and Society in Reformation Europe*, ed. E.I. Kouri and Tom Scott (London: MacMillan, 1987), 289–310.

[56] Oecolampadius, Bullinger, and Calvin had all used this passage to validate their arguments. For Oecolampadius, see Baker, "Church Discipline or Civil Punishment," 8;

should be told "to the church."[57] However, Erastus suggested that "to the church" actually meant "to the council."[58] This "council" was the magistrate rather than a church council. Erastus followed Zwingli here, who found that the city council was more than competent to make decisions on behalf of the church, although Erastus's unwillingness to perceive any separation between church and state was perhaps even stronger than Zwingli's.[59] Erastus allowed that Christians, if they were living in a non-Christian land (among "Turks or papists"), could set up an independent civil jurisdiction, like the Jewish Sanhedrin under the Romans.[60] However, were the magistrate Christian, this aspect of Matthew 18 no longer applied. Erastus here interpreted Matthew 18 through the lens of 1 Corinthians 6, where Christians were enjoined to settle their grievances amongst themselves rather than taking them before the courts of the heathens.[61] When proper Christian magistrates ruled, however, their

for Bullinger, see ibid., 13; for Calvin, see John T. McNeill, ed., *John Calvin: Institutes of the Christian Religion*, trans. Ford Lewis Battles (Philadelphia: Westminster, 1960), 4.22.2 & 3 (p. 1231).

[57] *Explicatio gravissimae quaestionis*, 26–29 (thesis 42). Whereas Zwingli considered the offenses discussed in Matthew 18 to be public, or sins against the whole church, Erastus considers them private grievances. Erastus took this from the line "if a brother sins against you." The key here is "against you," which is in the second person singular in the Greek "'εις σοι." Ironically, modern textual criticism is undecided as to whether this "against you" is actually part of the Greek text. Erastus suggests this passage is talking about the personal obligation of the individual Christian to forgive, and does not create an ecclesiastical mandate to punish offenses. Zwingli, alternatively thought the "against you" referred to the church corporately. E.J. Furcha and H. Wayne Pipkin, trans., *Huldrych Zwingli Writings*, 2 vols. (Pittsburgh: Pickwick, 1984), 1:227.

[58] *Explicatio gravissimae quaestionis*, 40 (thesis 52): "Tell it to the Church means nothing less than to tell it to the magistrate of your own people ..." (Dic Ecclesiae, non aliud significare, quam dic populi tui Magistratui ...). The Greek here is "'εκκλησια," which connotes "*the church* or *congregation* as a totality of Christians living in one place" in this passage. The range of meaning for "'εκκλησια," is quite large and does include the more general "assembly." (Bauer, *A Greek-English Lexicon*, 240–241.) This left Erastus room for interpretive play. Similar to his earlier conflation of "συναγωγη" with "συνεδριον" above, Erastus suggests "'εκκλησια" in this passage means "συνεδριον" as well. *Explicatio gravissimae quaestionis*, thesis 48.

[59] G.R. Potter, "Church and State, 1528: A Letter from Zwingli to Ambrosius Blarer (4 May 1528)," *Occasional Papers of the American Society for Reformation Research* (1977), 115. Zwingli states of the council: "if it reaches a conclusion, is there any reason why you should want a separate agreement from the church?" In this particular circumstance, Zwingli is more saying that the town magistrates are competent to decide for the church, rather than that the town council is itself the church.

[60] *Explicatio gravissimae quaestionis*, 62 (thesis 75).

[61] Ibid., 33–34 (thesis 47).

authority should not be duplicated. He argued that the church with the civil authority at its side had no need for excommunication: "We can now have no need to appoint for ourselves other judges and arbiters, besides the lawfully constituted magistracy."[62]

From Erastus's use of the concept of the Jewish Sanhedrin, it should be clear that biblical examples were crucial for Erastus. Erastus followed the Zurich tradition of interpreting New Testament practices through Old Testament analogies. Erastus offered the Passover celebration of the Jews as a guiding paradigm for present day Eucharistic practice.[63] Just as the Law of Moses did not prohibit anyone from partaking in the Passover because of sin, New Testament writers did not prohibit anyone from partaking in the Lord's Supper, since they could not void the Law.[64] The example of Christ confirmed Erastus's opinion, since Jesus ate the Last Supper with Judas, a manifest sinner, confirming Mosaic practice of an open Passover.[65] From these biblical examples Erastus concluded that "no baptized person is to be debarred from the Lord's table."[66]

Ultimately Erastus simply desired to avoid clerical whim in the control of the Eucharist. He knew from experience that earnest believers often suffered from church strife. His theses narrated the past tyranny of the Roman Church, and Erastus wanted no part in Olevianus's party's effort to reassert an analogous tyranny. Erastus displayed his implicit anticlericalism with the rhetorical question: "Can we hope for better terms, or greater moderation, from our modern men, than the world has experienced in their predecessors?"[67]

After receiving Beza's response, Erastus fortified his position with a voluminous *Confirmatio Thesium* which, at 280 pages, made up the bulk

---

[62] Ibid., 40–41 (thesis 52): "quemadmodum neque iudices & arbitros nunc necesse habemus nobis creare praeter legitimos magistratus."

[63] Ibid., 17–18 (thesis 25).

[64] Ibid., 18, 26–29 (theses 26, 42).

[65] Although the synoptic gospels appear to imply that Judas was present with Christ at the Last Supper (as Erastus likewise surmised), some patristic writers disputed this interpretation. The majority of patristic interpretation, according to Kenneth Hein, argued that Judas did in fact take part in the Last Supper, though he did so "unworthily." K. Hein, *Eucharist and Excommunication* (Bern: Herbert Lang, 1973) 38–50. Not surprisingly, Bullinger also advocated this position, as early as 1531. *Heinrich Bullinger Werke, 2. Abteilung Briefwechsel*, 1:213.

[66] *Explicatio gravissimae quaestionis*, 20 (thesis 30).

[67] Ibid., 60 (thesis 72): "An speramus nostrae aetatis homines meliores aut continentiores esse antiquis?"

of the printed *Explicatio Gravissimae Quaestionis*. The text lacked the vigor of the condensed theses but possessed all of its acerbity. Here is a listing of the book and chapter subdivisions with the chapter headings of the *Confirmatio*:

1. Preface (p. 67)
1.1 The definition of excommunication (p. 67)
1.2 On the degrees or parts of excommunication (p. 91)
1.3 Defense of the arguments against excommunication which are drawn from the Old Testament (p. 103)
1.4 Defense of the arguments which have been accepted from the New Testament (p. 111)
1.5 Confutation of the arguments of Beza which offer support for excommunication from the Old Testament (p. 126)

2.1 On [ritual] impurity of law and morals (p. 130)
2.2 Confutation of the arguments which have been made for excommunication from the new covenant (p. 152)

3.1 On the office and distinction of the magistrate (p. 159)
3.2 On the power of the Sanhedrin in the time of the Romans (p. 176)
3.3 Refutation of Beza's interpretation of the words of Christ: "Tell it to the Church." (p. 186)
3.4 Defense of the true interpretation of passage 1 Corinthians 5 (p. 211)
3.5 Confutation of the arguments for excommunication assembled from the passage of Paul in 1 Corinthians 5 (p. 232)
3.6 Concerning yeast (*fermentum*) [i.e., 1 Corinthians 5:6–8] (p. 240)
3.7 Defense of our understanding of yeast (p. 242)
3.8 Refutation of the arguments for excommunication out of private conviction and those drawn from 2 Thessalonians 3 (p. 247).
3.9 Refutation of certain other arguments for excommunication (p. 254)

4.1 On the presbytery (p. 258)
4.2 Defense of the arguments against the presbytery of excommunicators (p. 259)
4.3 Confutation of the arguments by which some suppose to establish their presbytery (p. 266)
4.4 Whether the Sanhedrin was a political magistracy (p. 275)
4.5 Confutation of the arguments on behalf of the presbytery cobbled together from the New Testament (p. 283)
4.6 Concerning the election of presbyters, from whose judgment they should be based, and when they were instituted (p. 285)
4.7 Whether the power of excommunication was in the hands of the presbytery (p. 294)

In the first lines of the preface, Erastus affirmed that excommunication or debarring people from the sacraments remained the topic in question; furthermore the present debate only considered individuals who possessed an understanding of the Christian faith, acknowledged their sinfulness, and nevertheless desired to take part in communion.[68] The first five books of the *Confirmatio* represented Erastus's reply to Beza, while the final book represented Erastus's replies to his Heidelberg colleagues.[69] Erastus's tone was markedly friendlier in his response to Ursinus compared to his rejoinder to Beza. At the end of the *Confirmatio*, Erastus's editor appended many letters from Zurich in support of Erastus.

Of particular interest in the *Confirmatio* is the first chapter of the third book entitled "On the Office and Distinction of the Magistrate." Here Erastus repeatedly asserted the unitary nature of political authority, based on both rational and biblical arguments, with lines such as:

> Since God, they say, hated all disorder, and wanted all things to be ordered in decency and propriety, he would have considered two heads in one body to be a monstrosity. Hence, in the Christian community he does not want there to be two distinct magistrates of equal power ruling the entire community. ... In summation, in a Christian state there is one magistrate, to whom is committed by God the external government of all things which belong either to civil life or to the life of Christian piety; that the right and authority of rule and jurisdiction has not been conceded to ministers or to any others.[70]

[68] *Confirmatio Thesium*, in *Explicatio Gravissimae Quaestionis*, 67.

[69] Bonnard, *Thomas Éraste*, 83–85.

[70] *Confirmatio Thesium*, in *Explicatio Gravissimae Quaestionis*, 161–162: "Deus, aiunt, cum oderit omnem ʿαταξιαν, & omnia velit ordine decenti & ʾευσχημονως fieri, duo in uno corpore capita ponere monstrosum putavit. Hinc in civitate Christiana non voluit duos esse magistratus distinctos aequali potestate totam civitatem regentes.... Summa est, Magistratum in Christiana Repub[lica] unicum esse, cui a Deo commissa sit gubernatio externa rerum omnium, quae vel ad civilem, vel ad piam & Christianam vitam pertinent: ius et autoritatem imperandi ac ius dicendi neque ministris neque aliis ullis concessum esse."

While the argument is rational and biblical, it relied more on the precedent of the Israelite state of the Old Testament than on the example of the nascent Christian community of the New Testament. Erastus argued, "Not a word may be produced from all of the books of the Old Testament which sanctions such a dual *imperium*, political and ecclesiastical."[71] After this blanket repudiation of dual authority he offered a proof of his claim with a summary history of the Israelite state from Moses to the Hasmoneans. This chapter is followed by a review of the power of the Sanhedrin in the Roman period. Erastus asserted that the Sanhedrin originally exercised jurisdiction over both sacred and political affairs. However, around the time of Christ most of the political authority passed into the hands of the Romans, leaving the Sanhedrin with ruling authority only over religious affairs. Nevertheless, it retained the power of the sword, that is, the right to inflict corporal punishments on malefactors, which is more associated with political authority, even as the Romans usurped some of the Sanhedrin's political competence. In Erastus's view, even if its jurisdiction had contracted, the Sanhedrin remained in essence a legitimate political magistracy.[72]

Despite his continued trumpeting of the superiority and indivisibility of political authority, Erastus remained rather anti-Erastian, in popular parlance, in his willingness to allow *any* political authority to establish religious policy. He struck something of a non-Erastian tone when he asserted: "In another [state], if perhaps the magistrate holds a false creed, the division of jurisdictions may in some sense appear tolerable."[73]

Not unlike the original theses, Erastus's views in the *Confirmatio* were chiefly based on his reading of Scripture, on this occasion fortified by a study of Josephus and the church fathers in addition to a more limited

[71] Ibid., 163: "Constat primum, nullum posse in omnibus libris testamenti veteris verbum ostendi, quo duplex istud imperium, Politicum & Ecclesiasticum approbetur."

[72] Ibid., 179–180: "Dixi Gabinii tempore, antequam Romani suos praesides Hierosolymis haberent, Synedrium habuisse potestatem de politicis & sacris rebus pariter iudicandi. At tempore Pilati aliorumque talium Praesidum, pars maxima huius potentiae ad Romanos transiit: ac relicta ipsi est de solis rebus ad religionem attinentibus iudicandi facultas. Haec autem non erat iurisdictio ecclesiastica, ut vos hodie à Politica discernitis: sed Politicae, quam prius totam possederat, pars erat. Nam ius gladii, carceris, plagarum, retinebant, quae vos ad ecclesiasticam potentiam pertinere negatis. Summa est, Magistratus erat legitimus & politicus quamvis non de omnibus causis, ut prius, sed de certis solum cognosceret."

[73] Ibid., 162: "In alia, in qua videlicet Magistratus falsam tuetur sententiam, certo quodam modo tolerabilis videri fortasse possit divisio rectionum."

knowledge of scholastic authorities. He does not reveal explicit dependence on many prior theologians or political theorists. He was aware of the earlier controversy within the French Reformed tradition associated with Jean Morély, who denied the presbytery power over excommunication, and noted with irony that Morély had been excommunicated by the Genevan Church for his views.[74] Erastus also cited the support of Peter Martyr Vermigli for his general conception of the unitary nature of political authority, but he conceded that Vermigli's view of the role of elders was quite different than his own. With the exception of the odd mention of Thomas Blarer of Constance and the Wurttemberg theologians' rejection of the dual order of presbyters, the work is relatively thin on references to sixteenth-century events or works.[75]

The main contention of Erastus's work was that prohibiting Christians from taking part in the sacraments had no biblical justification. This discovery had a decisive impact on his understanding of church discipline in general and church-state relations in particular. It is important, however, not to lose sight of Erastus's central concern: excommunication itself was the primary topic of his theses and their defense. Inherently related to excommunication was the institutional structure of church discipline. Likewise, any question of who should properly exercise discipline in a Christian commonwealth begged the question of the relationship between church and state. The development of Erastus's thought in the *Explicatio gravissimae quaestionis* can be compared to throwing a rock in a pond. The initial splash made by the rock was Erastus's decisive rejection of excommunication. The first surge caused by the splash was his reinterpretation of church discipline—though in line with the conventional Zurich model. The final wave created by the splash was his interpretation of church-state relations. In the conventional understanding of Erastianism, his ideas of church-state relations, viz., his denial of the validity of an independent ecclesiastical jurisdiction in a Christian state and the concomitant empowerment of the magistrate over the church, have been taken to epitomize his thought. Seen from within the context of the controversy, these "Erastian" ideas were not his central argument, but were the posture that he was driven to take in his attempt to refute the Gnesio-Calvinists' assertion that church discipline was mandated by divine law and was a mark of the true church. As Johann Heckel com-

[74] Ibid., 69–70.
[75] Ibid., 172–173, 291.

mented, "on the search for support for his view, he found a truly epoch-making juristic distinction."[76] Even here, however, Erastus was not essentially more radical than his Swiss predecessor Wolfgang Musculus. Erastus drew from him the dictum that "nature denies two authentic governments in the same people, whereof one is not to be subject to the other."[77] The force of Erastus's theses was directed at undercutting the rationale for an independent consistory to police morals; not recognizing the autonomous jurisdiction of the church vis-à-vis the state was simply a means to further this argument.[78]

To what extent was Erastus original and why did he become the most famous or infamous representative of the general Swiss-German view of church-state relations? As has been commonly observed, the notion that there can only be one legitimate sphere of power within a Christian state was not new with Erastus and flowed from the thought of Zwingli, Bullinger, and Musculus. Erastus's thought also shared some similarity with that of Peter Martyr Vermigli, whom he acknowledged.[79] Erastus was working within this tradition and the continuity of his thought with his forerunners' positions was more marked than his novelty. However, Erastus did frame his argument in a way which made both his Calvinist detractors and his later English partisans recognize that a line had been crossed and that Erastus's formulation represented a new type of challenge.

A key difference between Erastus and his predecessors was his polemical intensity. To a certain extent this polemical escalation flowed naturally from the genre of the works. Erastus, a master of the disputation, arranged his work in argumentative theses which sharpened the contrast between his views and those of his disciplinist colleagues. Whereas Bullinger's *Decades* and Musculus's *Loci Communes* offered rambling

[76] Johannes Heckel, "Cura religionis, Ius in Sacra, Ius circa Sacra," in *Festschrift Ulrich Stutz zum siebzigsten Geburtstag* [Kirchenrechtliche Abhandlungen 117–118] (Stuttgart: Ferdinand Enke, 1938), 292: "Auf der Suche nach Beweisen für seine Ansicht fand er nun eine wahrhaft epochemachende juristische Distinktion."

[77] *Explicatio gravissimae quaestionis*, introduction, [A5^r]: "Natura negat, (inquit Musculus) in eodem populo duas authenticas gubernationes, quarum una non sit alteri subiecta." See Wesel-Roth, *Thomas Erastus*, 110–112.

[78] It is important to remember Erastus's context and that his theses assumed a Christian magistrate. On other occasions he seemed to suggest that the precise church-political matrix was an issue of *adiaphora*.

[79] See John Patrick Donnelly, *Calvinism and Scholasticism in Vermigli's Doctrine of Man and Grace* (Leiden: Brill, 1976), 188.

textbook treatments which did not as a rule impose as strong a reading on the topics under consideration, Erastus's theses were intentionally posed in a confrontational manner. Erastus's presentation was a stake directed at the heart of the Calvinist disciplinary regime. Beza and Dathenus sensed this rhetorical and theological gap between Bullinger and Erastus and complained bitterly about Erastus's wholesale repudiation of their entire disciplinary system.[80] Thus, it was not by accident that later English divines focused on Erastus as a source of inspiration, nor that seventeenth century Presbyterian critics identified him as a figure who could perhaps be attacked without repudiating the entire German-speaking Swiss Reformed heritage.

A second difference was Erastus's assault on the concept of excommunication *in toto*. Whereas it had been common among the Swiss to leave definitive excommunication in the hands of secular authorities and in a de facto sense make excommunication a dead issue, they still tended to more or less accept the concept of excommunication even if in a severely limited form. Since consistorial discipline with excommunication was cherished by their Genevan brethren, with whom they wanted to maintain cordial relations, the general tendency of their rhetoric was to regard the specific form of discipline as a matter of adiaphora. While the Zurich and Bernese church leaders might have worked assiduously to curb the expansion of Calvin's model outside of Geneva, which they did successfully in the case of the Vaud and attempted to do in Heidelberg, they still did not want to demonize their coreligionists. As we have seen, Erastus went far beyond this and boldly proclaimed that the entire concept of excommunication was without theological justification or biblical merit. This impolitic assertion seems to have limited Erastus's appeal in Heidelberg in the 1560s, as men like Ursinus, who agreed that the conditions were not propitious for the erection of consistorial discipline, nevertheless could not stomach Erastus's sweeping repudiation of so much of the conventional wisdom.

Closely related to this point was Erastus's rejection of the claim that presbyterial authority was founded upon divine right. For Erastus, presbyterial authority was only an ad hoc arrangement for jurisdictions that were not blessed to live under a Christian sovereign. In making this argument, he elevated the vision of ancient Hebrews living under monarchy as the apposite model for how church-state relations should oper-

[80] Discussed below.

ate in a Christian society. This naturally relates to a further contribution of Erastus, which was his exposition of an alternative hermeneutical basis for the Zurich-Bern vision of church-state relations. Zwingli and Musculus had previously intimated that the kings of the ancient Israelites were appropriate models for contemporary Christian princes. Erastus buttressed this assertion with an investigation of the role of the Sanhedrin in Jewish life in the era both immediately prior to and after the time of Christ, based on a close reading of Josephus. Given that his seventeenth-century followers Thomas Coleman, John Selden, and John Lightfoot were formidable Hebrew scholars, Erastus's treatise and his reply to Beza offered these followers a powerful historical counter-argument to wield against the *de jure divino* claims of the advocates of presbyterial discipline.[81] While Erastus may have been inspired in part by one of the sixteenth century's greatest Hebraists in Pellikan and, in turn, inspired some of the seventeenth century's greatest Hebrew scholars to adopt a similar position, his own opinions were apparently based on Greek and Latin language sources rather than an intimate knowledge of Semitic texts.

Viewed from the perspective of the social history of ideas, Erastus's thought displayed a marked continuity with two powerful pre-Reformation tendencies. His vision of church-state relations largely reflected that of the cities and towns of pre-Reformation Switzerland and southwestern Germany. These communities had been usurping ecclesiastical jurisdictions before the Reformation and the acceptance of the Protestant gospel merely consolidated this process.[82] Thus, while there may have been notions borrowed from such theorists as Marsilius of Padua in Erastus's thought, Erastus's Swiss civic heritage supplied the animating force to his theory.[83] The novelty of Erastus is that, rather than delivering power over the church into the hands of a quasi-republican city council, the Heidelberg context pushed this transfer into the hands of the Christian prince. Since both types of government were dominated by a thin layer of individuals at the top of the social hierarchy, the difference between the Swiss canton and the German principality was not perhaps as large

[81] See *Confirmatio thesium*, in *Explicatio gravissimae quaestionis*, 176–186; 269–283. See Johann P. Sommerville, "Hobbes, Selden, Erastianism, and the History of the Jews," in *Hobbes and History*, ed. G.A.J. Rogers and Tom Sorell (London: Routledge, 2000) 168–174.

[82] See Moeller, *Imperial Cities and the Reformation.*

[83] On the influence of Marsilius on Bullinger and the Swiss, see Walton, "Der Streit zwischen Thomas Erastus und Caspar Olevian," 234.

as one might conventionally imagine. Bullinger and Gwalther, along with Erastus, felt that this model of church discipline was equally applicable to a principality.

A concomitant force was also evident in the writings of Erastus—anticlericalism. Recent research has established how pervasive anticlericalism was in southwestern Germany on the eve of the Reformation.[84] For many of these Germans, one of the primary components of the "freedom of the Christian" was the liberation from clerical tyranny. This pre-Reformation sentiment survived as a driving force in Erastus's thought. Related to this theme was Erastus's reprise of the early Protestant rhetorical strategy of contrasting the church's rules and traditions, "the laws of man," with the clear teaching of the Bible. Ironically here, Erastus made the Calvinist church leaders, rather than the Catholic authorities, the purveyors of corrupted and tyrannical tradition. The original impulse of Erastus's "Erastianism" was not to grant the Leviathan state dominion over the church, but to preserve Christian liberty from state-sanctioned clerical oppression.

Strife in Heidelberg and Beyond

In Erastus's estimation, a five-man cadre drove the movement to establish a church consistory on a Genevan model in Heidelberg: Zuleger, Olevianus, Dathenus, Ehem, and Konrad Marius.[85] The only one of these men to have undertaken proper theological studies was Dathenus. The other four were more properly legal scholars by education, though both Zuleger and Olevianus had at least logged a few months at Calvin's feet in Geneva. With his leading position in the church, Olevianus headed the disciplinist party, leading some to dub the group "Olevianists." Even the usually mild Ursinus judged that Olevianus "reigned" over Zuleger, Ehem, and the elector himself.[86] Although he served as the chief agitator for the independent consistory and obviously cared deeply about its implementation, Olevianus did not take up the pen himself to advocate the system or refute Erastus and Sylvan. The Bohemian Zuleger, who

[84] See Peter D. Dykema and Heiko A. Oberman, eds. *Anticlericalism in Late Medieval and Early Modern Europe* [*SMRT* 51] (Leiden: Brill, 1993).

[85] Erastus to Bullinger, Nov. 21, [1569], StAZ, E II 361, fol. 77.

[86] "Causa est, quia Olevianus Zulegerum, hic Ehemium, hic Josiam [Frederick] regit." Ursinus to Crato, Nov. 9, 1575. Sudhoff, *C. Olevianus und Z. Ursinus*, 393, Press, *Calvinismus und Territorialstaat*, 250.

became the president of the church council and grew into a formidable player at court, was with or ahead of Olevianus at every step. The two appear to have been the primary instigators behind the controversial iconoclasm campaign of 1564–1565. With Zuleger, Olevianus, and Marius all ensconced on the church council, it is clear where their chief strength lay. The cooperation of this trio had its origins in their days as law students in Bourges, where they participated in the underground Huguenot church.[87] The jurist Ehem had by this point yielded his university position to serve at court. He was a fixture of Palatine politics for decades and even returned to Heidelberg as chancellor during the regency of Johann Casimir. Wesel-Roth offered something of a Machiavellian interpretation of Ehem's role in this process, and went so far as to suggest that the later "terror" policies of the church council, which stifled the internal dissent, were useful to Ehem as it gave him a free hand in external political affairs.[88] The interventionist Palatine foreign policy on behalf of the Dutch and French Reformed communities and the Calvinist disciplinist urge were clearly related phenomena, but they did not necessarily follow each other in lock step. Marius was likewise a committed Calvinist who also happened to be Ehem's brother-in-law.[89] Dathenus was a stirring preacher and tireless organizer who was credited with fomenting iconoclasm in the Netherlands and whose intemperate rhetoric would later provoke the wrath of William the Silent.[90] As this conflict reached its high point, Dathenus took the lead in representing the cause of the Palatine disciplinists to foreign Reformed churches and may have briefly eclipsed Olevianus as the leader of the disciplinist faction. This was a tight, genuinely Calvinist group that was also passionately committed to assisting the struggle of their Reformed brethren in France and the Netherlands.

Though the theological faculty favored the Calvinist vision of church discipline over the Zurich system, it is important to note that the impetus for adopting a purer Calvinist system came more from within the upper echelon of the church itself rather than from the university. Nevertheless, the all-foreign theological faculty (one Frenchman, Boquin, and two Italians, Tremellius and Zanchi) played a significant role in promoting

[87] Goeters, "Olevianus als Theologe," 290–291.
[88] Wesel-Roth, *Thomas Erastus*, 65.
[89] Press, *Calvinismus und Territorialstaat*, 243.
[90] Phyllis Mack Crew, *Calvinist Preaching and Iconoclasm in the Netherlands, 1544–1569* (Cambridge: Cambridge UP, 1978); Johan Decavele, "Petrus Dathenus," in *OER*, 1:464–465; C.V. Wedgwood, *William the Silent* (New York: Norton, 1968) 195–198.

the disciplinists' aims. Both Boquin and Zanchi authored memoranda that favored the erection of consistorial discipline.[91] Tremellius's views are more difficult to discern, though his closest associations were with the disciplinists.[92] Along with writing on behalf of the Calvinist system, the foreigners' church in Heidelberg, where these theologians worshipped and ministered, served as the prototype for implementing the consistory model on the rest of the Palatinate. Indeed, these three served as the first elders in the foreigners' church consistory.[93]

As many contemporaries remarked, there was a split in support of the parties between the German and foreign populace in the Palatinate, with the foreigners (chiefly French and Netherlandish) lining up solidly in the disciplinist camp.[94] Of all the foreign groups, the Dutch were the most numerous and influential in the Palatinate. Dutch refugees had streamed into the Palatinate since the early 1560s. They possessed a large community at Frankenthal that would prove one of the most important refugee gatherings outside of Emden.[95] The Dutch presence was becoming so burdensome that Erastus quipped in a letter to Bullinger, "They should add to the litany: 'Save us from the Netherlanders, O Lord.' "[96] The sense of excessive Dutch influence became extreme in April of 1569 when Elector Frederick married the Baroness Amalie von Neuenahr zu Limburg, the widow of Hendrik van Brederode, one of the leaders of the Dutch revolt. Erastus heaped scorn on the marriage in a contemporary letter to Bullinger and thought it revealed the mani-

---

[91] Boquin's memorandum has not been identified among his printed works. "H. Zanchius ad Illustrissimum Principem Fridericum III. De Excommunicatione," *Operum theologicorum* ([Geneva?]: Stephanus Gamonetus, 1605), 7(2):139–147. Zanchi's position can also be observed in his letter to Johannes Wolf in *Hieronymi Zanchii Bergomatis, Theologi Clarissimi, Epistolarum Libri Duo* ... (Hanau: Antonius, 1609), 63–64. Burchill has argued that Zanchi, like Ursinus, "sought to maintain the middle ground." Burchill, "Girolamo Zanchi: Portrait of a Reformed Theologian and His Work" *SCJ* 15 (1984): 201.

[92] One circumstantial piece of evidence for Tremellius's likely pro-disciplinist position is that Pigafetta waited until he had become rector to launch his accusations against Erastus. See below.

[93] Erastus to Bullinger, July 8, (15)69, StAZ, E II 346a, fol. 551^{v}: "Ecclesiam instituerunt Gallicam, qualis olim Argentinae erat: in qua iam Seniores instituti sunt, Boquinus, Tremelius, Zanchus." Benrath, "Die Korrespondenz zwischen Bullinger und Thomas Erastus," 119.

[94] Horn, "Johann Sylvan," 251–257; Wesel-Roth, *Thomas Erastus*, 60. Alternatively, Horn notes that the Polish students tended to favor Erastus.

[95] Schaab, *Geschichte der Kurpfalz*, 2:101.

[96] Erastus to Bullinger, Feb. 2, 1569, Zurich, Staatsarchiv des Kantons Zürich, MS E II 346a, fols. 549–550: "Man solt in die Letanei gesetzt haben/ à Niderlandris, libera nos Domino, sagt iener."

fest hypocrisy of the disciplinists for matching the pious elector with this young, luxury-loving widow.[97] This scandalous marriage, tying one of the highest ranking princes to someone below his station, was a clear revelation of the strength of the Dutch-disciplinist party in Heidelberg.

There were a number of significant individuals who adopted a moderate stance on the church discipline question or whose positions have not been investigated in depth. For example, one would not have expected that the noted Philippist Lutheran theologian Victorinus Strigel, who had only joined the university and church council in 1567, would have been naturally inclined to support the Geneva program. His death in June of 1569 robbed the anti-disciplinists of a potential ally.

It is likewise difficult to categorize Ursinus's position as a straightforward endorsement of the disciplinist cause. The controversy itself unnerved Ursinus, and he attempted to remain above the partisan fray. As a true student and spiritual heir of Melanchthon, Ursinus has been the subject of much debate regarding whether he should ultimately be labeled a "Lutheran" or a "Calvinist." Often assessed merely between the poles of Wittenberg and Geneva, he remained in much closer contact with Bullinger and company than with Calvin and Beza.[98] Though history has rightly recognized Ursinus as the most perspicacious theologian of the Heidelberg Reformed, he never possessed the personal influence there that Calvin exercised in Geneva, or Melanchthon exercised in Wittenberg—a fact he himself bemoaned.[99] He had given up his position on the university faculty to dedicate all his labors to training pastors at the *Collegium Sapientiae*. He was not a member of the church council and never played a large role in church politics.[100] Ursinus was a retiring personality whose small tolerance for controversy had already been exhausted. After the Maulbronn colloquy, he was extremely reluctant to step into theological conflict as he demonstrated at Amberg to the

[97] Erastus to Bullinger, March 6, 1569, StAZ, E II 361, fols. 14–14av. Press, *Calvinismus und Territorialstaat*, 253 and Benrath, "Die Korrespondenz zwischen Bullinger und Thomas Erastus," 116–117. The "Bildnis des Kurfürsten Friedrich III. des Frommen von der Pfalz und seiner beiden Gemahlinnen Maria von Brandenburg-Kulmbach und Amalia von Neuenahr" can be seen at the Haus der Bayrischen Geschichte (http://www.hdbg.de/).

[98] Benrath, "Briefe des Heidelberger Theologen Zacharias Ursinus," 96–97.

[99] Benrath, "Briefe des Heidelberger Theologen Zacharias Ursinus," 98. Cf. Peter Lillback, "Ursinus's Development of the Covenant of Creation: A Debt to Melanchthon or Calvin?" *Westminster Theological Journal* 43 (1981): 247–288.

[100] Burchill, "On the Consolation of a Christian Scholar," 573.

disappointment of Frederick. In the controversy over church discipline, one has the sense that his personal sympathies were on the side of the anti-disciplinists, but that he could not endorse the extremes of Erastus's position. The discord that the protracted controversy had sown in the young church both depressed and enraged Ursinus. Erastus considered Ursinus a close friend, as he revealed in a later letter of recommendation to Abraham Musculus in Bern. Erastus proclaimed of Ursinus, "no one who lives under the sun is dearer to me," but he also stated, "he has his peculiar customs, which are not approved of by all."[101] Regarding Ursinus's "peculiar customs," Erastus was perhaps referring to his melancholy cast, his perpetual complaining, and his tendency to withdraw from worldly affairs. At any rate, Erastus was no doubt disappointed that he did not receive Ursinus's full support, and relations between the two men apparently grew tense during the controversy.[102]

In fact, Ursinus opposed both factions in the conflict over church discipline. He was angry that the disciplinist church leaders were pushing their vision of an enhanced disciplinary regime at an inopportune occasion. Yet he was angrier still with their espousal of an interventionist foreign policy on behalf of the French and Dutch Protestants. On the very eve of Withers's doctoral defense, Ursinus sent a memorandum to the elector both lamenting the fact that the church was provided with "inept pastors" and that the church council was "torn, discordant, dreaming of an untimely discipline." He further decried their neglect of their primary vocation and declared that they were "more concerned with war than with peace."[103] A year later Ursinus was still despondent about the state of the Palatine church. Ursinus not only poured his scorn upon the "new schemes" of the disciplinists, but he also faulted Erastus himself and his group of partisans in a letter to Johannes Crato von Krafftheim. "Erastus is the head of the faction against ecclesiastical censor: his followers are

[101] Erastus to A. Musculus, Nov. 23, (15)77. Autograph, Zofingen, no. 1.53: "Putavi, neminem sub sole vivere, qui amicior mihi esset." "Sed suos habet mores peculiares, qui non omnibus probantur."

[102] In his preface to the *Explicatio gravissimae quaestionis*, Erastus mentions giving his theses to be judged by an individual "I esteemed to be as dear a friend to me as was living" (*quo mihi amiciorem vivere neminem putabam*), [A6^v]. This comment would seem to refer to Ursinus, especially in view of Erastus's comment to Abraham Musculus quoted above.

[103] "Monita D.D. Ursini Friderico III. Electori proposita per Steph. Cirlerum camerae secretarium 1568 26. Maii," in Kluckhohn, *Briefe Friedrich des Frommen*, 2(2):1053–1055. "Senatum ecclesiasticum esse lacerum, discordem, immaturam disciplinam somniantem, quique hoc tempore magis bello quam pace sit occupatus" (p. 1054). See Press, *Calvinismus und Territorialstaat*, 264; Visser, *Zacharias Ursinus*, 147–170.

Xylander, Sylvan, [Johann] Willing—this one indeed an unlearned and arrogant demagogue; they infect many in the school and among the ministers."[104] Such a comment to their mutual friend Crato supplies the background to understand Erastus's contemporaneous exclamation: "Ursinus rages, although he does not differ much from us. Were he not insane, he would be able to agree with us."[105]

On the question of church discipline, however, Ursinus did not agree with Bullinger and Erastus, or with Olevianus for that matter. At the request of the elector, Ursinus wrote a brief "Judgment on Ecclesiastical Discipline and Excommunication" that most commentators have assessed as having come down between the two camps.[106] Though he rejected Erastus's outright repudiation of the power of the keys and dismissed many of the proof texts with which Erastus supported his position, he clearly did not see church discipline as the panacea that his Calvinist colleagues did. Unlike Erastus and the Zurich theologians, he did think that the church had a role to play in discipline, which could be exercised along the consistory model. He did not think that this body should be independent of state control, however, and also thought that excommunication itself should be extremely rare. In short, Ursinus considered church discipline to be quite biblical in theory but that its implementation should be restricted only to the most exceptional cases. While Erastus obviously recognized their disagreement, he both respected Ursinus's response and felt that the gap between them was less than that

[104] Zacharias Ursinus to Crato, Nov. 3, 1569. Quoted in J.F.A. Gillet, *Crato von Crafftheim und seine Freunde: Ein Beitrag zur Kirchengeschichte*, 2 vols. (Frankfurt/M., 1860–1861), 2:498–500 (no. 34) and Bonnard, *Thomas Éraste*, 80 (with the key section translated from Greek into Latin): "Erastus caput factionis est contra censuram ecclesiasticum (εκκλησιαστικην); asseclae Xylander, Sylvanus, Villingus, et hic quidem δημηγορος indoctus et superbus."

[105] Erastus to Bullinger, Nov. 21, [1569], StAZ, E II 361, fol. 77: "Ursinus furit, quamquam à nobis param absit. Nisi insaniret, posset nobis convenire." Discussed in Visser, *Zacharias Ursinus*, 152. Erastus also made an off-hand comment in a letter to Volcher Coiter revealing some strain with Ursinus: "Causam irae Ursinus nullam habuit," Aug. 28, n.y. [ca. 1570–1575], Basel, Öffentliche Bibliothek der Universität Basel, MS G2 II 37, fol. 11. This remark suggests that Ursinus's displeasure with Erastus had been widely communicated amongst the larger Crato-Ursinus circle.

[106] Zacharias Ursinus, "Judicium de Disciplina Ecclesiastica et Excommunicatione: Ad Electorem Fridericum III. Pium, Anno 1569," in *Opera Theologica*, 3:801–812. Wesel-Roth, *Thomas Erastus*, 59; Visser, *Zacharias Ursinus*, 151–154; Burchill, "On the Consolation of a Christian Scholar," 573–574. Ursinus's position can also be observed from his catechetical lectures which in no way agreed with Erastus's position. *The Commentary of Dr. Zacharias Ursinus on the Heidelberg Catechism*, 440–463.

of others who had opposed him.[107] He was also encouraged that Ursinus did not want to give the consistory jurisdiction over excommunication with no governmental oversight. Derk Visser has emphasized that though Ursinus did take up a position against Erastus, he was soon reconciled to him, and unlike Olevianus and his partisans, he never broke off communication with Bullinger.[108] Many years later Erastus reported to Gwalther that Ursinus's opinion on church discipline had moved further from the Gnesio-Calvinists, but that he feared making this public.[109]

While the anti-disciplinists were clearly isolated within the church hierarchy, they were well represented at court and within the university.[110] With good reason, past accounts have viewed Erastus as the linchpin of the anti-disciplinist faction. With his position at the university and his relationships within the church and at court based on his former position on the church council, he was a natural focal point for the opposition. Though most of the top clerics and university theologians were in the disciplinist camp, the opposition also had support within the church, if in general from somewhat disaffected pastors.

The most highly placed cleric on the side of the anti-disciplinists was the court preacher Johannes Willing. He played his most prominent role in Palatine politics in the period preceding the Augsburg diet of 1566, and he remained on especially good terms with Count Palatine Johann Casimir. Though Erastus expressed confidence in his ability and his character, most historians have suggested that personal ambition drove his passion for the anti-disciplinist cause. After the fact, Sylvan alleged that Willing had egged on the entire opposition movement in an attempt to replace Olevianus as head of the church.[111] Eventually, Willing

[107] Erastus to Grynaeus, Jan. 24, [1570], Basel UB, G II 4, fol. 278: "Scripsi nuper, me respondisse Bezae, et tribus aliis, Boquino, Zancho, Ursino. Hic à nobis minimum dissentit in rei substantia."

[108] Benrath, "Briefe des Heidelberger Theologen Zacharias Ursinus," 97; Visser, *Zacharias Ursinus*, 154.

[109] In the context of composing a new confession, Erastus asks Gwalther: "Vellem te ipsi scribere, ut in Confessione scribenda non misceat negocium Excommunicationis, quae fit exclusione à sacramentis, ne novae oriantur turbae. Scio eum rem intelligere. Sed quia semel contradixit ferociter, non vellet videre erravisse." Erastus to Gwalther, Nov. 15, 1577, Zurich, Zentralbibliothek, MS A 49, 310–311.

[110] See Appendix A for faculty roster as of Dec. 22, 1568.

[111] Sylvan to Erastus, Heidelberg, [October] 1570, Heidelberg, Universitätsarchiv Heidelberg, MS A-160/10, fol. 179. Printed in Hans Rott, ed. "Neue Quellen für eine Aktenrevision des Processes gegen Sylvan und seine Genossen," *Neues Archiv für die Geschichte der Stadt Heidelberg und der rheinischen Pfalz* 8 & 9 (1910 & 1911): 14–16: "Clarum est,

would lose his high standing in the church through his intrigue with the anti-disciplinists. He does not appear to have been involved in the Antitrinitarian affair and died of natural causes before the resolution of Sylvan's case.[112]

Johann Sylvan stood out as the most theologically astute cleric among the anti-disciplinists.[113] Little is known about Sylvan's early life other than the fact that he seems to have been born in the South Tyrol, in modern Italy. After studies at the University of Vienna where he took a licentiate in theology, Sylvan took employment as a court preacher in the service of the bishop of Würzburg. Thus Sylvan was born, educated and spent much of his early professional life within the old church. This commitment, however, would not endure. Sylvan was an open and reflective person for whom the quest for theological certainty must have seemed something like peeling off the layers of an onion in a perpetual quest for purer truth. Such intellectually malleable individuals like Sylvan found themselves conversion prone in this highly charged confessional era, and he in fact would travel a path from Catholicism to Lutheranism to the Reformed faith and, ultimately, Antitrinitarianism. He desperately wanted to reverse the final step, but his judges would not oblige.

While in the employ of the bishop of Würzburg, Sylvan came under the influence of Lutheran preaching at the diet of Regensburg. His conversion to Lutheranism followed after he had been charged with the task of defending the Catholic view of justification. He left the Catholic diocese of Würzburg and found refuge in Lutheran Württemberg. The Swabians were originally uncertain whether his conversion was genuine, but a printed confession of faith served to vouch for his sincerity.[114] He did not tarry long in the Lutheran camp, though. One of his first Protestant works was an attack on images, the underlying assumptions of which

---

et Willingum mera ambitione eo venisse quo ampliorem haberet materiam exagitandi senatum ecclesiasticum." Summarized in Burchill, *The Heidelberg Antitrinitarians*, 99.

112 Willing was relieved of his duties on the church council and resigned his position as court preacher in the spring of 1569. He first took a position at the *Peterskirche* in Heidelberg, where he replaced another anti-disciplinist Adam Neuser. He was then transferred to Bretten and later became Johann Casimir's court preacher in Kaiserlautern until he was released from this position in the spring of 1572. He died on July 10, 1572. Benrath, "Die Korrespondenz zwischen Bullinger und Thomas Erastus," 118, 137–140. See Seeling, *Johannes Willing (1525–1572)*.

113 Regarding Sylvan's life, see Horn, "Johann Sylvan," 219–310; Burchill, *The Heidelberg Antitrinitarians*, 21–27; Karlheinz Blaschke, "Johannes Sylvanus," *OER*, 4:132.

114 Brenz originally deemed his *Bekenntnis* "too harsh," and it had to be modified to please the Württembergers. Burchill, *The Heidelberg Antitrinitarians*, 29.

appeared to share more with Reformed thought than Lutheranism, and soon he found that he disagreed with the Lutheran interpretation of the Lord's Supper and particularly the doctrine of ubiquity. Fortunately for Sylvan, his doctrinal difficulties coincided with the Palatinate's turn to the Reformed faith, and pastors of his caliber had little difficulty finding employment in Frederick's church. He seems to have been placed in Kaiserslautern in early 1563, where he had something of a stormy relationship with his parishioners. They did not take kindly to his unilaterally renaming their children at the baptismal font to prevent giving the child a saint's name—proving that the disciplinists had not quite cornered the market on excessive zeal. Matthaeas Vehe-Glirius, the future Antitrinitarian and source of an entertaining account of the trip to Speyer that would prove their undoing, served as his deacon in Kaiserslautern. Since Sylvan's presence was increasingly required for theological and diplomatic tasks from the center of Heidelberg, he was transferred to Heidelberg, then more suitably assigned the post of superintendent at nearby Ladenburg. Christopher Burchill has compared his position to that of Ursinus, who like Sylvan was requested by the elector to compose a written opinion on the issue of church discipline.[115]

Another leader of the anti-disciplinist movement was the Heidelberg cleric Adam Neuser. We have already discussed his activities with reference to his possible participation in the authorship of the Heidelberg Catechism. Neuser's origins are even less certain than Sylvan's, though it is known that he was from Brandenburg-Ansbach, and it has been suggested that he studied with Wolfgang Musculus in Bern.[116] Neuser was on good terms with the Swiss in general, and the Bernese in particular, as many students from Bern lodged in his home in Heidelberg. Though he did not possess an illustrious academic pedigree, contemporaries judged him an able theologian. In fact, the university senate had favored appointing him to the third chair of theology over Olevianus, though the elector overruled them.[117] Later a rivalry with Olevianus would become evident, though it would be premature to suggest that it festered from 1561 onward. A theologian of some talent, Neuser purportedly defended the anti-disciplinist position at Withers's doctoral

[115] Horn, "Johann Sylvan," 240; Burchill, *The Heidelberg Antitrinitarians*, 32, 86. He also refused to baptize one child since the chosen godfather "sei ein turck, ein Judt." Sylvan's views can be fairly clearly perceived in his letter to Johannes Wolf, Sept. 1, 1568, published in Horn, 297–300; Synopsis in Burchill, *The Heidelberg Antitrinitarians*, 77–78.

[116] Burchill, *The Heidelberg Antitrinitarians*, 107–111.

[117] Ibid., 113.

disputation. His opposition to the plans of the church council likely was the root cause of his demotion from his position at the *Peterskirche*. His new job, serving under Olevianus at the *Heiliggeistkirche*, no doubt only added to his growing sense of alienation. It was also alleged that Neuser was overly fond of alcohol, a claim that critical historians accept. Even more so than in the case of Sylvan, Neuser must have realized by this point that his career in Heidelberg had run its course, and he was looking to relocate long before his Antitrinitarian beliefs were exposed.[118]

The anti-disciplinists' real strength did not lie in the church but at court and in the university. While the theological faculty was more or less behind the disciplinists, the anti-disciplinists predominated on the arts and medical faculties.[119] In addition to Erastus, the medical professor Sigismund Melanchthon (1537–1573) actively resisted the disciplinary regime, even refusing to take a seat on the consistory when it was eventually put in place in 1573. On the arts faculty, Wilhelm Xylander and Simon Grynaeus were solidly in Erastus's camp, while the other faculty members do not seem to have played an active role in the controversy.[120] Xylander's facility as perhaps the premier scholar of classical Greek in the empire was an obvious asset.[121] The instructor at the preparatory arts *Paedagogium*, Christoph Schilling, who later became caught in a turf war between the church council and the university, and the *Dionysianum* praeceptor, Timotheus Mader, were both associates of Erastus, which likely explains the level of hostility they later incurred from the disciplinist regime.[122] The university provided a safe haven for Erastus and later proved its loyalty by electing him rector of the university in the midst of the Antitrinitarian affair.

Erastus possessed a long list of allies at court. Though they were a clear majority on the high council, the most influential of all the councilors,

[118] Ibid., 107–108. Neuser's facility in the local dialect may have also enhanced his popular appeal. Alting, *Historia de ecclesiis Palatinis*, 102–103 (ch. 60).

[119] Unlike the later conflict in England, in the Heidelberg controversy the jurists did not play a leading role.

[120] Regarding Xylander, see Fr. Schöll in *ADB*, 44:582–598.

[121] After Xylander's death Erastus discussed his desire to have his annotated translation of the New Testament published. Apparently Xylander's interpretation of the key N.T. proof texts for church discipline (especially Matt. 18) was very favorable to Erastus's position. I have not been able to discover whether Xylander's translation was ever published. Erastus to Grynaeus, Sept. 14, (15)77, Basel UB, G II 4, fol. 209.

[122] Wesel-Roth, *Thomas Erastus*, 74; Burchill, "Die Universität zu Heidelberg," 243. For Mader, see Dagmar Drüll, ed., *Heidelberger Gelehrtenlexikon 1386–1651* (Berlin: Springer, 2002), 364–365.

Ehem, was not on their side. According to Volker Press, the chief steward Pleikard Landschad, the marshal Christoph von Gottfart, the justice of the peace Hartmann Hartmani, and the chancellor Christoph Prob all opposed the Calvinist disciplinary effort. Likewise, Frederick's secretary Stephan Cirler was especially close to Erastus and backed his resistance. Even the Count Palatine Johann Casimir, who frequently engaged in military efforts on behalf of the French and Dutch Protestants, rejected the disciplinists' aims. When one surveys the impressive support the anti-disciplinists possessed, it is not difficult to understand how confident they were that the elector would not make any radical innovations.[123]

The storm over church discipline raged through the summer and into the fall of 1568 in Heidelberg. By October an effort was underway to suppress the controversy. A letter from Erastus to Elector Frederick recounts an effort to confiscate the transcriptions of his theses in the students' possession. Alarmed that he was being portrayed as the troublemaker, Erastus defended himself by explaining the evolution of the controversy. He asked rhetorically why he should not be able to write, since he only sought the truth in harmony with the Scriptures. Erastus reported that he had sent the theses to Bullinger and Beza for their judgment but that he had not distributed them widely. However, the theses had circulated farther than he had realized. He belatedly sent an exemplar to Frederick, when he learned that a copy had made it into the elector's hands without his preface. Erastus mooted his intention to translate the theses into German so the prince could see for himself their mildness and scriptural integrity. Erastus entreated the elector not to believe that he sought to stir up dissention with the theses but that he had only sought the truth in humility.[124]

Apparently Erastus's effort succeeded in preventing his work from being confiscated, but he could not halt the effort to limit public debate on excommunication. With the elector's blessing, the theology faculty of the university took action to quiet the situation on October 14, 1568 by disallowing faculty from outside disciplines from taking part in theological disputations. This is sometimes described in the literature as the

[123] Press, *Calvinismus und Territorialstaat*, 249; Benrath, "Die Korrespondenz zwischen Bullinger und Thomas Erastus," 119; Wesel-Roth, *Thomas Erastus*, 60.

[124] Erastus to Friedrich, Oct, 6. [1568]. The letter exists in two copies: Heidelberg, Universitätsbibliothek, MS Cod. Pal. germ. 839, fols. 62–63 and Karlsruhe, General-Landesarchiv, Kopialbuch 961, fols. 108–114. Both manuscripts are apparently scribal copies, though the Heidelberg exemplar has a brief postscript in Erastus's hand.

prince's "*hofbefehl*" or at other times "silence order" on the question of church discipline, though it is not manifestly clear how extensive this injunction was.[125] Accepting this directive went against the grain of normal university politics, as universities strove to preserve their liberties from princely interference. The senate's protocol indicates a fair amount of discord over the proposed limitation. The rector equivocated on the policy, declaring: "No one was to mix themselves in theological disputations, unless to the extent that the laws permit it, and if perhaps some ambiguity should arise in these things, the judgment of the prince may be sought."[126] From Erastus's perspective, it was a completely illegitimate and one-sided policy, as the disciplinists, who largely controlled the pulpits, evidently felt empowered to address discipline in their sermons—though not beyond certain limits, as we will see. From Erastus's later correspondence it seems clear that this prohibition was either taken to mean that all public debate of controversial theological topics should cease, or that later a more extensive electoral order was issued effectively demanding silence on the church discipline question.[127] In any event, early modern governments had limited tools at best to suppress the exchange of ideas, and the jockeying for position between the parties continued, though in a more muted fashion.

Around the time efforts were being made to quash the controversy in Heidelberg, information about the dispute was streaming to Zurich, Geneva, and other Reformed communities. Erastus had sent copies of his theses to Bullinger, Johannes Haller in Bern, and, eventually, Beza that fall. He received a very warm response from Bullinger which did

[125] UAH, A-160/9, fols. 88v–89r. Excerpts with analysis in Winkelmann, *Urkundenbuch der Universität Heidelberg*, 2:131. See Wesel-Roth, *Thomas Erastus*, 55; Horn, "Johann Sylvan," 253; Hautz, *Geschichte der Universität Heidelberg*, 2:79–81; Benrath, "Die Korrespondenz zwischen Bullinger und Thomas Erastus," 115–116; Burchill, "Die Universität zu Heidelberg," 241.

[126] UAH, A-160/9, fol. 89r: "Tandem post multam disceptationem M.D. Rector ad hunc modum interloquibatur: probo ne quis disputationibus theologicis se misceat, nisi quatenus legibus id permittitur, et si quae forte in iis oboriatur ambiguetas, iudicium illustiss. principis requiratur."

[127] Erastus mentions a specific prohibition by the elector against distribution of his theses in a letter to J.J. Grynaeus, March 20, [1570], Basel UB, G II 4, fols. 279–280. The Schaffhausen student Johann Jetzler had sent a letter home to Konrad Ulmer saying: "Interea, dum haec geruntur, hac de controversia est in schola et Ecclesia silentium: quonium utrique parti imperavit Elector." Dec. 10, 1568, quoted in Horn, "Johann Sylvan" 253 (in note). See also Erastus to Bullinger, April 9 and 18, (15)71, quoted below in note chapter 7, note 53.

not necessarily endorse the extremes of Erastus's position, but let Erastus know in no uncertain terms that the Zurich theologians supported him.[128] Erastus would not find a sympathetic hearing in Geneva. Beza had evidently already seen the original version of the theses, apparently sent to him by Withers himself.[129]

While the controversy temporarily cooled, or at least began to move underground in Heidelberg into the winter of 1569, it was only beginning on the international level. Erastus complained that the elector's effort to silence the controversy was being used to the advantage of his opponents. Boquin, Ursinus, and Zanchi had all put forward counterarguments to Erastus's theses.[130] Neuser may also have contributed a report on church discipline to the elector, and Sylvan composed his own treatise on excommunication, which appears to have been widely circulated within the Palatine church.[131] Beza objected to Erastus's theses, and while Bullinger worked to influence the Palatine court, he also sought to ease the tension between Erastus and Beza.[132] Beza was exasperated with Erastus, as he revealed in a letter to Bullinger: "Would that Erastus would

---

[128] Bullinger to Erastus, Zurich, Oct. 17, 1568. *Explicatio gravissimae quaestionis*, 350–351: "A postremis verò meis ad te datis, mox accepi Theses tuas, insuper & Tractationem de Excommunicatione. Legi, & avidè quidem. Dedi legenda D. Wolphio, Lavatero, Hallero, Zuinglio, & imprimis Gualthero, & Simlero &c. Placent illa nobis. Neque enim existimamus negotium coenae Dominicae implicandum huic negotio. Diu cum Anabaptistis nostris contendimus hac de re, ostendimus Ecclesiam veram posse esse, et dici Ecclesiam, quae excommunicatione hac careat. Rursus tamen contendimus disciplinam esse debere in Ecclesia, ac satis esse, si ea administretur à magistratu. Interim nunquam damnavimus Ecclesiam Genevensem, quae suam habet disciplinam. Nos si talem inducere vellemus in nostras Ecclesias, perderemus certò has citius, quàm servaremus. Vide quid in Confessione nostra hac de re scripserimus. Sentimus nos praeterea vobiscum, non facere ad aedificationem Ecclesiarum Palatinatus, neque ère vel bono fore Principis, si talis instituatur disciplina, id iest, Excommunicatio, qualem nonnulli volunt: quos optaremus diligentius apud se expendere illud Apostoli: Data est mihi potestas ad aedificationem, non destructionem &c. Multa sanè sunt hic, maximè exulceratissimo hoc tempore consideranda. Breviter, tecum, mi Domine, & frater, sentimus. Multum haec caussa nos exercuit."

[129] Beza to Bullinger, Oct. 31, 1568, *CB*, 9:180–183: "Scripsit ad me non ita pridem D. Erastus, se commentatum esse quaedam de excommunitione, quae brevi esset ad me missurus. Paulo post ecce quasdam ad me theses, numero centum et amplius, ad me mittit Heydelberga studiosus quidam Anglus, nullo addito nec edito scriptoris nomine. Eas quum in manus sumpsissem, statim Erasti esse conjeci, sed perlegere non potui, adeo mihi ab ipso initio displicuerunt."

[130] Erastus to Bullinger, Feb. 2, 1569, StAZ, E II 346a, fols. 549–550. In this letter Erastus also notes that Beza is contemplating a response, though Erastus doubts that he will follow through with it.

[131] Burchill, *The Heidelberg Antitrinitarians*, 123 (for Neuser), 71 (for Sylvan).

[132] Bullinger to Beza, March 13, 1569, *CB*, 10:55–57 (no. 661): "Perge tu vere fraterne

be content to dissent concerning the use and need of excommunication, but not to overthrow the thing itself, contriving it to be a human thing or also a tyranny."[133]

After some months Beza likewise responded to Erastus's theses. This manuscript would eventually appear under the title *Pious and Moderate Tract concerning True Excommunication and the Christian Presbytery* (Tractatus pius et moderatus). Evidently Beza was in no hurry to send the tract to Erastus.[134] In September still Erastus "marveled that Beza had not sent it to him" despite the fact that Beza's response had been finished in July.[135] Bullinger did receive Beza's repudiation of Erastus's views in late July. He was clearly distressed by Beza's tract and asserted that he did not want to see it published but hoped to keep the disagreement private. While responding diplomatically to Beza, Bullinger lamented that the question of discipline had become tied to the Lord's Supper and also bemoaned the influence of Netherlandish exiles in the Palatinate.[136] Erastus would not see Beza's response until November of 1569, and he accused Beza of bad faith in withholding his rebuttal. Beza attempted to explain his actions, citing the need to first vet his work with his colleagues and his desire not to further inflame the Heidelberg scene by making his rebuttal widely available. Beza extended a hand of friendship to Erastus, but also implored him to stay within the limits of his own profession,

cum D. Erasto conferre. Scio esse qui frigidam suffundunt. Sed ne audieris tales. Dominus bonae causae non deerit, si modeste et prudenter agamus. Deus dissipet contentiones et dissidia."

[133] Beza to Bullinger, August 8, 1569, *CB*, 10:151–153 (no. 692): "Utinam Erastus noster contentus fuisset de usu et necessitate excommunicationis disserere, non autem rem ipsam convellere, quasi humanum aut etiam tyrannicum commentum, quod ita esse nunquam illi concedam, nisi longe firmiora protulerit argumenta."

[134] Theodore Beza, *Tractatus Pius et Moderatus de vera Excommunicatione, & christiano Presbyterio* ... (Geneva: Jean Le Preux, 1590); Beza to Bullinger, July 25, 1569, *CB*, 10:134–135 (no. 685). "Respondi ad D. Erasti Theses, et responsum Heidelbergam misi, quod curabo etiam tibi describendum. Neque id, ut spero, tibi caeterisve fratribus displicebit." Beza had, however, made his opinion known to Erastus in a letter prior to April, 1569. Erastus to Bullinger, April 13, [1569], Zurich, Zentralbibliothek, MS F 62, fol. 203. For an analysis of the *Tractatus*, see Tadataka Maruyama, *The Ecclesiology of Theodore Beza: The Reform of the True Church* [THR 166] (Geneva: Droz, 1978), 108–122. The publication of Beza's *Tractatus* is discussed in the epilogue below.

[135] Jan Lasicki to Beza, Sept. 22, 1569, *CB*, 10:193–195.

[136] Bullinger to Beza, August 1, 1569, *CB*, 10:140–141 (no. 687): "Legam libenter quae respondisti ad Theses nostri Erasti. Nollem ego publicata esse spero privato te scripto ista agere.... Mea quidem sententia potest in Ecclesia justa contitui disciplina, ut interim Coena Domini libera maneat omnibus illis, qui juxta Pauli doctrinam probarunt, neque convertatur in poenam."

and thus to withdraw from the church discipline discussion.[137] Erastus by no means gave Beza's response a sympathetic reading and wrote back what can only be described as a howler of a letter savaging Beza for the emptiness of his self-justification. Given the fact that Beza had earlier enjoined him to keep this a fraternal discussion, Erastus was particularly galled that Beza had not directly communicated with him, the very person with whom he had a difference of opinion. While Erastus was thus robbed of the potential benefit from Beza's fraternal censure, Beza had "armed his enemies against him." Erastus boldly proclaimed that he found Beza's refutation lame and also marveled at how much the champions of presbyterial oversight disagreed with one another. He informed Beza that he would refute his tract and that he would concentrate on separating the spheres of civil and ecclesiastical authority. In fact, Erastus must have already completed his *Confirmatio thesium*, the bulk of which was a response to Beza's critique, a couple of weeks prior to writing this letter. Though Beza repeatedly sought to reconcile with him, Erastus would spurn these gestures for over a decade.[138]

While Erastus and Beza penned the most prominent theological works in the controversy, the leaders of the Zurich church also attempted to influence the Heidelberg conflict. Bullinger and the Zurichers entered the fray on the anti-disciplinist side by sending two direct appeals to the Elector Frederick himself and addressing the issue at the core of the controversy in a number of theological works.[139] The Zurich opinion found little purchase with the disciplinist leaders who were now driving Palatine religious policy. Nevertheless, the leaders of the Palatine church wanted to maintain good relations with the Swiss Germans, and

[137] Beza to Erastus, December 18, 1569, *CB*, 10:245–247. Clearly Erastus and Beza exchanged multiple letters in 1568 as is revealed in Beza's correspondence with Bullinger and in Beza's preface to his *Tractatus pius et moderatus de vera Excommunicatione* (see below). Ironically the only letter which has been preserved from that year is Beza's essay-type letter to Erastus concerning astrology.

[138] Erastus to Beza, January, 1570, *CB*, 11:29–35: "Nunc cum adversarios meos armasti, et tela illa tua mihi ignota esse voluisti, re ipsa confutas quae verbis affirmas. Verisimile est alia fuise agitata consilia, de quibus me iam pridem aliquid audivisse non ignoras. At Deus videt iniustos hominum conatuas, nisi cum eis abuti statuit ad suam gloriam suorumque salutem. Cur, cum mittebas non duobus verbis seu dimidio verus mihi indicabas quod to iam innanibus verbis frustra studes excusare?" Erastus discusses receiving Beza's response and commencing his *Confirmatio thesium* in a letter to Bullinger, Nov. 21, 1569, StAZ, E II 361, fol. 77. Their eventual reconciliation is discussed in the epilogue.

[139] The letters are printed in *Stimmen aus dem Schweizerischen Reformationszeitalter über die Exkommunikation oder den Kirchenbann* (Bern: Hallersche Buchdruckerei, 1839). See Wesel-Roth, *Thomas Erastus*, 57–58; Bonnard, *Thomas Éraste*, 160–166.

dispatched Zuleger on a diplomatic mission to Zurich and Bern in early 1569 to make them more amenable to the disciplinist program. The mission was not surprisingly a flop, as can be discerned from the contemporary correspondence of Bullinger in Zurich and Haller in Bern, and relations between Heidelberg and the Swiss Germans soured markedly. Dathenus also endeavored to separate Bullinger from his attachment to Erastus and his "impious paradoxes."[140] In the meantime, the Heidelberg Calvinists began to repudiate their Zwinglian allies, and even prohibited the publication of Bullinger's *Decades* in Heidelberg due to the alleged theological errors it contained.[141] Not surprisingly, Zurich and Bern remained behind Erastus. Bullinger composed a strident response to Dathenus later in 1570, which may be the most remarkable document of the church discipline controversy. In it he outlined the long continuity of the Zurich-Bern position on church discipline and threw his weight solidly behind Erastus. Given Erastus's known contribution to the Palatine Reformation, Bullinger rebuked Dathenus for not treating Erastus in a more collegial manner. While Bullinger sided with Erastus, he nevertheless did not explicitly endorse Erastus's complete repudiation of excommunication.[142] The letter left Dathenus both stung and perplexed. Dathenus described the letter to Beza as being "gentle and friendly" but not lacking "teeth and spines." Dathenus seemed to fathom Bullinger's position but resented what seemed to be the Zurich effort to "judge" the Palatine church. It continued to bemuse Dathenus that Bullinger was defending Erastus so doggedly given the significant gap in their perspectives, as he commented: "I don't know how it is possible to reconcile his opinion with Erastus's theses."[143] Throughout the 1560s the Zurich church had been a chief source of support and council for the Heidelberg Reformed, but this close connection evaporated in the discipline controversy. The Heidelberg repudiation of the Zurich legacy echoed abroad; the synods of La Rochelle and Emden endorsed the organization of the Dutch and French churches along more explicitly Calvinist lines.[144]

[140] Dathenus to Bullinger, May 9, 1569, quoted in Bonnard, *Thomas Éraste*, 61.

[141] Erastus to Bullinger, May 22, [1569], StAZ, E II 361, fol. 38: "Clàm dehortantur quos possunt ab emptione Decadum hic excusorum quia tres magni in eis errores habeantur: de praedestina[tione], de descensu Christi ad inferos: de disciplina Ecclesiastica."

[142] Bullinger to Dathenus, June 1, 1570, printed in *Explicatio gravissimae quaestionis*, 355–367. See Benrath, "Die Korrespondenz zwischen Bullinger und Thomas Erastus," 122.

[143] Dathenus to Beza, Nov. 5, 1570, *CB*, 11:290–294 (no. 809): "Caeterum, quomodo ille suam sententiam cum Erasti thesibus conciliare possit, non video."

[144] Discussed more fully in the epilogue.

In the summer and fall of 1569, despite the fact that the attempt to institute consistorial oversight had little popular support, the disciplinists had already won over the elector and were moving ahead with plans to institute their system.[145] In the midst of this bitter controversy Erastus slipped out of town to celebrate his sister-in-law Lavinia's marriage with Johann Jakob Grynaeus, the brother of his close friend Simon Grynaeus. This match ended up solidifying a very productive alliance between the two families. Upon Erastus's return, he found the city in a state of excitement over a recent sermon by Olevianus on the story of Jesus and the ten lepers from Luke 17. In this passage, after healing the lepers, Jesus had enjoined them to "Go and show yourselves to the priests" to demonstrate that they had been healed and thus made ritually clean. According to Erastus's rather colored account, Olevianus had used this passage as a proof text to establish the principle that "ministers have the authority to exercise judgment over morals." Evidently the spectacle was so extreme in length and acerbity that Olevianus was brought before the prince's council, where he was admonished to act with greater prudence.[146] A week later Erastus recounts Olevianus made another unpleasant public scene with the Chancellor Prob and his son-in-law Gerhard Pastoir and accused Prob of discrediting him with the prince. Erastus commented that people were beginning to question Olevianus's sanity, and assessed, with no little *Schadenfreude*, that "what it has taken him eight or nine years to build, he has torn down completely with one sermon."[147]

---

[145] Erastus to Bullinger, July 8, (15)69, StAZ, E II 346a, fol. 551^{v}: "Adversarii nostri apud Principem videntur obtinere quod volunt: ii tanto odio flagrant in omnes illos, quos cupiditati suae opinantur resistere velle, ut à sceleratis artibus non abstineant, quo calumniis, metu, terrore, minis obruant, quos causa vincere nequeunt.... Consiliarii omnes, nobiles, ignobiles, populus, aula, adversantur: illi tamen fortiores sunt omnibus. Dicuntur collecturi principio manum, et ex illa electuros seniorem unum aut duos: accedentibus aliis, plures. Cogent autem accedere hoc modo. Non patientur alios accedere ad Coenam: nec baptizabunt liberos suos cuiquam, nisi prius promittat se coniuncturum se caetui suo sancto. Quid futurum sit nescio: boni nihil expecto." Later an exasperated Erastus wrote again to Bullinger concerning the disciplinists' minority position but overweening influence with the elector: "Non filios, Non Consiliarios, qui ei, uno excepto Ehemio, constanter adversantur omnes. Non nobiles, Non doctos, non plebeios aud[it]." Jan. 1, (15)70, StAZ, E II 361, fol. 17.

[146] Jan Lasicki to Beza, Sept. 22, 1569, *CB*, 10:193–195 (no. 706): "Invectus est quidem Olevianus ante paucos dies in eos principis consiliarios qui rei tam laudatae resistunt, adeo ut lachrymas ex oculis concionantis manantes viderimus. Verum ea re non nisi animos illorum adversum se concitavit. Imprudentiae eum accusant, quod ignarus rerum in Palatinatu, id urgeat, quod fieri non possit, universa plebe omnino refragante."

[147] Erastus to Bullinger, Oct. 10, 1569, StAZ, E II 361, fols. 16–16^{a}: "Eteni[m] Olevianus, ut est impotentis ingenni homo et furiosi cereb[ri] .16. Sept. concionem habuit non ultra

From Withers's promotion in 1568 into the winter of 1569–1570, the Heidelberg church and community were riven with dissent over church discipline. Both camps had formidable supporters. To this point, though the disciplinists had the inside track with the elector, it seemed their highhanded and inept tactics might undermine the effort to institute consistorial discipline. Erastus even optimistically quipped that "Our excommunication will kill its mother in delivery, before it sees the light of day."[148] Ironically the indiscretions of the anti-disciplinists themselves in the coming year would create the context in which the disciplinists would be given a free hand to remake the Palatine church.

---

quartam horae partem, de 10. leprosis, volens ex eo probare, Ministros habere potestatem exercendi iudicia de moribus. Hac re valde pertubati auditores, ut qui scirent eum nunquam ferè minus sesquihora c[on]cionari, varie fuerunt affecti. Admonitus Princeps, qui iam paratus erat exire ad venationem, vocatum ad se obiurgavi[t.] Sequenti Dominica in cathechistica concione, conversus, ad Cancellarium eiusque generum, palam conquestus est immani clamore et ululatu mendaciis se ab ipsis apud principem deformatum: et ita in illos debacchatus dicitur, ut nunquam sic in Verrem Cicero dixissem putetur. Existimant omnes eum non fuisse mentis compotem, ita foedè et turpiter egisse dicitur. Certè, si quid his octo novemve annis aedificavit, una illa concione totam destruxit." See Hollweg, *Neue Untersuchungen*, 1:140; Wesel-Roth, *Thomas Erastus*, 60; Press, *Calvinismus und Territorialstaat*, 120.

[148] Erastus to Bullinger, Jan. 24, [1570] StAZ, E II 361, fol. 33: "Nostra excommunicatio enecabit, puto, matrem suam parturientem antequam in lucem prodeat."

CHAPTER SEVEN

THE WATERSHED

> If they win, we will have a new Spanish Inquisition.
>
> Heinrich Bullinger to Johannes Haller, 1569

> I encountered more hatred at that time on account of the disputation regarding excommunication from my friends than I had experienced in the hatred of enemies on account of the Lord's Supper.
>
> Erastus to Abraham Musculus, 1577

The controversy over church discipline had split the Heidelberg intellectual community into opposing camps. The disciplinists enjoyed the support of the theological faculty and the church council and seemed to have the inside position with the elector. Alternatively, the majority of the non-theological faculty at the university aligned against the disciplinists, as did most of Frederick's non-ecclesiastical advisors including the majority of the high council and a few disenfranchised pastors. Though most observers thought that the elector favored the Genevan system, to this point he had taken no decisive action. The stalemate was broken when the disclosure of the existence of an Antitrinitarian cell within the Palatine church at the Imperial Diet at Speyer forced the elector to act. The Antitrinitarian debacle had broad consequences. On the imperial level, it was a public relations nightmare for the elector and for the Reformed communion in general. Within the Palatinate, the Antitrinitarian affair discredited the anti-disciplinists' cause, and the pro-discipline party would not resist using it as a justification to hound the former allies of the Antitrinitarian pastors. Finally, it was a personal tragedy for the protagonists Johann Sylvan and Adam Neuser, as well as their friends who were linked to them in the later investigation. The Antitrinitarian affair served as the hinge point of Elector Frederick III's late reign. It was likewise the watershed event of Erastus's life and would decisively reorient his future career.

Before the Antitrinitarian affair transformed the landscape of the Palatine intellectual community, a controversy had erupted surrounding the appointment of Petrus Ramus to the faculty of the University of Heidelberg. The Ramus controversy served as a prelude to the Antitrinitarian affair and is instructive since the forces lined up roughly in the same formation as in the conflict over church discipline. In this preliminary round of conflict, the anti-Ramist party, which was largely one and the same as the anti-disciplinist party, carried the day. Flush from this limited victory, the opponents of the Calvinist disciplinary system would be discredited in the Antitrinitarian debacle. The aftershocks of this controversy continued until Frederick's death and included an inquest to determine if Erastus himself was a heretic. Nevertheless, the time of crisis was not completely barren for Erastus and his family, as Erastus developed a close friendship with Johann Jakob Grynaeus.

The Ramus Episode

When Petrus Ramus (Pierre de la Ramée, 1515–1572) arrived in Heidelberg in late 1569, he entered a community which was already deeply divided over the issue of church discipline.[1] The reception of Ramus in Heidelberg would be instructive both of the strength of traditional Aristotelianism at the university and of how the divisions in Heidelberg continued to spread along nationalistic lines. If Ramus was not the most original philosopher of the sixteenth century, he may well have been the most provocative. In his master's theses at the University of Paris, he launched an attack on Aristotelian logic which led him to be viewed by many as an enemy both of sound philosophy and religion. Though his own logical system retained many Aristotelian features, he was largely branded a wholesale enemy of the Stagirite in contemporary polemics. After a brief period of persecution, Ramus became professor and then dean of the Collège Royal in Paris through the patronage of King Henry II. Ramus's conversion to the Reformed faith made his position in

[1] We lack an up-to-date, full-length biographical treatment of Ramus. See Charles Waddington, *Ramus (Pierre de la Ramée): sa vie, ses écrits et ses opinions* (Paris: 1855); Walter J. Ong, *Ramus, Method and the Decay of Dialogue* (Cambridge: Harvard UP, 1958); Skalnik, *Ramus and Reform*; Howard Hotson, *Commonplace Learning: Ramism and its German Ramifications, 1543–1630* (Oxford: Oxford UP, 2007).

France untenable during the early Wars of Religion, and he toured German lands in the late 1560s. After stops in Strasbourg, Zurich, and Basel—where he was particularly favored and in turn lauded the city and its medical revolutionary Paracelsus—Ramus came to Heidelberg in the fall of 1569.[2]

It must have immediately struck some of the court advisors and soon Elector Frederick himself that here was a golden opportunity to adorn the university with not only a renowned Parisian master, but a Calvinist to boot (though Calvin himself would have regarded Ramus as a Nicodemite for his reluctance to publicly identify himself with the Reformed cause). Regarding Ramus's religious views, Peter Bietenholz has quipped, "His Protestantism may have been sincere enough, but his doctrinal convictions clearly were less profound than his penchant for controversy."[3] Controversial or not, the famed Ramus had seemingly fallen into Heidelberg's hands after Strigel's premature death had left a vacancy on the faculty of arts. Approximately sixty of the foreign students appealed directly to the elector to appoint Ramus to Strigel's vacant chair. Ramus likewise enjoyed considerable favor at court, especially from the young prince Christoph. The decision was thus made to appoint Ramus, and Frederick instructed the university that as "Petrus Ramus is especially famed on account of his teaching and ability, we have gracefully intended to appoint him to an 'extraordinary' professorship of Ethics for a period, together with the enjoyment of the unused stipend that accompanies the post."[4] This effort, however, ran headlong into the opposition within the university. The rector protested that Ramus had neither applied for a position at the university nor had he been nominated by the

---

[2] I refer to his panegyric *Basilea* ([Lausanne], 1571). Cf. Peter G. Bietenholz, *Basle and France in the Sixteenth Century: The Basle Humanists and Printers in their Contacts with Francophone Culture* [THR 112] (Geneva: Droz, 1971), 156–158. For a comparison of Paracelsus and Ramus, see R[eijer] Hooykaas, *Humanisme, Science et Réforme: Pierre de la Ramée (1515–1572)* (Leiden: E.J. Brill, 1958), 105–112 and 121–124.

[3] Bietenholz, *Basle and France*, 154.

[4] UAH, A. 160/9a fol. 85^{v}. This brief excerpt is transcribed in Drüll, ed., *Heidelberger Gelehrtenlexikon 1386–1651*, 463. Moritz Benedikt Cantor's "Ramus in Heidelberg" offers a close reading of the university records, but exhibits no awareness of the pre-existing tensions in Heidelberg. Cantor, "Ramus in Heidelberg," *Zeitschrift für Mathematik und Physik* 3 (1858): 133–143. See also Kees Meerhoff, "Bartholomew Keckerman and the Anti-Ramist Tradition," in *Späthumanismus und reformierte Konfession: Theologie, Jurisprudenz und Philosophie in Heidelberg an der Wende zum 17. Jahrhundert* [Spätmittelalter und Reformation 31], ed. Christoph Strohm et al. (Tübingen: Mohr Siebeck, 2006), 169–206.

faculty according to the stipulations of their charter. The professors argued that his appointment would likewise undermine the integrity of their curriculum. Frederick opted to strong-arm the faculty and permitted Ramus to lecture on Cicero's *Oratio pro Marcello* in the faculty of arts at an hour when the lecture hall was not used.[5] The university grudgingly accepted this arrangement as long as it was clear that Ramus would not treat logical questions and specifically not Aristotle. German members of the student body spared no effort to derail his first lecture on December 13, 1569. The agile Ramus continued unflapped and allegedly won over much of his audience. This fragile compromise came to an end when Ramus finished his lectures on Cicero and promised to take up new lectures on dialectic soon. This caused a new round of complaints from the university, as the senate feared that Ramus was going to turn the philosophical basis of the entire curriculum on its head. The university bluntly asked the elector to abandon either Aristotle or Ramus and requested that he write the universities of Leipzig or Wittenberg for advice. Frederick apparently blinked at this juncture, and Ramus elected to leave Heidelberg shortly

[5] Erastus to Bullinger, Jan. 1, (15)70, StAZ, E II 361, fol. 17: "Vide quid egerint. Nuper per artes et factionem conatus est Ramus i[rre]pere in scholam. Non successit, proinde apertè agere coeperunt Zulegerus et sui. Perfecerunt tandem, ut legerit et legat, invita et protestant[e] tota schola, se non consentire quod omnino contra suas leges statut[a] et privilegia fieret. Non est inscriptus apud Rectorem: nec admonit[us] inscribi voluit: ac legit publicè: quod ab initia huius scholae in hunc diem usque auditum non est. Legit in facult[ate] artium. Non licet hoc nisi nomen dederit Decano. Nihil factum est. Interim Princeps [jura]vit quo[mod]o principes solent, se servaturum nostras leges. Quae tolerari possent omnia, si non esset is Ramus, contra quem, ut depravatorem omnium bonarum artium malignum et hominem ineruditum ac vanum, omnes Christiani [or]bis docti, maxime Itali ac Galli scripserunt. A Rege fransciso in publico Parisiensi Parlamento ad Triremes fuit iustè condemnatu[s] et libri eius incendio destinati, sed Lotharingici Card. ope servatus fuit. Inurit ma[c]ulam scholae nostrae, quam vix porro [deluet] multis annis Niceus. Nisi palàm restitisset, aeterna infami[a] digna esset. Sed isti quidvis possunt ac volunt. Iam ante dicimu[r] perpetui novatores. Quid nunc dicant de nobis, non audeo scribere. Summa est, apud Germanos perdidimus, quicquid habuimus existimat[ior]is." Erastus to Bullinger, Jan. 24, [1570], StAZ, E II 361, fols. 33^{r}–33^{v}: "Ramus per factionem quandam opera Zulegeri f[u]ltus à Principe impetravit, ut contra expressas leges Academiae legere inceperit publicè magna sua infamia. Coactus deinde est maiore turpitudine desistere, homo valde impudens et ambitiosus. Hodie indicavit mihi per suum quendam, cupere se mecum colloqui de Excom[munication]is negocio, cum hactenus totum se Adversariis tradiderit, atque palàm in lectione Orat[ionis] Ciceronianae pro Marcello ad emerendum favorem quorundam Excom[munication]em laudarit, homo nunquam bonus. Ego cum eo, si venerit, amicissimè, sed cautissimè agam. Quippe suspicio est subornatum venire."

afterwards.[6] Ramus returned to France, where he was murdered in the St. Bartholomew's massacre two years later.[7]

In constructing a list of Ramus's supporters and detractors, it becomes clear that Ramus's reception in Heidelberg was largely determined by the partisan rivalries that had arisen in the wake of the church discipline controversy. The church council president Zuleger was one of Ramus's chief backers; he advanced Ramus's appointment at the university on behalf of the elector but compromised it by trying to circumvent the faculty senate. Count Palatine Christoph supported Ramus, and as the controversy wore on, Frederick himself became increasingly committed to Ramus's cause. James Good has suggested that the other backers of Ramus were Olevianus, Boquin, Franciscus Junius (François du Jon), and Johannes Alting. Olevianus's role in this controversy has not been fully explained. Given that the supporters of Ramus were Olevianus's close associates, Olevianus likely was a proponent of Ramus's appointment. In any case it would have been unusual for Olevianus to have sided against Zuleger. It is even possible that Olevianus had studied under Ramus in Paris.[8] Olevianus's theological method has often been characterized as Ramistic, though recent scholarship has questioned this contention.[9] Given that Olevianus's close associate Beza was not at all enamored with Ramus or his philosophy, Olevianus's natural affinity in this matter was not clear. Since Ramus lodged with Tremellius and Ramus remembered him most fondly, we might tentatively place him in the Ramus camp

[6] Erastus to Grynaeus, Jan. 24, [1570], Basel UB, G II 4, fol. 278: "Ramo interdictum est lectionibus publicis. Invita Acadamia, et quidem contra leges eiusdem opera Zulegeri iussus fuit à Principe legere. At magno suo dedecore coactus postmodum est loco cedere. Qui abitionem ante festinabat, nunc cum à nullo retinetur ne quidem cogitare aliquid de profectione videtur." Erastus to Grynaeus, March 20, [1570], Basel UB, G II 4, fols. 279–280: "Ramus hinc iam abiit, spe sua frustratus. Eum Schegkius noster libro edito sic delineat imò sic depingit, ut post hac, spero, neminem sua sophistica et vix credibili impudentia sit decepturus facilè."

[7] Winkelmann, *Urkundenbuch der Universität Heidelberg*, 2:132–133; UAH, A. 160/9a fols. 83–94, 99–103, 102–106; Christopher Burchill, "Die Universität zu Heidelberg," 1:235–236; Waddington, *Ramus*,199–207; James I. Good, *The Heidelberg Catechism in its Newest Light* (Philadelphia: Sunday School Board of the Reformed Church in the United States, 1914), 109–112; Wolgast, *Die Universität Heidelberg*, 41–42; Sudhoff, *C. Olevianus und Z. Ursinus*, 331–333.

[8] This is the suggestion of Press, but it is not included in conventional biographical accounts of Olevianus (e.g., Sudhoff, Goeters, Bierma). Press, *Calvinismus und Territorialstaat*, 248.

[9] Bierma, *German Calvinism*, 162–168. Unfortunately, Bierma does not discuss Ramus's Heidelberg episode. It should be noted that Erastus blamed Zuleger rather than Olevianus for engineering Ramus's appointment.

without evidence to the contrary. Just as in the case of the Calvinist system of church discipline, Ramus's support was with the church council and the theologians, though his cause may not have been as uniformly popular among them as the Calvinist vision of church discipline. His main opponents were the German members of the arts and medical faculties.

Not surprisingly, Erastus was chief among Ramus's detractors. That Erastus's reaction against Ramus was so vociferously negative was in large part due to the depth of his own devotion to Aristotelian philosophy. However, the manner in which Ramus was packaged to the Heidelberg academics, that is, as an ally of the disciplinists who was being foisted on the university against their will, was at least as significant in fueling his negative reception as his philosophical position. Ramus's brash style did not win him many friends among the German faculty either. All of these factors were visible in Erastus's correspondence.[10] He claimed that Ramus's appointment was an illegal scam engineered by Zuleger. He also possessed an extremely low opinion of Ramus's learning and character. In a letter to Gwalther, Erastus wrote, "You have written rightly. He is completely French: that is, slippery, inconstant, arrogant, rash, most ambitious. He is a plague on the liberal arts, of which he is marvelously thoroughly ignorant."[11] Ramus attempted to approach Erastus, but Erastus was extremely apprehensive of interacting with him; Ramus was already the enemy in Erastus's eyes. Later Ramus informed Gwalther of his quarrel with Erastus: "When I was in Germany, I discussed church discipline with Erastus who attributed all authority in that sphere to the Christian prince, an opinion that I could not approve."[12] While in Heidelberg,

[10] See above notes 5 & 6.

[11] Erastus to Gwalther, March 24, (15)70, StAZ, MS E II 345, fols. 689–690: "Ramus hinc iam abiit, postquam turbant quantum potuit plus mult[ ] debuit. Recte scribis, Gallum esse totum: hoc est, lubricum, inconstantem, arrogantem, temerarium, ambitiosissimum. Pestis est bonarum artium quarum est omnium ad miraculum usque ignarus: Licet aliquibus propter loquentiam suam cum impudentia vix credibili coniun[ ] aliter persuaserit. At testantur omnes omnium artis regionum doct[ ] qualis sit: in primis autem nunc Schegkius in libro contra e[um] edito. Ipsius temeritatis exemplum scripsi arithmeticum a[d] D. Lavaterum virum optimum et doctissimum: quod fortè [mi]hi tunc in mentem venit. In disciplina dissentit à Ge[ne]vensibus ut dissentiat. Opinio eius est fatua mixturam debere ex omnibus Rerumpub. speciebus: Pleraque tamen tu[rbae] concedit, à qua etiam Ministros vult eligi."

[12] Ramus to Gwalther, July 23, 1571, quoted in Skalnik, *Ramus and Reform*, 114: "De Disciplina Ecclesiastica dum in Germania essem, sum collocutus cum Erasto, qui principi christiano totam hanc provinciam attribuebat, quod sane probare non potuit...."

Ramus took interest in the question of church discipline and reportedly wrote a brief tract on the matter that refuted Erastus's opinions.[13]

Was Erastus's hostility toward Ramus inevitable and irreversible? Not likely. In fact, they had much in common and could have, perhaps should have, been allies if events had evolved differently. The same might be said for Erastus's friend Xylander who shared Ramus's interest in Euclidean geometry. Ramus was not as profoundly anti-Aristotelian as commonly conceived or as perhaps his own rhetoric would lead one to believe. Ramus also befriended Erastus's patron Bullinger and was generally closer to the Zurich theologians than the Genevans. While in Basel, Ramus exposed the latent Lutheranism of the *antistes* Simon Sulzer—a person for whom Erastus likewise possessed nothing but scorn. And if Ramus had praised Paracelsus, he uttered these words before Erastus had taken on the task of refuting Paracelsus. But what is staggeringly ironic given the turn of events in Heidelberg was that Ramus himself did not approve of the presbyterial system of church discipline and supported the more congregational model advocated by Jean Morély. Here Erastus was not in direct agreement with Ramus, but at least they both opposed Beza's program.[14] Ramus later cooperated with Bullinger in trying to preserve freedom for Zwinglian ideas in the French Reformed church.[15] Between Erastus's prejudgment and Ramus's provocative style, however, there was little room for a meeting of the minds of these two significant Reformed philosophers. Though Erastus could not conceptualize it at the time, he was perhaps the biggest loser in making Heidelberg inhospitable for Ramus.

Erastus was not Ramus's only detractor nor was he the first to be exasperated by the quirky Frenchman. Clearly the majority of the professors and most notably the arts faculty were up in arms over the affair. Chief among these was the Greek linguist Xylander, one of Erastus's closest allies. Self-interest was no doubt an important factor in Xylander's case, since he had been slated by his colleagues to move into the Ethics chair.[16]

[13] Bonnard, *Thomas Éraste*, 86; Beza to Bullinger, Nov. 13, 1571, *CB*, 12:221 (no. 871): "Omitto haec, in quam, et illud ipsum urgeo de quo nunc agimus. Erasti dogma Consistorium et exommunicationem semel evertentis, sic P. Ramo displicuit, ut quum Heidelbergae esset, libellum etiam adversus eum scripserit, cuius exemplum brevi habiturum me spero."

[14] In fact, Beza would make precisely the charge that Ramus favored the cause of Erastus after Erastus had more or less conspired to run him out of town. Bietenholz, *Basle and France*, 154.

[15] Skalnik, *Ramus and Reform*, 114–115; 137–143.

[16] Winkelmann, *Urkundenbuch der Universität Heidelberg*, 2:132.

The voice that may well have proved decisive against Ramus, however, came from outside the university. While formerly on the faculty, Ursinus, to lessen his workload, had resigned his chair in favor of Zanchi. In the heat of the controversy, the elector once again turned to Ursinus for a written recommendation. This time Ursinus sided with Erastus and the ethnic Germans who had resisted Ramus's appointment. Ursinus opposed Ramus's teaching, in the words of Perry Miller, because "Ramus omitted essential steps in procedure, confused dialectic with rhetoric, and was irreverent to Aristotle."[17]

The Ramus affair suggested that despite the mischaracterization of Heidelberg as a "third Geneva,"[18] in reality it remained much more of a "second Wittenberg" in terms of its general philosophical orientation and the independence of its instructors from clerical domination. Differences on the Lord's Supper aside, Heidelberg was still a German university much like Wittenberg or Tübingen. Christopher Burchill has argued that the Ramus controversy revealed that the faculty did not want to lose their reputation "as a stronghold of a Melanchthon-influenced Aristotelianism."[19] The Ramus affair likewise proved that the ethnic German, Philippist-Zwinglian faction was still capable of winning a battle against the Calvinists and that the autonomy of the university faculty could not be totally bullied by court maneuvers. In the event, anti-disciplinists' victory in the Ramus episode, rather than being a harbinger of future success, would prove to be their swansong. The disclosure of an Antitrinitarian cell in the midst of the anti-disciplinist faction would bring an end to their influence.

The Heidelberg Antitrinitarians

Antitrinitarian ideas of different origins had been in the air in Heidelberg throughout the 1560s. Most would have known the story of the most important sixteenth-century Antitrinitarian, Michael Servetus, who was executed in Geneva in 1553. While Servetus was not the only thinker to

[17] Zacharias Ursinus, *Bedencken, ob P. Rami Dialectica und Rhetorica in die schulen einzufuhren, an Pfalzgraff Friedrich Churfurst den III gestellet durch Zachariam Ursinum im Jar 1570 als Ramus solches in der Universität zu Heydelberg zuthun für hette* (Magdeburg: Wilhelm Ross, 1586); Perry Miller, *The New England Mind: The Seventeenth Century* (New York: MacMillan, 1939; reprint, Boston: Beacon Press, 1961), 152.

[18] I.e., after Leiden.

[19] Burchill, "Die Universität zu Heidelberg," 236.

raise doubts about the scriptural foundations of the Trinitarian dogma, his work was the most influential, and his execution, after Calvin's willing participation in the trial, the most notorious.

While Bullinger had supported the Genevans' decision to execute Servetus, it is worth noting that the Swiss Germans were less vigilant in defending the orthodox doctrine of Christ than Calvin and the Genevans. A number of Italian dissenters of questioned orthodoxy lived productive lives in Germanic Switzerland.[20] The difference was perhaps more a factor of theological perspicacity than pure toleration (though the latter was perhaps in play in Basel). Calvin, having greater experience with Antitrinitarians, perceived the gravity of the challenge to orthodox Christology more readily than Bullinger.[21] As discussed in the prologue, Lelio Sozzini, considered the second father of Antitrinitarianism by many, lived peacefully within the walls of Zurich with Bullinger's blessing. His decisive contribution to radical thought came in the form of a commentary on the first chapter of the Gospel of John in which he denied the pre-existence of Christ and conceptualized him as a human on whom God had bestowed divine qualities. Fausto Sozzini (1539–1604), Lelio's nephew, further developed and spread his uncle's views.[22]

Though Geneva was more militant in defense of the Trinity, the same mysterious force that drew Servetus to Geneva also beckoned Valentino Gentili (d. 1566), Gianpaolo Alciati (d. 1565), and the apostle of late sixteenth-century Antitrinitarianism, Giorgio Biandrata (1516–1588). While these men and their ideas were repudiated in the heartland of the Reformed movement, Antitrinitarian ideas found more receptive audiences among the Protestant communities of Poland and Transylvania. In the case of the Heidelberg Antitrinitarians, the influence initially flowed east to west rather than west to east. Heidelberg became a popular destination for Polish students after Reformed Protestantism began to be favored over Lutheranism in Poland. Disputes concerning the nature of the Trinity had festered there in the 1560s, and naturally Polish students brought the controversies with them to Heidelberg. Many of these

[20] E.g., Celio Secondo Curione, Fausto Sozzini, and Pietro Perna, as well as the Savoyard Sebastian Castellio—the exception to this generalization being Valentino Gentile's execution in Bern.

[21] See Rotondò, *Calvin and the Italian Anti-Trinitarians.*

[22] The work in question, Lelio Sozzini's *Brevis explicatio in primum Johannis caput*, was not published in his lifetime. Cf. John Godbey, "Fausto and Lelio Sozzini," in *OER*, 4:90–92.

Polish students boarded with none other than Erastus.[23] Radical ideas also entered Heidelberg by means of Italian dissenters, who also frequented Erastus's home. Among those of suspect orthodoxy who made Christological questions a matter of discussion in Heidelberg were Stanislaus Pharnovius, Martin Seidel, Pietro Perna, and Simone Simoni.

The most important of these radicals was Simoni of Lucca, who had attempted to land a position on the Heidelberg faculty in 1568. Prior to coming to Heidelberg, Simoni had been the first and only professor of medicine at the Geneva Academy. Renowned as an Aristotelian philosopher, Simoni was an exceedingly difficult personality who was perennially in trouble with the Genevan consistory. Uncertain of his future there, Simoni elected to depart from Geneva before the situation deteriorated further. He arrived in Heidelberg in December 1568 in the midst of the church discipline controversy. Having been a frequent target of the disciplinary regime in Geneva, Simoni quite naturally fell in with the anti-disciplinist party in Heidelberg.[24] It seems likely that Simoni and Erastus were on fairly good terms.[25] Simoni had earlier written the preface to Erastus's response to Jakob Schegk's treatise on ubiquity.[26] Like Erastus, Simoni was also an anti-Ramist. However, no correspondence between the two men survives, and Erastus did not frequently mention him in his correspondence with others. Simoni's sojourn in Heidelberg was limited; either because of his radical views or simply because all the chairs were occupied, he was unable to land a permanent position at the university.[27] After departing from Heidelberg, he would join the faculty of

[23] Horn, "Johann Sylvan," 257; Theodor Wotschke, "Christoph Thretius: Ein Beitrag zur Geschichte des Kampfes der reformierten Kirche gegen den Antitrinitarismus in Polen," *Altpreussische Monatsschrift* 44, Heft 2 (1907): 152–210.

[24] Maag, *Seminary or University*, 27–28; Tedeschi, "The Cultural Contributions of Italian Protestant Reformers in the Late Renaissance," 133, 145. Tedeschi writes, "Simoni's encounters with Genevan officials for blasphemy, lapses in discipline and inobservance of the cult fill the pages of the Consistory records."

[25] In fact, their association would form part of Antonio Francesco Pigafetta's accusations against Erastus. UAH, A-160/10, fol. 153^r. Discussed below.

[26] See chapter 5.

[27] Simoni had compared Genevan church discipline to the Spanish Inquisition, a metaphor which Bullinger and Erastus would later pick up on (see the epigram). *CB*, 10:245–247. It is possible that the venom that came to the surface in the Ramus affair had its origins in Simoni's stay in Heidelberg. It seems unlikely that Simoni formally joined the university. He is mentioned in the university records on May 12, 1568 (UAH, A. 160/9 fol. 64^v; see also Winkelmann, *Urkundenbuch der Universität Heidelberg*, 2:130). Horn suggested that Simoni "read Aristotle," but he did not clarify *where* he lectured. Burchill notes that "Hier allerdings konnte die Universität kein Entgegenkommen zeigen, da alle Stellen besetzt waren" (Burchill, "Die Universität Heidelberg," 235). However, a letter

the Lutheran University of Leipzig. Oddly enough, this sometime radical returned to Catholicism and died a member of the Society of Jesus. That not all of Simoni's conversions were judged to be authentic by his contemporaries can be assessed by the title of a work written by a fellow Italian: *The Confession of Faith of Simone Simoni of Lucca, first a Catholic, then a Calvinist, later a Lutheran, finally a Catholic again, but always an Atheist.*[28] Simoni had a critical influence on the Heidelberg developments, since he challenged some of the basic philosophical and theological assumptions of the dissident party at this timely juncture. For example, he argued from the basis of Aristotelian physics that creation *ex nihilo* was illogical since "from nothing comes nothing." Simoni had also embarked on the line of inquiry which had led the Sozzinis to a radical position when he insisted that Christ was "begotten, not made." The one man who gave Simoni's ideas a sympathetic hearing was Johann Sylvan.[29]

That certain members of the anti-disciplinist group began to move toward Antitrinitarianism was due in large measure to Sylvan's intellectual curiosity and to the deep sense of alienation that he and Neuser felt within the Palatine church. The background of this reorientation was the constant wrangling over Christological questions in the Eucharistic debates. If Simoni's ideas had led Sylvan to question some features of received Trinitarian dogma, his attempt to refute the Antitrinitarian position pushed him over the precipice. For some months the Polish Reformed leaders Jan Lasicki and Christoph Thretius had been searching for a qualified theologian to refute the Antitrinitarian works that were causing such turmoil in Poland. After no Genevan theologian agreed to the job, Josias Simmler of Zurich took on the task, but by most accounts his effort was not satisfactory.[30] After seeking a qualified theologian anew in Heidelberg and being turned down by Ursinus, Lasicki was able to recruit Sylvan for the assignment. Just as Sylvan's attempt to defend the

from Sylvan to Johannes Wolf from April 1, 1569 documents his "expulsion" from the university. Burchill, *The Heidelberg Antitrinitarians*, 96; Bonnard, *Thomas Éraste*, 73–74; Beze to [Simoni], *CB*, 10:104–110 (no. 675).

[28] Tedeschi, "The Cultural Contributions of Italian Protestant Reformers," 133. The book was written by Marcello Squarcialupi, whose judgment of comets was published alongside Erastus's in the volume *De Cometis dissertationes novae* (Basel: Leonard Ostein, 1580) (See the bibliography).

[29] Our knowledge of the Simoni-Sylvan connection rests on the contents of a letter from Sylvan to Johannes Wolf, from May 5, 1569 (printed in Horn, "Johann Sylvan," 302–303). See also the analysis in ibid., 256; Burchill, *The Heidelberg Antitrinitarians*, 17, 96.

[30] Josias Simmler, *De aeterno Dei filio* (Zurich, 1568). See Dán, *Matthias Vehe-Glirius*, 24.

Catholic faith had precipitated his conversion to an evangelical view of justification, it was in his attempt to refute Antitrinitarianism that he became an Antitrinitarian. To enable Sylvan to undertake the refutation, Lasicki supplied him with books of the Antitrinitarians Adam Pastor and Biandrata. In May 1570 Sylvan began his task by conducting an investigation of the proof texts for the Trinitarian dogma. He did not find texts either in the Old or New Testament, however, that definitively taught the doctrine, so he requested the advice of the Old Testament professor Tremellius. Tremellius's reply that he could not supply sure proof texts for the Trinitarian dogma from the O.T. confirmed Sylvan's growing doubts about the Trinity. Rather than refuting the Antitrinitarians, he wrote a tract which supported Biandrata's position entitled: *True Christian Confession of the Ancient Faith of the One True God and of Messiah Jesus of the True Christ, against the Three-Person Idol and the Two-Natured False Deity of the Antichrist, Diligently Assembled from God's Word.*[31] Sylvan was not alone in these radical opinions; Neuser shared them as well. Sylvan's former deacon Vehe-Glirius and Jakob Suter were also influenced by these radical conversations. Knowing that their beliefs would not be accepted in the Palatinate, Sylvan and Neuser made plans to emigrate.

Sylvan and Neuser traveled a short distance up the Rhine to the Speyer Imperial Diet on July 10, 1570, in hope of making contact with the representative of the prince of Transylvania to secure the opportunity to emigrate to the only European land where Unitarianism had official legal standing.[32] At the diet, they attempted to pass a letter to none other than Biandrata, the personal physician of John Sigismund II Zàpolya. This letter proved their undoing. The Palatine authorities demanded it from the Transylvanian ambassador who instead handed it over to Emperor Maximilian.[33] The letter revealed the heretical opinions of Sylvan and Neuser, as well as their desire to immigrate to territory under the suzerainty of the Ottoman Sultan. Maximilian was scandalized by the letter and turned it over to the elector with the words, "Now you see what follows from your Zwinglian and Calvinist teaching."[34] Sylvan and Neuser's attempt to gain freedom of conscience created a state crisis.

[31] Horn, "Johann Sylvan," 261–262; Dán, *Matthias Vehe-Glirius*, 25–26; Burchill, *The Heidelberg Antitrinitarians*, 26, 87–88; Williams, *The Radical Reformation*, 1231–1235.

[32] On the complicated religious situation in Transylvania, see Williams, *The Radical Reformation*, 1099–133.

[33] The machinations behind this decision are discussed in Horn, "Johann Sylvan," 266 and Burchill, *The Heidelberg Antitrinitarians*, 98–99.

[34] Horn, "Johann Sylvan," 266.

The consequences of this scandalous affair were immediate. Sylvan was soon arrested with his young associate Vehe-Glirius.[35] Warned of his impending arrest by Simon Grynaeus, Neuser eluded capture and slipped out of town in women's clothing. While Sylvan would have to wait two years to learn his final judgment, Frederick was agitated enough by the debacle to take definitive action on the question of church discipline. Wanting to reestablish control over the Palatine church, the elector issued the "church discipline edict" (*Kirchenzuchtedikt*) on July 13, 1570.[36]

Consistorial Discipline Established

Despite the high level of animosity between the various factions, the political leadership of the Palatinate had been moving toward a compromise solution that would basically establish a consistorial system within the bureaucratic structure of the Palatine state. A new edict over church discipline had been in preparation throughout the spring of 1570. The basic contours of this program were worked out in advance, and hints of its implementation emerge in Erastus's correspondence from that period. Apparently the church leaders had hoped to institute their new system by Easter. Erastus marveled in a letter to Bullinger that Olevianus had taken a new interest in administering the Lord's Supper. Erastus commented, "The reason he has acted like this in this matter is that he swore to certain individuals that he would not administer the sacraments before he has obtained his domination. For he is the chief preacher, and has been empowered by the prince to exercise tyranny."[37] While Erastus's account

[35] Erastus to Bullinger, July 18, [1570], StAZ, E II 345, fol. 730: "Capti sunt nuper, id est ante paucos dies, concionatores tres aut .4. nomine imperatoris, ut fertur. Certi enim nihil dum potui cognoscere. Inter hos unus est Joh. Sylvanus. Dicuntur voluisse ad Regem Ungariae Stephanum proficisci et ab eius Legato conditionem petivisse. Re detecta coniecti sunt in carcerem. Ipsi hac videntur ratiocinatione usi: Ecclesiastici Senatores non ferent Excommunicationem suam oppugnantes, cum iam dimittere aliquos eam ob rem coeperint. Nos autem tales esse norunt. Proinde tempore iniquissimo forte nos pellent. Praestat ergo, ut in tempore nostris rebus consulamus. Caeterum in Imperio propter confessionem nostram locus nobis relictus nullus est. Nec in Helvetia multum spei: alibi linqua deest. Superest igitur Transylvania, ubi tametsi Princeps pravas tuetur opiniones, multae sunt Ecclesiae purae."

[36] Horn, "Johann Sylvan," 264–267; Wesel-Roth, *Thomas Erastus*, 62.

[37] Erastus to Bullinger, April 1, [1570], StAZ, E II 361, fol. 59: "Novi nihil interea accidit. Quamvis enim nostri constitutum haberent pridie Paschatis aliquid inchoare, non tamen ausi sunt tentare. Administravit cœnam Olevianus: atque haec prima est Sacramentorum administratio, dum est in Ministerio. Semper dicere solitus est, sanissum ad

is manifestly hostile to Olevianus, its underlying narrative is credible; it would have been in keeping with someone of Olevianus's convictions to have abstained from the public celebration of the sacraments until a purer church order had been established. Viret and Calvin before him had both withdrawn from celebrating the Lord's Supper due to lack of proper discipline.[38] Another sign of the relative strength of the disciplinist party within the church came with the removal of the formerly influential court preacher Willing from his post in Heidelberg in early 1570. In May, and thus prior to the proclamation of the edict, Dathenus could report to Beza that church discipline had been introduced "without difficulty" in the villages and countryside of the Palatinate; however, the resistance among the burghers, university, and court obstructed its introduction in Heidelberg itself. Erastus and his allies were still working to retain a role for the magistrate in church discipline, which can be dimly discerned from Dathenus's opaque remarks.[39]

The proclamation of the church discipline edict in July represented a qualified victory for the disciplinists in their effort to install more effective oversight of morals in the Palatine Church.[40] The document reflected an attempt to construct a measure of consistorial oversight within the framework of a territorial state church. It prescribed the ordination of overseers (*Aufseher*) in all localities who would meet weekly, as possible, with the local minister to discuss pastoral concerns. Sinners were to be called before this body and admonished in a "constructive fashion" as

Evangeliz[andum] non ad baptizandum, licet mentiretur, cum et ego unus ex mittentibus fuerim, ut praeclare sciam, quo[mod]o sit [r]eceptus. Sed ut hunc locum Pauli intelligit, ita pleraque intelligit. Ineptus homo nescit Hebraismum esse: atque interim se Paulo comparare audet. Hoc est in causa facti sui, quod quibusdam iuravit, se Sacramentum nullum administraturum, priusquam Dominatum obtinuerit suum: quod iam factum est."

[38] Bruening, *Calvinism's First Battleground*, 163, 251.

[39] Dathenus to Beza, May 23, 1570, *CB*, 11:140–142 (no. 772): "Quod ad disciplinae ecclesiasticae constitutionem attinet, experimur re ipsa illam non difficulter oppidatim et pagatim posse introduci, sed quominus hoc factum sit hactenus, sola fere haec civitas, quae propter cives et Academiam habet et Aulam, atque proinde infinitorum hominum partim levium partim etiam impiorum hospitium est, obstitit." Later in the same letter he discusses the obstructions of Erastus: "Medicus qui se teneri videt, hoc unum agit, ut formula aliqua disciplinae constituatur, sed tamen quae prorsus sit politica et qua pro abstentione et excommunicatione, ecclesiasticisque ex verbo Dei admonitionibus, delatio quaedam impoenitentium ad Magistratum constituatur. Nos, quod nostri est officii, agimus et speramus Deum nobis adfuturum."

[40] *EKO*, 14:52–54 and 436–441: Goeters entitles this document the "Edikt über die Einhaltung der Polizeiordung, die Einrichtung der Kirchendisziplin und der Classicalconvente und die Verbesserung des Almosens vom 13. Juli 1570."

often as necessary regarding how to amend their ways. If admonitions alone did not produce the desired repentance, the malefactors "would be, in a friendly manner and with Christian modesty, suspended from the Lord's Supper until they had displayed improvement, so that the celebration of the Holy Sacrament would be protected as far as possible."[41] However, the ministers and elders were not to regard these individuals as enemies. Likewise, ministers were explicitly enjoined not to attack these individuals from the pulpit. Definitive excommunication remained something of a magisterial affair; "obdurate" (*halstarrig*) sinners were to be reported in writing through governmental channels so they could be properly punished.

The decree contained a number of provisions to blunt the potentially sharp edge of consistorial discipline. It explicitly says that the district overseers were to be changed yearly to avoid "tyranny." Illegitimate births and other violations of sexual propriety were to be reported to the local bailiff (*Schultheiß*), but the order seems to assume that such illegitimate children would be baptized and recorded in the parish registers. It prescribed that communion must be held "at minimum every two months" and ordered the announcement of communion eight to fourteen days prior to its celebration. It also outlined three offenses—blasphemy, drunkenness/gluttony, and neglect of church services—for which one could be fined. The document instituted a monthly district-wide gathering of clergy, teachers, and pastoral candidates (*vleissigen studiern*) which would concern itself with collective study of Scripture, controversial theological topics, and the censure of morals. With this feature the program aspired to something along the lines of the Genevan Venerable Company of Pastors but also displayed practical similarities with the regional Zurich synods.[42] All in all, the document was moderate and cognizant of the difficulties of implementing such a program in a rural society. It also foresaw the need for close cooperation of the overseers with the local officials.

Like any successful compromise, neither party could have been completely enthusiastic about the decree. It fell short of the Gnesio-Calvinist ideal in that definitive excommunications would have to be approved by

[41] *EKO*, 14:438. "Und also sie freundtlich mit christlichen bescheidenheit von des hern disch biß zu erzeigenden besserung abmanen, damit die entheiligung der heiligen sacramenten soviel muglich verhutet werde." See the analysis in Anneliese Sprengler-Ruppenthal, *Gesammelte Aufsätze zu den Kirchenordnungen des 16. Jahrhunderts* [Ius ecclesiasticum 74] (Tübingen: Mohr Siebeck, 2004), 194–196.

[42] *EKO*, 14:54.

the magistrate. As Baker commented, "Olevianus won his presbytery but not his presbyterianism,"[43] and in a sense the mode of discipline that was established was perhaps closer to Ursinus's vision than anyone else's. Nevertheless, even if this reform did not represent a fully autonomous system of consistorial oversight, it certainly was significant progress towards protecting the sacrament through the suspension of notorious sinners. Despite the fact that the edict contained much that he had railed against in his theses, Erastus actually welcomed the new policy. As it maintained a clear role for the magistrate in the discipline process, he considered the decree tolerable.[44] He also contended that the disciplinists had achieved less with this directive than they had been theoretically granted with the church order of 1563.[45] He remained concerned about the specific individuals guiding the system and the potential misuse of the power in their hands. "This one thing is worrisome," mused Erastus, "that those who are admonished, if they are not seen by the elders in taking a vow of repentance, [they] are secretly ordered to abstain from the Lord's Supper."[46] The fact that the government delayed the public proclamation of the edict in Heidelberg until November 21, 1570, alongside contemporary observations from Erastus and Dathenus, confirms the impression that the new disciplinary regime was generally unpopular in the Palatine capital.[47]

An additional step in the development of consistorial discipline came with the electoral "Instruction" (*Bericht*) of April 25, 1571.[48] While some scholars have seen a great contrast between this document and the earlier church discipline edict, the continuities are more marked than the radical innovations. The contrast between the two documents apparently stems from their origins. While we are not well informed about the composition of the texts, the church discipline edict reads like a carefully crafted

[43] Baker, "In Defense of Magisterial Discipline: Bullinger's 'Tractatus de Excommunicatione' of 1568," 1:142.

[44] Erastus to Bullinger, August 8, 1570, StAZ, E II 345, fol. 691: "Puto Principis edictum de Excommunicatione propediem excudendum quo facto exemplum mox mittam. Tolerabile mihi videtur, ..." Against Wesel-Roth, it is difficult to construe the *Kirchenzuchtedikt* as a victory for Erastus. Wesel-Roth, *Thomas Erastus*, 63; [Goeters] in *EKO*, 14:53.

[45] Erastus to Bullinger, Sept. 21 [1570], StAZ, E II 361, fol. 61.

[46] Erastus to J.J. Grynaeus, Nov. 29, [1570], Basel UB, G II 4, fols. 300–301: "Unum hoc displicet, quod admonitos, si non videantur resipiscendo voto Seniorum respondere, clam iubeatur à mensa Domini abstinere."

[47] Wesel-Roth, *Thomas Erastus*, 70.

[48] *EKO*, 14:450–455. "Bericht der Pfarrer und Theologen der Kirche und Universität zu Heidelberg über das kurpfälische Kirchenwesen vom 25. April 1571."

consensus document that likely was worked out at the highest levels of the Palatine administration.[49] In short, it was perhaps the most proactive disciplinary regime which the high council would authorize. The "Instruction," alternatively, would appear to be the church council's self-conception of what a truly Reformed church should look like in structure and discipline. However, the degree to which this "Instruction" reflected official state policy is unclear. Even J.F. Gerhard Goeters, the last century's leading scholar of the constitutional history of the Palatine church, was at a loss to determine whether this "Instruction"—which was not printed—was legally enacted. Nevertheless, the two texts share basically a common vision. Perhaps the biggest difference between the two documents was that now the consistorial-classical model was asserting itself in the "Instruction" and beginning to break free from the administrative structure of the Palatine state. In this proposal the disciplinary regime took on a more recognizable Calvinist structure—though classic Calvinist terminology was still not fully employed.[50] This document further articulated the disciplinary regime and established a four-tiered system of consistorial-classical oversight in the Palatinate, with the basic consistory of elders and clerics (*versamlung der eltesten*) at the local level, a monthly gathering of local clergy (*vierwöchische versamlung der kirchendiener*), a yearly district gathering (*versamlung der eltesten*), and finally a territory-wide gathering as called by the elector (*allgemeine versamlungen*). Here, as in the previous document, the now more clearly defined consistory had power to suspend someone from the sacrament. In neither document, however, was the consistory given a clear mandate to excommunicate a recalcitrant sinner autonomously. In both occasions the "convent" was enjoined to collaborate with the local bailiff. Whether or not this enactment signaled the definitive triumph of the church council's drive to establish consistorial discipline remains contested. With many qualifications Goeters concluded, "the order represents the final victory of the presbyterial-synodal system in Electoral Palatinate, combined closely with the territorial prince's state church."[51] Alternatively Paul Münch has

[49] Wesel-Roth has suggested that Prob and the other anti-disciplinist councilors likely had a large role in the document's composition. Wesel-Roth, *Thomas Erastus*, 62.

[50] None of the cognate terms for "presbytery," "consistory" and "classis" appear in this document. There is a document, whose legal status was not fully clarified by Goeters, which bore the label "Officium Presbyterorum." This text likewise does not use the term "presbyter" internally, but rather speaks of "Eltesten." *EKO*, 55–56, 448–450.

[51] *EKO*, 14:56.

stressed the Palatinate's deviation from Reformed norms by not having participation of lay elders at the monthly gatherings and the general fact that the Palatine church remained firmly connected to the secular political order. Münch curtly surmised that, "Despite the reception of individual Reformed constitutional elements," the Palatine church "possessed quite a different church organization."[52]

While Erastus had found the first disciplinary degree palatable, he had nothing but disdain for the further innovations of the church council. His letters from this era are brimming with sarcastic and despairing comments about the new regime. After reading what was perhaps a draft of the "Instruction," Erastus marveled at the arbitrariness of it all and rued, "The sum is they do what they want, what comes into their heads."[53] The coming years would reveal that legal proclamations were not the only avenue available to the disciplinists for pursuing their vision of a pure church. Benrath's assertion that "the opponents of Erastus, after their partial victory on the field of theory and legislation, sought the complete victory in ecclesiastical reality" aptly describes the situation of the Heidelberg church after 1571.[54] In fact, the retention of something of the authoritarian form of a German state church with a powerful church council, which was effectively an arm of the state, may well have enhanced the disciplinists' position in the late years of Frederick's reign. As J. Neville Figgis commented, "The discipline was in fact Erastian in the worst sense of the word. It was imposed by the civil power at the bidding of foreign influence within and without the State, against the wishes of the great majority of the people."[55] Unfortunately for Erastus, his anti-disciplinist partisans would supply the test cases for the system in the early years of the new disciplinary regime.

[52] Münch, *Zucht und Ordnung*, 107.

[53] Erastus to Bullinger, April 9 & 18, (15)71, StAZ, E II 361, fols. 18–18[a]: "Res nostrae sunt, ut semper, ridiculae nimirum, gubernantib[us] omnia homin[ibus] imperitis, adolescentalis, oratorib[ius] novis, ut ille ait. Instituerunt passi[m] Seniores suos: et quotidie formas cudunt novas. Etiam in hoc Pr[es]byterio orta est controversia super loco .1. Tim. 5. peccantem cora[m] omnibus argue: volentib[us] Oleviano et similib[us] illum etiam peccatorem voc[a]ri, qui vel monitus vel sponte peccare desierit, et poenitenti[a] ductus mores emendarit, aliis negantibus. Res theologis scholae proponi debuit. Quid actum sit nec dum resciscere potui. Principis mandatum habet, ne quam publicè traducant: ipsi autem eos qui lapsi fuerunt, et sponte in viam redierunt, publicè nihilominus proclamant [etc.] cum ne illos quidam publicare Lex eorum sinat, qui sœp[e] moniti vix tandem resipiscere cœperunt. Summa est agunt quod volunt, et quod in mentem venit volunt: à Principè quidvis impetrare se posse dum vident."

[54] Benrath, "Die Korrespondenz zwischen Bullinger und Thomas Erastus," 123.

[55] Figgis, "Erastus and Erastianism," 76.

The church discipline controversy had not only been a struggle between disciplinists and anti-disciplinists within the church and university, it has also been a direct power struggle between the high council and its formerly subservient committee, the church council. After the release of the edict in 1570, in practical terms the church council seems to have been empowered to pursue its own agenda for the Palatine church in a much more assertive fashion than it had been allowed in the 1560s. The Palatine church, state, and academy were often at odds during the remainder of Frederick's reign, with the animosity becoming particularly acute between the church council and university. By the mid 1570s, the earlier generation of Upper German councilors such as Chancellor Prob had passed from the scene and often were replaced with eager proponents of Genevan discipline and an activist foreign policy, such as Count Ludwig von Sayn-Wittgenstein or Dietrich Weyer.[56]

Rumors

With a new disciplinary regimen coming to fruition and with one leading anti-disciplinist in jail and another on the lam, the early 1570s were shaping up to be a difficult period for Erastus in Heidelberg. His spirit was not broken, and he soon embarked on a new major academic project with the refutation of Paracelsus (see chapter 8). He continued to agitate against the Genevan form of church discipline, and, despite the elector's prohibition, apparently sent his theses off to anyone whom he thought might give them a sympathetic reading.[57] There are many hints in Beza's correspondence to indicate that Beza's refutation had circulated quite widely as well. While Bullinger had also demanded that the controversy

[56] Press, *Calvinismus und Territorialstaat*, 251, 258.

[57] For example, Erastus had entered into correspondence at this time regarding scientific topics with the Nuremberg physician Joachim Camerarius II, who was a part of the Crato-Ursinus circle. Erastus happily shared his theses with him as well. Erastus to J. Camerarius II, May 30, [1571], Erlangen, Universitätsbibliothek Erlangen (Trew Sammlung), MS no. 2: "Ei ego libentius theses meas de Excommunicatione ante biennium conscriptas (contra quas Adversarii mei superos et inferos, Gallos et Germanos frustra incitarunt. Tota Genevensis Ecclesia communicatis consiliis per Bezam infelicissime refutare tentavit, ut aliorum conatus miseriores sileam) tradidi. Fortasse proderit tandem homines aperire oculos, nec usque ad extremum caecutire." Gaspar van der Heyden, superintendent of the Dutch refugee church in Frankenthal, also marked the spread of Erastus's theses and tried to acquire Beza's response. Maximiliaan Frederik van Lennep, *Gaspar van der Heyden, 1530–1586* (Amsterdam, 1884), 224–225.

be kept private and Beza concurred, it was difficult to completely contain the controversy—especially with Beza's open encouragement of Puritans like Thomas Cartwright and William Travers, who were likewise agitating for presbyterial discipline.[58] In view of the friction of this period, it is remarkable that the leaders of the Zurich and Genevan churches managed to maintain their effectual cooperation. While they endeavored to offer a common front to the outside world, strains in their relationship were visible along the margins.

One of the first deviations from the public stance of unanimity came from the Zurich side in the spring of 1570 when Gwalther printed his *Homilies on the Book of Luke*, which touched on the subject of discipline and drew the attention of the Calvinists in Heidelberg and Geneva.[59] Beza wrote a conciliatory letter to Gwalther lamenting the long-running feud in the Palatinate and suggesting that he would read Gwalther's work in a fraternal spirit. Beza nevertheless bristled that anyone would dare to label the Genevan church "tyrannical" or compare the "sacred presbytery" with the Spanish Inquisition.[60] A few days later (and prior to the discovery of the Antitrinitarians), Gwalther sent an angry letter to Beza expressing his outrage that the publication of Bullinger's *Decades* had been prohibited in Heidelberg. He also noted that Erastus was being accused of "extreme impiety" and that his rejection of excommunication led to "atheism."[61] Relations between Zurich and Geneva remained tense in this period, and Bullinger was particularly perturbed to hear the rumor that Beza was considering publishing his refutation of Erastus. It was especially galling to Bullinger to learn this news secondhand from

[58] In fact, Thomas Cartwright matriculated at the University of Heidelberg with Richard Smith in January of 1574 (Toepke, *Die Matrikel der Universität Heidelberg*, 2:68). William Travers's work in favor of presbyterial discipline was published in Heidelberg that year. W. Travers, *A full and plaine declaration of ecclesiasticall discipline owt off the word off God and off the declininge off the churche off England from the same* ([Heidelberg]: [Michael Schirat], 1574).

[59] Rudolf Gwalther, *In Evangelium secundum Lucam homiliae CCXV* (Zurich: Froschauer, 1570). Jan Lasicki to Beza, Heidelberg, April 1, 1570. *CB*, 11:104–108 (no. 758): "Audio Gualterum theologum Tigurinum nescio quid in suis Lucam homiliis contra excommunicationem scripsisse. Quod hic cum applausu ab his legitur, qui oderunt hanc Christianam disciplinam."

[60] Beza to Gwalther, May 29, 1570, *CB*, 11:149–152 (no. 775).

[61] Gwalther to Beza, June 6, 1570, *CB*, 11:157–162 (no. 778): "D. Bullingeri Decades, quas prius illic suo idiomate excudi curarant, iam quidam illorum aperte damnant, fortassis illas cum aliis nostris libris proscripturi, etiam ubi regnum suum stabilierunt. D. Erastum extremae impietatis accusant (quod crimen te in illo nunquam deprehendisse puto). Et Atheismum dicunt eorum sententiam qui exclusionem a Coena non concedant."

someone who had heard it from Sulzer, of all people.[62] Bullinger bluntly asserted that he did not want to see Beza's work published.[63] In one of Gwalther's letters to Beza from that summer, he ironically inverted the traditional Calvinist discourse of scandals by blaming the "atrocious scandals" besetting the Palatinate on the effort to institute consistorial discipline—the Calvinist remedy for such conduct.[64] In February of 1571 a disheartened Bullinger wrote, "Concerning discipline and Erastus, I am not able to add to the things which Gwalther and I have already written you. I wish that this controversy had never begun."[65]

While Beza and the leaders of the Zurich church were able to press on in their joint cooperation, the deep fissure between the leaders of the Reformed community in Heidelberg would never be far from their minds in the coming years. A particularly interesting exchange of letters between Bullinger and Beza can now be understood when seen in the light of a previously unnoticed letter from Erastus's correspondence. Beza seems to have first received some indication from Nikolaus Zurkinden in Bern that Erastus was contemplating publishing his confutation of Beza's defense of presbyterial discipline.[66] It is not clear whether Beza took any immediate action on the basis of this knowledge, but later in 1572 Beza reported to Bullinger that Erastus was scheming to have his theses printed by someone going to study in England.[67] Bullinger wrote

---

[62] Interestingly, Erastus had also permitted Sulzer to see his theses. Erastus to Grynaeus, March 20, [1570], Basel UB, G II 4, fols. 279–280.

[63] Bullinger to Beza, July 19, 1570, *CB*, 11:211–215 (no. 790): "Unde nuper vehementer admiratus sum, cum ex Germania alius quidem vir praeclarus ad me scribens inter alia diceret: 'Narravit mihi nuper vir non fluxae fidei audivisse se a Doctore Sulcero Basiliensi Bezam in suis ad se literis scriptis minitari, scripto in publicum edito, impugnaturum se theses D. Erasti impietatemque eius detecturum.' "

[64] Gwalther to Beza, August 3, 1570. *CB*, 11:253–258 (no. 798).

[65] Bullinger to Beza, Feb. 2–3, 1571. *CB*, 12:27–32 (no. 818): "De disciplina et D. Erasto nihil possum illis addere quae antea ad te per Gualtherum et me sunt scripta. Vellem contentionem illam nunquam fuisse coeptam. Atque utinam bene et sopita, et disciplinat optime coepta, felicissimumque sortiatur finem."

[66] [Zurkinden] to Beza, Bern, September 16, 1571. Printed in Gillet, *Crato von Crafftheim und seine Freunde*, 2:513–514 (no. 47); *CB*, 12:179–181 (no. 859): "Quidam nuper Heydelberga huc venit et retulit, Erastum confutationem cudere nescio cuius tui consilii de disciplina ecclesiastica restauranda." The Bernese scholar Benedict Aretius had been in Heidelberg that summer as part of an unsuccessful effort to recruit Ursinus to the Lausanne Academy. It is likely he passed this information on to Zurkinden. Aretius's presence in Heidelberg and his return to Switzerland is documented in Erastus to Bullinger, Aug. 5, [1571], StAZ, E II 361, fol. 78.

[67] Beza to Bullinger, June 17, 1572, *CB*, 13:135–138 (no. 923): "Aliunde ad me scribitur, et quidem a viro fide digno, quendam istinc in Angliam profisciscentem studisse ut Erasti theses excuderentur."

back and basically told Beza that he did not know of any Englishman or anyone traveling to England who was endeavoring to print Erastus's theses.[68] A few months later Beza lamented, "would that Erastus would also be content to pursue his medical career rather than to spread his theses" and added that he was "most certain" the rumor concerning them, likely a veiled reference to Erastus's intent to publish them, was true.[69] Beza was right.

Earlier that year Erastus had sent a letter to Zurich students Rudolf Gwalther II and Rudolf Zwingli, who were making their way from Emden to England, in which he tentatively explored options for printing his theses abroad. These students' names reveal immediately that they were the veritable princes of the Zurich Reformation. Rudolf Gwalther II was the son of the future Zurich *antistes* Rudolf Gwalther and likewise, via his mother Regula Zwingli (1524–1565), the grandson of the great Reformer. His first cousin Rudolf Zwingli had an equally illustrious pedigree as the grandson of both Huldrych Zwingli and Heinrich Bullinger.[70] The students studied in Heidelberg for over a year prior to heading north to continue their education at Cambridge. Erastus's letter to the pair represents a trial balloon, and a hesitant one at that. Erastus sent his emended theses with a new preface to the students. The new preface (not the one which was eventually published with the *Explicatio gravissimae quaestionis*) was apparently intended to introduce the controversy but also to remove any specific references to the Heidelberg context. Erastus suggested that the treatise be presented as coming from a Spaniard in England, a fairly transparent attempt to link the tyranny of clerically controlled excommunication with the repression of the Spanish Inquisition. Erastus wanted the text to appear anonymously as he did not want anyone to be prejudiced

[68] Bullinger to Beza, July 12, 1572, *CB*, 13:165–167 (no. 932): "Multo autem iam tempore nullus Anglus, quod ego quidem sciam, apud nos apparuit, et nullus a nobis in Angliam discedens Erasti theses secum abstulit ut eas excudi curaret. Neque nos ulli descriptas dedimus. Neque scio si eas quisquam apud nos praeter me unum, habeat descriptas."

[69] Beza to Bullinger, Sept. 24, 1572, *CB*, 13:192–195 (no. 944): "Utinam quoque Erastus sua medicina contentus malit, quam suas illas theses serere, et quidem cum vestrae Ecclesiae praejudiciis. Quod enim at te de illis scripsi, certissimum est."

[70] Rudolf Zwingli was the son of Huldrych Zwingli II (1528–1571) and Anna Bullinger (1530–1565). Erastus had discussed hosting him in Heidelberg in a letter to Bullinger from Jan. 1, (15)70, StAZ, E II 361, fol. 17. Erastus reported their arrival to Gwalther, March 24, (15)70, StAZ, E II 345, fols. 689–690. The cousins had inscribed at the university on March 25, 1570. Toepke, *Die Matrikel der Universität Heidelberg*, 2:54.

for or against it because of its author.[71] Finally, he left it to the judgment of good and prudent men[72] as to whether the publication of his theses would serve the well-being of the church.

This letter reveals a good deal about Erastus's mindset in the immediate wake of the Antitrinitarian debacle. He was unbowed and perhaps a little reckless. He had seriously considered leaving Heidelberg, and as he was highly sought after as a physician, he had options.[73] It is almost as if Erastus is thinking aloud in the letter; he was not confident the time was right to publish his theses, but he clearly hoped that someone would find them so compelling as to insist on their publication. Erastus was in an uncomfortable position at this juncture, since Bullinger presumably did not want him to publish his theses. At the same time, he felt defenseless since his opponents had triumphed and were now all too happy to allow the heretical accusations against his partisans to adhere to him too. The trip of the young Zurich students had coincided closely with the Synod of Emden (October 1571). In a contemporaneous letter to Hardenberg, Erastus revealed that he had learned indirectly from the students that two

[71] Erastus to Rudolf Gwalther (II) and Rudolf Zwingli, Jan 24, 1572, Zurich, Zentralbibliothek (Thesaurus Hottingerianus), MS F 42, fol. 74: "Mitto vobis emendationem thesium, quas vos intelligo ex M. Timotheo exemplari transcripsisse: quod cum meo contuli, multisque in locis, ut videbitis, mutilum reperi. Mitto autem ideo, ut et vos integras habeatis: et aliis non mancas tradere cogamini (Facilè namque fero, ut petentib[us] concedatis.) Deinde ut, siquidem aliquem constitutum hoc habere cognoveritis[ ] ut eas excud[ere], sic non possitis impedire, saltem ut integrae excusae prodeant curetis. Ante omnia verò praefationem, quam Timotheus habet, suppri[m]i cupio. Non enim utilè est Ecclesiae intellegere qui in nostris naevi haereant. Aliàs non [multum] laborem si correctà emendatèque absque illa praefatione publicentur. Verum est, quod non puto tempestivum nunc esse, sed tempus puto commodius expectandum. Principis nostri optimi constitutio sic temperata est, ut à nemine temerè abiici posse censeam: quod ponentes quoque vestri iudica[tur]: Misi literas hasce [ad] D. Albertum Hardenbergium, et D. Gerardum Mortaingne: quem vos scribitis àb Hispano in Anglia no[m]i[n]ante oratum fuisse, ut theses meas curaret excudi. Velim vos Hispanum illum, quisquis est, (sive bonus, ut puto, sive malus, quod nolim, est.) de re tota commonefacere, eique theses correctas, ut earum correctionem ad vos nunc mitto, tradi. Misi correctionem unà cum his literis ad D. Gerhardum: eumque oravi, [verso] ut et has vobis literas transmittat, et correctionem unà quoque reddi curet, si prius ipse legerit, atque etiam transcripserit. Summa est. Nolim hoc tempore theses edi, nisi viri boni et prudentes (iu)dicent è[ ]s esse Ecclesiae. Deinde ut unde proponatur cupio, nulla personarum facta mentione, ac praefatione illa sublata: ut iudicia ho[minu]m sint libera, nec vel pro me vel pro aliis ex affectione pronuncient." The "Timotheus" mentioned in the letter is likely Timotheus Mader.

[72] Apparently Albert Hardenberg and Gerard de Mortaigne (as above).

[73] A contract had been worked out for Erastus's return to his previous position of personal physician to the counts of Henneberg, though the Henneberg Lutheran pastors evidently were not in favor of this development. Wesel-Roth, *Thomas Erastus*, 69.

of the delegates to the synod from the Palatinate had defamed him and his opposition to the disciplinary regime and were spreading the rumor that he was infected with the Arian heresy.[74] Erastus briefly surveyed the history of the controversy to Hardenberg and vociferously defended himself from the charge of heresy. Given that Erastus had not arranged the clandestine publication of his theses with the students prior to their departure, it could be that it was Erastus's exasperation at the rumors swirling about him that drove him to contemplate printing his theses.

The letter apparently made it through and presumably traveled back to Zurich with the younger Gwalther, where it was eventually gathered among the papers of his father. It seems that a voice of moderation prevailed, and Erastus's theses were not printed at this juncture. Beza must have been apprised of these developments from someone in England or Emden—though not likely Hardenberg.[75] This episode is tinged with personal tragedy, as one of the addressees of the letter would never receive it; the young Rudolf Zwingli was already dead when Erastus wrote the letter. While on the surface Bullinger seems either poorly informed or perhaps willfully ignorant, there was perhaps too large a time gap between his late grandson's departure for England and Beza's cry of alarm for Bullinger to associate the study tour of the cousins with an attempt to publish Erastus's theses. In any event, Erastus was not acting like a man who had a dark secret to hide, and thus perhaps more than anything else, this one piece of evidence makes it seem unlikely that Erastus was harboring a guilty conscience over the Antitrinitarian affair or his own alleged Antitrinitarian beliefs.

Resolution of the Antitrinitarian Affair

While Heidelberg had grown uncomfortable for Erastus, the situation was desperate for Neuser and Sylvan. After his flight, Neuser attempted to make his way to Transylvania. He made it as far as Debrecen in Hungary before abandoning the effort.[76] Relying on the assumption that his wife had destroyed all his incriminating manuscripts and hoping for leniency,

[74] Erastus to Hardenberg, [ca. Nov. 1571-Jan. 1572], Lambeth Palace Library, MS 2010, fols. 152^{r}–153^{v}.

[75] Hardenberg was not one of Beza's correspondents, and in any event one expects Hardenberg would have been too much in Erastus's debt for his efforts to secure Hardenberg's return to Bremen to have betrayed his confidence.

[76] Before the Speyer episode, he had taken a leave of absence and traveled as far as

he returned to Palatine territory and subsequently was taken into custody in Amberg.[77] He would soon learn that his hopes were misplaced. After having been returned to Heidelberg and subjected to torture, Neuser made a full confession to the authorities. With the likely complicity of the Palatine official Hartmann Hartmanni, however, Neuser made his escape from the Heidelberg dungeon on May 14, 1571. He first traveled to London and Paris and later made a secret visit to his family in Palatine territory. After a mildly successful stint as a pastor among the Unitarians in Poland, Neuser moved south into Hungary, eventually crossing into Ottoman territory with the object of publishing a defense of his radical views. Suspected as a spy, he was taken into custody by the Ottoman officials. Upon his arrival in Istanbul, he was circumcised according to Islamic custom. It has been frequently alleged that he became a Muslim, though his continued interest in questions of Christian theology—if from a radical standpoint—would seem to belie this notion.[78] He died in Istanbul in 1576, and his legend would be fodder for sermon illustrations for decades.[79]

Sylvan's story would not have such a relatively happy ending. Even though he soon repented of his Antitrinitarian convictions, offered to write a recantation for publication, and satisfied Zanchi and Tremellius of the sincerity of his repentance, he was not released from prison. At the moment when Erastus had anticipated Sylvan's discharge, Frederick ordered him moved from Heidelberg to a harsher confinement in Mannheim.[80] Two days before Sylvan's public trial, Erastus had no idea

---

Bratislava before abandoning this resettlement attempt on account of his ignorance of the Hungarian language.

[77] Erastus to Bullinger, Oct. 29 [1570], StAZ, E II 345, fols. 741–742: "De Sylvano et sociis nil habeo certi, quam quod scribere dicitur ille confutationem in carcere plenam et solidam. Si Dns. quod spero animum eius mutavit, poterit praestare multum, quia et doctus est, et cum hoc morbo laboravit penitius horum nebulonum sensa percepit, quaeque argumenta magis valeant apud ipsos expertus est Author primus, Adamus, heri vesperi adductus est Amberga. Puto nos tam finem aliquem huius rei prospect[uros]. Gaudeo, quod saltem non spargi pestilentissimus faetor iam possit, comprehensis omnibus conscii eius horribilis erroris."

[78] It is noteworthy that Erastus had already concluded that Neuser was "not an Arian but a Mohammedan." Erastus to Bullinger, May 27, (15)71, StAZ, E II 361, fol. 19. "Accidit aliud hic malum Quoniam .14. huius nostri evasit Adamus non Arianus, sed Mohametanus: nec dum captus est, quod quidem sciamus. Metuo ne in Poloniam evadat, aut in Italiam ac Venetiis cum Turcis familiaritate contracta traiiciat in Graeciam."

[79] Burchill, *The Heidelberg Antitrinitarians*, 12–13, 107–111.

[80] Erastus to Bullinger, Sept. 21 [1570] StAZ, E II 361, 61: "De Silvani ac sociorum rebus nihil certi possum scribere: nec possum absque periculo aliquo sciscitatis.

what fate awaited his friend.[81] On December 23, 1572 after a closed trial, Sylvan was beheaded on the Heidelberg marketplace in front of the *Heiliggeistkirche*. Considering the fact that the animus that the disciplinists had held against Sylvan had driven his apprehension and prosecution, his last words were, appropriately, "Forgive my enemies."[82]

The justice of Sylvan's execution has been much debated over the centuries and regarded as a blemish on the reputation of Frederick and the Heidelberg Reformed. Whether or not the penalty was justified—and

Audio tamen Electorem eum sua confessione praeclarè satisfecisse. Si in consilium ego adhiberer, dimittendum ante non esse suaderem, quam scripto publice errorem damnavisset ac confutavisset. Aiunt liberatum fuisse p[ ] si non expectatus fuisset reditus illius qui profugit in Transil[van]iam." Erastus to Bullinger, Nov. 2, [1571], StAZ, E II 361, fols. 74ʳ–74ᵛ: "De captivis nostris reliquis ita rem habere intelligo. Sylvanus post exhibitam confessionem scriptam, et collationem inter ipsum et Theologos, Zanchum, et Tremilium, habitum, quibus omninò satisfecisse ore scriptoque dicitur, certis conditionibus putabatur liberandus, assentientibus Consil[iariis] Supremis omnibus. At Princeps instigatus à nescio quibus praeter omnem omnium expectationem abduci Manhemium in carcerem tetriorem noctu iussit, insciis Consiliariis omnibus. Iste moerore confertus in duplicem incidit Quartanam: ex quibus graviter laborat. Et cum in loco sit natura humido, paludoso, et adiacente Rheno, valde vereor, ut non periclitetur. De confessione, et conversione ipsius sincera non dubitant, qui cum eo egerunt, Theologi. Nec ipse detrectat, imo cupit, ut audio, publicè excudi, ut toti mundo de resipiscentia eius constet. Nihilominus cum ab omnibus aliis veniam impetrarit, liberari ex carcere nondum potuit. Suspicor odium nunc gliscere, quod sibi disputatione de Disciplina illa comparavit. Rogatus ante biduum de duob. scripturae locis quid sentirem, ex tempore respondi rectè an non rectè vos cupio iudicarebet uxorem cum 5. liberis in ista rerum cantate sine marito [et] patre viventibus in summa mendicitate." Analyzed in Burchill, *The Heidelberg Antitrinitarians*, 45.

[81] Erastus to Bullinger, Dec. 21, 1572, StAZ, E II 361, fol. 20: "Res nostrae eodem ferè modo habent, nisi quod videntur pro co[mmun]i sorte omnium in peius vergere. Audio post biduum Silvanum sistendum iudicio publico. Sed quale iudicium sit futurum, qui nominati sint iudices, plane ignoro. Si vera sunt, quae audio, atrocissimè in Deum et homines peccavit. Sed quae in hac causa vera sint aut ficta, postea, puto, intelligemus." Summarized in Burchill, *The Heidelberg Antitrinitarians*, 46.

[82] Erastus to Bullinger, Jan. 13, [1573], StAZ, E II 361, fol. 31. Printed in Rott, "Neue Quellen für eine Aktenrevision," 252: "Silvanus capite multatus in foro die 23 Decembr. pie fertur mutuus. In errore se ultra 12 septimanas non fuisse eumque serio detestatum esse dicunt. Quae praeterea crimina intentata sunt, constanter negavit. Post orationem, cum iam cervici gladius immineret, *Herr*, dicitur oravisse, *verzeuch meinen feinden*. Formam judicii affirmant plerique his in locis inauditam fuisse. Qualis fuerit, nec scio nec scrutor. Hoc publice audimus ex consil. neminem omnino aut assentire voluisse aut etiam scisse aliquid certi de facto." On Dec. 23, 1572, Zanchi had written Crato: "De Sylvano, cui tandem propter dictas et scriptas in deum blasphemicas amputatum fuit caput, credo ab aliis te factum esse certiorem. Obiit pie et christiane. Deo sit laus. Invocavit enim dominum Jesus, ut etiam olim Stephanus. Sic suos ad se eripit e vado Dominus." Rott, "Briefe des Heidelberger Theologen Zacharias Ursinus aus Heidelberg und Neustadt a.H," 91.

authorities lined up on both sides, with a preponderance in favor of the death penalty—modern scholars have recognized that the decision was dictated by *raison d'état*. Erastus thought such a harsh penalty unnecessary given Sylvan's repudiation of his heretical beliefs, though by that point Erastus possessed limited influence at the Heidelberg court. Zanchi and Tremellius were also inclined to mercy and their testimony convinced the high council to recommend Sylvan's release. Beza counseled for severity, however, citing the precedent of Servetus as well as imprudent leniency shown to Biandrata, Gentili, and Alciati, who had been released after insincere repentance only to further spread their heresy. Dathenus and Olevianus offered similar arguments, and Olevianus also acted to prevent Sylvan's children from attending the Palatine schools.[83] Bullinger had advocated mercy but simultaneously considered Sylvan's death justified. The crucial voice, however, was that of Elector August of Saxony who thought that Sylvan's crimes merited a capital penalty.[84] Given that the Sylvan-Neuser affair had humiliated the Palatinate on the imperial level and had added fuel to the Lutheran case that the Palatine confession was heretical and subversive, Elector Frederick found it expedient to demonstrate the orthodoxy of his state's religion through the severity of his justice. Arguments for and against clemency were tossed about for weeks. When the actual trial arrived the verdict was predetermined: the executioner's block had been erected the previous day.[85] Sylvan's death was an *auto-da-fé* for state and confession.

Lingering Hostilities in the Reformed Community

The sacrifice of Sylvan did not bring closure to the festering antagonisms within the Palatine church. Two associates of Sylvan, Vehe-Glirius and Suter, would long be imprisoned without any demonstrable involvement in Sylvan and Neuser's scheme. Even though Vehe-Glirius would later become an important radical theologian in his own right, he claimed that his decision to accompany the fateful duo to Speyer had been motivated

---

[83] Burchill, *The Heidelberg Antitrinitarians*, 36–37; Alternatively, Xylander strove to get a Bible and other books to Sylvan in prison. Wundt, *Magazin für die Kirchen- und Gelehrten-Geschichte des Kurfürstenthums Pfalz*, 1:177.

[84] Rott, "Neue Quellen für eine Aktenrevision," 2, 34–38; Horn, "Johann Sylvan," 278–279; Burchill, *The Heidelberg Antitrinitarians*, 39–47.

[85] Burchill, *The Heidelberg Antitrinitarians*, 51.

by his desire to see the elephants at the imperial diet.[86] The church leaders now felt empowered to ferret out other miscreants, and given how wide heretical ideas had spread among the anti-disciplinist faction, one could well understand why the church leaders wanted to use consistorial discipline to purify the community and build a confessional consensus. Alternatively, Erastus and his associates felt that their past misdeeds had already been confessed and adjudicated; thus, the heightened scrutiny of their actions could only be seen as a malevolent and vindictive drive by the ecclesiastical leaders to destroy their opponents. This effort began with action against some of Erastus's closest associates and ended with potentially deadly accusations against Erastus himself.

A new round of hard feelings erupted in the spring of 1573 on account of the treatment of Erastus's allies Simon Grynaeus and Timotheus Mader. As Erastus reported to Bullinger, "Our excommunicators on the 20th or 21st of this month suspended Doctor Grynaeus and Master Timotheus Mader from the Lord's Supper for no reason." Erastus saw this as nothing more than a proxy battle in the long-running conflict: "Because they cannot hurt me, they endeavor to serve an evil turn on my friends."[87] Like Erastus himself, Grynaeus's contacts with the two leading Antitrinitarians were substantial enough to make him a suspect. Grynaeus in fact conceded that he had warned Neuser of Sylvan's arrest. Erastus's protégé Mader, however, was accused of complicity in the affair without much credible evidence to back up the assertion. Regardless, Mader and Grynaeus were suspended from communion prior to Easter in March of 1573. The fact that Mader and Grynaeus were excommunicated years after their alleged misdeeds, and after their friend Sylvan's ashes had been spread over the Neckar, spoke volumes for the depth of animos-

[86] Burchill, *The Heidelberg Antitrinitarians*, 166–167.

[87] Erastus to Bullinger, March 23, 1573, StAZ, E II 361, fols. 55r–55v. Printed in Rott, "Neue Quellen für eine Aktenrevision," 2: "Excommunicatores nostri 21 et 20 huius interdixerunt coena Doct. Grynaeo et D.M. Timotheo Madero, nulla de causa. Cum fuisset captus Silvanus et praeterveheretur vineam D. Grynaei, forte visi sunt ab eo, et rogati, ut Adamo indicarent suam captivitatem. Ipsi, qui ob id peti putarunt, ut auxilio eis esset, officium fecerunt. Pro ea re Electori, Scholae, omnibus aliis satisfecerunt ante 2 ½ annum. Nunc revocant, quod tam diu silentio praeterierunt. Sed quia mihi nocere non possunt, amicis male facere student." Erastus to Bullinger, July 31, 15(73), StAZ, E II 345, fol. 697. Printed in Rott, "Neue Quellen für eine Aktenrevision," 3: "Excommunicatores nostri strenuè pergunt, innocentissimum hominem Timotheum Maderum obliquè insimulare studuerunt (apertè non sunt ausi) Arianismi, de quo errore eum numquam cogitavisse tam credo, quam scio supra terram elatum solem diem efficere."

ity that the disciplinists harbored against Erastus's circle. Mader narrated that Olevianus had come to him personally and asked him to abstain from the sacrament for the sake of conscience. Mader had protested this action with the elders and even appealed his case to the elector, but it still took months before he was grudgingly allowed to return to communion.[88] Erastus complained that it was hardly Mader's conscience but only that of Olevianus himself that was troubled.[89] The Mader episode is an important window into the actual implementation of church discipline on ground. It seems the chief issue for Olevianus was genuinely the proper regard for the Lord's Supper, as opposed to using suspension to effect the reform of morals—though the issues were intimately connected. Thus, the Heidelberg clerics instituted a proactive disciplinary regime which required parishioners to clear themselves with the clergy prior to receiving communion. Once they had fallen from grace, they had to obtain the ministers' approval before returning to communion.[90] For Erastus, the suspension of Mader was a perfect confirmation of the clerical tyranny of excommunication that he had prophesied. Erastus complained bitterly about this development to Bullinger, who in turn cajoled Beza to rein in his allies in Heidelberg. The cases of Mader and Grynaeus thus became something of a rallying cry against the tyranny of the Calvinist disciplinary system.[91]

---

[88] Letter of Timotheus Mader, Nov. 11, 1573, UAH, A-160/10 fols. 47^{v}–48^{v}; Erastus discusses the appeal to the elector in a letter to Bullinger, July 31, 15(73), StAZ, E II 345, fol. 697.

[89] Erastus to Bullinger, Nov. 6, 15(73), StAZ, E II 345, fol. 699: "Maderis negocium tandem finitum est. Post sexta supplicationem impetravit, ut mentiretur Olevianus dicens, Maderum propter metum propriae conscientiae à coenu abstinuisse. Quae p[otes]t esse maior impudentia? Rogarunt, non sine minis, ut, si non propter propriam suam, propter ministrorum conscientiam abstineret. Postea causam extorquere nullam potuit. Tandem audit hoc quod dicit. Sed ista est Disciplina nostra."

[90] Erastus to Bullinger, Sept. 21, [1573], StAZ, E II 361, fols. 60–60^{a}: "Ad nostra venio: in quibus unum hoc certum est, nihil s[er]vare. Urget Maderus noster causam suam: sed nemo est, qu[i] respondeat . . . . nullam porrò admi[t]tendum ad Coenam D[omi]ni, qui se non indicaverit antea Sacerdoti. Sic impudenter revocant, quod summo vix labore potuimus, ipsis etiam consulentibus, ex Ecclesia ext[ur]bare. In summa nihil eos contradictionum in dictis e[t] factis pudet? Cur id faciant, quaeris? Ut clam possint insusurrare omnibus, damnatum, qui à coena Domini prohibeatur nisi redeat cum Ministris in gr[ati]am."

[91] Rott, "Neue Quellen für eine Aktenrevision," 1–4; Burchill, *The Heidelberg Antitrinitarians*, 49, 122; Wesel-Roth, *Thomas Erastus*, 73; Benrath, "Die Korrespondenz zwischen Bullinger und Thomas Erastus," 125; Walton, "Der Streit zwischen Thomas Erastus und Caspar Olevian," 221.

The developments in Heidelberg remained an open sore in relations between Zurich and Geneva. Beza inadvertently rubbed salt into the wound with the 1573 publication of a volume of his letters, which touched upon the Heidelberg controversy.[92] The fact that this volume was altered shortly after its publication created a scholarly conundrum that Bietenholz attempted to tackle by arguing that Beza had likely pulled one of the letters to avoid offending Erastus. The letter in question (no. 41) was Beza's response to Dathenus from February 6, 1571, though Dathenus's name was omitted from the text.[93] The letter contained Beza's counsel on the Heidelberg affairs and had been written in the aftermath of Dathenus's receipt of a very hostile letter from Bullinger.[94] Bietenholz theorized that the offending section was Beza's advocacy for the death sentence for Sylvan, and thus that Beza's "intolerance" had its "limits."[95] In the light of Erastus's correspondence it seems clear that Bietenholz over-interpreted the letter. While there was a fair amount in the collection that might annoy Bullinger or Erastus, the death sentence included, the most obvious gaffe was the fairly transparent discussion in the letter about Bullinger, the "venerable old one," and Gwalther, the "other one," which Erastus quickly saw through.[96] Apparently the edition was hurriedly retracted and another letter substituted in place of the letter to Dathenus.[97] While Beza and Bullinger maintained their effective cooperation, the episode further poisoned Erastus's feelings regarding Beza.

---

[92] Theodore Beza, *Epistolarum theologicarum Theodori Bezae Vezelii, liber unus* (Geneva: E. Vignon, 1573). As the discussion below will clarify, there are two versions of this book. See *CB*, 14:xiii–xx.

[93] Beza to "N" [Dathenus], Feb. 6, 1571, *CB*, 12:33–36 (no. 819).

[94] Discussed above in chapter 6.

[95] Peter G. Bietenholz, "Limits to Intolerance: The Two Editions of Beza's *Epistolae Theologicae*," *Bibliothèque d'Humanisme et Renaissance* 35 (1973): 311–313. See also Bonnard, *Thomas Éraste*, 91.

[96] Erastus to Bullinger, Sept. 21, [1573], StAZ, E II 361, fols. 60–60[a]. "Vidi lib. 1. Epist. Bezae nunc editum, in qu[o] tacitè, non tamen ubique obscurè, me perstringit. Verum d[e] hoc ubi perlegero." Erastus to Bullinger, Nov. 6, 15(73), StAZ, E II 345, fols. 699[r]–699[v]: "Puto te legisse Epist. Bezae editas: et intellegissa cum alia tum quae .41. scribit de sene quodam, hoc est, Bullingero, et altero, hoc est, Gualthero. Loquitur autem de literis, quas ad Illustriss. Principem tu, Gualth. et Wolfius scripsistis de hac disceptatione." The quotation that Erastus found troubling was: "De boni illius et venerandi senis literis recte omnino statuisti. Nec enim, si hic culpa est, illi proprie imputanda est, sed alteri qui ut fervidior est, ita est etiam audacior, ne quid acerbius dicam" (Letter "41," thus Beza to [Dathenus], Feb. 6, 1571, *CB*, 12:33–36 (no. 819)).

[97] Letter "41" in the altered edition is letter no. 831 in the modern edition of Beza's correspondence. *CB*, 12:99–101. See also the discussion in *CB*, 15:9.

Much of the friction in the Palatinate during this period was between the church council and the university, and a number of the conflicts can be viewed as skirmishes in the long-running feud over church discipline. Perhaps the most noteworthy piece of resistance was Sigismund Melanchthon's refusal to take a seat on the consistory. As participation of elders from the university was an integral part of the system of consistorial discipline, Melanchthon's action, though couched in deferential terms, was a provocative rejection of the disciplinary regime.[98] Sadly, Melanchthon died later that year, removing another moderate from the scene and depriving Erastus of an ally. A more passive form of defiance came when Xylander and Erastus refused to attend the university banquet in Beza's honor during his 1574 visit to Heidelberg.[99]

A more significant showdown came over the administration of the Heidelberg *Paedagogium* in 1574. This preparatory academy had been jointly administered by the church council and the university. The church council wanted to reform the institution and first suggested replacing the current director Christoph Schilling, who was currently engaged in a bitter struggle with his fellow Silesian instructor Johann Jungnitz. Both Schilling and Jungnitz can be placed fairly within the larger Crato-Ursinus circle, though Schilling had become something of a protégé of Erastus by this point.[100] While the move against Schilling can be viewed as another attack on one of Erastus's partisans, the animosity between Schilling and Jungnitz possessed a personal dimension outside the boundaries of the anti-disciplinist/disciplinist struggle. There are also hints in the sources that the action against Schilling was well-grounded, viz., that the aspiring physician was more interested in his medical studies than his teaching duties. While the university sought to reconcile Schilling and Jungnitz, the church council wanted to be done with the two and install their own candidate, Bertoldt Rivius from Frankfurt. However, the university was outraged when it learned that Rivius did not even possess a M.A. When the situation came to a head, the church council president Zuleger bluntly declared to the university:

[98] UAH, A-160/10, fols. 4–11; Wesel-Roth, *Thomas Erastus*, 71–72; Press, *Calvinismus und Territorialstaat*, 248; Burchill, "Die Universität zu Heidelberg," 240–241.

[99] Wesel-Roth, *Thomas Erastus*, 74; *CB*, 16:209–202 (no. 1161).

[100] See the Correspondence Register. Schilling composed the epigram "In inventores auri potabilis" which was published with Erastus's *De auro potabili* (See the bibliography). Jungnitz would later join the university faculty and would serve as one of Ursinus's literary executors. For Jungnitz, see Drüll, ed., *Heidelberger Gelehrtenlexikon 1386–1651*, 343–344; for Schilling, see *ADB*, 31:253–255.

"You can do what you want; we will move ahead, and the one who is the strongest, God will help."[101] Zuleger's assessment of church council's strength proved correct; it gained the elector's sanction to take over sole administration of the *Paedagogium*, but in doing so it relinquished the annual support that was due to pass to the institution from the university bursar.[102] With the resolution of this conflict over the *Paedagogium*, the wheel had turned full circle, and church hierarchy once again regained the upper hand in Heidelberg, which Heshusius previously had lost during the conflict over the Lord's Supper.

The Pigafetta Inquest

In 1574 the stakes would be raised when Erastus himself, the head of the anti-disciplinist party, was accused of Antitrinitarianism and subjected to a heresy inquest. Erastus's accuser was an Italian physician and anatomist named Antonio Francesco Pigafetta.[103] Pigafetta was a man with problems of his own. He had been charged with incest and other indiscretions by one of the leaders of the Heidelberg church and only lashed out at Erastus after being imprisoned himself. Beyond his moral infractions, Pigafetta was dissatisfied with his professional position in Heidelberg as a physician at the city hospital. He had hoped to secure a prestigious post on the university faculty, rather than only being called in for infrequent anatomical demonstrations. Pigafetta no doubt knew Erastus and his circle well since Erastus was by all accounts close to the Italian exiles in Heidelberg and Basel; his wife Isotta was, after all, Italian. It is likely that Pigafetta came to resent him and held Erastus responsible for his inability to land a university post. Erastus was apparently interested in securing the chair for either Simone Simoni or, more likely, his close friend Simon Grynaeus, so he may well have obstructed efforts to appoint Pigafetta.[104]

[101] UAH, A-160/10 fol. 119^r: "Ir müget thun waß Ihr wellet: wir wollen fortt fahren, und wer der starkst ist, denn würdt gott helffn." Burchill, "Die Universität zu Heidelberg," 243–244.

[102] UAH, A-160/10 fols. 103^r–132^v; J.G. Hautz, *Die erste Gelehrtenschule Reformirten Glaubensbekenntnisses in Deutschland oder Geschichte des Pädagogiums zu Heidelberg unter dem Kurfürsten Friedrich III. von der Pfalz in den Jahren 1565–1577* (Heidelberg, 1855), 17–36; Burchill, "Die Universität zu Heidelberg," 243–244.

[103] For a brief word on Pigafetta's medical activities, see Vivian Nutton, "Humanist Surgery," in *The Medical Renaissance*, 96; idem, "The Wittenberg Anatomy," in *Medicine and the Reformation*, 14.

[104] Wesel-Roth, *Thomas Erastus*, 76–77.

Pigafetta's festering resentment was revealed in his first action against Erastus. Before accusing Erastus of Antitrinitarianism, he had lodged a formal complaint with the university in late 1573, when Erastus was still rector, that Erastus had called him a "surgeon" in print.[105] This affront was perhaps more of a perceived than an intended insult. In the text in question Erastus had described Pigafetta as "the distinguished anatomist Dr. Antonius Franciscus Pigafetta, of Vicenza, the most felicitous surgeon of the Elector Palatine." That Erastus meant little harm here can be discerned by the fact that he also labeled his more accomplished friend Volcher Coiter, whom he clearly respected, an "anatomist and surgeon" in the same book.[106] The conventional wisdom that Erastus had intentionally belittled Pigafetta seems overdrawn.[107] Rather than using the term as a condescending designation for a less formally educated practitioner, in this case Erastus employed "surgeon" as an alternative title for one skilled in anatomy. The larger context of the quotation revealed that Erastus had actually described Pigafetta in a courteous manner, but Pigafetta was nevertheless rankled by the label "surgeon." As he had been received in the university matriculation list as a doctor of medicine, it is clear that Pigafetta wanted to be acknowledged by the more prestigious title.[108] He asserted that he had neither studied surgery nor was employed as a surgeon by the elector and demanded an apology. He was not satisfied.[109] It is no doubt a sign of Erastus's waning influence at court that the elector attempted to appoint Pigafetta to a chair in medicine just a few weeks

[105] UAH, A-160 / 10 fol. 47^r: "Placuit celeberrimo D.D. Thomae Erasto in quarta suarum disputationum Antiparcelsicarum nuper edita parte: me Palatini Electoris Chirurgu felicissimum vocare. Hoc a factum vel imprudenter, utinam vel me honoraret, persuadere mihi nullo modo potuit."

[106] Thomas Erastus, *Disputationum de nova medicina Philippi Paracelsi Pars Quarta et Ultima* (Basel: Pietro Perna, 1573), respectively, 69, 31. Note as well that a letter from Erastus to Pigafetta survives. Erastus to Pigafetta, Heidelberg, March 5, 1572, printed in *Disputationum & Epistolarum Medicinalium volumen* (Zurich: Johannes Wolf, 1595), 2^v–4^r. Erastus also referred to Pigafetta in a friendly fashion in a letter to Coiter and acknowledged that he was a medical doctor as well as a skilled anatomist. Erastus to Volcher Coiter, Aug. 28, [ca. 1572–1574], Basel UB G2 II 37, fol. 11.

[107] Cf. Nutton, "Humanist Surgery," 96; Rott, "Neue Quellen für eine Aktenrevision" (1911) 5: "Sicherlich war das eine von vielen kleinen Bosheiten Erastens gegen den welschen Spitalarzt."

[108] In the entry from 1573: "Antonius Franciscus Pigafetta, Vincentinus, medicinae doctor, 27 Aug." Toepke, *Die Matrikel der Universität Heidelberg*, 2:67.

[109] UAH, A-160 / 10 fol. 47^r. Erastus's explanation appears in UAH, A-160 / 10 fols. 50^r–52^v.

after Pigafetta had initiated this public feud with Erastus. The university declined to act on the proposal, however.[110]

In a desperate maneuver, Pigafetta accused Erastus of Antitrinitarianism, of causing a schism within the Palatine church, and of being the head of a "horrendous monster of hypocrisy."[111] The timing of the accusation, with the recent retirement of Chancellor Prob and with initiation of Tremellius's rectorate at the university, suggests that Pigafetta's case was a carefully engineered plan that must have enjoyed the cooperation of the disciplinist hierarchy.[112] Pigafetta outlined a rather complex conspiracy that portrayed Erastus as leading a subversive network including Simon Grynaeus, Xylander, Cirler, and Schilling. Pigafetta claimed Erastus had been protected by his friends on the high council and by his support among the nobility and had had continuous contact with individuals of dubious orthodoxy including Simoni and Perna. He also alleged that Erastus was fond of the opinions of Kaspar Schwenckfeld and that Pigafetta himself had given Erastus a book by the same. Many of these heretical notions had purportedly been discussed in Erastus's sauna. On this basis, Pigafetta denounced Erastus as an impious man who cared little for church services and claimed that Erastus had said that even a Turk could be saved if he performed good works. He also alleged that Erastus inclined to the quasi-Adoptionist Christology advocated by writers like Erastus's school-era friend Lelio Sozzini.[113] Were one to give credence to Pigafetta's accusations, it would suggest that Erastus was a spiritualist in the mode of a Sebastian Franck. It is clear that not only the disciplinist church leaders, but also the elector himself, initially took these charges very seriously. On the basis of Pigafetta's accusations, Frederick wrote Elector August of Saxony to urge him to launch a parallel investigation into Simoni's orthodoxy.[114] While Erastus was treated with considerable respect during the inquest, his two university colleagues Mader

[110] UAH, A-160/10 fols. 76^{v}–77^{r}.

[111] UAH, A-160/10 fol. 150^{r}.

[112] Wesel-Roth, *Thomas Erastus*, 77.

[113] UAH, A-160/10 fols. 145–180. The primary list of accusations against Erastus and the subsequent interrogation of Pigafetta from Jan. 8, 1575 are located at fols. 149^{v}–155^{r}. Fols. 177–180 are printed in Rott, "Neue Quellen für eine Aktenrevision," 9–17. Rott summarizes the remainder of the affair on pp. 5–9. Some of the key passages omitted by Rott are transcribed below. See also Wesel-Roth, *Thomas Erastus*, 76–78; Burchill, *The Heidelberg Antitrinitarians*, 49, 122.

[114] Kluckhohn, *Briefe Friedrich des Frommen*, 2(2):788–790.

and Simon Grynaeus were again handled roughly. Both were ordered imprisoned, and later the elector sought to fire Grynaeus—a move the university successfully resisted.

As provocative as Pigafetta's accusations were, neither he nor any of Erastus's enemies could produce any tangible proof that Erastus himself had advocated an Antitrinitarian position. Erastus does not appear to have felt particularly threatened by Pigafetta's claims, but became embittered as the process wore on.[115] Erastus defended himself before a university panel which met in the Heidelberg Castle on February 25 and 26, 1575 and effectively distanced himself from the rumored rampant heresy of the Italian exile community.[116] Even after the first hearing, it became clear that Pigafetta's assertions could not be substantiated, and the elector declared that Erastus would have to be forgiven and Pigafetta returned to confinement in chains.[117] The inquest began to shift away from Pigafetta's more fanciful claims toward Erastus's known extensive

[115] Erastus to Grynaeus, Jan. 4, (15)75, Basel UB, G II 4, fol. 206: "Pigafetta nunc atrocissima mihi intentat crimina: talia, inquam, ut, si vera sint, dignus censear, qui vivus excorier. Sed per Dei gratiam nihil me moverunt eius calumniae." Erastus's later mood is illustrated by his letter to Josias Simmler, April 2, (15)75, Zurich, Zentralbibliothek (Thesaurus Hottingerianus), MS F 59, fol. 484: "Miramini fabri impudentiam, nec sine causa: miraremini multò magis, si, quae nostri hic faciunt, videretis. Puto certè odio, acerbitate, corde felleo superare fabriculum. Unum enim hoc praecipuè dolere ipsis videtur, quod ii, quos adisse cœperunt, non simul corpore et anima in sempiternis cruciatibus aeternum vivant. Actionis, quam adversus me, benè de se meritum instituerunt, partem descripsi, sigillatim omnia nec scribere potui, nec recitare nunc debui. Unum tantum dicam, nihil eos ne nunc quidem omittere, postquam se pudefactos sic vident, ut sordeant magis quam unquam antea, quo mihi molestiam creent. Sed Princeps Illustriss. mihi clementer promisit, se porrò non auscultaturum accusationibus, quin me audiat. Incredibilis est malitia, audacia, impudentia, hominum illorum, hypocrisi sua apud optimum Principem omnia tegentium scelera sua."

[116] UAH, A-160/10 fols. 167^{r}–167^{v}: "Et primo interrogatus D. Erastus, an novisset Petrum Pernam, Simonem Simonium, & alium quendam Italum, & an sciret illorum aliquem esse infectum Arrianismo. Reddit mihi prorsus numquam constitit horum aliquem, inbutum esse Arriana haeresi. Pernam aliquando aegrotantem curavi & hac occasione in eius amicitiam veni, atque ex eo tempore familiariter nos coluimus. Postea Perna typis excudit librum quendam Ochini, in qu[o] sunt quidam errores, de quibus cum a me admoneretur, r[ed]dit, se de re Basiliensibus satisfecisse. Simonium non scivi esse in unius prius 1/quartam scriptum contra Genevenses proposuit. Postea aliquoties ad me scripsit de rebus philosophicis. De theologicis vero ne verbum quidem ullum unquam, & D. Zanchum post modum mihi narravit ipsum insimulari arrianismi, qui ego neque affirmo neque nego. Ad Italum quod attinet, is huc veniens commendatus mihi fuit, ut medicus vocari, ipsum aliq[uo]ties, ad coenam, sed numquam venit. De hydrope semel, de rebus vero theologicis nihil unqu[am] cum ipso contuli."

[117] UAH, A-160/10 fol. 167^{v}.

prior contacts with the Heidelberg Antitrinitarians.[118] In the course of the inquest, Erastus admitted to numerous indiscretions with members of the Antitrinitarian party, but steadfastly denied the more serious accusations. He conceded that he had suspected the Antitrinitarian opinions of Sylvan and Neuser before their discovery and had known of their desire to immigrate to Transylvania.[119] He also admitted to having received a heretical manuscript from Martin Seidel, which he had given to Seidel's brother with instructions to destroy it, rather than handing it over to the church council. Given the lack of substantive evidence against him and the palpable malice on the part of Pigafetta, the inquest exonerated Erastus of the most serious charges. Erastus was faulted for distributing his theses on excommunication and allowing students to copy them after the elector had restrained the parties from pursuing the conflict. The elector ordered Erastus not to speak or write against the official teaching of the Palatine church again and enjoined him to make peace with his adversaries.[120] However, the verdict was also a vindication for Erastus in that he was "pronounced innocent and freed of all improper suspicion."[121] Unlike Heshusius some fifteen years before, the elector spared Erastus from a more severe penalty and allowed him to remain at the university. This was a merciful act, since Erastus had taken a position in direct opposition to the Heidelberg Catechism in his theses and, to a certain degree, had covered up his friends' heretical activities. That he was allowed to stay in Heidelberg perhaps owed in equal measure to his past relationship to the elector, his status as a sought-after physician, the relative autonomy

[118] UAH, A-160/10 fol. 169^{r}: "De qua haeresi apud theologos et senatum ecclesiasticum in suspitionem venerat non ita pridem, atque adeo non tam propter D. Pigafettae maledica scripta & criminationes, quam propter amicitiam & consuetudinem qui ipsis olim cum Johanne Sylvano & Adamo Nesero...."

[119] UAH, A-160/10 fol. 177^{v}. Printed in Rott, "Neue Quellen für eine Aktenrevision," 11: "Ad quae in summa D. Erastus respondit, Sylvanum non solum sibi suspectum fuisse Arianismi, sed apud se Photini blasphemias contra filiam dei laudasse, Arium in eo reprehendisse, quod patribus Nicaenis nimium concesserit atque etiam consilium de sua in Transylvaniam profectione aperuisse, a quo se etsi se eum dehortatum dicat tamen non satis erat, eum cum Sylvano de re tanti momenti agere cum vel princeps vel alii amici fuerint admonendi, ut hominem tam dira cogitantem in officio retinuissent."

[120] UAH, A-160/10 fol. 180^{r}. Printed in Rott, "Neue Quellen für eine Aktenrevision," 16–17; Press, *Calvinismus und Territorialstaat*, 252; Walton, "Der Streit zwischen Thomas Erastus und Caspar Olevian," 218–219.

[121] UAH, A-160/10 fols. 169^{r}–169^{v}: "Verum tantum abfuit, ut aliquid in D. Erasto deprehensum sit, ut postea illustrissimus Princeps in scripto 29. Aprilis Universitati in arce praesentibus omnibus Academiae professoribus praeter ipsum D. Erastum, qui ob morbum adesse non poterat, praelecto et communicato D. Erastum, innocentem pronunciaverit et omni sinistra suspicione liberaverit." Hautz, *Geschichte des Pädagogiums*, 25.

of the university, and Erastus's own stature as a major intellectual figure. He also possessed influential allies abroad. One has little doubt that if Erastus had been serving on the Geneva Academy, he would have been sent packing. As Volker Press aptly surmised, "Erastus had indeed deftly pulled his head out of the noose, but through the events his influence had fallen to zero."[122]

The "Excommunication" of Erastus

Sometime during this era Erastus had withdrawn from publicly communing in the Heidelberg church. Whether this was from his own initiative or at the behest of the Palatine clergy is not known, but Erastus was only restored to communion after a series of complicated diplomatic actions at Easter in 1576. When we view Erastus's case in conjunction with other celebrated opponents of discipline such as Jean Morély, Philippe Berthelier, and Caspar Coolhaes, it appears the surest way to be excommunicated in the Calvinist tradition was to challenge the legitimacy of the practice itself. Since Erastus made little reference to the action in his correspondence and the consistory records that might have recorded it apparently have not survived, it is unlikely that Erastus's alleged "excommunication" can be fully comprehended. Many questions remain unexplained regarding this episode: Was it the major public ban or the minor suspension from the sacrament? Did Erastus's own truculence and passive resistance contribute to the length of his absence from the Lord's table? To what degree was the elector himself aware of Erastus's "excommunication" and did he approve of it?

The chief unanswered question regarding Erastus's suspension from communion is when it started: the absolute time range for the action is 1570–1575.[123] Considering the difficulties his friends faced in those years and the more serious allegations leveled against him, his separation from the disciplinist dominated church does not seem to have troubled him excessively. While it is not impossible that Erastus was suspended as early as 1570 when scandalous rumors concerning his orthodoxy were

[122] Press, *Calvinismus und Territorialstaat*, 252: "Erast hatte zwar geschickt seinen Kopf aus der Schlinge gezogen, aber durch die Ereignisse war sein Einfluß auf den Nullpunkt gesunken."

[123] Bonnard, *Thomas Éraste*, 100–102; Wesel-Roth, *Thomas Erastus*, 68–69, 142; Benrath, "Die Korrespondenz zwischen Bullinger und Thomas Erastus," 125; Rudolf, "Die Kirche in Heidelberg nach den letzten Briefen Bullinger-Beza," 100; *CB*, 15:160.

already abroad, it is perhaps more likely that his removal from the sacrament came later, as it would have been quite unusual for someone as prominent as Erastus to have lingered in this state for so many years.[124] The summer of 1573 is another possibility for the beginning of his suspension, as at this juncture the Heidelberg clergy seem to have implemented a proactive system for church members to be approved to take communion (discussed above in the Mader affair), and it is difficult to imagine Erastus seeking Olevianus's permission to commune. It is perhaps most likely, however, that Erastus's separation from the church only occurred with the accusations of Pigafetta and thus was effected in the first months of 1575. There would have been more than enough scandal associated with Erastus at that point for the elders to have requested that he withdraw from communion. While there is no hard evidence to exclude an earlier date, it strikes me as unlikely that Erastus would have complained so bitterly about the suspension of Mader and Grynaeus in 1573 if he likewise had already been banned. It also makes sense that Erastus might not have thought to mention the suspension from communion in his correspondence while he was facing the more serious prospect of a heresy inquest. What perhaps made the situation protracted was that quite early on Erastus was declared innocent by the elector and the university tribunal. Ironically, even though Pigafetta's accusations had proven insubstantial, the Pigafetta affair seems to have crystallized the suspicions regarding Erastus's orthodoxy in the eyes of the church leaders. Apparently the judgment of the university inquest was not a sufficient resolution for the church leaders, and this episode is yet another example of institutional discord in Heidelberg. Finally, Erastus's determined resistance to the church's power over excommunication was a major impediment. Since Erastus did not in essence recognize the consistory's authority to ban him, achieving reconciliation became a significant challenge. How could he in good conscience make a public repentance with a humil-

[124] For example, Erastus may be speaking obliquely of an attempt to discipline him in this letter. However, he implies that his purgation was successful on this occasion. Erastus to Bullinger, August 8, 1570, StAZ, E II 345, fol. 691: "Excommunicationis negotium de quo initio tantum quaerebatur, prospere cecidisset, nisi Cacodaemon excitavisset organa quaedam sua, et Arianismum, imò Photinianisimum potius, interspersisset. Quoniam amicus ego fui illorum, quibus pestilentissimum hoc virus instillavit Diabolus, in suspicionen per meos hostes veni, quasi eidem dogmati ego quoque assensus fuissem. Sed purgavi me, ut spero, eo modo, ut Deo iam ante, deinde omnibus aequis hominibus satisfecerim."

iating acceptance of the consistory's authority? Were he to do this, he would be guilty of the monstrous hypocrisy that Pigafetta had alleged.

While we know little about Erastus's initial withdrawal from communion, there is abundant evidence concerning the efforts to get him reinstated. There was a broad effort from 1574 onward to restore peace within the Heidelberg church. Bullinger had been particularly distressed by the state of the Heidelberg church during the last months of his life, and pleaded with Beza to restrain the highhanded maneuvers of Olevianus. Bullinger complained in great detail about the persecution of Erastus and Mader, the disciplinists' alienation of Prince Ludwig and the nobility, and that Olevianus had even refused to have a civil discussion with Johann Jakob Grynaeus when he attempted to intercede on his brother Simon's behalf.[125] Beza was rather stung by the letter and seems to have particularly resented Bullinger's swipe that Olevianus respected Beza above "other mortals." While conceding that Olevianus could be excessively sharp in judgment and lacked a certain gentleness in his passionate nature, Beza recoiled at the blame that was projected in his direction and also faulted Erastus for essentially treating him as an enemy during his visit to Heidelberg.[126] Beza nevertheless took action and composed a letter to Olevianus urging him to moderation.[127] After Bullinger's death in September, his successor Gwalther took the lead in advocating on Erastus's behalf and found a willing dialogue partner in the new Palatine chief steward Count Ludwig von Sayn-Wittgenstein.[128]

Beza was also intimately involved in the effort to restore peace in the Palatinate. Beza's repeated efforts to reconcile with Erastus were as noteworthy as Erastus's continued rebuff of his overtures. Erastus had broken off contact with Beza and allowed his protégé Johann Jakob Grynaeus to handle his communications with him. Ironically the later fruitful cooperation between Beza and the future head of the Basel church was to some

[125] Bullinger to Beza, April 25, 1575, *CB*, 16:74–80 (no. 1129); translated into German in Rudolf, "Die Kirche in Heidelberg nach den letzten Briefen Bullinger-Beza," 100–102. See Bonnard, *Thomas Éraste*,101; Wesel-Roth, *Thomas Erastus*, 74–78.

[126] Beza to Bullinger, June 8, 1575, *CB*, 16:110–114 (no. 1139); translated into German in Rudolf, "Die Kirche in Heidelberg nach den letzten Briefen Bullinger-Beza," 103–104.

[127] Beza to Olevianus, early June, 1575, *CB*, 16:107–109 (no. 1138); translated into German in Rudolf, "Die Kirche in Heidelberg nach den letzten Briefen Bullinger-Beza," 105.

[128] Bullinger had begun this process the previous spring. See Bullinger to Count Ludwig von Wittgenstein, March 12, 1574, printed in Gottlieb Friedländer, *Beiträge zur Reformationsgeschichte* (Berlin, 1837), 261–264. See Wesel-Roth, *Thomas Erastus*, 79–81.

extent based on their effort to heal the rift with Erastus.[129] Erastus deeply resented that Beza had in effect acted to empower the disciplinist leaders and then tried to play the role of a neutral peacemaker in Heidelberg. Erastus exclaimed of Beza's entreaties: "Phooey with the empty apology." Beza made repeated attempts to see Erastus during his visit to Heidelberg in early 1576, and Erastus continued to keep him at bay.[130]

The efforts to reconcile Erastus with the Palatine church came to fruition in April of 1576. There is a fascinating letter from Erastus to Gwalther from this era which documents his pessimism at reconciling with the church. In Erastus's view, he had remained silent for six years and had even endorsed the elector's edict concerning church discipline, but the disciplinist church leaders still asked for more from him. At the moment where the negotiations appeared to have been at a standstill, Erastus was called to see Count Wittgenstein, who brokered a settlement with Daniel Tossanus and a group of ministers and elders for Erastus to return to good standing in the Heidelberg church.[131] The letter does not

[129] It is thus interesting to observe an exasperated Beza referring to Grynaeus with derision in a contemporary letter to Bullinger (*CB*, 16:74–80 (no. 1129)). His view of Grynaeus would undergo a complete transformation, and already by 1576 he found Grynaeus a most useful partner in Basel (*CB*, 17:142). Beza would later dub Grynaeus "the great." F. Weiss, "Johann Jakob Grynaeus" in *Basler Biographien* (Basel: B. Schwabe, 1900), 194.

[130] Erastus to Grynaeus, Jan. 27, (15)76, Basel UB, G II 4, fol. 195: "Pacificatorem se tunc constituerat, ut adversarios meos me inscio, contr[à]que datam fidem, quantum potest contra me armat et incitat: et ut videre mihi eius tela non liceat, cavet. Excusat postea, non se debuisse in aliena Ecclesia imperium exe[rcer]e, aut pacificationem tentare. Pfui der losen entschuldigung. Quasi non liceat instituere quamvis, ubicumque agat, qui doceri cupit." Another letter (Erastus to Gwalther, Feb. 7, (15)76, ZBZ, A 49, fols. 299–300) outlines Beza's visit and includes Erastus's rather comical excuses for refusing to see Beza including Erastus's suffering from painful gas. Erastus discusses his annoyance at Beza's reconciliation efforts in a letter to Grynaeus, [ca. March, 1576], Basel UB, G II 4, fol. 264. See also Beza to Grynaeus, May 15, 1576, *CB*, 17:62–66 (no. 1191).

[131] The first half of the letter is printed in Wesel-Roth, *Thomas Erastus*, 144–145. Erastus to Gwalther, April 19, (15)76, ZBZ, A 49, fols. 301–303: "Ecce verò postquam haec scripsissem, à Comite vocatus ostendit binas mihi literas à te scriptas; quibus ab eo petas idem hoc, quod à me petis: addita commemoratione multarum rerum aliorum. Ego ei, praestante D. Cancellario, quae iam scripsi, respondi, per me non stetisse, quo minus aliter de nobis loquerentur homines: me privatim neminem scientem offendisse: si aliter a me factum indicaretur, satissfacturum: quam graviter ego sim offensus antea, dum profanum, diabolicum, fanaticum, impium, pacis turbatorem, honestatis osorem publicè me traduxerit (quae tamen nec verbo nec facto ultus fuerim) ipsos novisse: quid porrò apud Principem superiore anno fuerit actum, non esse ipsis ignotum: et proinde me non posse deprecari, quod nunquam commiserim. Huius g[ener]it multa inter nos acta sunt, die palmorum postridie [April 16] vocatis Ministris tribus Tussano, Reckio, Mylio, et duob. Senioribus, iussi sumus alteri alteris indicare, quod cuperemus

indicate that Erastus had to belie his own beliefs to return to communion. It does suggest, much to Erastus's consternation, that leading clerics such as Tossanus were still none too convinced of his orthodoxy. Despite these reservations, Erastus returned to communion at Easter in 1576 and seems to have been basically satisfied with the reconciliation that had been achieved.[132]

The major holdout for Erastus's full reconciliation was his old adversary Olevianus. While Erastus had been cleared by court and university and had been received back into the church, Olevianus refused to renew a fraternal relationship with Erastus. Olevianus had three pieces of circumstantial evidence against Erastus that made it impossible to accept his innocence. First, Erastus had kept Neuser's piece against the Gospel of John in his house for an entire year. Second, Sylvan's letters contained obscure passages that seemed to impugn Erastus. Finally, Sylvan had sought to transmit some manuscript pages to Erastus from jail.[133]

---

emmendari. Respondi, me privatim de Ministris nullis, praeterquam Oleviano queri. Petere autem me, ut hoc mihi facere liceat, quod Dominus iussit. Si pati velint, gr[ati]as me Deo acturum. Si nolint, Deo me rem, ut hucusque fecissem, commisurum: nec ob id cum aliquo litigaturum. Ibi Tussanus, me admitti [s]alvis eorum conscientiis posse. (Sed ita tum loquebatur, ad si suspicari se fateretur me Arianum esse: attamen quia probari id non posset, debere Ecclesiam mihi neganti credere) Quis porrò et qualis Hypocrita sit iste Tussanus, non ego tantum, sed alii multi iam pridem perspexerunt. Reliqui duo g[ener]alia attulerunt. Itaque pax haec facta est: ut esse apud tales potest. Ad me quod attinet, nihil amplius peto. Etsi enim laesum me scio etiam ab aliis, tanta non fuit tamen laesio illa (aut tanti saltem ego non aestimavi) ut propter eam mihi litem iudicarim movendam: quod ipsis omnibus dixi. Nec visum est tempus est locus cum Tussano expostulare. H[o]c mihi sufficit, mihi non esse metuendam repulsam. Caetera Domino curae erunt. Haec est summa actorum. Spero me die Paschatis ad Domini mensam iterum iturum. Quaeso igitur te, ut aliis DD. meis istic idem hoc indices. Non enim dubito, quin hac de re variè sint homines locuturi et scripturi. Res autem sic habet praecisè, ut dixi: non aliter." See also the letter from Gwalther to Beza, April 4, 1576, *CB*, 17:89–92 (no. 1195).

132 Ursinus to Josias Simmler. April 22 (Easter), 1576, printed in Benrath, "Briefe des Heidelberger Theologen Zacharias Ursinus," 131–132: "Hodie Dn. Erastum rursus vidi accendentem ad Coenam Domini magna mea laetitia." See Rudolf, "Die Kirche in Heidelberg nach den letzten Briefen Bullinger-Beza," 106. Erastus to Grynaeus, June 10 (Pentacost), (15)76. Basel UB, G II 4, fol. 197: "Reconciliationem, quam optabam, obtinui: ea conten[tus] sum, plura non quaero." The context of this letter suggests that he may have been speaking of Beza, though its timing suggests his general reconciliation with the church.

133 Erastus to Grynaeus, Sept. 22, 1576, Basel, Öffentliche Bibliothek der Universität Basel, MS G I 33, fols. 10–11: "Paucis diebus post certior fio, bonos viros quosdam reconciliationem inter Olevianum et me tentare coepisse per D. Simonem fratrem. Summ[e] petitionis eorum fuit haec, ut me Olevianum pro fratre habere test[ifi]carer, et, quia innocentiam meam illustiss[im]o Principi et Consiliariis p[ro]bavissem, ipsum orarem, ut suspicionib[us] missis in gr[ati]am me recip[ia]t. Ne verò nulla de causa haec peti putem,

Erastus, not surprisingly, was irate that Olevianus still regarded him with hostility, although Erastus's behind-the-scenes comments on Olevianus hardly reveal a cordial disposition toward Olevianus either. The situation prompted continued hand-wringing for the leaders of the Zurich and Geneva churches.[134] The hard feelings between Erastus and Olevianus had morphed from a theological disagreement into a straightforward feud, which would outlive the reign of Elector Frederick.

Even though the university inquest exonerated Erastus, and even though leading clerics other than Olevianus accepted his innocence from the more serious charges, we might still ask to what degree it was likely that he harbored Antitrinitarian sentiments. Here again there is a divide in the historiography. Most writers familiar with Erastus's entire career and his larger theological corpus do not think Erastus was inclined to heresy. Wesel-Roth, Figgis, Walton, and Benrath fall in this category.[135] Alternatively, other writers such as Burchill and Press, both of whom who were expertly informed on the circle of Heidelberg dissenters, have suggested that Erastus may well have toyed with these radical ideas himself.[136] Burchill has followed Erastus's disciplinist accusers in suggesting that through reading between the lines of Erastus's correspondence with Sylvan and comparing this material with Sylvan's letter to Biandrata, "It was clear that Erastus had been troubled by exactly the same problem as the other members of the group."[137] Even if one does not read such evidence to imply that Erastus seriously entertained doubts about the Trinity, one can hardly suppose that he never took part in such radical conversations. The long list of his theologically unreliable friends and associates included Sozzini, Simoni, Perna, and Seidel, among others. That dissenters beat a path to his door suggests that they found the company inside to their liking. And while Dathenus had no doubt over-

addiderunt, non defuisse Oleviano causas agendi, quod egit. Causas recensuisse audio tres. Prima est, quod librum Adami adversus Evangelium Joh[annis] per anni spacium domi meae habuerim. Alterum, quod literis ad Silvanum scriptis quaedam contineantur obscura, quae aptari huc poss[e] videantur. Tertia, quod idem Silvanus nescio quas schedas ex carcere ad me scripserit, quae penes ipso sint etc." Erastus responded to each of the charges in the subsequent text of the letter.

[134] Gwalther to Beza, Oct. 11, 1576, *CB*, 17:187–193 (no. 1220).

[135] Figgis, "Erastus and Erastianism," 76; Wesel-Roth, *Thomas Erastus*, 67; Walton, "Der Streit zwischen Thomas Erastus und Caspar Olevian," 219; Benrath, "Die Korrespondenz zwischen Bullinger und Thomas Erastus," 123.

[136] Burchill, *The Heidelberg Antitrinitarians*, 49; Press, *Calvinismus und Territorialstaat*, 252.

[137] Burchill, *The Heidelberg Antitrinitarians*, 49.

stated the case in alleging that Erastus's views on church discipline fostered atheism, the manner in which Erastus minimized the role of the visible church in his writings on excommunication did tend in a spiritualist direction.

Nevertheless, if Erastus had genuinely been an Antitrinitarian, it is difficult to believe that his enemies could not have produced evidence against him.[138] Likewise, one cannot ignore the basic point that he never made any recorded affirmation of Antitrinitarian beliefs, and for the remainder of his life frequently confessed his avid endorsement of orthodox Trinitarian dogma—so frequently perhaps that the contrast between his attestations before and after the Antitrinitarian affair may smack of protesting too much.[139] A month after the disclosure of Neuser and Sylvan, Erastus wrote Bullinger a letter in which he confessed his belief that "Scripture teaches that God is one substance, three persons. This I believe piously however it is possible, since I am not able to know fully, I am not anxious to know."[140] This letter may have been written for the censors as much as Bullinger, but it has an authentic ring of someone who knew the limits of theological knowledge. It also agreed with a letter he wrote to Albert Hardenberg in defense of his orthodoxy in which he claimed that he had read little on the question of the Trinity from either orthodox or heterodox authors.[141] Of particular interest is a later letter to an unidentified recipient in which he attempted to explain why he had never

---

[138] Wesel-Roth, *Thomas Erastus*, 67–68.

[139] For example, only after the Sylvan affair did Erastus commence to end his letters with formulaic expressions such as: "Deus opt. max. servet nos ab omni malo, propter unigenitum filium suum Dominum nostrum Jesum Christum. Amen." Erastus to Gwalther, Sept. 24, (1573), ZBZ (Hot.) F 38, fol. 274.

[140] Erastus to Bullinger, August 8, 1570, StAZ, E II 345, fol. 691: "Si qua unquam quaestio fuit de qua disputandum nobis minimè putarem, haec ipsa est: et quaecumque Dei essentiam attingunt. Scio enim ineffabiliter minus esse comparabiles captum nostrum et infinitam Dei maiestatem, quam si punctum non visibile comparetur cum mundo, non uno, sed mille, imò millies mille mundis. Non potest quisquam nostrum intelligere quid nostra sit anima, qua sumus, quod sumus: quomodo ergo intelligemus quatenus pateat Divina essentia? Deum esse unum substantia, trinum personis, docent Sacrae Literae. Haec ego credo piè, quomodo sit scire cum non satis possim, scire non laboro. Equidem non puto ullam esse temeritatem audaciorem, quam si homuncio conetur Christi Dei potentiam et Maiestatem cancellis ingenii sui includere, potestatemque Servatoris sui circumscribere." Transcription following Bonnard, *Thomas Éraste*, 100.

[141] Erastus to Hardenberg, [ca. Nov. 1571-Jan. 1572], London, Lambeth Palace Library, MS 2010, fols. 152^{r}–153^{v}: "Sed Deo est gratia, quod sceleratè impieque mentiuntur, quicunque me de Articulo Trinitatis vel dubitavisse aliquando dicunt. Nulla vel Orthodoxorum vel haereticorum nostri temporis scripta de hac re legi, praeter Jacobi Schegkii ex Simleri libellos: quos mihi summè probatos fuisse novit Deus."

corresponded with the famed humanist Andreas Dudith.[142] Various Poles, in particular Jan Lasicki, had often urged him to initiate a correspondence with Dudith. Erastus was receptive to the idea until he heard rumors that Dudith inclined toward Arianism. At this point, Erastus must have calculated that he had had enough heterodox friends for one lifetime. Thus to protect himself, he did not write Dudith. Erastus added:

> For you know how that worthless Olevianus attempted to make me a defendant of this same crime: although from no error or sin in my entire life have I been more alien. I scarcely think that any man has ever lived who ever doubted the article of the Sacred Trinity less than me.[143]

After being assured of Dudith's orthodoxy, Erastus did strike up a correspondence with him. The fruit of their friendship was two collections of treatises on comets in the wake of the famous comet of 1577.[144]

---

[142] Andreas Dudith attended the third session of the council of Trent as Bishop of Knin in Dalmatia. He made a strong impression at the council with his passionate speeches advocating the concession of the cup to the laity. He later was named Bishop of Pécs (Fünfkircken). While in the service of the Habsburgs in Poland, he left the church and married. After a flirtation with Unitarianism, Dudith embraced Protestant doctrine through the efforts of Crato. Gillet, *Crato von Crafftheim und seine Freunde*; Pierre Costil, *André Dudith Humaniste Hongrois 1533–1589: Sa Vie, son Oeuvre et ses Manuscrits Grecs* (Paris: Société D'édition "Les Belles Lettres," 1935); Hebert Jedin, *Geschichte des Konzils von Trient*, 4 vols. (Basel: Herder, 1948–1975), 4(1):172, 343; idem, "André Dudith," in *Dictionnaire d'histoire et de géographie ecclésiastiques* (Paris, 1912–) 14:988–990.

[143] Erastus to [Theophil Mader?, Christoph Schilling?], Heidelberg, March 26. 1577, SUB Bremen, 8, fols. 250–252. (See also the partial German translation in Hollweg, *Heinrich Bullingers Hausbuch*, 277, in note.) "Intelligo etiam ex tuis hospitium tibi dedisse g[e]n[er]osum et illustr[em] virum D. Andream Duditum: cuius ego virtutem, et doctrinam ante multos annos mireficè audivi praedicari. Invitatus saep[i]us fui à Polonis [In margin: et imprimis à Dn. N[icolo] Lasizio], ut ad eum literas darem: nec ego ali[e]nus ab ea re fui. Metui tamen, cum occasio nulla scribe[n]d[um] offerretur, ne vir tantus vel amicitiam et observantiam meam aspernaretur, vel aliter factum meum interpretaretur. Itaque me continui: nec multo post audivi eum in suspicionem aliquam venisse, quasi Arii Dogmati faveret. Etsi verò putarem iniuriam fieri viro tanto ingenio, iudicio, tantaque doctrina et pietate praedito, timidiorem tamen ea me res facit. Scis enim quam sceleratè Nebulo ille Olevianus eiusdem criminis reum me facere tentarit: cum à nullo errore et peccato in omni mea vita alienior fuerim. Vix puto vivere ullum hominem, qui minus me de articulo Trinitatis Sacrosantae unquam dubitarit. Quare sic mecum r[ati]ocinabar, si tibi intentare audent scelus tam nefarium, (de quo nulla creatura ex me verbum ullum audivit aut factum aliquis vidit, ex quo vel suspicio probabilis posset nasci) quid non audebunt de longius dissitis mentiri? Attamen cum de re ipsa nil mihi constiterit, et ne nunc quidem constet aliquid, optima sperare volui, (et iam etiam spero) nihil tamem faciendum mihi censui, quod Adversariis meis nequissimis occasionem pr[ae]beret suam improbitatem excusandi. Quis enim ego sum alià[s] ut n[on] vehementer gaudere debeam, si tanto viro plac[uis]se iudicer?"

[144] Thomas Erastus et al., *De Cometis dissertationes novae clariss. Vivorum Thom. Erasti, Andr. Dudithij, Marc. Squacialupi, Symon. Grynaei* (Basel: Leonard Ostein, 1580);

No definitive judgment can be offered concerning Erastus's orthodoxy at this point. It does not seem likely that he would have continued to campaign against the anti-disciplinists, had he been harboring such a dangerous secret. His continued agitation against the Calvinist vision of church discipline suggests that the issue which had become an obsession for Erastus was excommunication itself rather than a hidden Antitrinitarian agenda. From the surviving evidence, it seems clear that Erastus was never an active Antitrinitarian like many of his friends. However, there were apparently theological works he mentions in his correspondence that are not known to have survived, and thus we cannot judge their contents, though none bears such a provocative title as Sylvan's assault on "*the Three-Person Idol and the Two-Natured False Deity of the Antichrist*."[145]

In considering the magnitude of Erastus's engagement with the Antitrinitarian movement, it is appropriate to note the dissimilarity between his situation and that of Neuser and Sylvan. Unlike the two clerics, Erastus possessed a secure position at the university from which he could snipe at his disciplinist rivals. His enemies had no direct influence over his professional career. In the late 1560s, Erastus was not threatened with the potential loss of income and future prospects that the clerical members of his party faced. Even if Erastus had been expelled from Heidelberg, he could always earn a lucrative salary as a court physician elsewhere. Unlike Erastus, Neuser experienced firsthand the difficulty of landing another clerical job without a letter of reference from his past position. Erastus was a man of options, not of desperation, and he actually counseled his friends to beware of becoming too personally invested in the conflict.[146] Similarly, when one considers Erastus's life history, it stands in sharp contrast with Sylvan's. Whereas Sylvan had

---

Andreas Dudith et al., *De Cometarum Significatione Commentariolus* (Basel: Pietro Perna, 1579). See C. Doris Hellman, *The Comet of 1577* (New York: Columbia UP, 1944).

[145] The works are mentioned letters to Johann Jakob Grynaeus and Bullinger. Erastus mentions an "Antilogias Catechismi" (Nov. 29, [1570], Basel UB, G II 4, fols. 300–301 and Feb. 2, [1571], Basel UB, G II 4, fol. 282) and a "de Methodo Theologica Sententia" (Aug. 5, (15)77, Basel UB, G II 4, fols. 203–204). The *Antilogias catechismi* may be a coded expression for his *Explicatio gravissimae quaestionis* (or perhaps the *Confirmatio thesium* section of the work), his anti-Paracelsian disputations, or may simply refer to a work by someone else. In a letter to Bullinger he writes: "Antilogias catecheseos, ordinationis et theologorum vos iam accepisse puto; transmissum enim nuper est vasculum affini meo, in quo cum aliis quibusdam rebus ac suppellectile aliqua huius scripti exemplum inerat." Erastus to Bullinger, Oct. 29 [1570], StAZ, E II 345, fols. 741–742.

[146] Erastus to Sylvan, June 21, (1569), Amberg, Staatsarchiv Amberg, Religions-und

migrated from one religious conviction to another, the evidence suggests that Erastus remained faithful to a single vision of Christian truth his entire adult life. In short, Erastus did not feel the social pressure of the controversy as intensely as Neuser and Sylvan, and his personality profile would suggest that he was much less conversion prone than someone like Sylvan. When all these factors are taken together, it appears unlikely that Erastus positively espoused an Antitrinitarian position. If he had doubts, he had the discretion to keep them private.

Erastus and Johann Jakob Grynaeus

In Erastus's later life his fortunes would become increasingly intertwined with Basel's Grynaeus clan. The first famous Grynaeus in Basel was the humanist Simon Grynaeus (1493–1541), who had labored to establish the Reformed church in Basel after Oecolampadius's death.[147] Erastus was connected to the branch of the family descending from Simon's nephew Thomas Grynaeus.[148] Erastus's relationship with Thomas's sons Johann Jakob and Simon would be of critical importance for the confessional history of both Heidelberg and Basel. A foreshadowing of this alliance can be seen in a letter from Erastus to Thomas Grynaeus from the early 1560s in which Erastus suggested that Simon should come to Heidelberg where he could receive an academic appointment and that Johann Jakob should take his doctorate in Heidelberg rather than Tübingen.[149] Simon did take a position in Heidelberg and remained there as Erastus's partisan and trusted friend, becoming the joint targets of the wrath of the Heidelberg disciplinists in the 1570s. Johann Jakob, on the other hand, followed the advice of his mentor, the "Lutheranizing" Basel *antistes* Sulzer, and studied in Tübingen with Jakob Andreae. The events

Reformationswesen, MS no. 67, fol. 130. Printed in Rott, "Neue Quellen für eine Aktenrevision," 61. Summarized in Burchill, *The Heidelberg Antitrinitarians*, 13.

[147] Rene Teuteberg, "Simon Grynaeus," in *Der Reformation verpflichtet: Gestalten und Gestalter in Stadt und Landschaft Basel aus fünf Jahrhunderten* (Basel: Christoph Merian Verlag, 1979), 29.

[148] Thommen, *Geschichte der Universität Basel, 1532–1632*, 359; Carl Roth, "Stammtafeln einiger ausgestorbener Basler Gelehrtenfamilien," *Basler Zeitschrift für Geschichte und Altertumskunde* (1917): 393–403. Thomas Grynaeus took a position on the Basel faculty in 1537 before moving on to a pastorate in Rötteln in the Markgrafschaft of Baden.

[149] Erastus to Thomas Grynaeus, April 4, [ca. 1562], Basel UB, G II 4, fol. 266.

of the late 1560s, however, would bring Johann Jakob under Erastus's influence and make him receptive to a Reformed interpretation of the Lord's Supper.[150]

Thomas Grynaeus died in 1564, making it necessary for Johann Jakob to rapidly bring his theological studies to completion. Through the guidance of Andreae, it was determined that Grynaeus would defend doctoral theses on ubiquity. Grynaeus failed in his first attempt to defend these theses.[151] After this disappointment, the disconsolate Grynaeus passed through Heidelberg where he discussed his dilemma with Erastus and Zacharias Ursinus. It takes little imagination to envision how these Reformed thinkers may have used this opportunity to undermine Grynaeus's faith in the Lutheran teaching of ubiquity.[152] Nevertheless, in December of 1565 Johann Jakob was able to return to Tübingen and successfully defend his doctoral theses.[153]

In the short run, Grynaeus remained in the Lutheran camp and continued to be favored by Sulzer, who appointed him to Grynaeus's father's former position as church inspector in the village of Rötteln (by modern Lörrach) in the Markgrafschaft of Baden-Durlach near Basel. Grynaeus only came into close contact with Erastus after he married Erastus's sister-in-law, Lavinia de' Canonici, who had been residing with Erastus in Heidelberg. From this point Erastus and Grynaeus became intimate associates and academic collaborators. More than one hundred letters from Erastus to Grynaeus preserved in the Basel University library document their close relationship. These letters suggest a hierarchical relationship, with the senior Erastus keeping Grynaeus busy seeing his works through press, shipping him provisions, and handling financial transactions, while Erastus periodically extended Grynaeus a measure of fatherly advice and a good deal of money.

[150] Weiss, "Johann Jakob Grynaeus," 162–163; Hans R. Guggisberg, *Basel in the Sixteenth Century* (St. Louis: Center for Reformation Research, 1982), 45–48. For Sulzer, see Amy Nelson Burnett, "Simon Sulzer and the Consequences of the 1563 Strasbourg Consensus in Switzerland," *ARG* 83 (1992): 154–179.

[151] *Disputatio de Maiestate hominis Christi: deq[ue] vera et substantiali corporis et sanguinis eius in Eucharistia, praesentia. In qua … Praeside … Iacobo Andreae, Ecclesiae & Scholae Tubengensis Praeposito & Cancellario … Ioannes Iacobus Grynaeus pridie nonas Februarias [Feb. 4]* … (Tübingen: Ulrich Morhart, 1564; VD 16 A 2589).

[152] Weiss, "Johann Jakob Grynaeus," 162–163. Wilhelm Xylander was also in attendance.

[153] *Capita Disputationis ordinariae, de Maiestate hominis Christi: deqve vera et substantiali corporis et sanguinis eius in Eucharistia, praesentia. A Iacobo Andreae* … (Ioannes Iacobus Grynaeus … respondebit) … (Tübingen: Ulrich Morhart, 1564; VD 16 A 2504).

Traditionally, Grynaeus's conversion to a Reformed interpretation of the Lord's Supper has been credited to his relationship with Erastus.[154] Although we lack a full investigation of Grynaeus's conversion to a Reformed perspective from a study of his own writings, we receive some sense of the nature of the transition from Erastus's letters to Grynaeus. In these letters Erastus consistently and persuasively espoused the Reformed interpretation of the Lord's Supper and belittled Sulzer and the south German Lutherans.

The doctrine that Erastus attacked most sharply in his correspondence with Grynaeus was the Lutheran teaching of ubiquity. Erastus lumped ubiquity with speculative theological issues that had little value. Whereas ubiquity had no straightforward scriptural foundation, it was manifest in the scriptures that Christ ascended into heaven. Thus, Erastus argued, the clear scriptural text must take precedence over philosophical speculation. Like a good Zwinglian, Erastus emphasized that the purpose of the Lord's Supper was to give thanks for Christ's act of redemption. He concluded that the Lutherans were happy to debate the fine points of the Lord's Supper while they missed the heart of the matter, which was true piety. In this regard, Erastus concluded that the whole idea of ubiquity of the flesh of Christ was a fiction and a monstrosity.[155]

Perhaps more critical than Erastus's refutation of Lutheran doctrine was his careful attempt to alienate Grynaeus from his former Lutheran teachers. He warned Grynaeus to beware of Andreae, whom Erastus called a "bird," and suggested that if he wrote to Grynaeus, he should either not respond or think it over ten times.[156] No doubt it was more difficult to drive a wedge between Grynaeus and his mentor Sulzer. To achieve this goal Erastus combined judicious praise of Grynaeus with an assault on Sulzer's character in which he portrayed Sulzer as a

[154] Weiss, "Johann Jakob Grynaeus," 164; Max Geiger, *Die Basler Kirche und Theologie im Zeitalter der Hochorthodoxie* (Zollikon: Evangelischer Verlag, 1952); 40; Gottlieb Linder, *Simon Sulzer und sein Antheil in der Reformation im Lande Baden sowie an den Unionbestrebungen* (Heidelberg, 1890), 147. See also Kaspar von Greyerz, "Basels kirchliche und konfessionelle Beziehungen zum Oberrhein im späten 16. und frühen 17. Jahrhundert," In *Schweizerisch-Deutsche Beziehungen im Konfessionellen Zeitalter: Beiträge zur Kulturgeschichte 1580–1650*, ed. Martin Bircher et al. (Wiesbaden: Otto Harrassowitz, 1984), 227–252.

[155] Erastus to Grynaeus, Sept. 18, [ca, 1573], Basel UB, G II 4, fol. 290. "De usu potius coenae disputarent homines isti, quibus adeo cordi est Religio, quam de carnis Christi fictitia et monstrosa illa ubiquitate."

[156] Erastus to Grynaeus, Feb. 22, (15)73, Basel UB, G II 4, fol. 181.

deceptive hypocrite.[157] By 1574 Erastus could rejoice that Grynaeus had finally come to recognize Sulzer's real intentions. Nevertheless, Erastus counseled Grynaeus to remain wary in dealing with Sulzer.[158] Erastus prophesied that Grynaeus would be the healer of the Basel church, which Oswald Myconius had initially established only to have Sulzer tear it asunder, according to Erastus's partisan reading of Basel Reformation history.[159]

While a definitive assessment of Erastus's impact on Grynaeus cannot be drawn from these sources, the fact that these letters coincided with Grynaeus's initial break with Sulzer in October of 1573 suggests that his influence was significant.[160] It appears that Grynaeus's alienation from Sulzer was a two-stage process, with 1573 representing the first fissure in their relationship. Initially, Sulzer seems to have taken a conciliatory stance toward Grynaeus and even assisted Grynaeus's assumption of his own position on the Basel theological faculty in 1575.[161] Grynaeus and Sulzer became determined opponents only after the introduction of the *Formula of Concord* in the Markgrafschaft of Baden in 1577.[162] From all appearances, Erastus's encouragement and intellectual support played a significant role in winning Grynaeus as the champion of the Reformed confession in Basel. Grynaeus would later play a critical role in bringing Basel back into full alliance with the other Swiss-Reformed churches and in reestablishing the Reformed faith in the Palatinate after a Lutheran interlude.

[157] Ironically, Peter Patiens would say much the same about Grynaeus—that he had "honey in his mouth and gall in his heart." Linder, *Simon Sulzer*, 148.

[158] Erastus to Grynaeus, Nov. 15, 1574, Basel UB, G II 4, fol. 187 (added to a letter from Nov. 13 on fol. 186).

[159] Erastus to Grynaeus, March 25, [1578], Basel UB, G II 4, fol. 297: "Spero enim Deum per te vulnus istius Ecclesiae, quod Miconius primum designavit, Sulzerus postmodum impressit, et adhuc, ne coalescat, fovet, imò dilacerat, sanare velle."

[160] Linder, *Simon Sulzer*,147; Weiss, "Johann Jakob Grynaeus," 165. Especially if Basel UB G II 4, fol. 290 is correctly ascribed to 1573. In this case, Grynaeus's remonstrance to Sulzer that to embrace ubiquity one must give up the ascension nearly flows directly from Erastus's pen.

[161] Letter from Sulzer to Kasper Herwagen, Councilor of the Markgraf, regarding Grynaeus's transfer to Basel from his pastorate in Rötteln is printed in Linder, *Simon Sulzer*, 98–99.

[162] Linder, *Simon Sulzer*, 148; Weiss, "Johann Jakob Grynaeus," 167–169; Amy Nelson Burnett, *Teaching the Reformation: Ministers and Their Message in Basel, 1529–1629* (Oxford: Oxford UP, 2006), 134–135.

Conclusion

The year 1570 proved to be the watershed of Erastus's career in Heidelberg. From that point until Elector Frederick's death, Erastus, his supporters, and his Zwinglian vision of the Christian faith would be on the defensive. The Reformation of the Palatinate became fully "Calvinist" due to that party's victory in the controversy over church discipline. The Calvinist triumph was in no small measure facilitated by the Antitrinitarian fiasco. Because of his strong position at the university and his personal prestige, Erastus was able to weather the storm though his position was at times perilous. The disruption of his engagement in church affairs brought more time for scholarly pursuits. In the coming years he would reorient his career and find new opportunities to demonstrate both his academic talent and his religious orthodoxy.

Although the Calvinist faction did not accomplish all their aims in their quest to establish a consistory of elders fully independent of state control in the Palatinate, the Genevan vision of church discipline clearly triumphed over the Zurich model. The victory of the Calvinist model of discipline in Heidelberg symbolized the growing dominance of the Genevan paradigm of the Reformed faith over that of Zurich in the international Reformed movement. The Genevan ascendancy would continue to increase in the coming decades so that by the early seventeenth century the theological character of the international Reformed movement became increasingly Calvinist (e.g., doctrine of predestination and the marks of the church, but not uniformly so on the doctrine of the Lord's Supper). However, minority strains remained within the larger Reformed movement. The ideas of Erastus and the other advocates of the "single sphere" model of church-state relations continued to circulate in Reformed circles and would arise with renewed force in seventeenth-century England. These developments will be treated in the epilogue.

PART III

NEW SCHOLARLY DIRECTIONS AFTER 1570

CHAPTER EIGHT

ANTIPARACELSICA

> With God's help, I have finished the first part of the work against Paracelsus.... If a Swiss person wrote evil (however, I do not yet believe that he was Swiss), then a Swiss person has refuted him, if not well, at least truly.... For I solemnly swear to you, that neither Arius, nor Photinus, nor Muhammad, nor other Turk, nor any heretic who has [ever] lived was more heretical than this most pestilential magician.
>
> Erastus to Heinrich Bullinger

> The lost art of Medicine—recovered by Paracelsus—had an eternally sure foundation, against which all the gates of Hell cannot prevail, let alone the trashy books which Erastus, with his blind, stubborn adherents, has vomited forth against God and the truth.
>
> Benedictus Figulus on Erastus[1]

The year 1570 and the Speyer Imperial Diet marked a turning point in the life of Erastus. In addition to fulfilling his duties as professor of medicine and practicing physician, Erastus spent the first half of the 1560s shaping and defending the Reformed confession in the Palatinate. Although he had written several Latin medical and philosophical treatises, only one appeared in print prior to 1569.[2] For the remainder of his tenure in Heidelberg, Erastus invested most of his time in scholarly pursuits. The first project he took on, his four-volume refutation of the work of Paracelsus, would bring him both fame and infamy in the history of science.

As a humanist physician with deep reverence for classical medical texts, Erastus was appalled by the medical revolutionary Paracelsus,

[1] Benedictus Figulus [aka Benedikt Töpfer], "Dialogus, Alexandri a Suchten ...," in *Pandora Magnalium Naturalium Aurea Et Benedicta, De Benedicto Lapidis Philosoph. Mysterio* (Strasbourg: Lazarus Zetzner, 1608), 89: "Ich geschweig die Lumpenbücher so Erastus sampt seinen blinden/ verstockten und verfluchten Adhaerenten wider Gott unnd die warheit außgespreyet hat." English translation: *A Golden and Blessed Casket of Nature's Marvels*, trans. [Arthur Edward Waite] (London, 1893), 134–135.

[2] Thomas Erastus, *Ratio Formandorum Syllogismorum* (Basel: J. Oporinus, 1565).

who sought to discard all prior medical knowledge. Although Paracelsus had hardly concerned him before this point, Erastus was personally acquainted with Paracelsus's most important early opponents and thus well-placed to refute Paracelsus. Johannes Crato von Krafftheim, Heinrich Bullinger, Johann Jakob Grynaeus, and others aided Erastus in assembling his four volumes of anti-Paracelsian disputations (*Disputationum de medicina nova Philippi Paracelsi pars prima-quarta*, hereafter referred to as *De medicina nova*, 1–4).[3] After reviewing Paracelsus's vast corpus, Erastus unleashed a comprehensive attack on the religious, philosophical, and therapeutic bases of Paracelsus's medical program. Since Erastus's thinking differed from Paracelsus's at every turn, Erastus's effort to refute him supplies a salutary contrast which allows Erastus's unstated assumptions to become visible. Written at the nadir of his time in the Palatinate, Erastus used his attack on Paracelsus to secure a place among the medical elite of the Holy Roman Empire and to demonstrate his own theological orthodoxy. This chapter will focus on the manner in which Erastus portrayed Paracelsus and why he found Paracelsus's natural philosophy so profoundly heretical.

The Historical Background of Erastus's Opposition to Paracelsus

The sixteenth century was a period of great intellectual ferment. The invention and spread of printing in the mid-fifteenth century magnified the Renaissance cultural renewal that had taken hold in Northern Europe around the turn of the century. Without the proliferation of printing presses in Germany, it would have been impossible to imagine that Martin Luther's revolt would have ever turned into such a tremendous mass media event. The Protestants were not the only beneficiaries of movable type. Elizabeth Eisenstein has asserted that the advent of print

[3] *Disputationum De medicina nova Philippi Paracelsi Pars Prima: In qua, quae de remediis superstitiosis & Magicis curationibus ille prodidit, praecipue examinantur (Basel: Pietro Perna, [1571]); Disputationum de nova Philippi Paracelsi medicina Pars Altera: In qua Philosophiae Paracelsicae Principia & Elementa explorantur* ([Basel]: Pietro Perna, 1572); *Disputationum de nova Philippi Paracelsi Medicina Pars Tertia* ([Basel]: Pietro Perna, 1572); *Disputationum de nova medicina Philippi Paracelsi Pars Quarta et Ultima* (Basel: Pietro Perna, 1573; hereafter collectively cited as *De medicina nova*, with the respective volume designated with an Arabic numeral). See also the translation of *De medicina nova*, 1 (without the appendix), Franz Josef Schmidt, ed., *Disputationen über die neue Medizin des Philippus Paracelsus* (Hamm: self-published, 1978).

enabled the rediscovery of antique culture to turn into a "permanent renaissance."[4] This recovery of classical knowledge also had a profound impact on medical studies. The fundamental basis of all learned European medical knowledge—Muslim, Christian, and Jewish—had been the Greek medical authors of the ancient world. The classics of ancient medicine were the *Hippocratic corpus* associated with, though not all authored by, Hippocrates of Cos (ca. 460–ca. 377 BC) as well as the even more voluminous writings of Galen of Pergamum (ca. 130–ca. 200 AD). Galen assimilated and structured the medical knowledge of the ancient world to such a degree that the title "Galenism" can basically stand for the conventional wisdom in learned medicine from late antiquity into the early modern era. In the early medieval era, medical knowledge fared no better than other types of secular learning in the general cultural decline pejoratively referred to as the Dark Ages. Only a few of the antique medical texts remained in circulation. With limited access to the classics of ancient medicine and restricted knowledge of Greek, Western Europeans would eventually find alternatives in the great medical compilations of Arab-Islamic civilization which entered Western Europe from the twelfth century onward. Admittedly, it is rather crude to speak of the Arab-Islamic medical tradition as a monolithic entity. Two of its most famous representatives, Avicenna (Ibn Sina, 980–1037) and Rhazes (Razi, d. 925), were Persians; the translator Johannitius (Hunayn ibn Ishaq, d. 837) was a Nestorian Christian from southern Iraq; and the great Aristotelian philosopher-physician Averroës (Ibn Rushd, 1126–1198) was from Moorish Spain. Avicenna's *Canon*, a great medical sourcebook that distilled the classics of the ancient world into a manageable system, became far and away the favorite medical textbook of the Latin West. Learned medieval Christian practitioners remained largely within the medical tradition founded by Hippocrates and Galen; however, this tradition was mediated to the West primarily through Arabic sources such as Avicenna.[5]

[4] See Elizabeth Eisenstein, *The Printing Revolution in Early Modern Europe* (Cambridge: Cambridge UP, 1983), 111.

[5] Lawrence I. Conrad, "The Arab-Islamic Medical Tradition," in *The Western Medical Tradition 800 BC to AD 1800*; Vivian Nutton, "Medicine in Late Antiquity and the Early Middle Ages," in *The Western Medical Tradition*; idem, "Medicine in Medieval Western Europe, 1000–1500," in *The Western Medical Tradition*; Nancy G. Siraisi, *Medieval and Early Renaissance Medicine* (Chicago: University of Chicago Press, 1990); idem, *Avicenna in Renaissance Italy: The Canon and Medical Teaching in Italian Universities after 1500* (Princeton: Princeton UP, 1987).

The dominant position of Arabic medicine in the West was to change during the late Renaissance. First, a revival of Greek letters beginning in Italy in the early fifteenth century became widespread by the second half of the century. This revival of Greek coincided with the development of printing. The first complete works of Galen in Greek hit the fairs in 1525 and the *Hippocratic Corpus* would follow the next year. The new proliferation of knowledge of Greek, combined with the availability of a wider array of texts, transformed medical knowledge in the sixteenth century. When historians speak of the "medical Renaissance" of the sixteenth century, it is primarily this recovery of ancient learning that they have in mind. In general this medical Renaissance was text-oriented and deferred to the authority of the classics like the other "humanisms" of the period. The medical Renaissance's privileging of Greek texts has led some scholars to suggest that the phenomenon should actually be more properly labeled medical "Hellenism" as opposed to simple medical humanism.[6] Many of the scholars of the period, including Erastus, cultivated a certain disdain for the classic Arabic medical texts that had been favored in the high medieval and early Renaissance period.[7] While this revival of the Greek medical knowledge of the ancient world was at the heart of the medical Renaissance, the movement did venture beyond the simple assimilation and recapitulation of ancient medical knowledge. Girolamo Fracastoro put forward his intuitively perceptive "seeds of disease" theory, which in some senses presaged the later discoveries of Robert Koch and Louis Pasteur. Andreas Vesalius published his epochal work of anatomy *De humani corporis fabrica* in 1543 with the Basel publishing house of Johannes Oporinus, Erastus's biographer and publisher. Beyond the real advances represented by these figures and other luminaries such as Jean Fernel, Gabriele Falloppio, and Giambattista da Monte, what is most striking is the degree to which these individuals remained within the larger Galenic paradigm. Fracastoro's innovative theory of disease was largely derived from Galen and other ancient sources. Even Vesalius, the person with the best claim to be a true innovator, remained largely within Galenic conceptions of anatomy and physiology and did not overturn the notion of inter-ventricular pores, a bequest of Galen which was critical to the faulty understanding of the circulation of blood.

[6] See the introduction to A. Wear, R.K. French, and I.M. Lonie, *The Medical Renaissance of the Sixteenth Century* (Cambridge: Cambridge UP, 1985), 8.

[7] See chapter 2 regarding Erastus's role in the revision of the University of Heidelberg's medical statutes and early anatomical instruction in Heidelberg.

In short, the sixteenth century did experience a distinct medical Renaissance; however, the parameters for this renewal were largely determined by ancient Greek medical texts.[8] The "medical revolution" awaited future centuries.

Protestants were active participants in this "medical Renaissance." Only a few years after Luther nailed his *Ninety-five Theses* to the castle church door in Wittenberg, his younger associate Melanchthon began the project of setting forth a distinctly Protestant natural philosophy based largely on Aristotle, Plato, and Galen at the University of Wittenberg.[9] Although Luther had early rejected what he considered the pernicious influence of Aristotle on theological studies, Luther himself, and Melanchthon to an even greater degree, still considered the ancient Greeks to be the highest authorities in questions of natural philosophy. With a basis of a Protestant biblical theology and humanist study of the classical texts of natural philosophy, the Wittenberg curriculum served as a model for other central European universities such as Marburg, Jena, Tübingen, and later Heidelberg. This new Protestant tradition did not represent a radical break with the scholastic past, but a reorientation brought on by changes in theological assumptions and a rapid incorporation of humanist methodology. Within this Protestant-humanist intellectual drift, there was a natural sympathy for the program of medical Hellenism. For example, Johannes Crato von Krafftheim, a prized pupil of Luther and Melanchthon, traveled to Padua to study medicine, where he eventually served as an assistant to Giambattista da Monte, one of the most influential of the medical humanists, before embarking on his own illustrious career as imperial physician. As Vivian Nutton has shown, Melanchthon himself had a tremendous impact on the development of the Wittenberg anatomy and incorporated these medical insights into his conception of human nature.[10] In a word, there was no conflict between the medical Renaissance and Protestantism; rather, Protestant Germans were avid participants in the renewal of ancient medical knowledge.

[8] Regarding Fracastoro's originality or lack thereof, see Vivian Nutton, "The Seeds of Disease: An Explanation of Contagion and Infection from the Greeks to the Renaissance," *Medical History* 27 (1983): 1–34. Andrew Wear, "Medicine in Early Modern Europe 1500–1700," in *The Western Medical Tradition 800 BC to AD 1800*, 207–361, cf. especially the "chronological table" on pp. 207–213.

[9] Kusukawa, *The Transformation of Natural Philosophy: The Case of Philip Melanchthon*.

[10] Nutton, "Wittenberg Anatomy," in *Medicine and the Reformation*, 11–32.

While the medical Renaissance was still in its early phase, Paracelsus (1493/94–1541) proposed a more radical overhaul of natural philosophy and medical practice. Born Theophrastus Bombastus von Hohenheim, sometimes with an extra name or two thrown in for good measure, Paracelsus was the true knight-errant of the medical Renaissance. Paracelsus advocated the abandonment of ancient authorities of natural philosophy and the development of a new experimental learning, which integrated themes from alchemy, natural magic, and a spiritualistic brand of Christianity.[11] Paracelsus's new philosophy made its public debut in his meteoric rise and fall at the University of Basel in 1527–1528, which was signaled by his unprecedented medical lectures in the vernacular and the perhaps legendary account of his burning of Avicenna's *Canon*.[12] After his fall from prominence in Basel, Paracelsus led an itinerant life, stopping for short sojourns here and there, depositing manuscripts far and wide. He died in relative obscurity in Salzburg in 1541.[13]

If Paracelsus had been underappreciated while alive, it was due in large part to the fact that his contemporaries did not know the full richness of his corpus, since few of his works were printed in his lifetime. His unconventional habits and difficult personality likewise made it nearly impossible for Paracelsus's medical contribution to be judged on its own terms. For all his limitations and quirks, he was, in the words of leading contemporary historian of pre-modern medicine Nutton, "the only innovative medical theorist of the sixteenth century."[14] He rejected the Galenic notion that disease was by definition an imbalance of the four humors and developed a theory that emphasized external causes of disease. In this theory, sometimes termed a parasitic conception of disease, an exter-

[11] Paracelsus's religiosity defies simple categorization. He is now generally considered something of a radical spiritualist reformer, though he never formally broke with the Catholic Church. See Ute Gause, *Paracelsus: Genese und Entfaltung seiner frühen Theologie* (Stuttgart: J.C.B. Mohr, 1993).

[12] Pagel, *Paracelsus* (see above n. 3), 19–22.

[13] Regarding Paracelsus's biography, see Udo Benzenhöfer, *Paracelsus* (Reinbek bei Hamburg: Rowohlt, 1997); Charles Webster, *Paracelsus: Medicine, Magic and Mission at the End of Time* (New Haven: Yale UP, 2008). See also the competent popular treatment in English by Philip Ball, *The Devil's Doctor: Paracelsus and the World of Renaissance Magic and Science* (New York: Farrar, Straus and Giroux, 2006). For a brief introduction to Paracelsus studies and concise bibliography, see Gerhild Scholz Williams and Charles D. Gunnoe, eds., *Paracelsian Moments: Science, Medicine, and Astrology in Early Modern Europe* [*SCE&S* 64] (Kirksville, Mo.: Truman State UP, 2002). See additionally the new collection of translated texts: Paracelsus, *Essential Theoretical Writings*, ed. Andrew Weeks (Leiden: Brill, 2008).

[14] Nutton, "The Seeds of Disease," 23.

nal agent would attack one particular organ. In Paracelsus's theory, this harmful agent was the disease itself rather than simply being the cause of disease. If his theory ran 180 degrees against the Galenists, so did his proposed therapies. He abandoned traditional remedies, which after all were intended to restore the balance of the four humors, in favor of new chemical medicines. His miracle drugs were perhaps even more dangerous than the traditional run of prescriptions based on herbs. In this case, Paracelsus's chemical medicine was important primarily for the stimulus that it gave to the emerging science of chemistry. Beyond his general stimulus to chemical medicine, in his emphasis on experiment and observation, seen for example in his path-breaking work linking certain diseases to the mining industry, he has rightly earned a prominent place in the history of medicine.

Paracelsus's works were to find a warmer reception in the second half of the sixteenth century than they ever had in his lifetime. A full-scale Paracelsian revival was afoot by the 1570s. Michael Toxites, Gerhard Dorn, and Adam von Bodenstein (son of the Reformer Andreas Karlstadt von Bodenstein) all worked feverishly to uncover Paracelsus's manuscripts and see them through press. The popularity of Paracelsus's writings was enough to spawn a veritable Paracelsian school in the later sixteenth century which featured new works in the Paracelsian tradition by authors such as Jacques Gohory (aka Leo Suavius), Alexander von Suchten, Petrus Servinus, and Oswald Croll, as well as a befuddling panoply of pseudo-Paracelsian texts. As we shall see below in the late sixteenth century, it became increasingly difficult to separate the "Paracelsian" from the genuine Paracelsus. As time progressed, the Paracelsian movement displayed a more pervasive Hermetic influence and a greater predilection for transmutational alchemy (chrysopoeia) than Paracelsus's own work had exhibited.[15] This school did not represent the establishment, but rather, the vibrant counter-culture in sixteenth-century natural philosophy. Though Paracelsus had clearly thrown down the gauntlet with his explicit rejection of Galen, Aristotle, and Avicenna, the two paradigms of medical theory were not always in conflict, and figures such as Theodor Zwinger and Johann Winther (Guintherius) von Andernach

[15] The fourteenth volume of the Sudhoff edition contains many such spurious works. For a fascinating look into the pseudo-Paracelsian world, see Joachim Telle, "'Von der Wahrheit der alchemischen Kunst': Der pseudoparacelsische Brieftraktat 'Vom Wunderstein' in einer frühneuzeitliche Verfassung," in *Resultate und Desiderate der Paracelsus-Forschung*, ed. Peter Dilg and Hartmut Rudolf (Stuttgart: Franz Steiner Verlag, 1993), 57–78.

sought to mediate between the competing traditions.[16] Alternatively, there were times when the divisions between the two schools of natural philosophy seemed absolute, as in Thomas Erastus's comprehensive rejection of the Paracelsian system.

Erastus published the first full-scale refutation of Paracelsianism at precisely the time when the Paracelsian revival was reaching a crescendo. He had not been the first to become alarmed by Paracelsian practitioners; an undercurrent of humanist criticism had already joined insinuations of heresy from orthodox Protestant medical scholars. As this excursus on anti-Paracelsianism will demonstrate, Erastus was closely connected to the major pre-1570 critics of Paracelsus. Every element of the anti-Paracelsian critique before Erastus would find its way into the text of Erastus's *De medicina nova*.

Anti-Paracelsianism before Erastus

Johannes Oporinus

Paracelsus's first major "critic," if we may use the term loosely, was his former amanuensis Johannes Oporinus (1507–1568), who later found fame as Basel's leading humanist printer. Oporinus had served Paracelsus during the height of Hohenheim's acceptance by Basel's humanist-oriented establishment in the late 1520s. Oporinus lived through Paracelsus's fall and abrupt departure from Basel (1528), and helped facilitate his master's resettlement in Alsace. After abandoning his medical studies, Oporinus was briefly engaged as a professor of classical languages at the University of Basel before he discovered his life work in printing, a career that was crowned by the printing of Theodor Bibliander's edition of the *Koran* (1543) and Vesalius's *De humani corporibus fabrica* (1543).[17]

Oporinus's influence on the Paracelsian revival of the second half of the sixteenth century was ambiguous. On the one hand, he was the

---

[16] See Allen G. Debus, "Guitherius, Libavius and Sennert: The Chemical Compromise in Early Modern Medicine," in *Science, Medicine and Society in the Renaissance: Essays to Honor Walter Pagel*, ed. Allen G. Debus (New York: Science History Publications, 1972); Carlos Gilly, "Zwischen Erfahrung und Spekulation: Theodor Zwinger und die religiöse und kulturelle Krise seiner Zeit," *Basler Zeitschrift für Geschichte und Altertumskunde* 77 (1977): 57–137 and 79 (1979): 125–233.

[17] Martin Steinmann, *Johannes Oporinus: Ein Basler Buchdrucker um die Mitte des 16. Jahrhunderts* [BBG 105] (Basel: Helbing & Lichtenhahn, 1967).

source for many of the Paracelsian manuscripts that eventually found their way into the famous Huser edition of Paracelsus's works. On the other hand, in a development that many Germanic Paracelsus scholars have viewed with scorn, he also composed a letter which detailed Hohenheim's lifestyle, cures, and vices.[18] Much remains uncertain regarding this letter, including when it was written (in 1555 or 1565) and to whom it was originally addressed. Although Johann Weyer has commonly been held as the addressee, the earliest extant manuscript version does not corroborate this fact.[19] At this juncture there is no consensus as to whether Oporinus's letter should be regarded as a *Schmähbrief* (slanderous attack),[20] as most pro-Paracelsian scholarship has seen it, or if it represented, in the words of Walter Pagel, "awe mingled with a measure of admiration and relief as after waking after a nightmare."[21] Despite its appreciation for Hohenheim's cures, the letter contains much information that could make it a fertile source for someone attempting to discredit Paracelsus. The allegations include an overly large appetite for drink, carousing among peasants, never being heard to pray, rejecting the pope and Luther as well as Galen and Hippocrates, and a general want of hygiene, which prompted Oporinus to refer to Paracelsus as "pig-like." Most damaging, as Sepp Domandl has suggested, were the parts of the letter potentially implicating Paracelsus in sorcery, including Oporinus's suggestion that Hohenheim's purse was always mysteriously full.[22]

There is every reason to expect that Erastus and Oporinus knew each other quite well. Although no correspondence between the two has survived, abundant surviving evidence suggests they had a strong connection with one another. Erastus studied at the University of Basel and was part of Oporinus's humanist milieu, corresponding with his

[18] Sepp Domandl, "Paracelsus, Weyrer, [*sic*] Oporin. Die Hintergruende des Pamphlets von 1555," in *Paracelsus. Werk und Wirkung. Festgabe für Kurt Goldhammer* [*SBPF* 13], ed. Sepp Domandl (Vienna: Verband der wissenschaftlichen Gesellschaften Österreichs, 1975): 53–70 and 391–392. Udo Benzenhöfer, "Zum Brief des Johannes Oporinus über Paracelsus: Die Bislang älteste bekannte Briefüberlieferung in einer 'Oratio' von Gervasius Marstaller," *Sudhoffs Archiv* 73 (1989): 55–63. Domandl reprints Daniel Sennert's 1629 Latin version. Benzenhöfer prints a 1571 manuscript version stemming from Gervasius Marstaller. For an English summary and assessment, see Pagel, *Paracelsus*, 29–31.

[19] Benzenhöfer, "Zum Brief des Johannes Oporinus," 61. The letter was addressed either to Weyer or Reiner Solenander or to both collectively.

[20] Domandl, "Paracelsus, Weyrer, Oporin," 53. Taking issue with Sudhoff's earlier negative assessment, Domandl also concludes that "Oporin war sicher ein begabter, sehr gebildeter und tüchtiger Mann." Domandl, "Paracelsus, Weyrer, Oporin," 67.

[21] Pagel, *Paracelsus*, 30.

[22] Domandl, "Paracelsus, Weyrer, Oporin," 53–55, 62.

associates Bonifacius and Basilius Amerbach, Martin Borrhaus, and Caelio Secundo Curione.[23] Moreover, a remark in a letter from Oporinus to Bullinger suggests that Erastus had corresponded with Oporinus.[24] Indeed this would be expected, since Oporinus was the publisher of Erastus's first philosophical work in 1565. The best piece of evidence that connects them is the biographical sketch of Erastus that Oporinus composed for Pantaleon's book of biographies (which was reproduced in chapter one). Thus, we know definitively that Oporinus had considerable knowledge of Erastus's early life.[25] Since Erastus was the junior member of this relationship and he mentioned Oporinus in both his printed works and correspondence, it would seem fair to assume that Erastus knew Oporinus equally well.

This connection raises the possibility that Erastus's conception of Paracelsus was dependent in part on conversations with Oporinus. Indeed, in a section of *De medicina nova* in which Erastus quoted Oporinus, he remarked that the characterizations came from Oporinus's "letters and his words."[26] Although we cannot exclude such a possibility, I judge it unlikely that Erastus had actually discussed Paracelsus's life and customs at length with Oporinus before the latter's death. I base this assessment on Erastus's apparent lack of interest in Paracelsus before 1570. This theory appears to be supported by the fact that Erastus was not able to produce any unique testimony from Oporinus in *De medicina nova*, but printed forty percent of the text of Oporinus's "Letter to Weyer" nearly verbatim. This perhaps suggests that he learned of Oporinus's opinions concerning Paracelsus only secondhand and after Oporinus's death in 1568.[27] Thus, we can in all likelihood exclude a firsthand transmission of Oporinus's opinions regarding Paracelsus to Erastus. It is not clear how Erastus received a copy of Oporinus's "Letter to Weyer," though it may have come through Grynaeus or Zwinger in Basel, Caspar Wolf or Bullinger in Zurich, or perhaps from Weyer himself. Although one may agree with Webster that "the Oporinus letter counts as a benign judgement" concerning Paracelsus, we shall see below that the manner in which Konrad Gessner and Erastus interpreted its content and employed it in their anti-

[23] See the Correspondence Register.

[24] *CO*, 18:241–242 (no. 3275).

[25] Pantaleon, *Prosopographia Heroum*, 3:545. See chapter 1.

[26] *De medicina nova*, 1:239: "Haec partim ex Oporini literis excepere, partim ex eius sermonibus annotare libuit."

[27] *De medicina nova*, 1:236–240. Concerning Oporinus, see also *De medicina nova*, 2:12.

Paracelsian propaganda was hardly benign.[28] Thus, whether or not Oporinus was attempting to slander his former master, his portrait became an important component of Erastus's attempt to assassinate Hohenheim's character.

Konrad Gessner

If Oporinus was an anti-Paracelsian by default, Konrad Gessner was also an enigmatic anti-Paracelsian. Gessner (1516–1565) is remembered as Switzerland's great early modern naturalist for such works as the *Historiae animalium* (1551) and for being the first modern bibliographer, with the *Bibliotheca universalis* (1545). Among his additional works was a collection of medical recipes titled *Thesaurus Evonymi Philiatri de remediis secretis* (1552), which also established him as a proponent of experimentally oriented chemical medicine.[29] Despite all that he had in common with the Paracelsians, however, Gessner was the most outspoken opponent of Paracelsus in the 1560s. His appreciation for chemical pharmacology aside, he was to become, in the words of Webster, "arguably the figure most responsible for determining the image of Paracelsus."[30]

Gessner's assault on Paracelsus was more of an attack on Paracelsus's peculiar customs and teachings than a critique of chemical medicine in general. This assault was not limited to Paracelsus but applied to other Paracelsians, such as Suchten, as well. Gessner's letters from the early 1560s are peppered with accusations and warnings concerning the sect of Paracelsian physicians.[31] To Joachim Camerarius II, Gessner

[28] Charles Webster, "Conrad Gessner and the infidelity of Paracelsus," *New Perspectives on Renaissance Thought: Essays in the History of Science, Education and Philosophy in Memory of Charles B. Schmitt*, ed. John Henry and Sarah Hutton (London: Duckworth, 1990), 15.

[29] For an English translation, cf. Konrad Gessner, *The Treasure of Euonymus* (London, 1559; facsimile reprint, New York: De Capo, 1969).

[30] Webster, "Conrad Gessner and the infidelity of Paracelsus," 13; Konrad Gessner, *Epistolarum Medicinalium libri III* (Zurich: C. Froschauer, 1577); Bernhard Milt, "Conrad Gessner und Paracelsus," *Schweizerische medizinische Wochenschrift* 59 (1929): 486–509; Gernot Rath, "Die Briefe Konrad Geßners aus der Trewschen Sammlung," *Gesnerus* 7 (1950): 140–170; 8 (1951): 195–215; Egon Helmich, ed., *Die Briefe Konrad Gesners an Crato von Krafftheim nach der Briefsammlung von 1566* (Düsseldorf: G.H. Nolte, 1938).

[31] E.g. Gessner to Crato, Zurich, Aug. 16, 1561. Gessner, *Epistolarum medicinalium*, fol. 1^{v}: "Oporinus Basileae olim discipulus Theophrasti, & familiaris fuit, is mira de eius cum daemonibus commercio praedicat. Astrologiam vanam, Geomantiam, Necromantiam, & huiusmodi artes prohibitas exercent. Equidem suspicor illos ex Druidarum reliquiis esse, qui apud Celtas veteres in subterraneis locis a daemonibus aliquot annis

had emphasized that the Paracelsians he knew were both unlearned and immoral.[32] An extreme example of his critique can be seen in a letter to Crato dated August 16, 1560, in which he concludes that Paracelsus was an "impious man, and sorcerer, who was clearly in league with demons."[33] Gessner's critique was thus fundamentally religious and contained two separate accusations. The first was that of magic, but not benign or natural magic; rather, conversation with demons. The second accusation suggested that the Paracelsians denied Christ's divine nature and were, therefore, a reprise of the Arian heresy. At best, then, Paracelsians were a sect of Antitrinitarians, at worst a group practicing pre-Christian sorcery.

The enigma of Gessner's rejection of Paracelsianism was that he paired this religious refutation with a call to defend the tradition of medicine represented by Galen and Hippocrates. This argument might represent a cogent line of reasoning if Gessner were a conservative desiring to defend all things traditional, but this was manifestly not the case. As mentioned above, in his *Treasury of Euonymus*, Gessner had spurred the trend toward innovation in chemical pharmacology and displayed a willingness to try secret remedies. In a letter to Johann Muralt he admitted that he had learned much concerning metals from Paracelsus, and that he himself used antimony, though infrequently.[34] It is difficult to comprehend Gessner's rejection of Paracelsian medicine, when he said, "I do not approve of their teaching and methods and also not their forbidden craft," since he had not fully spelled out what aspect of their medical therapy he rejected.[35] Thus, we are left with Gessner's clear rejection of Paracelsus on religious grounds and a seemingly ambivalent-to-positive opinion regarding Paracelsian pharmacology.

Since Erastus was from Baden in Switzerland and had ties to such Zurich notables as Bullinger, Konrad Pellikan, and Rudolf Gwalther, it seems almost inevitable that Erastus's and Gessner's paths would have

---

erudiebantur." Gessner to Didymus Obrecht, Zurich, March 18, 1560, Gessner, *Epistolarum medicinalium*, fol. 114^{v}: "Fuit is Paracelsus nostra memoria Magus, admirabilis homo, notus amicis quibusdam meis, a vicinis nostris Helvetiis oriundus, pervagatus magnum orbis partem. Chymia arte, quam ipse puto Spagyricam vocat, excellentissimus omnium, ita ut per eam metalla immutaret, argentum ac aurem faceret...."

32 Rath, "Die Briefe Konrad Geßners," 159–162.

33 Gessner, *Epistolarum medicinalium*, fol. 1^{v}.

34 Rath, "Die Briefe Konrad Geßners," 207–211.

35 Rath, "Die Briefe Konrad Geßners," 160, 162. Gessner to J. Camerarius, Jan. 27, 1565, Rath, 160: "Doctrinam et methodum eorum non probo neque artes illicitas quas medicinae exercendae necessarius aiunt ... Medicamenta vero eorum multa sane admiror."

crossed. Indeed, their paths did cross frequently, but, rather than becoming fellow travelers, it seems that they were often moving in opposite directions. For example, even if the theory that Erastus studied in Zurich before attending the University of Basel is correct, he would not likely have come into significant contact with Gessner, since this period would have been when Gessner was a Greek instructor at the Lausanne Academy (1537–1540). Later the two would have had the opportunity to meet in Basel, where Gessner received his M.D. in 1541, although the neophyte Erastus hardly would have been a peer to Gessner, who was already such an accomplished scholar that his reception of the doctorate from the Basel faculty was something akin to an honorary presentation.[36] As we saw in chapter one, when Erastus was a student in Bologna, he attempted to act as an intermediary between Gessner and the great Swedish naturalist Olaus Magnus. Since we do not possess the contemporary letters that passed between Erastus and Gessner, it is difficult to perceive how the episode eventually turned out, though the limited information we possess does not indicate they were on overly familiar terms at that juncture. Their acquaintance is further attested by Erastus's signature in Gessner's *Liber amicorum*, and the two extant letters of Erastus to Gessner reveal a degree of personal familiarity.[37] In later years when the two were on a more comparable intellectual level, even though Erastus was a medical professor, theological controversies absorbed much of his productive energy. However, Erastus did compose his "Letter concerning the Nature, Material, Origin, and Use of the Sandstone (*Lapis Sabulosus*), Which Is Found in the Rhenish Palatinate," a work hailed as the earliest independent publication in soil science, at Gessner's behest.[38]

[36] Eduard K. Fueter, *NDB*, 6:343.

[37] Richard Durling, "Conrad Gesner's *Liber amicorum* 1555–1565," *Gesnerus* 22 (1965): 134–159 (no. 15). Erastus's undated entry is signed "Thomas Erastus, Helvetius." Erastus to Gessner, April 11, (1557), StAZ, MS E II 361, fol. 56; Erastus to Gessner, Heidelberg, Sept. 17 1564, Zurich, Zentralbibliothek, MS Z VIII 119, fols. 1–18 (partially printed in Thomas Erastus, *Disputationum et Epistolarum Medicinalium volumen*, ed. Theophil Mader (Zurich: Johannes Wolf, 1595), fols. 90^r–105^v (no. 25)). Ironically, Erastus's letter from Sept. 17, 1564 was a treatise on the plague, the disease which would take Gessner's life the next year. Erastus had suffered the plague as a youth and published a vernacular tract on it as well. *Kurtzer Bericht für den gemeinen Mann/ wie er sich in disen sterbenden leuffen/ ohne sondern kosten mit Preservativen unnd Remedien verwaren und halten soll* (Heidelberg: J. Mayer, 1563). Cf. Wesel-Roth, *Thomas Erastus*, 2–3. Concerning the "Bericht," cf. Joachim Telle, "Die Pestschrift des Thomas Erastus," in *Bibliotheca Palatina. Katalog zur Ausstellung*, Textband, ed. Elmar Mittler (Heidelberg: Braus, 1986), 97–98.

[38] "Epistola de natura, materia, ortu atque usu lapidis sabulosi, qui in Palatinatu ad Rhenum reperitur," in *Explicatio quaestionis famosae illius, utrum ex metallis ignobilibus*

Erastus grasped the magnitude of Gessner's scholarly achievement and, upon learning of his death, composed a moving tribute to Gessner in a letter to their mutual friend Bullinger.[39] By the early 1570s when Erastus turned his attentions fully upon questions of natural philosophy, Gessner had been dead nearly five years. Arguably much of Erastus's best work is in the spirit of Gessner's naturalism and in some senses Erastus was to become Gessner's intellectual heir. This is manifestly the case with regard to Gessner's impact on Erastus's conception of Paracelsus. However, although we know Gessner wrote to Crato, Didymus Obrecht, Aldoph Occo, and others warning them of Paracelsians, there is no surviving evidence that he conveyed a similar admonition to Erastus. In the limited extant sources connecting the two during Gessner's lifetime, there is apparently no mention of Paracelsus. Thus, it appears that as in the case of Oporinus, Erastus did not experience his elder contemporary's opinions regarding Paracelsus directly. On the contrary, he encountered them as literary sources years after they were written.

Erastus did have direct access to Gessner's writings concerning Paracelsus. While he could have received a more than adequate impression of Gessner's opinion of Hohenheim from Crato or Camerarius, with whom Erastus was in communication at this time, Erastus was also able to access Gessner's papers through the assistance of Gessner's successor, Caspar Wolf.[40] Erastus's readers, in turn, benefited from his good connections and read a twenty-four line selection condemning Paracelsus from Gessner's letter to Crato from August 16, 1560, in the third volume of *De medicina nova*.[41] The rabid repudiation of Hohenheim's unortho-

aurum verum & naturale arte conflari possit, printed with *De medicina nova*, 2. See below. See Wolfgang Ziehen, ed., *Epistola de natura, materia, ortu atque usu lapidis sabulosi qui in Palatinatu ad Rhenum reperitur* (Aalen: Scientia Verlag, 1984).

[39] Erastus to Bullinger, Heidelberg, Jan. 1, 1566, StAZ, E II 361, fol. 10: "Valde perturbarunt nos literae tuae in ea parte, in qua D. Gesnerum mortuum scribis. Vir fuit summus, in laboribus perpetuus, ea praeditus humanitate et ingenii placiditate, qua vix alius quisquam. Deus ut nos quidem iudicamus, magnum lumen extinxit patriae. Vix multis saeculis extitit homo [t]ogatus, excipio Theologos, qui magis illustravit et ornarit patriam. Sed Dei consilia bona sunt, cogitationes nostrae sunt somnia. Valde amavi optimum, eruditissimum et sanctum virum, et cum gaudio, ubi Deo visum erit, eum cum aliis piis revidebo in Semperiternum. Amen."

[40] Wolf would later serve as the editor of the 1577 edition of Gessner's correspondence. Erastus was also in correspondence with the Zurich physician Taddeo Duni in the spring of 1571. See the Correspondence Register.

[41] What follows is taken from Erastus's text of *De medicina nova*, 3 (1572). The texts are virtually identical, with only two alternate readings in Erastus's version. In the 1577 edition of Gessner's letters "Alexandri a Suchten:" is read in the place of "N.N." Two lines

doxy and the accusation of magic contained in Gessner's letters were to become central features of Erastus's censure of Paracelsus.

Johann Weyer

One of the first writers to assail Paracelsus in print was Johann Weyer (1515–1588), court physician of Duke Wilhelm III of Jülich-Cleves and famed opponent of witch-hunts, whose controversy with Erastus on that topic will be investigated in the following chapter. Weyer studied at the University of Paris and should also be counted as a representative of the medical Renaissance. In both his appreciation for the medical authorities of antiquity and his disdain for anything that smacked of quackery, Weyer was a natural opponent of Paracelsian revival. The likelihood that Weyer was the recipient of the famous letter of Oporinus recalling Paracelsus's lifestyle suggests that Weyer had been following the advance of Paracelsianism from an early date.[42] It will be recalled that Oporinus's publishing house also printed every authorized Latin version of *De praestigiis daemonum* published in Weyer's lifetime.[43] Weyer was not alone in his opposition to Paracelsian practitioners, but part of a larger lower Rhenish circle of anti-Paracelsians including Gervasius

---

further, "Dei filium" is read instead of "filium Dei." There are also minor differences in punctuation, which I have not noted.

"His scriptis reperi propositiones a te missas nebulonis illius N.N. [Alexandri a Suchten:] de cuius in re medica, causis & curationibus morborum imperitia, ut nihil dicam, (neque enim opus est apud te). Vide quem nobis conspicuum filium Dei [Dei filium] faciat: non alium scilicet, quam spiritum mundi & naturae, eundemque corporis nostri (mirum quod non etiam asini ac bovis addit) qui artificio Discipulorum Theophrasti a materia seu corporibus elementorum separari potest. Si quis ipsum urgeat; dicet se Philosophorum sententiam retulisse, non suam. At qui ita recitat, ut laudet. Et scio alios quoque Theophrasteos talia suis scriptis aspergere, unde Christi divinitatem eos negare facile appareat. Ipsum quidem Theophrastum Arianum fuisse omnino mihi constat. Hoc agunt, ut Christum omnino nudum hominem fuisse persuadeant, nec alium in eo spiritum quam in nobis esse. Scio in Polonia & dudum Arianos multos fuisse, & nuper ab Italis quibusdam eo profectis ipsorum numerum augeri. Itaque & hanc ob causam, & ut artis medicae nostrae fundamenta ac methodum secundum Hippocratem & Galenum verissime traditam tuearis, oro te & hortor, vir doctissime, ut omnibus modis te illis calumniatoribus, magis, & Arianis opponas. Qua in re si quid ego etiam potero, non deero." *De medicina nova*, 3:14–15.

[42] See chapter 9 for literature on Weyer.

[43] George Mora et al. eds., *Witches, Devils and Doctors in the Renaissance: Johann Weyer, De praestigiis daemonum* (Binghamton, N.Y.: Center for Medieval and Early Renaissance Studies, 1991; hereafter cited as Mora, *Witches, Devils and Doctors*), lviii.

Marstaller, Rainer Solenander, and Bernhard Dessen von Kronenburg.[44] Weyer included this harsh rebuke of the Paracelsian sect in *De praestigiis daemonum*:

> They rail at the ancient and sacrosanct art of medicine, and slander and reject it, and bend their efforts to trample it underfoot, fabricating new principles and new expressions, which even they do not understand or defend by rational argument, content with the confused heap of useless words with which Paracelsus filled his writings. He vaunts that he is the monarch of medicine, discoverer of the true art; and as such do his followers regard him and worship and venerate him.[45]

The picture that Weyer presented was of Paracelsus as a would-be medical prophet who had rejected all previous medicine, and who now possessed a cult-like band of followers whom Weyer rejected as charlatans. Weyer, like other humanists such as Crato and Gessner, was put off by the deliberate obscurity of Paracelsian texts. Weyer was quick to assert, however, that he was not opposed to chemistry and that he employed chemical cures himself (including antimony). Weyer's position on chemical medicine was at best ambivalent, however, since he added that the "Paracelsians' eyes have been closed by the soot of Chemistry," leaving them vulnerable to Satan's exploits.[46] While leaving the door cracked for a positive role for iatrochemistry, Weyer's estimation of the learning and practice of Paracelsians was uniformly negative.

Although there were few direct references to Weyer in *De medicina nova*, it is clear from a letter Erastus sent to Bullinger on October 29, 1570, that the *De praestigiis daemonum* was one of the first things Erastus read concerning Paracelsus.[47] The magnitude of Weyer's influence on

[44] See Benzenhöfer, "Zum Brief des Johannes Oporinus."

[45] Quoted from Mora, *Witches, Devils and Doctors*, 154. Johann Weyer, *De praestigiis daemonum, et incantationibus ac veneficiis Libri sex* … (Basel: Ex Officina Oporiniana, 1568), 196: "quibus medicam artem veterem & sacrosanctam insectantur, calumniantur, reijciunt, pedibusque conterere satagunt, nova ementiti principia cum vocibus novis: quae nec ipsi quidem intelligunt, nec rationibus defendent, contenti verborum inutilium, quibus sua Paraclesus opplevit scripta, congerie & acervo. Hic se medicinae monarcham, veraeque artis inventorum iactat: talem illum quoque habent colunt & veneratur eius sectatores." For an assessment of the ebb and flow of Weyer's conception of Paracelsus, see Michaela Valente, *Johann Wier: agli albori della critica razionale dell'occulto e del demoniaco nell'Europa del Cinquecento* (Florence: L.S. Olschki, 2003), 109–134.

[46] Weyer, *De praestigiis daemonum* (1568), 200: "Paracelsistarum oculos fuligine chymico obductos."

[47] Erastus to Bullinger, StAZ, E II 345, fol. 741. The editions of *De praestigiis daemonum* vary greatly, with the trend being accumulation over time (and greater demonization of Paracelsus). For instance, the 1564 edition did not have the negative refer-

Erastus's image of Paracelsus has been obscured by their disagreement regarding witchcraft. Weyer has the curious distinction of being a chief source for Erastus's conception of Paracelsus as well as being himself the principal subject of one of the disputations of *De medicina nova*.[48] Erastus's correspondence with Bullinger and Joachim Camerarius II reveals that Erastus had seen letters from Weyer around the end of 1572 and that their disagreement concerning the punishment of witches was the source of a measure of antagonism.[49] Disagreements aside, Weyer did not hesitate to recognize Erastus's critique of Paracelsus in his 1577 edition of *De praestigiis daemonum*.[50] In fact, although Erastus opposed Weyer on his central passion, defending the accused from the charge of witchcraft, it would be difficult to suggest another sixteenth-century figure who influenced Erastus's natural philosophy as much as Weyer. Although Weyer cannot be considered an active collaborator on *De medicina nova*, Erastus knew Weyer's work well and eventually would make Weyer's image of Paracelsus as a medical false prophet a central theme of his refutation of Paracelsus.

Erastus's Decision to Refute Paracelsus

Although Erastus was personally connected to all of Paracelsus's major critics, in other ways he was an unlikely opponent of Paracelsus. Erastus had been brought to the University of Heidelberg in 1558 by the

ence to Paracelsus quoted above. The 1577 edition added the *Liber Apologeticus*, which has more anti-Paracelsian material. Michaela Valente offers side-by-side comparisons of many relevant texts. Valente, *Johann Wier*, 125–134.

[48] *De medicina nova*, 1:193–215. Erastus, however, did not mention Weyer by name in this disputation and would later employ the same tactic in his later *Repetitio disputationis de Lamiis* (Basel: Pietro Perna, [1578]). Erastus does mention Weyer on at least two other occasions in the work. *De medicina nova*, 1:187; 4:131. See below.

[49] The letters are discussed in detail in chapter 9. Erastus to J. Camerarius II, Jan. 31, [1573], UB Erlangen (Sammlung Trew), MS no. 6 and Erastus to Bullinger, Jan. 13, [1573], StAZ, E II 361, fol. 31.

[50] Concerning the opinions of Augier Ferrier, Weyer notes: "Hanc autem Ferrerii sententiam, eiusmodi nimirum effectus ex constanti & firma operantis persuasione consequi, modo patientis animus non reluctetur, erudite confutat ornatissimus vir D. Thomas Erastus in parte prima disputat. de nova Paracelsi medicina." *De praestigiis daemonum* ... (Basel: Ex Officina Oporiniana, 1577), col. 579. In his rebuttal of Leo Suavius (Jacques Gohory) in the *Liber Apologeticus*, Weyer states: "Tibi autem Leo Suavi, quum ad monomachiae conflictum in Paracelsi protectionem nimis pruriant unguiculi, cum doctissimo exercitatissimoque in hoc belligerandi genere Thoma Erasto philosopho, & antiquae

pro-alchemical Elector Ottheinrich, who had earlier employed the Paracelsians Suchten, Bodenstein, and Toxites and whose former residence in Neuburg was a major repository of Spagyrical manuscripts.[51] When Erastus was called to Heidelberg, he may have been known as an anti-astrological doctor, but not as an anti-Paracelsian. At that point, Erastus's medical reputation was based chiefly on his practice and not on his publishing activity. Erastus testified in a dedicatory letter to August of Saxony in the first volume of *De medicina nova* that he had come upon one of Paracelsus's writings some time previously when Paracelsus was not so famous, but that he had set it aside since he found it barbarous.[52] It was only when the "Paracelsian revival" reached a crescendo around the year 1570 with a spate of spagyrical publications that Erastus began to take note of Hohenheim again.[53] A survey of Erastus's earlier writings reveals no definitive mention of Paracelsus before he wrote *De medicina nova*. Although Erastus had many close connections to Hohenheim's contemporaries, he had shown practically no interest in Paracelsus's medical philosophy, much less his personal life, until he decided to undertake the refutation in the fall of 1570.

Erastus had displayed some interest, however, in Paracelsian pharmacology in the 1560s. The first issue that brought him into contact with Paracelsian medicine was the antimony debate. The introduction to the first volume of *De medicina nova* spoke of "heated dispute among some scholars over the power of antimony."[54] Rather than the later Parisian debate over antimony, Erastus apparently was speaking of the south German controversy whose key players were Achilles Pirmin Gasser and Lukas Stenglin. Both men worked in Augsburg and were the most visible opponents of Paracelsian pharmacology during this period.[55] Stenglin

medicinae patrono multis nominibus laudatissimo congredere, si quid verae philosophiae, quid artis medicae, quid animi aut virium in te resideat." *De praestigiis daemonum* (1577), col. 881.

[51] Telle, "Kurfürst Ottheinrich, Hans Kilian und Paracelsus," 130–146.

[52] *De medicina nova*, 1:aiiv.

[53] For a general (and none too sympathetic) overview of the Paracelsian revival, see Thorndike, *History of Magic and Experimental Science*, 5:617–651. Whereas Sudhoff could only find eleven editions of works by Paracelsus published in the 1550s, he was able to list ninety-four editions from the 1560s. Indeed, seventeen editions were printed in 1570 alone. Karl Sudhoff, *Versuch einer Kritik der Echtheit der Paracelsischen Schriften. I. Theil: Bibliographia Paracelsica. Besprechung der unter Hohenheims Namen 1527–1893 erscheinenen Druckschriften* (Berlin, 1894; reprint, Graz, 1958; hereafter cited as *Bibliographia Paracelsica*), 44–218.

[54] *De medicina nova*, 1:aiiv.

[55] Wlodzimierz Hubicki, "Alexander von Suchten," *Sudhoffs Archiv* 44 (1960): 54–

addressed the antimony question in a set of theses in 1566, which assessed the drug's usefulness as a purgative in strict Galenic terms. He concluded that antimony's toxicity was widely recognized, like mercury and other metals, and that its capacity for harm, in most cases, outweighed its therapeutic usefulness. While not directly assaulting Paracelsus, Stenglin noted antimony's novelty and suggested that some doctors might use it out of avarice or ignorance.[56] Erastus had likewise weighed in on the antimony debate, perhaps as early as 1563, in the closing sections of his book *On the occult powers of drugs*.[57] He also warned of antimony's toxicity but limited his critique to the drug itself. Erastus displayed none of his later vitriol against Paracelsus in the work. Since the book was not published until 1574, however, we cannot be sure that the brief chapter on antimony was written in 1563. Thus, while there is evidence that Erastus had passing knowledge of the fringes of Paracelsian medicine in the 1560s, his

63; *De medicina nova*, 3:13–60. Erastus received a manuscript of Gasser and Stenglin's censure of Alexander von Suchten's propositions from Balthasar Brauch of Schwäbisch Gmünd. These theses, rather than being the printed theses of Stenglin cited below, were likely the two sets of manuscript theses that Thorndike reviewed in the Vatican Library (Thorndike, *History of Magic and Experimental Science*, 5:640–641). Erastus's connection with Stenglin is documented in a letter from 1575; however, I have found no sources which prove a direct contact between them in the late 1560s. Erastus to Stenglin, Jan. 10, 1575, printed in Erastus, *Disputationum et Epistolarum Medicinalium volumen*, fols. 73r–76v (no. 22). Likewise, there is evidence for contact between Erastus and Gasser in the mid-1570s, but not before. Cf. Karl Heinz Burmeister, *Achilles Pirmin Gasser, 1505–1577: Arzt und Naturforscher, Historiker und Humanist*, 2 vols. (Wiesbaden: Guido Pressler, 1970), 193.

56 Lukas Stenglin, *Quaestiones III. Quarum primus est. An Stimmi seu Antimonium aergrotantibus citra noxam exhiberi possit* (Augsburg: Philipp Ulhard, 1566), theses 58 and 60; idem, *Apologia Adversus Stibii Spongiam, non ita dudum a Michaele Toxite* (Augsburg: Mathaeus Francus, 1569). Concerning Toxites's response, see Charles Schmidt, *Michael Schütz genannt Toxites: Leben Eines Humanisten und Arztes aus dem 16. Jahrhundert* (Strasbourg, 1888), 101–102.

57 Thomas Erastus, *De occultis pharmacorum potestatibus* ... (Basel: Pietro Perna, 1574). This work contains the only potential pre-1570 mention of Paracelsus by Erastus that I have found. I say potential, in that, although the text of the book was dated July 22, 1563, it was not printed until 1574. The book mentions a "Theophrastus" in the text once (p. 127) and likewise in the chapter dedicated to antimony. Otherwise the only other likely reference to Paracelsus comes in the title of Chapter 26, "Refutatio rationis, qua Paracelsici usum Stibii commendant" (p. 125). In my estimation, it is likely that this title was composed during the preparation of the book for publication in 1574, particularly since such practitioners are referred to as "Paracelsians," which would have been a novel category in 1563; whereas, it would have been common by the mid-1570s. Because the chapter itself does *not* include a personal attack on Paracelsus, which was a conventional part of *De medicina nova* and *De auro potabili*, I think that it is likely that the chapter was in fact written in 1563.

special concern for Paracelsus only commenced with the composition of *De medicina nova*.

Erastus made the decision to refute the teachings of Paracelsus while the imperial diet was being held in Speyer in 1570.[58] The first mention of Paracelsus in Erastus's correspondence comes out of the blue in a letter to Bullinger from October 29, in which he reports, "I am completely absorbed in reflection regarding confuting the most monstrous and absurd dogma of Paracelsus."[59] Activities at Speyer provided the impulse for Erastus to undertake the confutation. Erastus reported to Grynaeus that a conference had been held in Speyer with Crato and Heinrich Petri in attendance concerning the "life and vices of Paracelsus."[60] After the meeting, Crato wrote to Erastus and urged him to undertake the refutation of Paracelsus. Erastus also relates that Johann Hermann, personal physician to Duke August of Saxony, urged him to refute Paracelsian doctrine in toto.[61]

Having outlined his course of action, Erastus wrote his friends seeking their input on the project. Analysis of the work itself and Erastus's correspondence grants a clear picture of who supplied him with information. Erastus immediately turned to Bullinger for information regarding Paracelsus's personal life. With his position as head of the Zurich church and through his immense correspondence network, Bullinger was ideally located to channel any fruitful source material regarding Paracelsus's Swiss origins to Erastus. Erastus first asked Bullinger if he knew anything about a "von Hohenheim" family in Einsiedeln and what he knew of Paracelsus through Dr. Clauser. Very likely to Erastus's surprise, Bullinger was able to comply with his request by sending along his own reminiscence of meeting Paracelsus some forty years before (discussed below). Beyond his assistance in ferreting out Paracelsus's Swiss origins, Bullinger was also consulted by Erastus regarding the theological sections of the work as the project progressed.

In Erastus's contemporaneous correspondence, he singled out the imperial court physician Johannes Crato von Krafftheim (1519–1585) as the person who most strongly urged him to undertake a refutation of Paracelsus. Crato, one of the leading academic physicians of the age,

[58] See discussion in chapter 6. The diet was held May 22 – Dec. 11, 1570.

[59] Erastus to Bullinger, Oct. 29 [1570], StAZ, E II 345, fols. 741–742. See Appendix B, text no. 1.

[60] Erastus to J.J. Grynaeus, Nov. 29, [1571], Basel UB, G II 4, fol. 300^v. Quoted in full in Appendix B, text no. 2.

[61] *De medicina nova*, 1:aiiv.

served the Habsburg court from late in the reign of Ferdinand I and enjoyed an especially close relationship with the Emperor Maximilian II.[62] At some point Crato appears to have become extremely alarmed at the growing menace of Paracelsianism and by the late 1560s had become something of a leader of the opposition to Paracelsus.[63] He had been one of the first authors to lash out at Paracelsus in print, including a long diatribe against Paracelsus in the preface of his edition of Da Monte's *In Nonum Librum Rhasis ad R. Almansorem [...] lectiones*.[64] Paracelsus was not mentioned by name in this attack, however, due to the cunning maneuver of the printer Pietro Perna, who was also one of the chief printers of Paracelsus's works. Perna simply removed Paracelsus's name from the text. Even though Hohenheim's name was excised, as Carlos Gilly has argued, it was not difficult to discern the object of Crato's scorn.[65] Crato greatly encouraged Erastus's work; in fact, one receives the impression that Erastus was tapped to tackle a project that Crato did not have the time to do himself. Crato loomed large both in the pages of *De medicina nova* and in Erastus's letters to other individuals at that time. Unfortunately, no letters survive from Crato to Erastus with which we can directly assess Crato's encouragement of the project. We can discern, however, that Crato was content with Erastus's work when he commends the effort of "Noster Erastus" in later letters to

[62] Gillet, *Crato von Crafftheim und seine Freunde*; Marlene Jantsch, "Crato von Krafftheim," in *Gestalten und Ideen um Paracelsus* [*SBPF* 11], ed. Sepp Domandl (Vienna: Notring, 1972), 99–108; Howard Louthan, *Johannis Crato and the Austrian Habsburgs: Reforming a Counter-Reform Court* [Studies in Reformed Theology and History 2/3] (Princeton, 1994).

[63] Carlos Gilly, "'Theophrastia Sancta': Der Paracelsismus als Religion im Streit mit den offiziellen Kirchen," in *Analecta Paracelsica*, Joachim Telle, ed. (Stuttgart, Steiner, 1994), 431–432 (For a shorter English version of the article see: Carlos Gilly, "'Theophrastia Sancta'—Paracelsianism as a Religion, in Conflict with the Established Churches," in *Paracelsus: The Man and His Reputation, His Ideas and Their Transformation*, ed. Ole Grell (Leiden: Brill, 1998), 151–185); Webster, "Conrad Gessner and the infidelity of Paracelsus," 23; Ralf Bröer, "Friedenspolitik durch Verketzerung: Johannes Crato (1519–1585) und die Denunziation der Paracelsisten als Arianer," *Medizinhistorisches Journal* 37 (2002): 139–182. See also Charles D. Gunnoe, Jr. and Jole Shackelford, "Johannes Crato von Krafftheim (1519–1585): Imperial Physician, Irenicist, and Anti-Paracelsian," in *Ideas and Cultural Margins in Early Modern Germany: Essays in Honor of H.C. Erik Midelfort*, ed. Elizabeth Plummer & Robin Barnes (Aldershot, England: Ashgate, 2009), 201–216.

[64] Giovanni Battista da Monte (Montanus), *In Nonum Librum Rhasis ad R. Almansoren lectiones*, ed. Johannes Crato (Basel: [Pietro Perna & Heinrich Petri], 1562). Gilly reprints a long quotation from the work in "Theophrastia Sancta," 432, note 18.

[65] Gilly, "Theophrastia Sancta," 431–432.

Zwinger.[66] Erastus's correspondence to Crato from this time (1570–1573) has also not survived, perhaps because Crato was accompanying Emperor Maximilian II on his travels. The letters from Erastus to Crato that have survived, both from the 1560s and the later 1570s, do not concern Paracelsus. Nevertheless, in his correspondence with Bullinger, Heinrich Smet, and Joachim Camerarius II, Erastus reports having received letters from Crato encouraging the work. These lost letters must been the source for the quotations from Crato found in the pages of *De medicina nova*.[67]

What Erastus records from Crato is a reprise of Gessner's accusations, re-emphasizing the Paracelsians' ties to Arianism.[68] In the fourth volume of *De medicina nova* Erastus includes a quote from Crato saying that he had seen a book written some two hundred years earlier by a monk from Ulm that contained Hohenheim's medications.[69] Not only does this slander Paracelsus, but it also had the effect of distancing some positive elements of Paracelsian pharmacology from Hohenheim's person. Crato also supplied a lively account of Paracelsus's stay in Moravia, which will be discussed more fully below. Beyond the information he supplied, Crato's chief significance must be seen in his role as the project's catalyst and cheerleader.

Considering Crato's difficult life as an itinerant imperial physician, it is unlikely that he would have made an ideal collaborator for a multi-volume work. Into the void created by Crato's inaccessibility stepped Johann Jakob Grynaeus, Camerarius, Heinrich Smet, and to a lesser degree, Bullinger and Gwalther. Erastus referred to the project as "Paracelsica nostra" when speaking to these men who served as collaborators in proofing and critiquing the work.[70]

---

[66] Scholtz, *Epistolarum philosophicarum, medicinalium, ac chymicarum a summis nostrae aetatis philosophis ac medicis exaraturum, volumen*, cols. 237–240.

[67] Erastus to Camerarius, May 30 [1571], Erlangen UB (Sammlung Trew), MS no. 2; Erastus to Bullinger, April 9, (15)71, StAZ, E II 361, fol. 18. See the Correspondence Register.

[68] *De medicina nova*, 3:15–16. Regarding Crato and the accusation of Arianism, see Bröer, "Friedenspolitik durch Verketzerung," 142, 166–169; Wilhelm Kühlmann and Joachim Telle, eds., *Corpus Paracelsisticum: Dokumente frühneuzeitlicher Naturphilosophie in Deutschland, Der Frühparacelsismus* (Tübingen: Max Niemeyer, 2001, 2004), 1:473–474.

[69] *De medicina nova*, 4:300 (Crato quoted by Erastus): "Remedia quibus aliquando usus dicitur, non illius esse ex eo certus sum, quod librum vidi ante 200. fere annos a monacho quod a Ulmae scriptum, in eo eadem medicamenta, quae ille frustillatim nunc in has nunc in alias chartas sparsit, perspicue sunt perscripta. Nullum reperies in ullo Paracelsi libro medicamentum integrum in uno loco, spargit in diversas."

[70] E.g., Appendix B, text no. 9.

The humanist physician Joachim Camerarius II (1534–1598) of Nuremberg was an ideal person to help with the project, considering his broad humanist medical training and his ties to Crato and Gessner. Joachim Camerarius II was the namesake of his more famous father Joachim Camerarius the Elder (1500–1574), who was a leading humanist, confessional irenicist, and close associate of Melanchthon. After studying medicine with Crato in Breslau, Camerarius II likewise took his place as one of the most influential humanist naturalists of central Europe. Apparently Erastus and Camerarius II began to correspond only after Erastus undertook the anti-Paracelsian project. Erastus informed him of his researches and sent him volumes to review.[71] He even sought to persuade Camerarius II to talk his friend, the famous pharmacologist Pierandrei Mattioli (1500–1577), into undertaking an investigation of Paracelsus's pharmacology.

Erastus's key collaborator on the anti-Paracelsian project was Johann Jakob Grynaeus, who at that time was a pastor and superintendent in Rötteln in the Margravate of Baden outside of Basel. Grynaeus's most valuable asset to the anti-Paracelsian project was his proximity to Basel, where Paracelsus had experienced a memorable sojourn. Erastus charged Grynaeus with securing a printer for the project and also for digging up material on Paracelsus in Basel. Grynaeus served as Erastus's primary contact with the printer Perna and produced the indices for the work.

Three members of the faculty of the University of Heidelberg also supported Erastus's endeavor. It was only natural that Erastus's close friend and confessional ally Simon Grynaeus, Johann Jakob's brother, would aid Erastus. He was still a member of the arts faculty in the early 1570s, though he would later ascend to the more prestigious and higher paying medical faculty. Sigismund Melanchthon, the nephew of Philipp Melanchthon and occupant of the third chair of medicine at the Heidelberg University when the project began, was party to some of the discussions that lay behind the project.[72] Finally, Wilhelm Xylander, the academy's leading classical scholar and an ally of Erastus in university politics, wrote introductory poems in Greek and Latin for volume one.[73]

[71] Erastus to Camerarius, Erlangen UB (Sammlung Trew), MSS nos. 1–6. Erastus sent Camerarius greetings in a letter by Zacharias Ursinus dated May 3, 1567. This fact suggests that Erastus was keen to make Camerarius's acquaintance and perhaps gain entrance into the larger Crato intellectual circle. Rott, "Briefe des Heidelberger Theologen Zacharias Ursinus aus Heidelberg und Neustadt a.H.," 65.

[72] *De medicina nova*, 4:69, 182; Wesel-Roth, *Thomas Erastus*, 71.

[73] *De medicina nova*, 1:B2–B3; Wesel-Roth, *Thomas Erastus*, 66.

Aside from Crato and Camerarius, this entire group had previously cooperated with Erastus's attempt to resist the imposition of a consistory of elders in the Palatinate.

Disputations on the New Medicine of Philip Paracelsus

Erastus's anti-Paracelsian work was issued in four parts from 1571 to 1573. The first volume of *De medicina nova* does not bear a date on the title page and has generally been assigned the date of 1572, along with volume two, as they always seem to be bound together in library collections. However, since the autumn Frankfurt fair catalog confirms that volume one was already in print in 1571, we can confidently assign that year as the publication date.[74] Volumes two and three followed in 1572 and volume four in the fall of 1573.

In the first volume of *De medicina nova*, Erastus primarily dealt with the theological implications of Paracelsus's magical-astrological worldview. The subtitle of the book read: "In which the things concerning the superstitious remedies and magical cures he produced are chiefly examined." A list of the chapter titles grants a good indication of the range of the work:

1. On creation.
2. On the effective power (*virtute effectrice*) of miracles.
3. On imaginative powers, which the body exercises either in itself or in another.
4. On enchantment and its associated effects.
5. Certain things concerning the rotating intelligences of the celestial orbs.
6. Whether other natural and licit magic be permitted.
7. On the operation of magic, and on its types; whereby, on the efficacy of words, characters, images figures and other superstitious medications are disputed in great detail.
8. On *lamia* or *striges* [witches] things which are not un-useful to know.

[74] *Die Messkatalog Georg Willers*, 1:382. See note 3 for full publication information. From Erastus's letters from 1571, it is clear that he was obsessed to see the first volume appear at the fall Frankfurt fair. The main body of the book was finished on March 26, 1571 and the introduction is dated May 1. Erastus's personal letter to Elector August of Saxony explaining his dedication of the work was dated Sept. 9, 1571.

9. On magic of divination, and of its kinds; and also not a little on foreseeing.
10. On the heavens of the stars and their power and influence.
11. A little on the life and death of Paracelsus.[75]

In addition to the listed chapters, the book also included an appendix on pages 243–267, which addressed select topics that Erastus found particularly galling from Paracelsus's recently published *Astronomia Magna* (analyzed in detail below). Paracelsus was not always the target of Erastus's critique in the first volume, a phenomenon that has often confused scholars. For example as mentioned above, Erastus included a brief disputation on the punishment of witches in the book that was a response to Johann Weyer. This chapter had nothing to do with Paracelsianism per se beyond lumping Paracelsus in Weyer's category of learned magicians who were, according to Weyer, much more culpable for their crimes than ignorant witches.[76] Erastus also took on the Paracelsian notion that granted nearly unlimited powers to the imagination in the healing process. Using Aristotelian reasoning, Erastus rejected this notion that imagination could be an efficient cause for any natural effect. Using imagination, a person can only construct a mental image; imagination cannot impact physical reality.[77] Here Erastus was taking on the ideas of Pomponazzi and Avicenna as well as Paracelsus. As the list of chapter titles suggests, a primary focus of this first volume was astrology. Like his earlier anti-astrological works, his theologically driven desire to protect the honor of God occupied first place in his thought, though he paired this motif with arguments from experience. Hand-in-hand with Erastus's attack on astrology was a critique of natural magic. Here, too, Paracelsus was not the only target of the work; Erastus directly assaulted Marsilio Ficino himself. Erastus exclaimed,

> Would you think this man a priest of God ... and not rather the patron and high priest of Egyptian mysteries ... ? Certainly there have never lived under the sun ... more diligent worshipers of demons than the Platonists.[78]

[75] *De medicina nova*, 1:[β4].

[76] *De medicina nova*, 1, chapter 8, pp. 193–215: "De lamiis seu strigibus non inutilia scitu."

[77] *De medicina nova*, 1:78. See Pagel, *Paracelsus*, 316–317; Walker, *Spiritual and Demonic Magic from Ficino to Campanella*, 156–166.

[78] English quotation from Walker, *Spiritual and Demonic Magic from Ficino to Campanella*, 163. *De medicina nova*, 1:118: "An tu Sacerdotem Dei, qualis videri voluit, ac

It should not be surprising that Erastus also rejected the notion that amulets possessed special powers or that specific words might have a healing agency. The first volume of *De medicina nova* was thus a full-fledged attack on natural and demonic magic focused on Paracelsus, whom Erastus saw as the culmination of the tradition.

Part two of *De medicina nova*, "In which the principles and elements of Paracelsian philosophy are explored," as the subtitle proclaimed, was less oriented toward the magical-religious questions of volume one, but focused on a number of fundamental questions of pre-modern natural philosophy. The chapter headings included:

1. On the teaching and the teacher or master of Paracelsus.
2. On the true principles of natural things.
3. On the false principles of nature of Paracelsus.
4. On the elements of mixed things.
5. On the hidden seeds of things in the abyss of Paracelsian elements.
6. On mixture.
7. On the imperfection of certain mixtures, the generation and cause.
8. On generation.
9. On the Cabala and its types and parts, and whether it is in some way licit or not.[79]

The absolute impasse between Erastus's traditional Aristotelian scientific notions and Paracelsus's more innovative and often ad hoc approach was never more evident than it was here. Whereas the object of book one had ultimately been to reveal Paracelsus's "monstrous impiety," the purpose of book two was to demonstrate his "incredible ignorance and asinine rudeness."[80] Indeed, Erastus spent a great deal of energy simply asserting that Paracelsus lacked a rudimentary facility in philosophical discourse, as was evident in his misuse of terms. The chief subject of the second book was the refutation of Paracelsus's three-principle theory. Paracelsus's three principles—salt, sulfur, and mercury—played a central role in his chemical philosophy. These principles did not per se replace the four elements of fire, water, earth, and air as schematized by Empedo-

non potius Aegyptiorum sacrorum approbatorem & Antistitem esse putabis ita licenter in pietatem insanientem? Certum est, nullus sub hoc Sole (de Philosophis loquor) vixisse maiores & officiosiores Daemonum cultores Platonicis."

79 *De medicina nova*, 1:[ ]:(4v].

80 *De medicina nova*, 2:1.

cles. As Pagel has suggested, "They are rather principles within matter that condition the state in which matter can occur."[81] Erastus objected to Paracelsus's use of terms since he had labeled something a "principle" that seemed by definition to possess material existence. He rejected Paracelsus's contention that any substance could be reduced to a combination of salt, sulfur, and mercury if decomposed by heat.[82] Alternatively Erastus upheld the traditional four-element theory. He suggested that the properties of substances or composites, which Paracelsus credited to the innate principles, were nothing other than a factor of the specific mixture of the four elements in the substance. If Erastus found Paracelsus's quasi-material "principles" difficult, he had even less use for the tendency in some of Paracelsus's works to conceptualize "elements" as the non-material spirit that served as the guiding soul of a given substance. For Erastus, this notion represented an even greater misuse of conventional philosophical categories.[83] Erastus's critiques were well aimed. As Allen Debus commented, "Erastus had touched on a sore point when he attacked the work of Paracelsus in regard to the three principles. Paracelsus had not been at all lucid when he had spoken of the elements, the principles, and their interrelation."[84] Paracelsus's own contradictions on this matter perhaps also explain why Erastus took particular pains to address the more systematic presentation of Paracelsian element theory contained in Petrus Severinus's *Idea of Philosophical Medicine*, though without mentioning Severinus by name. Jole Shackelford has recently demonstrated that the Dane Severinus was the object of much of Erastus's critique of Paracelsian element theory.[85] Erastus rejected Paracelsus's chemical philosophy in toto and defended traditional Aristotelian concepts of elements, mixture, and change.

[81] Walter Pagel, "Paracelsus," in *DSB*, 10:309.

[82] Regarding this observation of Erastus, Debus remarked: "It is interesting that these were the most powerful arguments to be used by Robert Boyle against the principles in his *Sceptical Chymist* nearly a century later." Debus, *The English Paracelsians* (New York: Franklin Watts, 1966), 39.

[83] *De medicina nova*, 3, passim; Pagel, *Paracelsus*, 319–322.

[84] Debus, *The English Paracelsians*, 39.

[85] Petrus Severinus [Peder Soerenson], *Idea medicinae philosophicae fundamenta continens totius doctrinae Paracelsicae, Hippocraticae et Galenicae* (Basel: Heinrich Petri, 1571). Jole Shackelford, "Early Reception of Paracelsian Theory: Severinus and Erastus," *SCJ* 26 (1995): 123–135; idem, *A Philosophical Path for Paracelsian Medicine: The Ideas, Intellectual Context, and Influence of Petrus Severinus (1540/2–1602)* (Copenhagen: Museum Tusculanum Press, 2004). Severinus's reaction to Erastus's censure will be discussed below.

In a move destined to vex catalogers through the centuries, Erastus's publisher Perna also printed two independent works of Erastus and attached them as addenda to *De medicina nova*, 2. Since the first of these works, *Explication of this Famous Question, Whether it Is Possible to Produce True and Natural Gold out of Ignoble Metals by Art* (Explicatio quaestionis famosae),[86] appeared with its own dated title page, separate pagination and distinct signature numbers and since it was not mentioned on the title page of *De medicina nova*, 2, by rights it should be considered an independent publication. Appearing with the *Explicatio quaestionis famosae* was Erastus's important "Letter Concerning the Nature, Material, Origin and Use of the Sandstone, Which Is Found in the Rhenish Palatinate,"[87] which also has its own title page but continues the pagination of *Explicatio quaestionis famosae*. Against considering *Explicatio quaestionis famosae* an independent book, however, is the fact that it was manifestly issued with *De medicina nova*, 2, and the fact that the two works were listed in the table of contents of *De medicina nova*, 2. Since these two works did not treat Paracelsus in particular, I will not include them in my analysis of the *De medicina nova*.[88] Without going into detail, I will note that the *Explicatio quaestionis famosae* did attract a significant amount of attention in its day. It prompted the French alchemist Gaston DuClo (aka Claveus) to write his *Defense of Chrysopoeia* to counter Erastus's rejection of alchemical transmutation.[89] What is particularly interesting is that DuClo was hardly more enamored with Paracelsian *arcana* than Erastus himself. DuClo took pains to praise Erastus's general status as a philosopher, though he rejected what he saw as Erastus's premature and poorly informed refutation of the transmutation of metals in his *Defense of Chrysopoeia*. DuClo's work in turn elicited the criticism of Andreas Libavius, whom Gilly has called the "most important intel-

[86] *Explicatio Quaestionis famosae illius, utrum ex metalis ignobilibus aurum verum & naturale arte conflari possit* (Basel, Pietro Perna, 1572).

[87] See note 38 above.

[88] For an analysis of the contents of *Explicatio quaestionis famosae* and its place in the early modern alchemical debate, see the chapter "Erastus and the Critique of Chemical Analysis" in William R. Newman, *Atoms and Alchemy: Chymistry and the Experimental Origins of the Scientific Revolution* (Chicago: University of Chicago Press, 2005), 45–65.

[89] Gaston DuClo, *Apologia Chrysopoeiae et Argyropoeiae, adversus Thomam Erastum, Doctorem et Professorem Medicinae* (1598; reprint, Oberursel: Cornelius Sutorius, 1602). Regarding DuClo, see Lawrence M. Principe, "Diversity in Alchemy: The Case of Gaston "Claveus" DuClo, a Scholastic Mercurialist Chysopoeian," in *Reading the Book of Nature* [*SCE&S* 41], ed. Allen Debus and Michael Walton (Kirksville, Mo., 1998), 181–200.

lectual follower of Erastus."[90] While Libavius may have borrowed a few elements of his anti-Paracelsian critique from Erastus, he likewise did not shy away from finding fault with Erastus's chemical views. Libavius would debate the issue of transmutation with another anti-Paracelsian, Nicolas Guibert. These debates reveal that the chemical philosophy was not the proprietary territory of Paracelsians in the late sixteenth and early seventeenth centuries.[91]

In the third volume of *De medicina nova*, Erastus launched a broadside against the Paracelsian medical philosophy. Central to this volume was the fundamental difference between the Paracelsian and the more traditional conception of disease. As mentioned above, Paracelsus's conception of disease was one of the more innovative aspects of his medical theory. Rather than understanding disease in the traditional sense as the simple imbalance of the four humors, Paracelsus developed a conception of disease as a toxin or a parasite that attacked a particular organ or "seat" of disease. Erastus had little patience for this complete departure from the traditional conception of disease and thought it was ludicrous to consider disease a "created substance." Here Paracelsus had committed a most basic philosophical error in that he confused the cause of disease with disease itself. At no point did Erastus's philosophical categories blind him more from the potential utility of Paracelsian theory. In this book, Erastus also rejected the pervasive notion of the microcosm-macrocosm analogy in Paracelsus's works. Once again, far from restricting himself to the work of Paracelsus, Erastus also included a long refutation of Suchten's *18 Propositions* in *De medicina nova*, 3.[92]

The final volume of *De medicina nova* was the only one to deal extensively with actual questions of medical therapy. Its subtitle proclaimed its goal of being a book, *In which the True Method* (ratio) *of Curing*

[90] Gilly, "Zwischen Erfahrung und Spekulation," *Basler Zeitschrift für Geschichte und Altertumskunde* 77 (1977): 66.

[91] Nicolas Guibert, *Alchymia ratione et experientia ita demum viriliter impugnata & expugnata, una cum suis fallaciis & deliramentis, quibus homines imbubinârat: ut nunquam imposterum se erigere valeat* (Strasbourg: Lazarus Zetzner, 1603). Andreas Libavius, *Defensio et declaratio perspicua alchymiae transmutatoriae, opposita Nicolai Guiperti Lotharingi Ph. Med. expugnationi virili: Et Gastonis Clavei Iurisconsulti Nivernatis Apologia contra Erastum malé sartae & pravae* ... (Oberursel: Ex officina Cornelii Sutorii, 1604). See Bruce T. Moran, *Andreas Libavius and the Transformation of Alchemy: Separating Chemical Cultures with Polemical Fire* (Sagamore Beach, MA: Science History Publications, 2007); Newman, *Atoms and Alchemy*, 66–153.

[92] *De medicina nova*, 3:13–60. See Bröer, "Friedenspolitik durch Verketzerung," 175–178. See also Appendix B, text no. 12.

the Maladies of Epilepsy, Elephantitis or Leprosy, Dropsy, Arthritis and Colic Are Demonstrated and Paracelsianism Is Most Firmly Confuted. As is evident from the subtitle, Erastus discoursed here on various diseases, simultaneously critiquing Paracelsus and putting forward his own observations and theories. Although beyond the purview of this study, the volume offers a fertile field of investigation in determining the degree to which Erastus advanced the state of knowledge on select diseases. Owsei Temkin, one of the past century's foremost historians of medicine, applauded the advances made by Erastus in the description of epilepsy. It had been common to consider epilepsy a disease that caused loss of consciousness, making the entire body experience convulsions. Erastus broke with tradition and suggested that there might be forms of epilepsy that caused convulsions in only specific parts of the body. Being able to conceptualize a more limited form of epilepsy, Erastus distinguished between "perfect" and "imperfect" forms of epilepsy. From these observations Temkin concluded, "This simplified clinical classification represented a real advance over the elaborate and often artificial divisions of the preceding period."[93] Erastus has also been credited for recognizing the aura to be the sign rather than the cause of the onset of an epileptic episode—more than two hundred years before this became commonly accepted in Western medicine.[94] Though Erastus has sometimes been falsely labeled as a medical theorist with a "medieval" outlook due to his rejection of Paracelsus, Erastus's observations on epilepsy give us a brief glimpse of how original some of his medical contributions were.

Erastus's Reconstruction of the Historical Paracelsus

1. *Images of Paracelsus in* De medicina nova

One of the most enduring and often most entertaining aspects of Erastus's *Disputations* was its depiction of Paracelsus's life and customs for future generations. The fact that Erastus printed so many discrediting stories about Paracelsus caused him to be viewed as something of a pariah by early modern Paracelsians and by the Germanic founders of the history of medicine. Setting aside the hero worship of Paracelsus, one can

[93] Temkin, *The Falling Sickness*, 193. See also Pagel, *Paracelsus*, 327–329.
[94] William Richard Gowers, *Epilepsy and Other Chronic Convulsive Diseases: Their Causes, Symptoms & Treatment* (New York, 1885), 34.

appreciate that the unflattering stories that Erastus no doubt assembled for a polemical purpose hold in most cases genuine biographical kernels that should be seriously considered by scholars seeking to reconstruct Paracelsus's biography. Erastus assaulted Paracelsus not through misrepresentation and fabrication but through selection. Erastus may have been inclined to believe and report the worst of Paracelsus, but we have no reason to think that he was dishonest. Where we can verify his accounts with other sources, it is clear that he recounted the sordid tales he collected with great accuracy. Since the characterizations of Paracelsus by Gessner and Oporinus have already been discussed, they will not be addressed again in this section, even though Erastus incorporated their depictions in *De medicina nova*.

Erastus went to great lengths to collect information on Paracelsus. Around 1570, he asked his contacts in Switzerland to gather information regarding Paracelsus's family but was not able to connect Paracelsus to any living Swiss relative. This fact was some consolation to Erastus, who wanted to distance Paracelsus from his beloved homeland; as he writes in *De medicina nova*, "I can hardly believe he was Swiss."[95] Erastus incorrectly assumed that Paracelsus's given name had been "Philipp Bombast" and that he was born in Hohenheim in Southwestern Germany. He noted that Paracelsus had lived in the province of Carinthia in Austria for some years as a child. An unnamed source informed Erastus that Paracelsus had been castrated by a soldier when he was a young boy tending geese. Erastus suggested that this story corroborated Oporinus's claim that Paracelsus had shown little interest in women, but it ultimately seems too much calculated as a partisan insult to be credible. Later Paracelsus allegedly traveled to Spain, where he first learned magic, then chemistry. This account may represent the vestige of a pro-Paracelsian tradition that sought to connect Paracelsus with the tradition of the great Spanish alchemical theorists Ramon Lull and Arnold of Villanova.[96]

[95] *De medicina nova*, 1:237: "Helvetium fuisse vix credo."

[96] *De medicina nova*, 1:237–238: "Hoc in loco, narratum mihi est exectos ei testes fuisse à milite, dum anseres pasceret.... Eunuchum fuisse cum alia multa, tum facies indicant: & quod, Oporino teste, feminas prorsus despexit." A second castration story involved Paracelsus's testicles being removed by the bite of a boar. The examination of Paracelsus's skeleton has revealed the existence of certain female characteristics on his pelvis and cranium. This fact has led some scholars to suggest that Paracelsus may have suffered from a congenital hormonal imbalance related to the abnormal processing of androgens. A firm diagnosis of this condition would certainly shed light on Paracelsus's psychological state and his sexual history. See Herbert Kritscher et al., "Forensisch-

Johannes Crato von Krafftheim: Paracelsus in Moravia and Vienna

The most significant biographical gem that Erastus was able to uncover was a report by the Moravian nobleman Berthold V von Leipa (d. 1575), relayed to Erastus by Crato.[97] The story begins in the imperial chambers in Prague in 1570, where Crato was having a discussion with two other physicians of Emperor Maximilian, Giulio Alessandrini and Nicolaus Biese.[98] As they were talking the nobleman Berthold von Leipa approached them and told them a story of Paracelsus's misadventures in Moravský Krumlov.[99] Berthold recounted that his father, Johann von Leipa, had summoned Paracelsus to his bed because of Paracelsus's reputation in treating arthritis. Though Paracelsus attended Johann for some two years, he was not able to improve his condition. Other noble patients were not to be that fortunate. Paracelsus's treatment caused Berthold to lose sight in one eye and the medication he gave to the wife of Baron Johann von Zerotín caused her to break into seizures and promptly expire.[100] This disaster was enough to trigger one of Paracelsus's charac-

anthropologische Untersuchungen der Skelettreste des Paracelsus," in *Paracelsus (1943–1541): Keines andern Knecht* ... ed. H. Dopsch et al. (Salzburg: Anton Pustet, 1993), 53–61.

[97] *De medicina nova*, 4:159–160. Full translation and analysis in Gunnoe and Shackelford, "Johannes Crato von Krafftheim (1519–1585)," 210–212. The Leipa were a prominent Moravian noble house. Vladimir Zapletal, "Paracelsus-Tradition in der Tschechoslowakei," in *Gestalten und Ideen um Paracelsus*, 158–160; Augustin Tschinkel, "Paracelsus bei König Ferdinand I," in *Paracelsus—Werk und Wirkung* (Vienna, 1975), 340; Zedler, *Universal-Lexicon*, 16:1644–1645.

[98] Julius Alexandinus von Neustein (Italian, Guilio Alessandrini, 1506–1590), a personal physician to Emperors Ferdinand I and Maximilian II from Trent. Like Crato, Alessandrini was also ennobled by the Habsburgs and granted the title of Count Palatine. Along with being a noted Platonic philosopher, Alessandrini also translated the works of Galen from Greek into Latin. He engaged in a heated exchange in defense of Galen against Girolamo Argenterio. *NDB*, 1:197; Zedler, *Universal-Lexicon*, 1:1173; Christoph Wilhelm Kestner, *Medicinisches Gelehrten-Lexicon* (Jena, 1740; reprint, Hildesheim: George Olms, 1971), 26; M.A. Becker, "Die letze Tage und der Tod Maximilians II," *Blätter des Vereines für Landeskunde von Niederösterreich*, 11 (1877): 16–17. Nicolaus Biese (1516–1572) a Galenic physician from Ghent, who likewise served as personal physician to Maximillian II. Zedler, *Universal-Lexicon*, 3:1809; Kestner, *Medicinisches Gelehrten-Lexicon*, 112.

[99] Zapletal judged that Paracelsus's stay in Moravský Krumlov probably lasted five to six months. Zapletal, "Paracelsus-Tradition in der Tschechoslowakei," 161; Karl Pisa, *Paracelsus in Österreich* (St. Pölten/Vienna: Niederösterreichisches Pressehaus, 1991), 116–120.

[100] Likely Johanna von Pernstein (Johanka z Pernštejna, b. 1516, d. ?), daughter of Johann von Pernstein (Jan z Pernštejna, d. 1548), the wife of Johann III von Žerotín (Jan ze Žerotína, d. ca. 1558/60). Paracelsus must have journeyed to the Žerotín residence

teristic flights, this time into Hungary. Berthold also informed Crato that Paracelsus had written quite a lot in Moravský Krumlov—one of the volumes of the *Astronomia Magna* is in fact dated from that time—though Berthold added that he accomplished this in a drunken state.[101] Evidently Paracelsus was able to recover the manuscripts that he deposited in Moravský Krumlov, perhaps through the intervention of the emperor.

How does one assess such a tale? On the one hand, it was told some thirty years after the events that it purports to describe, and it was passed from Berthold to Crato and then to Erastus. Given the care with which Erastus handled other texts by his humanist colleagues, we can confidently assume that Erastus printed Crato's account accurately. On the other hand, it is the story of an eyewitness (or rather, a one-eyed witness) of Paracelsus's activities in Moravia. It correlates well with Paracelsus's known movements of the time and the individuals described were historical personages. Though the story of a dissatisfied patient as recorded by a disparager of Paracelsus, the account possesses a fundamental historicity and has been used by Paracelsus scholars, with less than direct acknowledgment, as a source for Paracelsus's activities in Moravia.[102]

In addition to Berthold's story of events which transpired in Moravia, Crato was also able to describe the circumstances of Paracelsus's supposed meeting with King Ferdinand in Vienna. This is one of two versions of the alleged meeting that we possess. The other is an utterly fanciful Czech account, *Colloquium Ferdinandi regis cum D. Theophrasto Paracelsus Svevo*.[103] In that version of events, despite the murderous opposition of the "learned physicians," Paracelsus treated the ailing king

---

in Strážnice, a Moravian city located near the current Czech-Slovak border. Zapletal, "Paracelsus-Tradition in der Tschechoslowakei," 161. Like the Leipa with whom they were intermarried, the Žerotíns were a prominent Moravian noble house and supporters of the *Unitas Fratrum*. See R.J.W. Evans, *Rudolf II and his World* (Oxford: Clarendon, 1973), 41–42.

[101] His "Beschlußrede" to the *Astronomia Magna* is dated from there on July 22, 1537. *PI*, 12:vi and 273.

[102] The basic work here is Zapletal's article, which contained no citations. A close reading of this work reveals a heavy dependence on the Crato-Erastus text. This reliance is rather ironic, as Zapletal had complained of Berthold's reminiscences, "die jedoch nun mehr verschwommen waren" (p. 162). Pisa (likewise without citations) brought much of Zapletal's content into his book. Zapletal, "Paracelsus-Tradition in der Tschechoslowakei;" Pisa, *Paracelsus in Österreich*.

[103] A. German translation of this Czech text is printed in Georg Sticker, "Ein Gespräch des Königs Ferdinand mit Paracelsus," *Nova Acta Leopoldina* 10 (1941): 267–279. Tschinkel critiques this translation in "Paracelsus bei König Ferdinand I." This story is also hinted at more faintly in the early seventeenth-century "Rhapsodia vitae Theophrasti

with potable gold and immediately improved his condition. After the successful cure, Paracelsus and the king sat down to dinner, during which Paracelsus discoursed on the requisite moral qualities of a successful alchemist. Paracelsus was fêted by the king and given a golden chain on his departure. About the only similarity between this Czech account and the one that appeared in Erastus's pages is the hostility between Paracelsus and the court physicians. In the Crato-Erastus text, King Ferdinand could smell a quack and denounced Paracelsus as a "lying and impudent impostor." Not content to conclude with Paracelsus's humiliation at the imperial court, the Crato-Erastus text added the additional insult: "Paracelsus always had traffic with Jews and the most vile men."[104]

Crato's version of this story was recorded earlier and possesses more historically verifiable details than the later Czech account. It is difficult to escape the conclusion that the Crato-Erastus text must be given priority over the *Colloquium* as an historical source. Both texts tell us more about the polarization of the Paracelsus image that had occurred by the late sixteenth century, however, than about any putative meeting between Ferdinand and Paracelsus. In the one account, Paracelsus was the heroic alchemist whose success at chrysopoeia clearly led his list of credits. In the other account, Paracelsus was a plain charlatan whose greatest offense was his refusal to enter a meaningful dialogue with Ferdinand's humanist physicians. Armed with the firsthand information from Berthold von Leipa, Crato was able to construct a distinct image of a shiftless, drunken, and deliberately obscure quack that harmonized perfectly with the other negative testimony that Erastus assembled and published.

Paracelsi." See Sven Limbeck, "Paracelsus in einer frühneuzeitlichen Historiensammlung: Die 'Rhapsodia vitae Theophrasti Paracelsi' von Peter Payngk," in *Analecta Paracelsica*, 1–58.

[104] *De medicina nova*, 4:160: "Semper illi negotium fuisse cum Iudaeis & vilissimis hominibus." Alternatively, the "Colloquium Ferdinandi regis cum D. Theophrasto Paracelsus Svevo" places an anti-Semitic comment in the mouth of Paracelsus. See G. Sticker, "Ein Gespräch des Königs Ferdinand mit Paracelsus," 275. For a recent assessment of Paracelsus's anti-Semitism, see Udo Benzenhöfer and Karin Finsterbusch, "Antijudaismus in den medizinisch-naturwissenschaftlichen und philosophischen Schriften des Paracelsus," in *Paracelsus und seine internationale Rezeption in der frühen Neuzeit. Beiträge zur Geschichte des Paracelsismus*, ed. Heinz Schott and Ilana Zinguer (Leiden: E.J. Brill, 1998), 96–109.

Heinrich Bullinger: Paracelsus in Zurich

Another significant account of Paracelsus's life was relayed to Erastus by Bullinger. Bullinger had likely met Paracelsus in 1527, when Bullinger had taken leave of his teaching position in Kappel to spend a few months hearing lectures under Zwingli in Zurich.[105] Some forty years later, Bullinger recounted to Erastus:

> I talked with him [Paracelsus] now and again about various things, also regarding theological and religious topics. But one would be hard pressed to fathom anything of piety from his words, but one could find a great deal regarding magic, though I do not know how he went about it. If you had seen him, you would not have said that he was a physician, but rather a teamster, and he was marvelously delighted by the companionship of teamsters. While he lived here at the Stork Inn,[106] he would observe teamsters arriving at the tavern, and the filthy man would eat and drink excessively with them. Sometimes he was so overcome by wine, that he would settle down on the nearest bench and sleep off his foul hangover. And then, [narrates Erastus], having interjected certain things concerning his habits and clothing, such as Oporinus's account also contains,[107] [Bullinger] concludes thus: In short, he [Paracelsus] was a dirty and vulgar man in every respect. He seldom if ever attended church services, and seemed to care little for God and holy things.[108]

[105] Bullinger was in Zurich from the middle of June until the middle of November. Blanke, *Der junge Bullinger*, 67; Bullinger, *Diarium*, 11.

[106] The "Hotel zum Storchen" continues to operate in Zurich. It is located at Weinplatz 2 across the Limat from the Grossmünster. Milt has also noted that its owner at that time remained loyal to the Catholic church. Bernhard Milt, "Paracelsus und Zürich," *Vierteljahrsschrift der Naturforschenden Gesellschaft in Zürich* 86 (1941): 322.

[107] An abridged version of the Oporinus letter immediately precedes these passages from Bullinger in *De medicina nova*, 1:238–239. The extracts highlighted Paracelsus's proclivity to drink, his tendency to sleep in his clothes, and his lack of conventional piety, and included an insinuation of practicing magic. See the translation of Erastus's paired down version of Oporinus's text by Jeremy Venema in Gunnoe, "Thomas Erastus and his Circle of Anti-Paracelsians," in *Analecta Paracelsica*, 146–148.

[108] *De medicina nova*, 1:239–240: "Contuli cum eo, inquit, semel & iterum de rebus varijs etiam Theologicis vel Religionis. Sed ex omnibus eius sermonibus pietatis nihil intelligere licuit, Magiae verò, quam ille nescio quam fingebat, plurimum. Si eum vidisses, non Medicum dixisses, sed Aurigam: & sodalitio Aurigarum mirificè delectabatur. Ergo dum viveret hîc in diversorio Ciconiae, observabat adventantes in hoc hospitium Aurigas: & cum his homo spurcus vorabat & perpotabat: ita nonnunquam vino sopitus, ut se in proximum scamnum collocaret, crapulam que fœdam edormiret. [Erastus's paraphrase follows] Deinde interiectis quibusdam de habitu & vestitu eius, qualia Oporinus etiam habet, sic concludit. [Bullinger's letter concludes] Breviter sordidus erat per omnia & homo spurcus. Rarò aut nunquam ingrediebatur coetus sacros, ac visus est Deum & res Divinas leviter curare." This quotation probably comes from a lost letter from Bullinger

Bullinger's account must be taken seriously since it is one of the few eyewitness accounts of Paracelsus we possess. However, it must be conceded that Bullinger's engagement with Paracelsus must have been brief. Likewise, the long time span between when he likely met Paracelsus (ca. 1527) and when he probably composed this reminiscence (late 1570) undermines this document's value as source. Still, given the general reliability of Bullinger and the account's congruence with other stories of Paracelsus, we must lend it at least a modicum of credence. Bullinger's report contained a clear insinuation of magic and a direct slight of Paracelsus's piety. These accusations, paired with Gessner's attacks, revealed unanimity in the Zurichers' assessment: Paracelsus had practiced forbidden black magic. This was the inescapable conclusion of the combined testimonies of Gessner, Oporinus, and Bullinger, as Erastus himself expressed in his reply to Bullinger after receiving his report: "It is certain that he was a magician and a confederate of demons."[109] Bullinger's account offered yet another testimony, from a person who was an unrivaled authority in Reformed circles, to the heretical nature of Paracelsianism.

Georg Vetter: A Companion of Paracelsus

If we are to believe Erastus, however, not only Paracelsus's enemies but also his friends alleged that he toyed with demonic magic. Although not necessarily as provocative as the stories from Crato and Bullinger, of equal interest is the testimonial by the purported travel companion of Paracelsus, Georg Vetter. Vetter had attended Paracelsus's lectures in Basel and served as his famulus ca. 1527–1528. Erastus recounted that Vetter had traveled with Paracelsus for over two years "through Austria, Transylvania and other regions." If Erastus's description is accurate, this would suggest that Vetter accompanied Paracelsus sometime during the period from 1537 to 1540. In the 1570s Vetter worked as a minister in a parish about forty kilometers from Heidelberg in Beerfelden in the Odenwald. His clerical status is evidenced by Toxites's dedication of the 1574 edition of Paracelsus's testament.[110] Vetter's testimony is particularly

to Erastus which was written between Oct. 29, 1570 and Jan. 3, 1571. See the German translation in Milt, "Conrad Gesner und Paracelsus" (1929), 488.

[109] Erastus to Bullinger, Jan. 3, 1571, ZBZ, F 62 fol. 204^{v}. See Appendix B, text no. 3.

[110] Sudhoff, *Bibliographia Paracelsica*, 156, 256. For a thorough reconstruction of Vetter's connections to the Paracelsian movement, see text no. 54 "Toxites, Michael an Georg Vetter" in Kühlmann and Telle, eds., *Corpus Paracelsisticum*, 2:297–320.

interesting, as it comes from someone who still claimed to be a supporter of Paracelsus. Not surprisingly, the information from Vetter's account largely mirrored the stories of Oporinus, Crato, and Bullinger, including the familiar charges of alcoholism and impiety. Expressed more strongly in the Vetter account, however, was an accusation of diabolical magic:

> Recently a most pious, learned, and industrious man, Georg Vetter—loving and devoted to Paracelsus—adamantly brought to my attention that [Paracelsus] was extremely devoted to impious magic and that he had befriended an evil spirit. "I feared nothing more," he said, "that when [Paracelsus] was drunk (which was frequently) that he would summon a troop of devils, which again and again he wanted to do by his special art; but at my request, he abandoned it. When I warned Paracelsus (when sober) that he made these utterances, which gravely offended God, and that the devil would render the final judgment upon his own servants, he responded that he would soon be singing for redemption."[111]

After the quotation, Erastus added the rhetorical comment that he was forced to accept Vetter's account because of Vetter's piety and genuine devotion to Paracelsus. He also included Vetter's comment that "The total time in which I lived with him, he did not discuss theology nor philosophy nor medicine besides surgery," which not only assaulted Paracelsus's piety, but also lowered him from the ranks of learned physicians to the more humble status of a surgeon.

While Vetter remains something of an obscure figure to modern scholarship, his connection with Paracelsus was genuine, making this text in all likelihood an authentic biographical fragment from a firsthand witness. Adding further credence to Vetter is the fact that we find the Paracelsian Toxites making a respectful inquiry with Vetter for information about Paracelsus's life and cures *after* the publication of these reminiscences.[112] Additionally, it should be noted that Erastus quoted his sources faithfully, if selectively, in *De medicina nova*.[113] With Vetter working in a nearby

[111] *De medicina nova*, 2:2: "Nuper mihi vir pius, doctus, industrius, D. Georg. Vetterus Paracelsi amans & stu[dio]sus, asserverantissimè affirmavit, eum Magiae nefandae perquam studiosum fuisse, & cacodaemonem haud aliter quàm socium nominare consuevisse. Nihil magis, inquiebat, metui, quotiens ebrius erat (erat autem frequenter) quàm ut agmina Diabolorum accerseret: quod saepenumero facere voluit (specium artis suae editurus) sed à me rogatus omisit. Cum sobrium monerem, ut missa isthaec facere, quòd Deum graviter offenderet, quodque ad extremum triste stipendium solitus esset persolvere famulis suis diabolus: respondebat, se non multò pòst receptui cantaturum esse."

[112] Kühlmann and Telle, eds., *Corpus Paracelsisticum*, 2:303. The letter from Toxites to Vetter was dated March 12, 1574.

[113] He clearly quoted Gessner and Oporinus with great accuracy. In my experience with comparing his citations from the works of Paracelsus, his quotations and translations

parish, Erastus would hardly have been in a position to fabricate or alter his testimony, especially given Erastus's own increasingly threatened personal reputation. It should also be noted that the most damning line, "that he was accustomed to call an evil spirit his friend," did not purport to be a direct quotation from Vetter but was Erastus's own interpolation. Despite these limitations, it is hard to escape the conclusion that Paracelsus considered himself to be an authentic *magus* and that his practice of these arts was enough to make a more conventionally pious associate very uncomfortable. If one lends a little additional credence to Vetter, it is possible to speculate that Paracelsus considered himself to be walking, and perhaps occasionally transgressing, the fine line between natural and demonic magic.[114]

Markus Recklau: Paracelsus in Upper Bavaria

Erastus also included the account of the court physician Markus Recklau, whose testimony attacked Paracelsus's medical reputation. Recklau, whom Erastus identifies as a personal physician of Ottheinrich and Frederick III, supplied Erastus with a noteworthy tale of Paracelsus's activities in upper Bavaria.[115] According to Recklau, Paracelsus was summoned to attend the wife of an Augsburg patrician named von Langenmantel, who was then residing in the town of Schongau on the Lech in the foothills of the Alps.

appear to be quite accurate. Jole Shackelford has also been able to find very precise excerpts from Severinus's *Idea medicinae* in Erastus's text. Shackelford, "Early Reception of Paracelsian Theory," 127–128; idem, *A Philosophical Path for Paracelsian Medicine*, 217–218.

[114] Erastus reiterates the claim of diabolical inspiration a few pages later. *De medicina nova*, 2:16. See also Kühlmann and Telle, eds., *Corpus Paracelsisticum*, 1:135, 598–599. For Paracelsus's own opinion regarding the possibility of Christian magic, see Arlene Miller Guinsberg, "Die Ideenwelt des Paracelsus und seiner Anhänger in Hinsicht auf das Thema des christlichen Magus und dessen Wirken," in *Von Paracelsus zu Goethe und Wilhelm von Humboldt*, 27–54.

[115] The existence of "Dr. Marx Rechklau" is documented by manuscripts in the Codex Palatinus Germanicus (Heidelberg, UB, MS Cod. Pal. germ. 193) and by an entry in the Tübingen matriculation of "Marcus Rechlau de Memingen" (Nov. 3, 1529) (*Urkunden zur Geschichte der Universität Tübingen aus den Jahren 1476 bis 1550* (Tübingen, 1877), 647). Erastus also references "D. Marcus Reccklaw" in *De occultis pharmacorum potestatibus*, 123. It would seem likely that he was related to Johann Recklau, who was a member of the church council under Elector Frederick III. Press, *Calvinismus und Territorialstaat*, 243.

Paracelsus was able to restore the appearance of health to the woman, but soon after his departure, she expired. From there he traveled down the Lech to Landsberg, Bavaria, where Recklau practiced medicine at that time. Recklau currently attended two noble patients of the von Pfeten family—one suffering from edema (dropsy), the other from consumption (phthisis).[116] Upon Paracelsus's advent, a local surgeon, Georg Rausner, informed Recklau that an illustrious physician had arrived who possessed the ability "to cure almost all serious diseases." With Recklau's approval, Paracelsus was taken to see the two noble patients. Recklau recounted that Paracelsus interrogated both himself and the noble relative of his patients in a most condescending manner. Paracelsus required Recklau to give a lengthy analysis of the patients' ailments, but after Recklau had finished his discourse, Paracelsus simply remained silent.

Later Paracelsus, the surgeon Raunser, and Recklau retired to a local tavern. While having a drink, Paracelsus allegedly spied the town's fine fountain, which spewed water high into the air. According to Recklau, Paracelsus declared the fountain to be a threat to public health. Paracelsus purportedly asserted, "If I were a doctor in this town, I would appeal to the magistrate to have this fountain destroyed, … lest the wind blow water into the faces of the women coming to market."[117] According to Recklau's account, Paracelsus left the next day without saying farewell to Recklau, his noble patron Sebald von Pfeten, or his patients. Recklau added the additional insult that he had been unable to elicit one word of Latin from Paracelsus's tongue.

The Recklau text also included an epilogue recounting Paracelsus's next malpractice, relayed to Recklau by the Paracelsian Johann Vogt. Upon leaving Landsberg, Paracelsus traveled the short distance to Munich, where he treated a certain "Monachus," an official in the kitchen of the Duke of Bavaria. The story alleges that the ducal physicians Dr. Panthaleon and Dr. Alexander Karthauser were already treating Monachus quite successfully. The patient was taken from their care and entrusted to Paracelsus, who treated the patient with mercury. When Paracelsus saw that his patient, rather than improving, was ebbing towards death, he fled to Austria, leaving his patient to die the next day.[118]

---

[116] The patients were the wife and sister of Sebald von Pfeten.

[117] *De medicina nova*, 3:213: "[S]i huius oppidi forem medicus, inquit, apud magistratum hoc agerem, ut fons iste tolleretur.… [N]e ventus mulieribus ad mercatum venientibus aquam in faciem impelleret."

[118] *De medicina nova*, 3:212–214.

As with Vetter, not enough is presently known of Recklau for us to assess this account, though with his purported prominence both as a court physician for the Palatine Wittelsbachs and as perhaps the city physician of Schongau, this question should yield to future research. The events described may have occurred during Paracelsus's travels in 1536, after the publication of *Grosse Wundarznei*, but standard biographical accounts of Paracelsus make no mention of a visit to Schongau or Landsberg.[119] It is no great revelation to learn that Paracelsus led a highly itinerate life. The events which occurred in Landsberg, the only ones which Recklau likely observed firsthand, are likewise described from the position of a practitioner understandably jealous of his own status as a medical authority. While much in Recklau's account might smack of professional rivalry, the quixotic figure he describes harmonizes well with the historical Paracelsus. One hopes that future research will shed more light on these obscure episodes.

Brief Accounts

Beyond these longer accounts, Erastus also included a number of shorter testimonies in the *De medicina nova* that likewise undercut Paracelsus's reputation as a medical practitioner and chemical innovator. Crato's assertion that Paracelsus lifted his innovative preparations from medieval manuscripts falls into this category.[120] In much a similar spirit is the comment of Balthasar Brauch of Schwäbish Gmünd that the physicians Hieronymus Schaller, Johann Magenbuch, and Wolfgang Talhauser had produced similar innovations in medical preparations, though they remained pious men and did not advance the ludicrous claim to be founding a whole new art.[121]

[119] E.g., Pagel, *Paracelsus*; Johannes Hemleben, *Paracelsus: Revolutionär, Arzt und Christ*, 2nd ed. (Frauenfeld: Verlag Huber, 1974); Charles Webster, *Paracelsus: Medicine, Magic and Mission at the End of Time* (New Haven: Yale UP, 2008).

[120] *De medicina nova*, 4:300. "Remedia quibus aliquando usus dicitur, non illius esse ex eo certus sum, quòd librum vidi ante 200. ferè annos à monacho quodam Ulmae scriptum." The text in question has been identified as *Von der Heiligen Dreifaltigkeit* (aka *Buchs der Heiligen Dreifaltigkeit* or *Liber sancte trintatis*) which was composed ca. 1410/19. Authorship of the piece is generally credited to a Minorite monk named Ulmannus. Herwig Buntz, "Deutsch alchimistische Traktate des 15. und 16. Jahrhunderts" (Doctoral dissertation, University of Munich, 1968), 34. See Joachim Telle, in *Lexikon des Mittelalters* (Munich: Artemis, 1983), 2:812–813; idem, "Ulmannus" in *Die deutsche Literatur des Mittelalters Verfasserlexikon* (Berlin: de Gruyter, 2004), 11:1574–1580.

[121] *De medicina nova*, 2:3. See Joachim Telle, "Wolfgang Talhauser: Zu Leben und Werk

Erastus also claimed to have testimony from the inhabitants of Basel who had witnessed Paracelsus in action. These men did not begrudge credit to Paracelsus in his treatment of ulcers, but they were less laudatory of his treatment of other maladies. Although Paracelsus at first seemed to have cured the printer Johannes Froben, the Baselers (including Erasmus) would quickly learn that his medications had negative side effects. In Erastus's assessment, Paracelsus's remedies were very powerful in expelling corrupted humors, but the vestiges of Paracelsus's medicaments that remained in the body proved most toxic. Erastus recounted the rumor, which he alleged had been corroborated to him by many, that everyone who consumed Paracelsus's drugs in Basel perished within a year.[122] In short, Paracelsus's cure was worse than the disease.

Though I have made some attempts to assess the potential reliability of these stories, my main interest here is to document how Erastus shaped the image of Paracelsus rather than embarking on a quest for the "historical Paracelsus." The representation that Erastus hammered home possessed seven basic features: (1) Paracelsus and his followers were dangerous heretics; (2) Paracelsus dabbled in demonic magic; (3) Paracelsus was unlearned and wrote in a most obscure style; (4) As a physician, Paracelsus was at best ineffective and at worst lethal; (5) Paracelsus was a drunkard; (6) Paracelsus was personally unreliable and prone to flight in difficult circumstances; (7) Though Paracelsus was a successful chemist, he was not as innovative or perhaps as independent as conventionally thought. Each of these basic points was to be found in more than one story, and most were made clearly enough that Erastus had little need to interpolate more. One exception is the charge of contact with demons. Though the theme was certainly present in the stories, Erastus spelled it out more explicitly than did his sources.

---

eines Augsburger Stadtarztes und seinen Beziehungen zu Paracelsus und Schwenckfeld," *Medizinhistorisches Journal* 7 (1972): 1–30; and Joachim Telle and Peter Assion, "Der Nürnberger Stadtarzt Johannes Magenbuch: Zu Leben und Werk eines Mediziners der Reformationszeit," *Sudhoffs Archiv* 56 (1972): 353–421.

[122] *De medicina nova*, 4:253. Erastus had been aware of these stories as early as 1570. Erastus to Johann Jakob Grynaeus, Nov. 29, [1570], Basel UB, G II 4, fols. 300–301. See also Kühlmann and Telle, eds., *Corpus Paracelsisticum*, 1:437, 511; Joachim Telle, "Paracelsus als Wunderheiler und Goldmacher in Basel: Zu dem Brief eines Ungenannten an Michael Neander (1575)," in *Medizin* und *Kultur*: *Ärztliches Denken und Handeln im Dialog zwischen Natur- und Geisteswissenschaften*, ed. Giovanni Maio and Volker Roelcke (Stuttgart: Schattauer, 2001), 13–32.

While Erastus emphasized these distinct points of Paracelsus's biography, whether his readers would have put them together as clearly as I have described is doubtful since Erastus scattered these biographical tidbits throughout the four volumes of *De medicina nova*. It is important to note that almost all of these accounts are given in the voice of a third party. This provided the rhetorical advantage of allowing the reports to appear more authoritative and Erastus to appear more objective. Nevertheless, Erastus was able to manage his sources in such a way as to put forward a coherent image of Paracelsus. By means of judicious selection, he was able to create his own composite narrative from the many eyewitness testimonies he included in the *De medicina nova*. The narrative Erastus crafted was an exhaustive attack on both Paracelsus's personal integrity and his professional competence.

Whether this narrative was persuasive to Erastus's contemporaries is another question. From the anecdotal evidence I have gathered, I can offer only a provisional assessment. On the one hand, Erastus's effort was apparently successful in convincing humanist physicians that Paracelsus was a disreputable character. Erastus's work quickly became a source for other anti-Paracelsian writers; for example, Bernhard Dessen von Kronenburg (1510–1574) incorporated biographical details from Erastus's work into his *Medicina veteris et rationalis* in 1573.[123] Similarly, Jean Antoine Fenot hailed the success of Erastus's exposé of Paracelsus's gross iniquity and false theory in his own critique of alchemy in 1575.[124] Later, academic physicians such as Andreas Libavius and Daniel Sennert who sought to mediate between Paracelsian and Galenic medicine tended to be most wary of Paracelsus's personal reputation.[125] Debus likewise has

[123] Bernhard Dessen von Kronenburg, *Medicinae Veteris Et Rationalis, Adversus Oberronis Cuiusdam Mendacissimi Atque Impudentissimi Georgii Fedronis, ac universae Sectae Paracelsiae imposturas, defensio* (Cologne: Johannes Gymnicus, 1573), 54, 90. This work actually appeared in print prior to the fourth volume of Erastus's *De medicina nova* (Die Messkatalog Georg Willers, 1:489, 518). Some of the details of Erastus's accounts also found their way into Christoph Gottlieb von Murr's "Litterargeschichte des Theophrastus Paracelsus," in *Neues Journal zur Litteratur und Kunstgeschichte* 2 (1799): 233–234.

[124] Jean Antoine Fenot, *Alexipharmacum, Sive Antidotus Apologetica, ad virulentias Iosephi cuiusdam Quercetani Armeniaci, evomitas in libellum Jacobi Auberti, de ortu & causis Metallorum contra Chymistas* (Basil: [Pietro Perna], 1575), 2: "Quod ad Paracelsum nequissimum illum attinet, eum cum tota sua falsa doctrina ad Erastum celeberrimum illum philosophum & medicum praestantissimum ablegamus, qui pro dignitate honorificè eum excipiet."

[125] See Bruce Moran, "Libavius the Paracelsian? Monstrous Novelties, Institutions, and the Norms of Social Virtue," in *Reading the Book of Nature*, 67–79; and Debus, "Guitherius, Libavius and Sennert: The Chemical Compromise in Early Modern Medicine."

argued that Erastus's critique had a major impact on the reception of Paracelsianism in England and made English scientists quite suspicious of him.[126]

On the other hand, Erastus's attack on Paracelsus's person does not appear to have had a major impact on the appeal of Paracelsian scientific ideas. For those who were inclined to look favorably on Paracelsus, Erastus's efforts smacked of partisanship and *ad hominem* overkill. This can be observed in the case of the English Paracelsian Richard Bostocke, who elected to write off his hero's alcoholism as a national defect:

> If Paracelsus some tyme woulde be dronke after his Countrey maner I can not excuse hym no more then I can excuse in some nations glottenie, in other pride, and contempt of all others in comparison of themselves, in others breach of promise and fidelitie, in others dissimulation, triflyng and muche babling, but lett the doctrine bee tried by the worke and successe, not by their faultes in their liues.[127]

What Bostocke was unwilling to concede was that Paracelsus's quirks and peccadilloes somehow invalidated his scientific achievement. To the contrary, the virulence of Erastus's attack on Paracelsus's person seemed to betray an a priori unwillingness to entertain Paracelsus's scientific contribution.

Levinus Battus (1545–1591), a medical professor of Rostock, likewise was not impressed by Erastus's assault on Paracelsus's personal integrity. Little is known of Battus, but since he considered Paracelsus the "Luther of medicine," one can confidently label him a Paracelsian.[128] In a letter from 1573, Battus took issue both with the ad hominem nature of Erastus's attack and his source base. Battus dismissed Vetter's account because he was such an obscure figure and the negative stories from Basel because they were likely written by Paracelsus's rivals. He argued

[126] Debus, *The English Paracelsians*, 49. See below.

[127] R.B. [Richard Bostocke], *The difference betwene the auncient Phisicke, first taught by the godly forfathers, consisting in unitie peace and concord: and the later Phisicke proceding from Idolaters, Ethnikes, and Heathen: as Gallen, and such other consisting in dualitie, discord and contrarietie* (London: for Robert Walley, 1585), Liiii.^{v}. Regarding Bostocke, see David Harley, "Rychard Bostok of Tandridge, Surrey (C. 1530–1605), M.P., Paracelsian propagandist and friend of John Dee," *Ambix* 47 (2000): 29–36.

[128] The claim that Paracelsus was the "Luther of medicine" has a long history. See the articles by Vivian Nutton and Bernhard Dietrich Haage in *Paracelsus: Das Werk—die Rezeption* as well as Andrew Weeks, *Paracelsus: Speculative Theory and the Crisis of the Early Reformation* (Albany: State University of New York Press, 1997). Battus likely introduced Paracelsian ideas to Tycho Brahe. See Shackleford, *A Philosophical Path for Paracelsian Medicine*, 63–65.

that Oporinus's letter hardly proved all that Erastus had attempted to draw from it and that Talhauser's and Magenbuch's excellence in chemical preparations did not detract from Paracelsus's honor. As for the claim that Paracelsus was not particularly learned or eloquent, Battus cited the adage of Celsus that medicines rather than eloquence cured diseases. Battus also resented that Erastus used dubious tactics in attacking propositions derived from the work of Severinus and then claiming victory over Paracelsus. Finally, he did not take Erastus's charge of diabolism seriously, because he thought that Paracelsus had made proper distinctions between natural and demonic magic in his writings and that Paracelsus's methods—the Kabbalah, chiromancy, physiognomy, the theory of signatures, and the art of the furnace—were not demonic but were derived from the light of nature.[129] In short, the obvious partisan slant made Erastus's work easier to dismiss, and a Paracelsian had little difficulty supplying a more sympathetic reading to the aspects of Paracelsus's life and teaching that Erastus had found so troubling.[130]

Erastus's representations reflected one side of the polarization of the image of Paracelsus in the late sixteenth century. Not unlike Luther, Paracelsus had been increasingly sainted by his admirers and demonized by his enemies. At the extremes of both positions, Paracelsus was no longer simply a radical medical innovator with a quirky personality, but rather a man imbued with either magical or demonic power.

2. *Erastus's Paracelsian Library*

Erastus was a diligent student of Paracelsus. With his location in Heidelberg close to the biannual Frankfurt fairs and through his good connections with the Basel printing trade, Erastus was able to gather nearly all of the editions of Paracelsus that had been published at the time he composed *De medicina nova*. In the introduction Erastus recounted that he had read 113 books of Paracelsus. Karl Sudhoff himself, the great cataloger and editor of Paracelsus's works, found this an impressive number because of its close approximation to the number of editions that he was

[129] Levinus Battus, letter to [Heinrich Smet?], March 12, 1573, printed in Heinrich Smet, ed., *Miscellanea ... Medica* (Frankfurt: Jonas Rhodius, 1661), 691–692. Note that this letter was written before the completion of *De medicina nova*, 4. For more on Battus and Smet, see Kühlmann and Telle, "Humanismus und Medizin," 277–281.

[130] Figulus also repudiated Erastus's critique of Paracelsian medicine with great vitriol and humor in "Dialogus, Alexandri a Suchten," 49–111 (especially pp. 67 ff.)

able to collect with imprints prior to 1571.[131] From analysis of the rough citations in the *De medicina nova*, it is clear that Erastus's claim was no idle boast. Erastus used all of Paracelsus's major works in composing his refutation. The table below offers an approximate tally of Erastus's references to Paracelsus's works. Given the imprecision of sixteenth-century citations, linking Erastus's oblique references to Paracelsus's titles leaves a number of question marks. Nevertheless the table substantiates the claim that Erastus knew Paracelsus's published corpus well. Secondarily it sheds light on which works most shaped Erastus's view of Paracelsus. Erastus cited Paracelsus's speculative philosophical works far more frequently than his more strictly medical works (e.g., far more citations from the *Astronomia Magna* than the *Grosse Wundarznei*). The exception to this pattern was the heavy citation of works on individual diseases that were treated in *De medicina nova*, 4. Another significant pattern was the heavy citation of works of questionable authenticity, especially the *Philosophia ad Athenienses*.

Figure 1. Erastus's Paracelsian Library. Table of the books of Paracelsus cited in Erastus's *Disputationum De medicina nova Philippi Paracelsi pars prima[-quarta]* (Basel, [1571]–73). Some of the alternate titles Erastus employed are included in parentheses.

Title of Paracelsian Work	Location in *Sämtliche Werke (PI)*	Number of Citations 1–2	3–5	6–10	10–15	15 +
Astronomia Magna (Philosophia Sagax)	I, 12					X
Auslegung ... Aphorismorum Hippocratis	I, 4	X				
Das Buch von den tartarischen Krankheiten (Liber de Tartaro)	I, 11			X		
De artis praesagae	I, 14	X ?				
De Guaiaco [or *Vom Holz Guajaco* I, 7]	I, 3	X ?				
De Gradibus	I, 4	X				
De inventione artium	I, 14	X				
De lunaticis	I, 14		X			
De modo pharmacandi	I, 4			X		
De peste	I, 8	X ?				
De thermis (Bäderbuchlein)	I, 2	X				

131 Sudhoff, *Bibliographia Paracelsica*, 217.

Title of Paracelsian Work	Location in *Sämtliche Werke (PI)*	Number of Citations 1–2	3–5	6–10	10–15	15 +
De vita longa	I, 3			X		
Elf Tractat vom Ursprung, Ursachen und Kur einzelner Krankheiten:	I, 1					
Von der Wassersucht			X			
De colico dolore (Kolik)		X				
Große Wundarznei (De Chirugiae)	I, 10			X		
Labyrinthus medicorum errantium	I, 11	X				
Herbarius (De Elleboro)	I, 2		X			
Liber meteororum (De Meteoris Ein Buch in zehn Capita)	I, 13					X
Neun Bücher Archidoxis	I, 3					X
Paragranum	I, 8					X
Der Paragraphen	I, 5			X		
Philosophia magna	I, 14	X				
Opus Paramirum	I, 9			[x]		X
De matrice [Paramiri Liber quartus de Matrice]				[x]		
Sieben Defensionen	I, 11	X				
Spitalbuch (Liber pro Hospital.)	I, 7		X			
Von den hinfallenden Siechtagen (De Caduco, Epilepsia)	I, 8					X
Von den Podagrischen Krankheiten (De podagra)	I, 1					X
Von den unsichtbaren Krankheiten und ihren Ursachen (De morbis invisibilis)	I, 9			X		
Von Purgieren	I, 4	X ?				
Pseudo-Paracelsian Works						
De lapide philosophorum	I, 14	X				
De occulta philosophia	I, 14		X			
De tinctura physicorum	I, 14		X			
Liber vexationum	I, 14	X				
Philosophia ad Athenienses	I, 13					X

Erastus's Rejection of Paracelsus's Religio-Philosophical Worldview

Recent scholarship has significantly enhanced our knowledge of the religious dimension of Paracelsianism. Andrew Weeks has provocatively argued that Paracelsus's religious speculation in fact lies at the heart of his scientific outlook.[132] Not only is Paracelsus's theological corpus receiving fresh attention,[133] but scholars such as Gilly and Webster have displayed the importance of the accusation of heresy in the early reaction to Paracelsian ideas among the intellectual circles of the Holy Roman Empire.[134] Until the Paracelsian revival had reached an advanced stage, however, there was little sustained reflection on the religious implications of his natural philosophy. The publication in 1570 of Bartolomäus Reußner's *A Short Explanation and Christian Refutation of the Unheard of Blasphemies and Lies, which Paracelsus has poured out Against God, His Word and the Praiseworthy Art of Medicine in the Three Books of Philosophy to the Athenians* inaugurated a new era in the reaction to Paracelsus with the study of theological implications of Paracelsian texts.[135] Ironically, Paracelsus's early religious opponents had not read his specifically theological corpus, the bulk of which existed only in manuscript in

---

132 Weeks, *Paracelsus: Speculative Theory and the Crisis of the Early Reformation*, passim.

133 For example, Katrin Biegger, *De invocatione beatae Mariae virginis: Paracelsus und die Marienverehrung* [Kosmosophie 6] (Stuttgart: Steiner, 1990); Hartmut Rudolph, "Paracelsus' Laientheologie in traditionsgeschichtlicher Sicht und in ihrer Zuordnung zu Reformation und katholischer Reform," in *Resultate und Desiderate der Paracelsus-Forschung*, ed. Hartmut Rudolph and Peter Dilg (Stuttgart: Steiner, 1993); Bruce T. Moran, "Paracelsus, Religion, and Dissent: The Case of Philipp Homagius and Georg Zimmermann," *Ambix* 43 (1996): 65–79; Dane T. Daniel, "Invisible Wombs: Rethinking Paracelsus's Concept of Body and Matter," *Ambix* 53 (2006): 129–142. See as well, Paracelsus, *Neue Paracelsus-Edition*, ed. Urs Leo Gantenbein (Berlin: de Gruyter, 2008–).

134 Gilly, "Theophrastia Sancta," 425–488; Webster, "Conrad Gessner and the infidelity of Paracelsus," 13–23.

135 Bartholomäus Reußner, *Ein kurtze Erklerung und Christliche Widerlegung/Der unerhörten Gotteslesterungen und Lügen/ welche Paracelsus in den dreyen Büchern Philosphiae ad Athenienses hat wider Gott/ sein Wort und die löbliche Kunst der Artzney außgeschüttet* (Gorlitz: Ambrosius Fritsch, 1570). Reußner, a city physician of Zittau (Lausitz), concentrated his attack on the Paracelsian conception of creation. Reußner was born March 11, 1532 in Lemberg where his father was a member of the city council. He practiced medicine in Breslau before becoming city physician in Zittau. He died on Oct. 23, 1572. Given Reußner's interests and locus of activity, it is difficult to imagine that he was not an acquaintance of Crato, through whom he easily could have come into contact with Erastus. I have yet to find a clear reference to Reußner in Erastus's work or correspondence. Christian Gottlieb Jöcher, ed., *Allgemeines Gelehrten-Lexicon* (Leipzig, 1750–1819) 3:2031–2032.

1570.[136] Thus, the late sixteenth-century theological reaction to Paracelsus was not a rejection of his religious writings per se, but an attack upon the religious implications of this natural philosophy.

Creation

Perhaps taking his cue from Reußner, Erastus opened his attack in the first volume of *De medicina nova* on the Paracelsian notion of creation. Before addressing Erastus's specific objections, it is fitting to outline the nature and difficulties of Paracelsus's theory of creation. Paracelsus taught that creation largely consisted of a divine or angelic separation of preexisting matter. The central question regarding the Paracelsian theory of creation, which has intrigued commentators since the sixteenth century, is whether this primeval material—which he alternatively called *materia prima, materia ultima*, and *mysterium magnum*—was itself created by God or whether it was uncreated.

Since Pagel was able to show that many of Paracelsus's ideas appeared to have been influenced by Gnostic conceptions, we might imagine that Hohenheim advocated the existence of uncreated matter before "creation," in line with the Gnostic tradition.[137] Passages in the Paracelsian corpus appear to bear out this Gnostic interpretation. For example in *Das Buch de Mineralibus*, Paracelsus taught that *materia ultima* was "bei Gott" in the beginning. From it, *materia prima* was made. Pagel argued that this passage clearly assumed that some type of primeval matter existed alongside of God at creation.[138] While this passage was the most positive affirmation of the existence of uncreated matter among the genuine works of Paracelsus, other passages could be adduced to argue that he definitely taught that God first created all matter. For example in *De Meteoris*—in a passage that did not directly address the question of primeval matter—

[136] Gilly, "Theophrastia Sancta," 434. Erastus likewise quotes from all of Paracelsus's major medical and natural philosophical works but displays no awareness of Paracelsus's unpublished theological works.

[137] Walter Pagel, "Paracelsus in the Neoplatonic and Gnostic Tradition," *Ambix* 8 (1960): 125–166; idem, "The Prime Matter of Paracelsus," *Ambix* 9 (1961): 117–135; Walter Pagel and Marianne Winder, "The Higher Elements and Prime Matter in Renaissance Naturalism and in Paracelsus," *Ambix* 21 (1974): 94–127.

[138] *Das Buch de Mineralibus, PI*, 3:34: "Nun ist das erst gewesen bei got, der anfang, das ist ultima materia, die selbige ultimam materiam hat er gemacht in primam materiam." One should note that judging this reference is further complicated by the fact that Paracelsus here spoke of "materia ultima" rather than "materia prima." Pagel, "Paracelsus in the Neoplatonic and Gnostic Tradition," 142.

he did say that each of the four elements have bodies which were made "from nothing."[139] Thus, the works in which Paracelsus's authorship is not questioned are ambiguous on the question of the createdness of prime matter.

The spurious works in the Paracelsian corpus speak with no more clarity on this issue than the authentic works. On the one hand, the *Secretum magicum* suggested that God created the *materia prima*.[140] On the other hand, the *Philosophia ad Athenienses*, a text labeled pseudo-Paracelsian by Sudhoff but widely accepted as authentic in the sixteenth century, offered a definitive affirmation of the pre-existence of uncreated matter.[141] Here our unknown author spoke of a *Mysterium magnum*

---

139 *Liber Meteororum, PI*, 13:134: "nun sollent ir aber wissen, das alle vier corpora der vier elementen gemacht seind aus nichts, das ist alein gemacht durch das wort gottes, das fiat geheißen hat." Pagel did not find this reference a definitive rejection of the pre-existence of matter, since Paracelsus was speaking here of a later stage of creation. Pagel, "Paracelsus in the Neoplatonic and Gnostic Tradition," 145–144 [*sic*].

140 Pagel, "Paracelsus in the Neoplatonic and Gnostic Tradition," 146.

141 Sudhoff treats the question of the authenticity of the *Philosophia ad Athenienses* in the introduction to *PI*, 13: xi–xiii. Sudhoff's first complaint against this text was the lack of manuscript attestation for it by its sixteenth-century editors. Neither its original publisher Theodor Birckmann nor Johann Huser, who included it in his authoritative collection, made any reference to a manuscript source. Sudhoff lamented, "Auch haben wir ausschließlich diesen Kölner Druck [of Birckmann] unserem Texte ... zugrunde legen müssen, da uns keine einzige handschriftliche Überlieferung dieser Schrift bekannt geworden ist." The second major complaint against the work stems from its fragmentary nature. It is obviously incomplete (e.g., it starts with the second "*paras*") and shows signs of having been worked over by an editor. The most obvious indication of the latter is the fact that the introductions refer to "the Prince Theophrastus" in the third person. Thus, Sudhoff considered it a work of questioned authenticity but did not rule out the possibility that the work might contain "einen echten Kern" which stemmed from Paracelsus. Later scholars have been more sanguine regarding its potential authenticity, and Josef Strebel regarded the text as a preliminary draft of the *Astronomia Magna*. Kurt Goldammer also raised objections to Sudhoff's earlier critique and referred to it as "die den echten Paracelsus gedankenreich paraphrasierende und interpretierende 'Philosophia ad Athenienses,'" though he still labeled the work "deutero-Paracelsian." Pagel often mined the *Philosophia ad Athenienses* as a source for "Paracelsian" ideas. With his extensive use of the work, Pagel appears to have been a de facto advocate of the authenticity of the *Philosophia ad Athenienses* even if he was forthcoming about the questions of its genuineness. Following Pagel, many Anglo-American writers have traced the impact of "Paracelsian" ideas in a broad sense, rather than limit their studies to works which can be concretely proven to have come from Paracelsus's pen. We can agree with Pagel and his followers that the work was universally regarded as "Paracelsian;" nevertheless, the fundamental reservations regarding the work's authenticity raised by Sudhoff have not been overturned. Given the fact that a later redactor edited the text and that it contains an apparent accretion of materials that are not in close harmony with the rest of Paracelsus's works, the *Philosophia ad Athenienses* cannot in the final analysis be regarded as a faithful representation of Paracelsus's own thought, however much it

from which all things were separated. Along with Paracelsus's sixteenth-century critics, Pagel asserted that it was clear that the *Philosophia ad Athenienses* taught that *mysterium magnum* was uncreated.[142]

It was precisely on the concept of uncreated prime matter that Erastus focused his attack. Like his patristic and scholastic predecessors, Erastus asserted that the proposition that God created the world *ex nihilo* was a non-negotiable item for Christians. He claimed that Paracelsus had expressly taught that the *mysterium magnum* was uncreated in *Philosophia ad Athenienses* and that Paracelsus did not believe in "creation" per se, but only in the "separation" of previously existing material. Erastus interpreted Paracelsus's theory of creation to be nothing other than the chaos that existed in the beginning of the world as described by Pre-Socratic philosopher Anaxagoras.[143] Erastus went on to claim that Paracelsus's teaching was actually much worse than Anaxagoras's since at least the Pre-Socratic philosopher had taught that this "separation" was accomplished by God; whereas, Paracelsus suggested that "mortal gods" had completed this process of separation.[144] Thus, Paracelsus had denied the fundamental principle of creation *ex nihilo* and, worse yet, had suggested that God employed daemonic powers to complete creation.

became an integral part of the "Paracelsian" heritage. Sudhoff, *PI*, 13:xii; Pagel, *Paracelsus*, 89–91; Kurt Goldammer, "Zur philosophischen und religiösen Sinngebung von Heilung und Heilmittel bei Paracelsus," in *Paracelsus in neuen Horizonten: Gesammelte Aufsätze* [*SBPF* 24], 343–357 (Vienna: Verband der Wiss. Ges. Österreichs, 1986), 353.

[142] *Philosophia ad Athenienses, PI*, 13:404–417. However, Pagel cannot prove that pseudo-Paracelsian author was definitely thinking in Gnostic terms in this passage. Pagel also noted the disagreement among Paracelsians regarding whether *materia prima* was uncreated. For example, Robert Fludd assumed that Paracelsus taught that the materia prima was uncreated, though Fludd himself preferred to think of it as created by God. Alternatively, both Heinrich Khunrath and Joseph Duchesne appear to have regarded the chaos as created. Pagel, "Paracelsus in the Neoplatonic and Gnostic Tradition," 143, 147–148.

[143] Anaxagoras of Clazomenae (ca. 500–428 BC) had rejected the notion of generation and passing-away. See G.S. Kirk et al., *The Presocratic Philosophers*, 2nd ed. (Cambridge: Cambridge UP, 1983), 352–384. It reveals much about Erastus's intellectual background that he connects this notion with Anaxagoras rather than the Hermetic tradition. Erastus no doubt knew Anaxagoras as mediated through Aristotle. He likely had passages in mind like this one from the *Physics* where Aristotle characterizes Anaxagoras's position with: "The upshot of all this is that everything must once have been mixed together and must have started changing at some point in time." Aristotle, *Physics*, trans. Robin Waterfield (Oxford: Oxford UP, 1996), 64 [203b].

[144] *De medicina nova*, 1:4. See the extensive discussion on this point with a long translation from Erastus in Kühlmann and Telle, eds., *Corpus Paracelsisticum*, 1:11–13.

Erastus rejected the theory of the *Philosophia ad Athenienses* and offered his own theory of creation that interpreted the Genesis narrative within Aristotelian categories. According to Erastus, there were two clearly distinguishable types of creation, both of which only God had the power to perform. The first kind was absolute creation—the creation of the world *ex nihilo*.[145] In Erastus's conception, in the first moment of creation all the *materia* on earth received their particular *forma* by God's command: "For in the same moment that he commanded that they should exist by his omnipotent word, he mixed and arranged the parts of the *materia* and also differentiated and adorned them with many potentials and dispositions so that the different and manifold *forma* appeared in the same moment."[146] This first moment of creation was described in the first sentence of Genesis: "In the beginning, God created heaven and earth." Being a good Aristotelian, Erastus had to clarify that here Moses must have included all the terrestrial elements, including water, air, and fire, in the word "earth." After the initial creation, "the earth (i.e., the mass of the elements) existed empty and void."[147] This "prime matter" of Erastus lacked the *forma* of later composite *materia* and was equally suitable to be molded into any one type of *materia* as another.[148]

Following the vocabulary of Genesis, Erastus was able to distinguish a second type of creation as well. The second type was a non-absolute creation, in which God made new compounds and creatures from the prime matter of his first act of creation. The most obvious example of this was the creation of Adam, whom Erastus noted was called a "creature" only when he received the spirit of life. Eve likewise was created when God formed her from Adam's rib. In this line of thought, something

[145] Of course, Aristotle himself had not taught creation *ex nihilo* but maintained the eternity of the world. For Aristotle's conception, the thought of the early church fathers, and the scholastic tradition, see respectively, G.E.R. Lloyd, *Aristotle: The Growth and Structure of his Thought* (Cambridge: Cambridge UP, 1968); Jaroslav Pelikan, "Creation and Causality in Christian Thought," *Journal of Religion* 40 (1960): 246–255; David C. Lindberg, *The Beginnings of Western Science* (Chicago, University of Chicago, 1992).

[146] *De medicina nova*, 1:11: "Etenim momento eodem quo, ut haec existerent, iussit, tam variè omnipotente suo Verbo materiae partes miscuit at temperavit, tamque multiplicibus potentiis & dispositionibus distinxit & exornavit, quam variae multiplicesque formae in eadem subitò apparverunt."

[147] Ibid., 7: "Disertè namque dicitur, terram, id est, elementorum massam, inanem & vacuam extitisse, hoc est, formis istis compositarum rerum caruisse, quae simul atque Deus esse iussit, eodem illo momento perfectae extiterint."

[148] Ibid., 15: "Quoniam potentia, quam tunc habuit solam, generalissima fuit, per quam ad rerum omnium creationem aequè idonea erat, ad nullam magis apta, quam ad aliam quamlibet."

must be called "creation" if it required divine agency for its existence. Erastus criticized what he described as the scholastic view of creation, which only viewed the first "type" of creation as creation per se; the second action of creating the various compounds of the world (i.e., the other five active days of creation) was only considered "adornment and definition" by God. Erastus placed two qualifications on this notion. First, to have been rightly considered a creation, the new creature or compound could not have originated out of its own innate power. Thus, when a seed grows into a tree, it is no "creation;" rather, the seed has simply developed out of its inborn potential. The second qualification was that it must have been made immediately and without movement or change.[149] In this second phase of creation, God transformed the *materia prima* of the first creation into composites: "Out of these elements before any alteration then," claimed Erastus, "the same workman created diverse kinds of things through his omnipotent word."[150]

Seen in the light of Erastus's interpretation of Genesis, Paracelsus denied both the initial creation *ex nihilo* as well as God's role in the secondary acts of creation in giving composite materials their set forms. The Paracelsian notion that angelic or daemonic forces were at work in this separation of matter troubled Erastus, and he surmised that Paracelsus had really believed that Christ was one of these minor deities but did not have the courage to say it. In this connection, he accused Paracelsus of Arianism in placing the son in a subordinate position to the father.[151]

This condemnation of Paracelsus's theory of creation, expressed as it was in an Aristotelian vocabulary, was ironic considering the fact that contemporary Paracelsians such as Dorn and Bostocke were hailing Paracelsus precisely for avoiding the pernicious influence of Aristotle and Galen. To them, Paracelsus had freed natural philosophy from the pagan ancient philosophers and had set forth a restored Christian natural philosophy.[152] Meanwhile, Erastus continued in the tradition of the scholastics in explaining the doctrine of creation with an Aristotelian vocabulary

[149] Ibid., 6–8.

[150] Ibid., 7: "Ex his elementis deinde nulla prorsus alteratione praegressa diversas rerum species omnipotente suo verbo creavit idem opifex."

[151] Ibid., 24.

[152] Gerhard Dorn, *De naturae luce physica ex genesi desumpta* ..., in *Theatrum Chemicum*, ed., Lazarus Zetzner (Strasbourg, 1659–1661); [Bostocke], The difference betwene the auncient Phisicke ... and the later Phisicke. On Dorn, see Kühlmann and Telle, eds. *Corpus Paracelsisticum*, 2:823–963 and Didier Kahn, *Alchimie et paracelsisme en France à la fin de la Renaissance (1567–1625)* [Cahiers d'Humanisme et Renaissance 80] (Geneva: Droz, 2007), passim.

and building a bastion around the concept of creation *ex nihilo*, though not restricting "creation" to solely *creatio ex nihilo*. Whereas Dorn and Bostocke regarded Paracelsus as the restorer of Godly natural philosophy, Erastus condemned him as "blinder than the heathens."[153]

Adam's Flesh and the Resurrection of the Body

At the 1571 Lenten Frankfurt fair, Erastus came upon a text which caused him to put the publication of the first volume of his anti-Paracelsian disputations on hold. This book was Toxites's *editio princeps* of Paracelsus's *Astronomia Magna oder die gantze Philosophia sagax der grossen und kleinen Welt*.[154] Erastus not only recoiled from the "horrible heresies" of the work, he also marveled that Toxites had been so "audacious" as to dedicate it to the pious Lutheran Elector August of Saxony. Erastus wrote a special refutation of the *Astronomia Magna* that he appended to the first volume of his *De medicina nova*.[155] He also dedicated the work to Elector August and wrote him a personal letter gently warning him of the numerous blasphemies contained in the *Astronomia Magna* and cautioning him of patronage seekers of ill-repute who would sully his glorious reputation.[156]

Whereas Erastus's critique of the *Philosophia ad Athenienses* had focused on Paracelsus's conception of creation, here Erastus objected to Paracelsus's anthropology and its broader theological implications. First, Erastus rejected the three-part division of human beings that Paracelsus had outlined in the *Astronomia Magna*. According to Paracelsus, a human consisted of three components: elemental, sidereal, and divine. This notion related the composition of humans—the microcosm—to the composition of the universe—the macrocosm. Conceptualizing humans in this manner had clear utility for medical therapy. For example, the part of humans that was made of elements would respond to chemical

[153] *De medicina nova*, 1:25: "quo videas ipsis Ethnicis coeciorem fuisse."

[154] A loose translation would be: Great Astronomy or the Complete Adept Philosophy of the Macrocosm and the Microcosm. Paracelsus, *Astronomia Magna: oder die gantze Philosophia sagax der grossen und kleinen Welt* (Frankfurt: Sigmund Feyrabend: 1571) [Sudhoff, *Bibliographia Paracelsica*, 219 (no. 131)]. For Erastus's reaction to the publication, see Appendix B, texts nos. 6 & 7.

[155] *De medicina nova*, 1:243–267.

[156] Erastus to Elector August von Sachsen, Heidelberg, Sept. 9, 1571. Sächsisches Hauptstaatsarchiv (Dresden), Geheim. Rat (Geheim. Archiv), Loc. 8523, Sechs unterschiedliche Bücher, Bd. 1; 1570–1574, fols. 186^r–187^v. See Kühlmann and Telle, eds., *Corpus Paracelsisticum*, 2:227–228; 471–473.

medicines. Likewise, the sidereal or celestial part of humans was the part that was most under the influence of the powers of the stars. Finally, there were spiritual maladies that could only be treated by the divine physician.

As successful as this division may have been in explaining how the microcosm was related to the macrocosm and likewise harmonized with Paracelsian medical theory, Erastus recoiled from the heretical implications of what he considered to be a three-substance anthropology and interpreted this theory as an attack on the traditional Christian belief in the resurrection of the body.[157] Unlike Platonic thought, which had emphasized only the existence of the immortal soul in the afterlife, the New Testament writers taught that the human person, a union of soul and body, would itself be resurrected at the last judgment. While later Christian writers incorporated the notion of an immortal soul into their theology, nearly all held that the body would itself be materially resurrected at the last judgment.[158] In Paracelsus's conception, however, only the divine part of humans could be received by God into paradise. Paracelsus termed this divine aspect alternatively "living flesh," "heavenly flesh," and flesh "from the holy spirit" and maintained that it was given to humans in baptism.[159] Paracelsus argued that only things which have their origin in God can return to God. Alternatively, neither the elemental nor even the celestial part of humans could be resurrected.[160] At death the elemental part of humans returned to earth, the sidereal to the stars, and the divine to God. Erastus interpreted what Paracelsus termed the elemental and sidereal dimension of humans to be nothing other than the human body.[161] Since such discussion suggested that actual human flesh could not be resurrected, Erastus concluded that Paracelsus's theory was a manifest denial of the Christian doctrine of the resurrection of the body. This

[157] Paracelsus did not speak of substances but of "parts" (*Theilen*) or "beings" (*Wesen*). *Astronomia Magna, PI*, 12:10.

[158] Oscar Cullmann, *Immortality of the Soul or Resurrection of the Dead?* (New York: MacMillan, 1964); Caroline Walker Bynum, *The Resurrection of the Body in Western Christianity, 200–1336* (New York: Columbia, 1995), 5–14. While St. Paul's discussion of the resurrection in 1 Corinthians 15 does emphasize the spiritual nature of the resurrected body (verse 12: "It is sown a physical body, it is raised a spiritual body"), it is also clear that he taught a continuity between the earthy body and the heavenly body (verse 53: "For this perishable nature must put on the imperishable, and this mortal nature must put on immortality."). Quotations from the *Revised Standard Version*.

[159] *Astronomia Magna*, PI, 12:308–309.

[160] *Astronomia Magna, PI*, 12:288: "doch so kompt nichts gen himel, weder der elementisch noch der siderisch leib, alein der mensch der ein geist ist und nemlich der geist der von got ist." *De medicina nova*, 1:245.

[161] *De medicina nova*, 1:251.

threefold composition could have been more readily harmonized with Christian theology if one understood Paracelsus to mean properties or qualities of the human body that corresponded to earthly, celestial, and divine existence. Since Erastus interpreted Paracelsus from the perspective of Aristotelian categories, however, Erastus insisted that Paracelsus must here be understood to refer to substances rather than qualities.[162] The fact that Paracelsus at other times taught that there were two bodies in man (mortal and immortal) rather than three parts (elemental, sidereal, divine) did not soften Erastus's criticism, since Paracelsus still maintained that the earthly body returned to earth while only the eternal body entered the kingdom of God.[163] Erastus offered the standard critique of the inconsistent and self-contradictory nature of Paracelsus's works and at one point counted the various ways that Paracelsus had divided the human person and exclaimed: "Thus you have a three-bodied monster of a man composed out of nine parts."[164]

Paracelsus would not have accepted this accusation of heresy but would have asserted that he too believed in the resurrection of the body. In the *Paramirum*, Paracelsus had taught that human flesh could not enter the kingdom of God until it was regenerated. Erastus conceded that Paracelsus's conception of the sanctification of human flesh necessary for it to enter heaven was fundamentally orthodox in the *Paramirum*.[165] However, Erastus argued that Paracelsus's teaching in the *Astronomia Magna* went beyond the bounds of orthodoxy. Here, rather than maintaining that human flesh had simply to be sanctified to enter paradise, Paracelsus suggested that humans must receive new spiritual

---

[162] In this light, it is interesting to observe Erastus's translation of Paracelsus's sentence, "So doch got zwei wesen im menschen gemacht hatt, das irdisch und das ewig und seind zusammen vermelet bis an die auferstehung?" with "Deus duas essentias in homine fecit, terrenam & eternam: quae coniunctae manent usque ad resurrectionem." In Erastus's translation, Paracelsus's "Wesen," which could suggest a number of nuances, has been translated with "*essentia*" which Erastus correlates with the Aristotelian category of "substance" or "'ουσια." *Astronomia Magna*, *PI*, 12:10; *De medicina nova*, 1:251.

[163] *De medicina nova*, 1:251.

[164] Ibid., 261: "Sic monstrum tricorporeum hominis habebis ex partibus novem compositum." Regarding the competing anthropological conceptions in Paracelsus's work, see H.C. Erik Midelfort, "The Anthropological Roots of Paracelsus' Psychiatry," in *Kreatur und Kosmos*, ed. Rosemarie Dilg-Frank (Stuttgart: Fischer, 1981), 67–77; Gause, *Paracelsus*, 85; Kurt Goldammer, "Paracelsische Eschatologie: Zum Verständnis der Anthropologie und Kosmologie Hohenheims," in *Paracelsus in neuen Horizonten*, 108; Dane T. Daniel, "Invisible Wombs: Rethinking Paracelsus's Concept of Body and Matter," *Ambix* 53 (2006): 129–142.

[165] *De medicina nova*, 1:248.

flesh by the agency of the Holy Spirit. Paracelsus thus distinguished between two types of flesh: "Adam's flesh," which could not enter paradise, and flesh incarnate through the Holy Spirit, which, since it had its origin in God, could return to God.[166] Paracelsus apparently attempted to reconcile a Neoplatonic notion of the migration of the incorporeal soul to the divine with the Christian notion of the resurrection of the body. Kurt Goldammer has suggested that Paracelsus was torn between a spiritualist-dualistic pneumatology and an authentic faith in the resurrection. This led Paracelsus to adopt what Goldammer has termed a "paradoxical compromise-formula."[167] Although Paracelsus offered a plausible, if paradoxical, reinterpretation of the doctrine of the resurrection of the body, Erastus asserted that such a spiritualistic interpretation of the resurrection of the body with "heavenly flesh" substituted for "Adam's flesh" was tantamount to an outright rejection of corporeal resurrection. Likewise, Paracelsus's application of this distinction between heavenly flesh and Adam's flesh to his understanding of Christ opened the door to extensive criticism of Paracelsus's Christology and soteriology.

Erastus's attack on Paracelsus's Christology began with the depiction of the Virgin Mary's role in the incarnation. What follows is the passage from the *Astronomia Magna* which Erastus found most unsettling:

> From the Virgin comes the new birth and not from woman. From this it follows, that the Virgin, from whom the new birth has proceeded and been born, has been a daughter of Abraham according to the promise and not from Adam; that is, she has been born from Abraham without male seed, in the power of the promise without all mortal nature. From the Virgin, who

[166] *Astronomia Magna, PI*, 12:306–310. Hartmut Rudolf suggests that this teaching was also present in Paracelsus's earlier theological work *De geneologia Christi*, a work which Rudolf maintains bears many resemblances to the later *Astronomia Magna*. Hartmut Rudolf, "Kosmosspekulation und Trinitätslehre: Ein Beitrag zur Bezeihung zwischen Weltbild und Theologie bei Paracelsus," in *Paracelsus in der Tradition* [*SBPF* 21], ed. Sepp Domandl, 32–47 (Vienna, 1980), 42.

[167] In contrast to Goldammer, Rudolf has asked whether Paracelsus actually held a negative view of the "earthly-material body." Rudolf suggests that it was the mortality of the body which Paracelsus held in low regard, rather than flesh and blood itself. I am inclined to agree with Goldammer that Paracelsus's notion is at least implicitly dualistic, since it would seem to preclude any real continuity between the "mortal flesh" which humans received as descendants of Adam and the "heavenly flesh" that they are given by Christ. The Paracelsian notion does not represent a simple material/immaterial dualism. For example, the sidereal part of humans is itself invisible, but, like the elemental body, it cannot be resurrected. Goldammer, "Paracelsische Eschatologie," 111; Rudolf, "Kosmosspekulation und Trinitätslehre," 43.

> thus is not from Adam, not from his seed, only out of his flesh, Christ was born, who was conceived by the Holy Spirit and was made incarnate from holy flesh, not according to the order of the mortal flesh, but according to the new birth which thus proceeds from the Holy Spirit. From this you should consider the fact that [he is] *out of* Adam's flesh in much the same way that you might consider wine which was stored in a vat; it is *out of* the vat, but it is not *of* the vat. From this it follows that that which is incarnate from the Holy Spirit is from heaven and will return again to heaven; that, however, which is not incarnate from the Holy Spirit, that will not return to heaven.[168]

To save Mary from the blemish of original sin, Paracelsus argued that Mary was not descended from Adam but rather from Abraham and was thus not born of Adam's seed, though he does not explicitly deny that she still possessed Adam's flesh.[169] Erastus did not follow the full subtlety of this point and asserted that Paracelsus taught that Mary's flesh was not derived from Adam and therefore she did not possess normal human flesh.[170] Here was a rare occasion where Erastus as a Reformed Protestant could criticize a Catholic motif in Paracelsus's thought. Erastus, however, chose not to dwell on the exalted view of Mary that undergirded Paracelsus's theory and focused instead on the fundamental Christological issue. Like Mary, Christ was not born of Adam's seed but was made incarnate by the Holy Spirit in Mary's womb. To illustrate this theory, Paracelsus claimed that Christ had only dwelt in Mary's womb as wine filled a barrel.[171] She had only been a channel for Christ's holy flesh; he became

[168] *Astronomia Magna, PI*, 12:308–309: "aus der jungfrauen gehet die neue geburt und nicht aus der frauen. aus dem folgt nun, das die jungfrau, aus der ausgangen und geboren ist die neu geburt, ein tochter ist gewesen von Abraham nach der verheischung und nicht aus Adam, das ist sie ist gewesen von Abraham on menlichen samen geborn, in kraft der verheischung on alle tötliche natur. aus der jungfrauen, die also von Adam nit ist, nit von seinem samen, nur aus seinem fleisch, ist geboren Christus, der empfangen ist vom heiligen geist und vom heiligen fleisch incarnirt/ nicht nach der ordnung des tödlichen fleischs, sonder nach der neuen geburt, die da gehet aus dem heiligen geist. darin verstanden aus Adams fleisch nich anderst, dann sovil als ihr verstehen möget von einem wein, der in ein faß gelegt wird, der ist auß dem faß, aber nicht vom faß. iezt folgt auf das, was von dem gist incarniert wird, das ist vom himel und kompt wider gen himel; das aber von dem geist nicht incarnirt wird, das kompt nit gen himel."

[169] *Astronomia Magna, PI*, 12:307–309. At first sight it might appear difficult to understand why Paracelsus had argued that Mary was not born of Adam's seed, since he also maintained that Christ received no flesh from Mary but was made incarnate by the Holy Spirit in Mary's womb. This answer to this puzzle is that Paracelsus had taught that both Christ *and* Mary bore human nature only as a covering. In this sense, Mary shares more in common with Christ than normal mortals. Gause, *Paracelsus*, 45.

[170] *De medicina nova*, 1:255.

[171] Paracelsus had earlier used this same analogy to illustrate how the Virgin Mary grew

incarnate in her, but did not assume her flesh.[172] Since Mary had not been born of Adam's seed and Christ did not assume flesh from Mary, it would seem that Paracelsus had double-insulated Christ from the taint of original sin. While Paracelsus denied that Christ received flesh from Mary, he taught that Christ possessed "holy flesh" made incarnate by the Holy Spirit. Here Paracelsus's conception is rather close to that of the radical reformer Melchior Hoffman, who also argued that Christ did not possess "Adamic flesh" but rather a purely celestial nature.[173]

In Erastus's view, to assert that Christ did not assume Adam's flesh was to say that he possessed some other type of flesh than that of normal humans; in short, that Christ was not truly human.[174] Erastus argued that not only did this clash with the Apostles' Creed, it also called into question whether Christ could have actually died for humans on the cross if he did not possess mortal flesh.[175] Thus, Paracelsus's attempt to apply his "spiritualist" natural philosophy to the doctrine of Christ necessarily called into question Jesus' ability to serve as an atoning sacrifice for humanity.

The idea that it was possible that all humans did not inherit their flesh from Adam led to many novel conceptions in Paracelsus's thought that Erastus considered to be strange heresies. Paracelsus taught that the blessed actually possessed two bodies: a mortal one, born of Adam's flesh, and an immortal one, made incarnate by the Holy Spirit. Following this distinction, he speculated that the apostles in New Testament times performed miracles by their "new bodies" rather than by their "old bodies." Such capacities did not only apply to the saints, and Erastus alleged that Paracelsus attributed immaterial bodies to nymphs, wild men, and giants.[176] Paracelsus had also suggested that the inhabitants of the New

in the womb of her mother St. Ann without receiving the stain of her fallen nature. Gause, *Paracelsus*, 44–45.

[172] *Astronomia Magna*, *PI*, 12:309: "aus der jungfrauen, die also von Adam nit ist, nit von seinem samen, nur aus seinem fleisch, ist geboren Christus, der empfangen ist vom heiligen geist und vom heiligen fleisch incarnirt/ nicht nach der ordnung des tödlichen fleischs, sonder nach der neuen geburt, die da gehet aus dem heiligen geist. darin verstanden aus Adams fleisch nich anderst, dann sovil als ihr verstehen möget von einem wein, der in ein faß gelegt wird, der ist auß dem faß, aber nicht vom faß."

[173] Williams, *The Radical Reformation*, 495, passim.

[174] *De medicina nova*, 1:247, 252. Interestingly it was precisely this "heretical" notion of Christ's flesh that Valentin Weigel found attractive. See Moran, "Paracelsus, Religion, and Dissent," 69.

[175] *De medicina nova*, 1:255.

[176] Ibid., 254; *Astronomia Magna*, *PI*, 12:113–114, 244–249, 362–363. See also *Liber de*

World were not necessarily descended from the Adam of Genesis but had perhaps descended from "another Adam."[177] Later Spanish writers vehemently condemned this notion of Paracelsus when grappling with the question of whether American Indians were fully human. Like Erastus, they also asserted that Paracelsus's suggestion, if followed to its natural conclusion, might well call into question the salvation of Western Christians as well.[178]

The final error that Erastus cited in reference to "Adam's flesh" was that Paracelsus's theories were an attack on divine omnipotence. Erastus distilled this charge from Paracelsus's description of how immortal bodies were created. According to Paracelsus, God the father had only been responsible for the creation of mortal flesh, like the flesh of Adam. However, the immortal flesh of those who enter heaven was created and given by Christ. Erastus considered the mere notion that God the father was unable to transform mortal flesh into immortal flesh an affront to divine omnipotence.[179]

Erastus adeptly and for the most part honestly ferreted out the latent heresy of Paracelsus's writings. That the first volume of *De medicina nova* was entirely devoted to the rejection of Paracelsus's religio-magical universe gives a fair representation in itself regarding the seriousness with which Erastus took this dimension of his task. Erastus was generally perceptive in his treatment of Paracelsus, but he was not charitable. Like Paracelsus's more sympathetic interpreter Bostocke, Erastus had been able to conceptualize ways in which the Paracelsian natural philosophy could be reconciled with an orthodox Christian position. Unlike Bostocke, however, Erastus chose to emphasize the cacophony and heterodoxy of Paracelsus's teachings rather than their unity and orthodoxy.

---

nymphis, sylphis, pygmaeis et salamandris et de caeteris spiritibus, in *PI*, 14:115–151. For an English translation, see Paracelsus, *Four Treatises*, ed., Henry E. Sigerist (Baltimore: Johns Hopkins, 1941; paperback ed., 1996).

177 *Astronomia Magna*, *PI*, 12:35: "und so mag ich nit underlassen, von denen ein kleine meldung zu tun, die in verborgenen insulen gefunden seind worden, und noch verborgen sind, das sie von Adam zusein geglaubt mögen werden, mag sichs nit befinden, das Adams kinder seind kommen in die verborgenen insulen, sonder wol zu bedenken, das dieselbigen leut von einem andern Adam seind; dan dahin wirt es schwerlich komen, das sie fleish und bluts halben uns gefreundt sein. und das ist auch wol zu gedenken, were Adam im paradeis bliben, es were villeicht ein anderer Adam worden, doch villeicht nit mit der bildtnus gottes, als dan die neuen insulen seind."

178 See Anthony Pagden, *The Fall of Natural Man* (Cambridge: Cambridge UP, 1982), 22–23.

179 *De medicina nova*, 1:254–255.

Erastus's Rejection of Chemical Pharmacology: De auro potabili

In early 1576 Erastus composed yet another refutation of Paracelsianism entitled *Disputation Concerning Potable Gold* (De auro potabili) which Perna would print in 1578.[180] The work set forth Erastus's own rationale for the independence of medicine as a secular pursuit and issued an attack on Paracelsus's chemical pharmacology. *De auro potabili* was written in a dialogue form like most of Erastus's works. On this occasion, however, even the Paracelsian interlocutor, the same "Furnius" (man of the furnace) from *De medicina nova*, did not refrain from taking shots at Paracelsus. Within the first twenty pages Paracelsus was assailed as "the first enemy of medicine" and labeled "magician, atheist, and pig."[181] Erastus had already committed himself to a universal rejection of Paracelsus in *De medicina nova* and he made no effort to present an even-handed treatment in *De auro potabili*.

Medicine as an Empirical Pursuit

Erastus took great pains in the book to distinguish his understanding of medicine as an empirical science from the prophetic-magical medicine of Paracelsus. What follows is Erastus's description of medicine, which will probably sound more like what one would expect from Paracelsus, according to textbook accounts of Paracelsus's attack on the obscurantism of the "scholastic" physicians. In Erastus's conception medicine had to have a basis in experience; it could not only be the study of classical texts. Thus, for a so-called medical Hellenist, he possessed a strong emphasis on the importance of observation. "The learning/doctrine of good physicians does not only consist in the knowledge of languages," asserted Erastus, "but is much more determined by the perception of causes, motions and the effects of nature."[182] Erastus described medicine as a craft and made a comparison between medicine and agriculture.

---

[180] Thomas Erastus, *Disputatio de auro potabili, in qua accurate admodum disquiritur, num ex metallis opera chemiae, concinnata pharmaca tutè utiliterque bibi possint* (Basel: Pietro Perna, 1578; reprinted, Basel: Conrad Waldkirch, 1584; hereafter cited as *De auro potabili*). I have used the 1584 reprint.

[181] *De auro potabili*, 6: "primus oppugnator medicinae" and 20: "magus, atheos, porcus."

[182] *De auro potabili*, 3: "Bonorum Medicorum doctrina non in sola linguarum notitia consistit, sed multo magis perspicientia causarum, motionum, & effectuum naturae definitur."

Indeed, the good doctor is like the industrious farmer. In both cases success only comes to the person who does the necessary work. Just as God would not send a harvest to the farmer who had not taken the effort to sow his seed, success in medical treatment depended upon the conscientious labors of the practitioner. Though both the farmer and the physician must ultimately give thanks to God as the ultimate provider of their success, it was God's intention that no positive results could proceed unless the farmer and the physician did their part.[183] Likewise, medical effects came through skill and effort, not through arcane or prophetic knowledge. Erastus made a clear epistemological distinction between theological and medical knowledge. In opposition to theological knowledge, which was known through divine revelation, medical knowledge had to be experienced in nature. The human need for medicine was not a product of incomplete theological understanding; rather, the continuing practice of medicine was a part of God's plan. Erastus argued that accepting the fact that medicine lay under the sovereignty of God also implied that there were limits to medicine's effectiveness. God had never intended all sickness to be curable.[184]

Erastus's vision of medicine as a scientific craft was accompanied by a deep appreciation for the antiquity of medicine. This long tradition was in part proven by the presence of doctors in the Scriptures. Since medical knowledge was experienced in nature, the body of medical knowledge grows over time. In this instance Erastus suggested a notion of cumulative advance or progress of medical learning and argued that the Paracelsians were simply foolhardy to reject centuries of medical learning.[185] Erastus portrayed Paracelsus as a reckless innovator who had abandoned accumulated wisdom of the physicians of antiquity to forge a new medical sect. Naturally this went against Erastus's reverence for medical tradition. Erastus continually complained about the audacity of Paracelsus, since he bragged that he was superior to all the physicians of antiquity. Of prime annoyance for Erastus were the new elements of Paracelsus, which Erastus thought to be clearly invalidated by experience and tradition. In this connection Erastus accused Paracelsus of being an atomist.[186]

[183] Ibid., 14–15.
[184] Ibid., 10–11.
[185] Ibid., 13.
[186] Ibid., 7.

The central picture that Erastus outlined was of Paracelsus as a medical false prophet. The claim of secret knowledge or new revelation was Erastus's *bête noir* and this arcane aspect is the lead motif of Erastus's Paracelsus image. When Erastus attacked Paracelsus, this arcane image occupied the central position. Erastus attempted to prove that no medical revelation existed in the present. Since the Paracelsians claimed to have new or secret knowledge, these concepts must simply derive from the devil.[187] Erastus thought that Paracelsus had claimed to know more about medicine than God had ordained for humans. To Erastus, Paracelsus's hubris was in clear contradiction of the Bible, and with something of a scholastic twist, Erastus asserted that Paracelsus had been guilty of a capital crime for claiming to know more than God had intended humans to know.[188]

Medicine and Nutrition

Erastus's reaction to Paracelsian metallic therapy was closely related to his Galenic theory of nutrition. Digestion in the strict Galenic sense was achieved when the food was transformed in the blood by inner heat. Erastus insisted that there was a direct connection between the power of nutrition and the power of medicine. This meant that unless a potential medicine had nutritional value, that is, that it could be digested, it could not serve a medicinal purpose. Erastus's scheme lies well within the tendency of Galenic theory to closely associate health with nutrition. Furthermore, Erastus distinguished between the *forma* of a sub-

---

[187] For example, when speaking of Christ's apparent approval of the vocation of physicians in his era, Erastus comments, "At Paracelsica nondum erat in Tartaro fabrica." Ibid., 10.

[188] Ibid., 19–20: "Caeterum qui vel cogitare apud se audet, Paracelsum Deo rectius statuisse, non tantum est impius, sed capitali supplicatio dignus." It should be noted that this charge is made by the interlocutor "Furnius." Gilly has recently focused attention on Erastus's "dear wish" to apply the death penalty to Paracelsians. Ironically, Erastus was here developing Weyer's claim that learned magicians who accessed demonic power warranted the death penalty more than gullible witches. (See Weyer, *De praestigiis daemonum*, book 6: "De magorum infamium, laminarum, et venificorum poenis.") To modern readers, Erastus in this case unhappily picks up Weyer's negative influence in stressing the culpability of literate magicians without embracing his more salutary call for clemency for uneducated female practitioners who rather naively thought they could access diabolical power (see chapter 9 below). While Erastus's assertion here is disquieting, it is essentially rhetorical. Carlos Gilly, "Capital Punishment for Paracelsians: A Dear Wish of Thomas Erastus," in *Magia, alchimia, scienza dal '400 al '700*, ed. Carlos Gilly and Cis van Heertum (Florence, Centro Di, 2002): 247–251.

stance and its *potentia* or *facultates*. In Erastus's conception there was a residue of *potentia* or *facultates* after the destruction of the *forma*. It was this residue which gives medicines their power. However, these *facultates* always depended on the *tota substantia* of the material from which they were derived. Erastus's view left little room for a significant role for chemists in the preparation of drugs. If a chemist could change the total substance of metals, metals might possess a wider pharmacological usage; however, humans are only able to mix and blend the substances that God has created. A chemist can purify a substance for use in medicines but cannot change the *tota substantia* of the *forma*. Thus, all potential medicines are very much restricted to their original form. The consequences of this very restricted understanding of chemical change based on Aristotelian distinctions had a severe impact on Erastus's receptivity to the pharmacological innovations introduced by the chemical physicians.[189]

Metallic Therapy

Although the book in which Erastus dealt with medicines made from metals is ostensibly about potable gold, the book is primarily preoccupied with the possibility of metallic cures and spends little time on the specific topic of *Trinkgold*. Erastus compared the substance of metals and the substance of humans within a traditional Galenic conception of temperament. Metals are naturally hard and dry, whereas the human body is soft and wet. For this reason the introduction of metals into the body could lead to a destruction of the harmony of the humors. This loss of harmony meant the loss of health in the Galenic system. Erastus also compared the material complexity of metals with that of the substance of the human body. Material complexity corresponded to the complexity of the form. While metals are chemically simple, the material complexity of human substance corresponds to the high position of humans in creation.[190]

After making his point concerning the differences between humans and metals, Erastus returned the argument to the question of nutrition. He suggested that such a complex being as the human cannot receive nourishment from completely simple substances such as metals. Not only were metals too simple, they were inanimate (non-organic), and all

---

[189] Ibid., 29–42.

[190] Ibid., 44–49. See Kühlmann and Telle, eds., *Corpus Paracelsisticum*, 2:522.

nutrients must stem from living material. Organic material can only be constituted from other organic materials. Metals were never alive, and therefore they cannot be nutritional. Since Erastus had already asserted the necessary interrelation between nutrition and medicine, it followed that non-nutritious metals have no proper medical use. The only apparent exception was the use of metals for the treatment of stomach ulcers. Erastus explained that medications for stomach ulcers were not normal drugs, since in this case the medicines were not actually digested. Rather, they only moved through the stomach, before passing undigested out of the body. While such a distinction might appear facile, the distinction was critical for a Galenist. Since metals were not digestible, they could not improve the patient's humoral condition, and therefore Erastus insisted that they should not be thought of as genuine medicines.[191]

It should be obvious from this discussion that Erastus has basically precluded the possibility of metallic drugs. He nevertheless continued with philosophical speculations concerning the characteristics of liquid metals. It appears that Erastus thought that metals were truly immutable. Thus, even if metals appeared to have undergone a temporary liquefaction, these liquid metals must return to their former dry condition. Since they must return to their normal solid state, liquid metals possess no great advantage over normal metals as drugs.

Erastus also engaged the theory that incorruptible metals like gold have a special ability to prolong human life. Although this theory is basically inconceivable from his philosophical standpoint, he entertained its possibility for the sake of argument. Once again he returned to his emphasis on nutrition. If gold is not digestible by our bodies, such a therapy made no sense, since the gold would have no opportunity to influence our bodies. If gold were digestible, however, it would also be corruptible, and thus it could not help the corruptible body. Thus, in Erastus's mind the popular fixation with discovering an alchemical elixir which would prove to be a universal panacea was completely irreconcilable with sound medical theory.[192]

De auro potabili offered both more and less to its readers than it advertised. It was not really the exhaustive investigation of potable gold that its title indicated. Alternatively, it contained a great deal of information on Erastus's overall philosophy of medicine. As a weapon in the anti-Paracelsian arsenal, it may have been even more effective than *De medi-*

[191] Ibid., 58–66.
[192] Ibid., 70–72.

cina nova since it was more narrowly focused on a key aspect of Paracelsianism's popularity without the extraneous biographical bits and the long digressions into theological questions. Likewise, its readers received a shrill warning concerning the false claims of the Paracelsians and heard a biblical rationale as to why Paracelsus's innovations were medical heresy rather than a longed for medical reformation.

The Impact of Erastus's Anti-Paracelsian Writings

Erastus's comprehensive repudiation of the Paracelsian system hardly stemmed the new wave of enthusiasm for the spagyrical master. Indeed, it is likely that Erastus's work only fanned the flames of the Paracelsian revival. New editions of Paracelsus continued to flow from the presses, and the academic establishment began to take Paracelsus's ideas more seriously. One beneficiary of this interest was Perna, the publisher of Erastus's anti-Paracelsian opus. Perna was an Italian exile who, along with favoring Paracelsians in his presses, had a penchant for dissident and heretical writers such as Sebastian Castellio and Bernardino Ochino.[193] Recent historians have made Perna out to be a signal example of late humanist radicalism with his promotion of "Paracelsianism, Hermeticism, and Heresy."[194] Given that publishing Erastus seemed to go against the grain of Perna's editorial policy, historians have speculated about what motivated Perna's decision. Antonio Rotondò suggested that he may have done it to keep his imperial printing privilege, since he may have feared that the imperial physician Crato was going to take action against him.[195] Given the fact that Perna had arbitrarily censored Crato's attack on Paracelsus in a book issued from his house, Rotondò's suggestion is not entirely implausible. Regardless of Perna's initial motive, there would seem to be no reason to think that Perna was compelled to print

[193] See Hans Rudolf Guggisberg, "Pietro Perna, Fausto Sozzini und die Dialogi quatuor Sebastian Castellios," in *Studia bibliographica in Honorem Herman de la Fontaine Verwey*, ed. Menno Hertzberger, 171–200 (Amsterdam, 1967), especially 177–179; Antonio Rotondò, "Pietro Perna e la vita culturale e religiosa di Basilea fra il 1570 e il 1580," in *Studi e ricerche di storia ereticale italiana del' Cinquecento*, 1:273–394 (Turin: Giappichelli, 1974), see especially, 363; Kühlmann and Telle, eds., *Corpus Paracelsisticum*, 2:729–733; Leandro Perini, *La vita e i tempi di Pietro Perna* [Studi e testi del Rinascimento europeo 17] (Roma: Edizioni di Storia e Letteratura, 2002).

[194] Gilly, "Zwischen Erfahrung und Spekulation," *Basler Zeitschrift für Geschichte und Altertumskunde* 77 (1977): 72.

[195] Rotondò, "Pietro Perna," 375.

additional works of Erastus. Given Erastus's struggle against the Calvinist disciplinary regime in Heidelberg, Perna may have seen Erastus more as a brother in dissent than as a fixture of the establishment. Sudhoff's assessment of 1894 that "Perna favored Paracelsianism solely on account of considerations of the book trade" more adequately captures the economic basis that no doubt influenced Perna's editorial decisions.[196] Given that Perna had a certain investment in Paracelsus, he likely calculated that an anti-Paracelsian work would foster debate and perhaps enhance the sales of his Paracelsian titles.[197] Though it is difficult to quantify the direct impact of Erastus's work, judging from the number of editions of Paracelsus's works, it appears Perna's investment in an anti-Paracelsian title only increased demand for further Paracelsian books.[198]

Though Erastus could not stop the spread of Paracelsianism, he made a definite impact on its reception. While Toxites might comment that Erastus's work had caused him to be "disdained" by learned society, he knew that Erastus's work had been read seriously by many.[199] Jole Shackelford has argued that Erastus's refutation of Paracelsus had a profound effect on the Danish Paracelsian Petrus Severinus (1540/2–1602). Severinus was the author of perhaps the most cogent synthesis of Paracelsian medical ideas. Although Erastus did not mention him by name, he attacked Severinus's ideas in *De medicina nova*, 2, by directly citing Severinus's text in order to refute him. Erastus was not as circumspect in his private correspondence. In a letter to Bullinger he exclaimed: "And now there is one who, by coloring impiety with pretty speech and defending absurdity (an abominable endeavor!), has dared to publish a book, the *Idea of Philosophical and Paracelsian Medicine etc.*,[200] by which he has deceived, deceives, and will deceive many people, etc."[201] In short, Erastus was alarmed by Severinus's book, since unlike Paracelsus's own work, it was both eloquent and internally coherent. Severinus was appalled in turn by what he considered an overly theoretical and sophistic attack by

[196] Sudhoff, *Bibliographia Paracelsica*, 247: "Perna pflegt den Paracelsismus natürlich allein aus Buchhändlerrücksichten."

[197] Rotondò, "Pietro Perna," 375.

[198] Sudhoff, *Bibliographia Paracelsica*, particularly, 60–365.

[199] Toxites to Leonhard Thurneisser, Dec. 7, 1576: "glerte leut Erastum darum verachten." Kühlmann and Telle, eds., *Corpus Paracelsisticum*, 2:448–451 (text No. 65); 454–456 (analysis).

[200] Severinus, *Idea medicinae philosophicae fundamenta continens totius doctrinae Paracelsicae, Hippocraticae et Galenicae*.

[201] Erastus to Bullinger, Nov. 2, [1571], StAZ, E II 361, fol. 74. See Appendix B, text no. 10.

Erastus, a "philosopher of words," on his view of elements, a theory that to Severinus's mind was not based on scholastic speculation but on the study of nature and experience of the furnace. Stung by Erastus's attack in the pages of *De medicina nova*, Severinus suggested that he would abandon the controversy if other authorities in Germany were impressed with Erastus's refutation.[202] Though Severinus defended himself convincingly in his private correspondence (and his friend Tycho Brahe likewise did not mind aiming a barb at Erastus),[203] he did not venture to counter Erastus's refutation in print. In fact, Severinus never published another work after his *Idea medicinae*. For all intents, Erastus had driven Severinus from the field.[204]

Debus likewise argued that Erastus's works had a significant impact on the reception of Paracelsian ideas in England. Debus noted that chemical medicine arrived in England without an explicit connection to Paracelsus, and by and large there was an openness to his chemical cures. Debus was convinced, however, that many learned Englishmen actually first learned of Paracelsus's larger medical philosophy from Erastus as opposed to directly from Paracelsus. He theorized that the chief reason Erastus's work received a ready reception in England was that it was written in Latin rather than Paracelsus's idiosyncratic German. This would seem to be a large claim to make on the basis of Erastus's *De medicina nova*, which was printed once and in Basel. Although the *De medicina nova* did not go into multiple printings, it was by no means rare and enjoys a wide distribution in modern European libraries. Regarding

[202] Shackelford, "Early Reception of Paracelsian Theory," 130–131.

[203] See Thorndike, *History of Magic and Experimental Science*, 5:656.

[204] In the mid-seventeenth century, Ambrosius Rhodius would return to Erastus's critique of Severinus in his *Disputationes supra Ideam medicinae philosophicae Petri Severini* ... (Copenhagen, 1643). See Shackelford, *A Philosophical Path for Paracelsian Medicine*, 377–402, especially 395–396. In his article on Severinus and Erastus, Shackelford suggested that Severinus's quotation, "we have suffered on the account of the theologians in these times," likely referred to the theologically oriented critique of Paracelsianism offered by Erastus and Johann Weyer. While this interpretation is not impossible, it must be remembered that while both Erastus and Weyer handled theological topics, neither was a theologian in a strict vocational sense. This point needs to be emphasized, since Erastus is often incorrectly described as a "professor of theology" in the secondary literature—a position he never held. We have also seen that because he was not a theologian, he was prohibited from discussing theological questions after the church disciplinary controversy. It is likewise worth noting that, their differences on Paracelsus aside, both Erastus and Severinus faced the hostility of Gnesio-Lutherans; in the controversy over the Lord's Supper, Erastus was actually allied with many of Severinus's Philippist co-religionists. Shackelford, "Early Reception of Paracelsian Theory," 131.

Erastus's impact in England, Debus has concluded, "the Paracelsian mystical universe was introduced by the way of a major attack on it, and with very few exceptions this alchemical cosmology became the object of distrust and suspicion during the Elizabethan period."[205] Erastus did not halt the flow of Mosaic philosophy to England, however, and Paracelsus eventually found avid disciples in England, such as Bostocke and Robert Fludd.

Erastus also had an impact on the reception of Paracelsianism in France. Among Erastus's most eager readers were, ironically enough, the Catholic theology faculty of the University of Paris. The fact that Erastus's name was on the *Index* does not seem to have undermined their interest in his anti-Paracelsian work. Didier Kahn has undertaken a thorough investigation of the fifty-nine theses against Paracelsus which the Sorbonne faculty issued on October 9, 1578. The vast majority of the theses, entitled "Impieties and Errors of Paracelsus, gathered from the books of the same and from Erastus and Dessen," stem directly from Erastus, with only a few from either Paracelsus's works or Dessen von Kronenburg. In short, the Parisian theologians endorsed Erastus's diagnosis of Paracelsus's heresy wholesale.[206] Debus was also able to uncover a number of French writers who were influenced by Erastus's work.[207] Erastus remained influential in France into the seventeenth century and had a significant impact on the thought of the famed mathematician and scientific impresario Fr. Marin Mersenne.[208]

An intriguing episode which revealed something of the changing fortunes of Paracelsianism in academia as well as the impact of Erastus's rebuttal of Paracelsus occurred in Basel with the promotion of Thomas Moffet under Theodor Zwinger (1533–1588).[209] Zwinger played a major

[205] Debus, *The English Paracelsians*, 49.

[206] Didier Kahn, "Cinquante-neuf thèses de Paracelse censurées par la Faculte de theologie de Paris, le 9 octobre 1578," in *Documents oubliés sur l'alchimie, la kabbale et Guillaume Postel: offerts, à l'occasion de son 90e anniversaire, à François Secret par ses élèves et amis, ed. François Secret and Matton Sylvain* [THR 353] (Geneva: Droz, 2001), 161–178 (The theses themselves are printed on pp. 170–178). See also idem, *Alchimie et paracelsisme en France.*

[207] See Allen G. Debus, *The French Paracelsians* (Cambridge: Cambridge UP, 1991). Among these, Nicolas Guibert and Toussaint Ducret deserve special mention. See the bibliography.

[208] Regarding Mersenne, see Robert LeNoble, *Mersenne ou Naissance du Mécanisme* (Paris: Librairie Philosophique J. Vrin. 1943), 211–217.

[209] Regarding Zwinger, see Gilly, "Zwischen Erfahrung und Spekulation." Erastus seems to have been on friendly terms with the medical professor Isaak Keller as well, though I have found no surviving correspondence between them. Erastus passed many greetings

role in the reevaluation of the medical philosophy of Paracelsus that occurred after 1570. Like Erastus, Zwinger's initial reaction to Paracelsus was negative. In an early work Zwinger used Paracelsus as an example of a braggart and had nothing positive to say about his medicine.[210] More significantly it appeared that Zwinger played a role in getting the Paracelsian Bodenstein expelled from the Basel medical faculty in 1564. Zwinger's opinion of Paracelsus was to change, however, ironically enough through his study of Hippocrates. By the late 1570s Zwinger had undergone a complete reversal of opinion regarding Paracelsus and was now corresponding with Paracelsians like Severinus and building his own chemical laboratory.[211]

The doctoral theses of the English student Thomas Moffet (1553–1604) in 1578 proved to be a contest between Zwinger's enthusiasm for Paracelsian medicine and his reluctance to make an enemy of Erastus. Moffet, who clearly allied himself with the Paracelsian faction, later earned renown as a pioneer in the field of entomology.[212] For these accomplishments, he was immortalized in a nursery rhyme ("Little Miss Muffet sat on a tuffet …"). Without the permission of the university, Moffet took the liberty of printing his doctoral theses, which amounted to a spirited defense of Paracelsianism as well as a stinging attack on Erastus.[213] Since Erastus had written the most famous rebuttal of Paracel-

to Keller by way of Grynaeus. Keller was likely close to the Grynaeus clan, as Samuel Grynaeus (son of Simon Grynaeus, the elder) served as his counsel in the financial scandal in which he was involved in 1579. Thommen, *Geschichte der Universität Basel, 1532–1632*, 214–217. Both Erastus and Zwinger were among the better known physicians in German-speaking lands and shared many common friends (Crato, Gessner, and Peter Monau). It would not appear likely that they had become acquainted during Erastus's school days in Basel, since Erastus was some ten years older than Zwinger and had already begun his medical studies in Italy before Zwinger enrolled in the university. Their surviving correspondence is meager (only four letter from Erastus to Zwinger and one from Zwinger to Erastus), likely due to the fact that Erastus delegated many tasks in Basel to Johann Jakob Grynaeus.

[210] He also indirectly congratulated Weyer for taking a position against Paracelsian medicine. See the letter from Zwinger to Weyer printed in Weyer's *De praestigiis daemonum* (1577), cols. 901–902.

[211] Gilly, "Zwischen Erfahrung und Spekulation," *Basler Zeitschrift für Geschichte und Altertumskunde* 77 (1977): 95–96; Kühlmann and Telle, eds., *Corpus Paracelsisticum*, 2:101–105; 756–757; 767–822.

[212] Thomas Moffet, *Insectorum sive minimorum animalium theatrum* (London, 1634). Diane Simpkins, "Thomas Moffett," in *DSB*, 9:440–441; Victor Houliston, "Moffet [Moufet, Muffet], Thomas [T.M.] (1553–1604)," *Oxford Dictionary of National Biography* (Oxford: Oxford UP, 2004).

[213] Thomas Moffet, *De anodinis medicamentis eorumque causis et usibus physica &*

sianism, it was natural for this young alchemist to attack Erastus, which he did with great zest. He criticized Erastus for his superficial refutation of Paracelsus, which dealt only with arguments over words and not the substance of Paracelsian therapy. Moffet asserted, "Erastus's authority is not so exalted today that he can dispense with these authors, who were experts in the particulars of these medicines, with one word."[214]

Unfortunately for Moffet, he had misjudged the degree of freedom of expression at the University of Basel, as well as Erastus's reputation in the Basel intellectual community. The medical faculty took action to censor Moffet for his work in which he "excessively belittles the physician Erastus and also attacks Galen." His theses were confiscated by the order of the faculty and he was forced to alter his work so radically that the edited version was only half as long as the original version. Naturally the personal attacks on Erastus were eliminated, as well as some of his more pointed critiques of the Galenic system.[215]

Moffet was greatly offended that his theses were suppressed and suggested that this would not have happened in mother England where academic freedom reigned.[216] Moffet would not remain silent concerning his distaste for Erastus's brand of Galenism and named his anti-chemical interlocutor "Philerastus" in a work published after Erastus's death.[217] On

medica consideratio in Theses aliquot digesta ... (Basel: Brylinger, 1578). See Blaser, Robert-Henri, "Ein mutiges Bekenntnis zu Paracelsus in Basel," in Paracelsus in Basel, 200–210 (Muttenz /Basel: St. Argobast, 1979). Also published in French as "Un rare temoignage de fidelite envers Paracelse a Bale: Les 'Theses de anodinis medicamentis' du medicin anglais Thomas Moffet (1578)," in *Current Problems in History of Medicine*, ed. R. Blaser and H. Buess (Basel: Karger, 1966), 502–512. Blaser includes translations of some of Moffet's assertions against Erastus.

[214] Moffet, *De anodinis*, thesis 97: "Verùm non tanta est Erasti hodie auctoritas, ut quae praedicti Authores in anodinis istis peculiaribus erant experti, ipse verbo unico dissolvat." See Blaser, "Ein mutiges Bekenntnis zu Paracelsus in Basel," 208.

[215] Gilly prints the medical faculty's decree regarding the theses on p. 109: "Decembris die 16. Thomas Moufetus Anglus disputaturus publice pro gradu, theses inscio Decano imprimi curavit in quibus Erastum Medicum nimis temere perstringebat et Galenum quoque insectabatur."

[216] Gilly, "Zwischen Erfahrung und Spekulation," *Basler Zeitschrift für Geschichte und Altertumskunde* 77 (1977): 110–111. Moffet recovered from his disappointment and remained in contact with Zwinger after leaving Basel.

[217] Thomas Moffet, "De Jure et Praesentia Chemicorum Medicamentorum," in *Theatrum Chemicum*, ed. L. Zetzner (Strasbourg, 1659). First published in Frankfurt in 1584, this work includes a dialogue between Philerastus (i.e., phil-erastus, representative of traditional Galenic medicine) and Chemista, an advocate of chemical medicine. Allen G. Debus, *The English Paracelians* (New York: Franklin Watts, 1966), 72; Shackelford, *A Philosophical Path for Paracelsian Medicine*, 253–255.

the other hand, it does not appear that Erastus was much agitated by Moffet's attack. At least he claimed that he was unconcerned by it after the theses had been suppressed. Erastus's primary response was gratitude that the Basel faculty would take such firm action on his behalf.[218]

Erastus was even more successful in implementing an anti-Paracelsian program at the University of Heidelberg. At the request of Frederick III, Erastus proposed an amendment to the faculty's bylaws that prohibited "sophistic and seditious disputations" (perhaps a veiled reference to the Paracelsians). More importantly, the amendment prohibited the use of "metal remedies out of mercury [or] antimony" by the university faculty. These two amendments would officially enter the medical faculty's bylaws under Ludwig VI and remain in effect until 1655.[219]

Conclusion

In the cases of both Erastus and Reußner, orthodox Protestant physicians were at least as exercised at the religious heresy of Paracelsianism as they were at the novelty of Paracelsian medical theory. This accusation of heresy had first been advanced by Gessner and Crato but was put forward in a much more definitive and explicit manner by Erastus. Like Reußner before him, Erastus directed much of his animus against the likely pseudo-Paracelsian *Philosophia ad Athenienses*. Thus, it is clear that the more Hermetic orientation of the pseudo-Paracelsian corpus made the reception of Paracelsian ideas by mainstream Protestant natural philosophers more problematic.[220] However, not only the Neo-Platonic or Hermetic themes irritated Erastus; Paracelsus's own idiosyncratic theological vision was equally distressing. In the case of the *Astronomia Magna*, Paracelsus had offered a radical reinterpretation

[218] Erastus to Grynaeus, Jan. 14, (15)79, Basel UB, G II 4, fol. 233. Grynaeus kept him informed of the affair and promised to send him a copy of Moffet's theses.

[219] Wesel-Roth, *Thomas Erastus*, 8; Stübler, *Geschichte der medizinischen Fakultät der Universität Heidelberg 1386–1925*, 61.

[220] Here I follow the suggestion of Webster that "A more hermetic view of the magus ideal of Paracelsus derives from the corpus of doubtful or spurious writings attributed to Paracelsus, and to the works of early Paracelsians, sources which have deeply influenced historical accounts of Paracelsus himself and which prove that the Paracelsian movement was swept up in the hermetic tide which engulfed Europe in the late sixteenth century." Charles Webster, *From Paracelsus to Newton: Magic and the Making of Modern Science* (Cambridge: Cambridge UP, 1982), 57. See also Kühlmann and Telle, eds., *Corpus Paracelsisticum*, 2:28.

of human anthropology, the nature of Christ's flesh, and the resurrection of the body. Although animated by a unique, largely biblical, spiritualistic vision, by almost any sixteenth-century standard, Paracelsus was a heretic many times over.[221] Although Erastus was generally an honest critic of Paracelsus, his tendency to examine Paracelsus's teaching through Aristotelian lenses compounded the difficulty of reconciling Paracelsus's natural philosophy with mainstream Protestantism. As Pagel asserted, "Erastus spared no effort in marshalling an imposing array of argument which must have appeared unanswerable to his colleagues."[222] While Erastus's work only offered a blunt "No!" to Paracelsus's entire system of natural philosophy, the end result of his exchange with the Paracelsian corpus was likely more productive. In delivering an acid critique of Paracelsus's religious and magical concepts, he paved the way for the future separation of Paracelsus's progressive medical and pharmacological ideas from their original heretical milieu through later writers like Andreas Libavius and Daniel Sennert.[223]

While Gessner's relationship to Paracelsian medicine has been characterized as ambivalent, there was no neutrality on Erastus's part. Gessner could label Paracelsus a magician and still say he approved of much of Paracelsian medicine. Although Erastus paid lip service to the virtues of chemical preparations, he was fundamentally closed to Paracelsian chemical therapy. At heart Erastus was a Galenist's Galenist who had an overwhelming preference for botanic medicines. In Erastus's conception, health was largely a matter of nutrition, and since he did not think metals were digestible, he concluded that they could not function as true medicines.[224] Thus, unlike Gessner's precocious willingness to try various cures, whatever their origin, Erastus was unreceptive to Paracelsian pharmacology for medical-philosophical reasons. Erastus could genuinely praise Paracelsus for reviving the "art of preparing and distilling," but by this he meant purifying substances to their undiluted essences, not chemical transformation.[225] Erastus comes close to totally rejecting the possibility of chemical change in *De auro potabili*, arguing that humans can only blend, mix, or purify what God has made, not transform one

[221] See Walker, *Spiritual and Demonic Magic from Ficino to Campanella*, 164.

[222] Pagel, *Paracelsus*, 330.

[223] See Debus, "Guitherius, Libavius and Sennert: The Chemical Compromise in Early Modern Medicine" and Bruce Moran, "Libavius the Paracelsian?" in *Reading the Book of Nature*, 67–79.

[224] *De auro potabili*, 22–29, 44–48.

[225] *De medicina nova*, 1:B.

substance into something different.[226] Thus, in comparison to Gessner, Erastus did not merely reject Paracelsus's alleged heresy and magic, but directly assailed chemical pharmacology.

Erastus's refutation of Paracelsus was most strident at the point where religion and medicine intersected, and the Paracelsus that most deeply animated Erastus was that of a medical false prophet. Weyer had sounded this theme of warning against medical false prophets earlier. After reviewing biblical passages in an attempt to assert the antiquity of medicine, Weyer had exclaimed, "And there is nothing here about the coming in the last days of the 'Monarch' and discoverer of medicine Theophrastus Paracelsus."[227] This may appear to be an elusive insight, given that Erastus himself employed theological arguments to make this point. Neither Erastus nor Weyer attempted to draw his medicine from the Bible, however. Rather, they maintained that the Bible upheld medicine as an ancient and independent vocation. In Erastus's conception, medicine is like farming in that results come from hard labor and skills are accumulated over time. Medical knowledge is not an issue of special revelation or secret wisdom, but must be garnered through observation.[228] Physicians such as Weyer and Erastus felt the fundamental integrity of medicine as a secular pursuit was threatened by the Paracelsian *arcana*. Here one may perhaps be surprised to find that Renaissance physicians such as Erastus and Weyer, who are sometimes labeled "schoolmen" or "medieval," employed the argument of experience against the Paracelsians. To defend his own tradition of medicine, Erastus portrayed the Paracelsians as a group of medical Gnostics who claimed divine illumination for their craft.

The sixteenth century was not an era of scientific revolution but of "scientific Renaissance." Various trends within the scientific Renaissance would stimulate the scientific revolution, but full-blown modern science with its use of hypotheses and insistence on quantification awaited the great virtuosi of the seventeenth century.[229] Both Erastus and Paracelsus have their place within this scientific Renaissance. Indeed Erastus, with his devoted medical Hellenism, in many senses was a more representative

[226] *De auro potabili*, 67–68.

[227] Weyer, *De praestigiis daemonum* (1568), 197: "Nihil hic de venturo in extremis diebus medicinae Monarchia & inuentore, Paracelso Theophrasto." Quoted from Mora, *Witches, Devils and Doctors*, 154.

[228] *De auro potabili*, 13–14.

[229] On these distinctions, see Debus, *Man and Nature in the Renaissance*.

figure of the medical Renaissance than Paracelsus. Paracelsus, however, as a great proponent of chemical experimentation and through his ability to theorize new conceptions of health and disease, was clearly a more significant force than humanists like Erastus in pointing toward the seventeenth century advances among individuals like Joan Baptista Van Helmont and Robert Boyle. Nevertheless, the tendency represented by Erastus, with its similar emphasis on observation and its more disenchanted and rationalistic view of the world, also represented a progressive trend in the history of medicine that Temkin and others have recognized. Even Pagel, perhaps Paracelsus's most adept modern expositor, conceded that "belief and personal religious experience formed the nucleus of Paracelsus's world, whereas superstition and credulity are but a sideline in Erastus's critical and logical reasoning."[230] Despite Erastus's proto-empirical tendencies, however, his Aristotelian-Galenic framework blinded him to some of the more innovative features of Paracelsus's system. Both Erastus and Paracelsus had their limitations, and both were more speculative than empirical thinkers.[231] Neither Erastus's Protestant vision of medical Hellenism nor Paracelsianism itself represented the future of medicine. Rather, the new medical and chemical innovations that arrived in the seventeenth century owed as much to the dialectical relationship between the two tendencies as to either trend individually.

Erastus's anti-Paracelsian works must not only be seen as an attack on Paracelsus but also as an attempt on Erastus's part to redefine himself. In this case the contrast between the standard depictions of Erastus in the history of science literature and in church historical accounts is instructive. For those who know Erastus from the perspective of the church discipline struggle, it would not be difficult to believe that he actually shared some of the radical opinions of the Antitrinitarians Johann Sylvan and Adam Neuser. Those who know him chiefly from the anti-Paracelsian works, however, have tended to view him as an unbending champion of religious and scientific orthodoxy. That Erastus was able to forge this orthodox image is no doubt a testament to his success in reinventing himself in the wake of the Antitrinitarian debacle. Ironically, the image that he was unable to secure in Heidelberg in the 1570s has largely triumphed in the historiography of science. It is particularly noteworthy that nearly all of the negative features of his portrait of Paracelsus were allegations

[230] Pagel, *Paracelsus*, 331.

[231] This is precisely the point regarding Paracelsus that Weeks has stressed in *Paracelsus: Speculative Theory and the Crisis of the Early Reformation*.

that had previously been lodged either against him or his close scholarly allies.[232] Thus, in tackling these accusations and pinning them one by one on Paracelsus, Erastus was apparently engaged in a bit of self-exorcism. It may well have been an unconscious process, but conscious or not, Erastus staked a claim to be far more orthodox than his condemned friends, and modern historians, with few exceptions, have believed him.

Afterword

Since an earlier version of this study was published in *Analecta Paracelsica*, Carlos Gilly has challenged some of its fundamental assertions in a learned short article.[233] In brief Gilly has argued that Erastus's motivation for refuting Paracelsus was likely a internal debate with Jakob Curio, his senior colleague on the medical faculty; that Crato was not a major inspiration for Erastus; and that Erastus was under no danger during the time that he undertook the refutation, so defending his own status should not be seen as a primary motivation of Erastus's anti-Paracelsian works. First, Gilly's discovery of the pro-Paracelsian / anti-Galenic position of Erastus's senior medical colleague is a significant contribution to our understanding of the Heidelberg context. While future researchers should probe this connection more fully, they will look in vain in Erastus's correspondence for evidence of a festering resentment toward Curio. Since Erastus was hardly reticent in his criticism of his colleagues in his letters, this gap is difficult to explain if Erastus had in fact been engaged in a long running feud with Curio. Thus, while a rivalry with Curio together with an implicit defense of Galenism might have been a factor in Erastus's decision to refute Paracelsus, it is difficult to see hostility with Curio as a primary motivator for opposing Paracelsus. Second, given the direct impact of Crato's anti-Paracelsianism on Erastus and the degree that

[232] Above, p. 303. The bulk of these charges would have been leveled against his heretical antidiciplinist partisans Neuser and Sylvan, though some of the accusations also concern Simon Simoni and Wilhelm Xylander. I have in mind the accusations of drunkenness against Neuser and Xylander, the denial of creation *ex nihilo* that was lodged against Simoni, the fascination with alchemy and magic, which was alleged of Sylvan, and the charge of the Arianism, which was lodged against almost all of Erastus's associates. When Neuser was in Istanbul, he would be accused of dabbling in magic in the attempt to produce money, a claim reminiscent of the stories of Paracelsus's full purse. See Horn, "Johann Sylvan," 256; Burchill, *The Heidelberg Antitrinitarians*, 18–19.

[233] Gilly, "Capital Punishment for Paracelsians: A Dear Wish of Thomas Erastus," 247–251.

Erastus emphasized Crato's involvement, it also seems Gilly has undervalued the significance of Crato's encouragement upon the project. However, I accept Gilly's critique that Crato's concrete influence on Erastus's decision to refute Paracelsus may have been amplified after the fact to capitalize on Crato's celebrity.[234] Whereas Erastus and Crato had not been in close contact prior to 1570, afterward Erastus can fairly be considered a member of the larger Crato circle. In short, the extant sources reveal a much more positive stimulus and encouragement from Crato for the anti-Paracelsian writings than Gilly allows and are nearly silent on any motivating hostility toward Curio. Finally, Gilly's assertion that Erastus's position was not in jeopardy in the early 1570s because of the influential backing of the Zurich church is belied by the tremendous hardship and persecution that Erastus and his associates faced from 1570–1576 as discussed in detail in chapter 7.

[234] Tilmann Walter has also noted that Erastus's self assertion of close connections with Gessner and Crato were part of his "rhetorical strategy." Tilmann Walter, "Paracelsuskritische Haltungen oder "Antiparacelsismus"?, 1570–1630," *Würzburger medizinhistorische Mitteilungen* 27 (2008): 381–408 (here p. 391).

CHAPTER NINE

CONCERNING WITCHES: ERASTUS'S DEBATE WITH JOHANN WEYER

> Erastus himselfe, ... is forced to confesse, that these Greeke words ... are most commonlie put for illusion, false packing, cousenage, fraud, knaverie and deceipt: and is further driven to saie, that in ancient time, the learned were not so blockish, as not to see that the promises of magicians and inchanters were false, and nothing else but knaverie, cousenage, and old wives fables....
>
> Reginald Scot on Erastus

Background

The debate between Weyer and Erastus on the punishment of witches came at a timely juncture in the history of witchcraft and witch-hunting. While the Western witchcraft paradigm had coalesced during the late Middle Ages, the great witch-hunts in which thousands of European men and women lost their lives were almost exclusively a civil legal phenomenon of the early modern era; indeed, the seventeenth century was the great century of witch-hunting.[1] Whereas thirty years ago it would have been common to consider the entire learned witchcraft paradigm an elite construct which was largely imposed from above on an unwilling populace, recent scholarship has greatly expanded our knowledge of the rise of the learned witchcraft paradigm and the dialectical nature of witch hunting. One of the key insights of modern scholarship has been to

[1] What follows is a revised and expanded version of the article "The Debate between Johann Weyer and Thomas Erastus on the Punishment of Witches," in *Cultures of Communication from Reformation to Enlightenment: Constructing Publics in the Early Modern German Lands*, ed. James Van Horn Melton (Aldershot, Hampshire: Ashgate Press, 2002), 257–285. This chapter includes the full quotations of the primary sources omitted from the previous published version.

For a competent overview, see Brian P. Levack, *The Witch-Hunt in Early Modern Europe*, 3rd ed. (Harlow, England: Pearson Longmans, 2006).

recognize the bottom up nature of many witchcraft accusations.[2] Academic scholarship has also gotten beyond some of the rather crude early assertions that the witch-hunt was an unrestrained clerical "war on women," or represented an attempt by male medical practitioners to eliminate their midwife competitors, though the sex-related nature of the crime of witchcraft remains a central preoccupation for research.[3] Finally, we know much more about the evolution of witchcraft beliefs in the late medieval period. The classic Western witchcraft paradigm only fully coalesced in the fifteenth century and represented an amalgam of accusations, many of which had previously been lodged against Cathars and Jews.[4] Once this paradigm had been established, inquisitorial manuals such as Heinrich Kramer's infamous *Malleus Maleficarum* and court personnel disseminated this conception of the crime of witchcraft, the chief components of which were the belief that witches entered into an illicit pact with the devil in order to access his powers and that they used their malevolent powers to engage in concrete magical acts intended to harm their neighbors (*maleficia*). Subsidiary components of this paradigm, which varied in prominence from region to region, included the witch's mark, night flights, use of familiar spirits or other demonic agents, and obscene acts with the devil to seal the diabolical pact. The notion that witchcraft was a clandestine conspiracy in which the devil's minions regularly assembled at the witches' sabbath was a particularly vital component of the witchcraft paradigm in central Europe.[5] By the seventeenth century, there was abundant anecdotal evidence that not only learned

---

[2] Robin Briggs, *Witches and Neighbors: The Social and Cultural Context of European Witchcraft* (New York: Viking, 1996).

[3] Among the more provocative studies are: Diane Purkiss, *The Witch in History: Early Modern and Twentieth-Century Representations* (London: Routledge, 1996); Lyndal Roper, *Oedipus and the Devil: Witchcraft, Sexuality and Religion in Early Modern Europe* (London: Routledge, 1994); and idem, *Witch Craze: Terror and Fantasy in Baroque Germany* (New Haven: Yale UP, 2004).

[4] These trends are manifest in Alan Charles Kors and Edward Peters eds., *Witchcraft in Europe 400–1700: A Documentary History*, 2nd ed. (Philadelphia: University of Pennsylvania Press 2001). Regarding the particular role of the infamous *Malleus Maleficarum* in this process, see Hans Peter Broedel, *The Malleus Maleficarum and the Construction of Witchcraft: Theology and Popular Belief* (Manchester: Manchester UP, 2003). For a challenging synthesis of early modern demonology, see Stuart Clark, *Thinking with Demons: The Idea of Witchcraft in Early Modern Europe* (Oxford: Clarendon Press, 1997).

[5] These topics are expertly handled in Richard M. Golden, ed. *Encyclopedia of Witchcraft: The Western Tradition* (Santa Barbara: ABC-CLIO, 2006).

inquisitors and court personnel knew the narrative of the stereotypical acts performed by witches, but that even young children had imbibed this construct.[6] On the eve of the Reformation, although witch-hunting itself was relatively infrequent, the intellectual apparatus that would make these bloodbaths possible had been fully articulated.

Both humanism and the Protestant Reformation offered new opportunities for intellectuals at least to question inherited medieval ideas of magic and witchcraft. This questioning was not limited to demonology, but at first chiefly concerned the perceived magical dimension of medieval Catholicism. Indeed, the criticisms of Erasmus were directed primarily against the superstitious ideas he saw *within* the church.[7] Erasmus also engaged in a limited critique of late medieval demonology. He was able to show that the idea of witches making a pact with the devil was a "modern" innovation. Nevertheless, the humanist assault on witchcraft was incomplete and as William Monter has concluded, "Renaissance humanism did not attack the central presuppositions of the system of witchcraft constructed by the Inquisition."[8]

Protestants were more adamant than humanists like Erasmus had been in their desire to root out the perceived unbiblical magic of medieval Catholicism. They rejected the many "false miracles" that had been associated with late medieval popular piety and even suggested that sanctioned clerical practices such as exorcisms were in actuality nothing more than black magic.[9] In this atmosphere it was at least conceivable that Protestants would reject the entire witchcraft paradigm as extra-biblical scholastic speculation. Protestants were not so quick to disbelieve in the reality of diabolical magic (although they naturally condemned it), as they were to repudiate the magical dimension of medieval Catholicism. The writings of Martin Luther reveal an essential ambivalence regarding the question of witches. He certainly believed that witches were real, but he displayed a measure of uncertainty regarding their powers.

[6] See, for example, the adolescent who attempted to employ witchcraft accusations to her advantage in David Warren Sabean's "The Sacred Bond of Unity: Community through the Eyes of a Thirteen-year-old Witch (1683)" in *Power in the Blood* (Cambridge, Cambridge UP, 1984), 94–112.

[7] Eire, *War Against the Idols*, see especially chapter 2, "Erasmus as a Critic of Late Medieval Piety," 28–53.

[8] E. William Monter, "Law, Medicine, and the Acceptance of Witchcraft, 1560–1580," in *European Witchcraft*, ed. E. William Monter (New York: Wiley, 1969), 57.

[9] Keith Thomas, *Religion and the Decline of Magic* (New York: Scribners, 1971).

Jörg Haustein, in fact, traced the roots of Protestant skepticism toward witchcraft to the work of Luther.[10] Nevertheless, Protestants did not decisively address the witchcraft question in the first half of the sixteenth century and, indeed, neither Luther, nor Zwingli, nor Calvin wrote what could be considered a major treatise on the subject.[11] In fact, the first six decades of the sixteenth century witnessed a general lull in the production of demonological writings, both among Protestants and Catholics.[12]

The full potential of Protestant skepticism and Erasmian humanism did not make their mark on witchcraft theory until the work of Netherlandish physician Johann Weyer (1515–1588). Weyer garnered his knowledge of occult and magical arts at an early age through an apprenticeship to Heinrich Cornelius Agrippa von Nettesheim. After studying at the University of Paris, he was employed as the court physician to Duke Wilhelm III of Jülich-Cleves.[13] His life's passion, however, was directed toward ending the cruel treatment of women accused of witchcraft. In 1563, he published the first edition of his masterwork, *De praestigiis daemonum* (On the Wiles of Demons).[14] Weyer's *De praestigiis daemonum* made him the most influential Protestant demonological writer of the sixteenth century. The work ranged far beyond the specific topic of the punishment of witches and presented an encyclopedic treatment

[10] "The continuity of Protestant thought, which leads ultimately to Weyer, does not begin with Brenz, but rather, is already present in Luther." Jörg Haustein, "Martin Luther als Gegner des Hexenwahns" in *Vom Unfug des Hexen-Processes: Gegner der Hexenverfolgung von Johann Weyer bis Friedrich Spee* [Wolfenbüttler Forschungen 55] ed. Hartmut Lehmann & Otto Ulbricht (Wiesbaden: Harrassowitz, 1992), 51.

[11] The idea that Calvinism had a special role in fomenting witch-hunting fervor was refuted by John L. Teal in "Witchcraft and Calvinism in Elizabethan England: Divine Power and Human Agency," *Journal of the History of Ideas* 23 (1962): 21–36.

[12] See Monter, "Law, Medicine and the Acceptance of Witchcraft," 59–69.

[13] Valente, *Johann Wier*; H.C. Erik Midelfort, "Johann Weyer and Transformation of the Insanity Defense," in *The German People and the Reformation*, ed. R. Po-Chia Hsia (Ithaca: Cornell, 1988), 234–261; idem, "Johann Weyer in medizinischer, theologischer und rechtsgeschichtlicher Hinsicht," in *Vom Unfug des Hexen-Processes*, 53–54; Carl Binz, *Doctor Johann Weyer, ein rheinisher Arzt, der erste Bekaempfer des Hexenwahns: Ein Beitrag zur Geschichte der Aufklaerung und der Heilkunde*, 2nd ed. (Berlin, 1896; reprint, New York: Arno, 1976).

[14] Johann Weyer, *De praestigiis daemonum, et incantationibus ac veneficiis Libri V* (Basel, 1563). Six Latin editions of *De praestigiis daemonum* were published in Weyer's lifetime (1563, 1564, 1566, 1568, 1577, and 1583). Weyer expanded the work over time and included answers to his detractors' objections. His general pattern was to add new material, and he only infrequently rewrote sections. I will cite all of the editions as *De praestigiis daemonum* and distinguish between them by including the year of publication in each reference. For an excellent English translation of the 1583 edition and a bibliography of Weyer's works, see Mora, *Witches, Devils and Doctors*.

of the devil, magic, and witchcraft. As such, the work served as a source book for other demonological writers. Weyer's motive was to undermine every conceivable foundation employed to apply the death penalty to witches. Weyer argued that the majority of those accused of witchcraft were deranged old women who suffered from an excess of melancholic humors. In this deranged state, they often dreamt up fantastic crimes that they confessed to inquisitors.[15] Furthermore, Weyer argued that the alleged witches were not capable of producing the *maleficia* or harm of which they were accused. Weyer possessed a severely limited view of what witches could achieve, even with demonic assistance, and declared that the crimes they confessed were in fact impossible. The centerpiece of Weyer's work was his attack on the notion of the pact with the devil, which Weyer claimed was "deceptive, foolish and of no weight."[16] He also claimed that the biblical proof texts generally cited to condemn the accused to the flames did not apply to contemporary witches. Weyer thus offered an exhaustive rebuttal of the traditional rationales for imposing the death penalty on witches.

Erastus's literary foray into the world of demonology did not come as a result of a lifetime's fascination with witchcraft, but was a response to Weyer's plea for humane treatment of witches. Erastus sympathized with Weyer's compassion for the senile old women who suffered in the persecution, but he felt Weyer had gone beyond the boundaries of Scripture in arguing for sweeping clemency. These two Protestant physicians found themselves most unlikely adversaries in the dispute.[17] They had much in common: they had mutual acquaintances, had both published with the famed humanist printer Johannes Oporinus in Basel, and were generally part of the same Rhenish-Protestant intellectual milieu. Beyond their confessional and occupational similarities, Weyer and Erastus also shared mutual disdain for Paracelsian medicine. I have previously argued that Weyer was a formative influence on Erastus's conception of Paracelsus. In the medical arena they were partisans, and Erastus cited Weyer to make his case against Paracelsus while Weyer was generous with his praise for Erastus's anti-Paracelsian work.[18]

---

[15] *De praestigiis daemonum* (1583), book 4, ch. 7. Mora, 183.

[16] *De praestigiis daemonum* (1583), book 3, ch. 3. Mora, 173.

[17] Regarding Weyer's religious confession, see Midelfort, "Johann Weyer and Transformation of the Insanity Defense," 238–239 and Jürgen Michael Schmidt, *Glaube und Skepsis: die Kurpfalz und die abendländische Hexenverfolgung, 1446–1685* (Bielefeld: Verlag für Regionalgeschichte, 2000), 139–140.

[18] See chapter 8. For Weyer's positive assessment of Erastus's anti-Paracelsian work, see *De praestigiis daemonum* (1577), cols. 579 and 881.

Unmasking the Controversy

Given their mutual friends and general agreement on most issues, it is not surprising that neither Erastus nor Weyer relished making an enemy of the other. The deference they showed to one another in the course of the debate has left a curious imprint on their dispute. Not only did they not demonize each other, a tactic that Jean Bodin would later employ in refuting Weyer, they refrained from even mentioning each other by name when refuting the opponent's position.[19] This fact alone has undermined the historical understanding of their interaction. For instance, the otherwise vigilant editors of a modern English translation of *De praestigiis daemonum* were oblivious to the fact that one chapter was written in direct response to Erastus and incorrectly assume at one point that Weyer was addressing Bodin's criticisms, when he was actually countering Erastus.[20] However, analysis of Erastus's correspondence and a close investigation of the text of *De praestigiis daemonum* reveal how much both Erastus and Weyer directly responded to the critiques of the other. At this point I will briefly outline the chronology of the Erastus/Weyer debate before turning to the actual content of the controversy.

Erastus was embroiled in the controversy regarding church discipline when he first turned his attention to the question of the punishment of witches. He wrote his first short treatise regarding witchcraft in late 1570.[21] This twenty-three page disputation refuting Weyer's appeal for

[19] Erastus does mention Weyer on at least two other occasions in his work. *De medicina nova*, 1:187; 4:131. Regarding Bodin's scandalous accusations, see Binz, *Doctor Johann Weyer*, 87.

[20] The editors only briefly mention Erastus as an opponent of Weyer and are completely unaware of Weyer's direct refutation of Erastus's criticisms. The title of the chapter in question is "Adversus caput praecedens obiectionum quarundam productarum confutatio." *De praestigiis daemonum*, book 6, ch. 22 [*sic*] in the 1577 edition (cols. 741–763); book 6, ch. 24 in 1583 (cols. 742–762). Weyer made a new addition to this chapter in 1583 from cols. 742–744. (In Mora, *Witches, Devils and Doctors*, 543–544, from "The kindly reader ..." to "... let us return to our main argument.") The most egregious error of the editors of *Witches, Devils and Doctors in the Renaissance* is that they allow their assumption that Weyer is refuting Bodin to influence the text itself. On page 544 they add Bodin's name in brackets when Weyer clearly appears to be answering Erastus. Later they even venture to insert Bodin's name into the text (without brackets!), even though Weyer does *not* mention Bodin here in the 1583 edition. Weyer, *De praestigiis daemonum* (1583), col. 744. See figure 2 for definitive proof that Weyer was responding to Erastus in this passage.

[21] Erastus to Heinrich Bullinger, Oct. 29, [1570], StAZ, E II 345, fol. 741^{v}. "Mitto interim vobis quaestionem ad idem ferme argumentum pertinentem, an sagae nostrae iure divino capitaliter peccant, examinandam. Rogatus à viro opt. et doctiss. adde etiam

clemency for witches was published as a chapter in the first volume of his anti-Paracelsian work *De medicina nova Philippi Paracelsi* in 1571.[22] After the publication of the treatise, Erastus's opinions attracted Weyer's notice. Although no correspondence between the two survives, other letters from Erastus's hand that have been preserved bear witness to the fact that they exchanged letters. That it was an animated exchange can be drawn from a letter written by Erastus in the spring of 1572 to their mutual friend Theodor Zwinger, a Basel physician. Speaking of critiques of his *De medicina nova*, Erastus related:

> But thus far I have received none that please me, ... with the exception of Weyer. He says that I do not think correctly concerning the punishment of witches and promises to refute me. God as my witness, if he does this, I will enjoy the greatest benefit. I have written him in as friendly a manner as possible, and have requested a debate, either privately or publicly. It makes little difference to me. If he would show me my error privately, I would not delay to admit it publicly.[23]

Although Erastus no doubt exaggerated his willingness to concede defeat, the desire to come to a mutual understanding and to avoid a public row was genuine. Nevertheless, Erastus was less than sanguine that such a rapprochement could be reached, as he revealed in a letter to the humanist physician Joachim Camerarius, II in early 1573:

piisimo [Johann Ewich?] scripsi, qui contra me sentit cum Wiero Medico in lib. *De praestigiis daemonum*." See also the contemporaneous letters to Johann Jakob Grynaeus (Basel UB, G II 4, fols. 287 and 282). These letters suggest that Erastus was using the 1568 edition of *De praestigiis daemonum*. That he had access to this edition is confirmed by the university's purchase of the volume in 1568. UAH A-160/8, fol. 7.

[22] This disputation is entitled "De lamiis seu strigibus non inutilia scitu" in the table of contents and is found in *De medicina nova*, 1:193–215.

[23] Erastus to Theodor Zwinger, Heidelberg, Easter [April 6, 1572], Basel, Öffentliche Bibliothek der Universität Basel, Fr. Gr. MS II 4, no. 93: "Sed huc usque nullum audivi, qui mihi gratificaretur (quod unicè tamen, cupio, pete, oro) excepto Wiero. Hic enim de Lamiarum pœnis me non recte sentire ait, probaturumque promittit. Deum testor, si fecerit summi beneficii loco habebo. Scripsi ei, ut amicius non possem, et ad defensionem seu privatam seu publicam cohortatus sum. Mea non refert utro malit modo. Si clam mihi errorem monstrabit, ego publicè fateri non cunctabor. Una enim veritas cum mihi proposita sit, ac me errare posse sciam, non dubitabo meliora docenti publicè agere gratias, et cuius opera p[ro]fecerim aliis indicare. Rog[o] igitur te, qui ingenio, iudicio, et doctrina vales plus aliis multis, ne confere nostra graveris ita, ut amicitiae nihil tribuas, publici boni solius rationem habeas. Reddam ego pro viribus beneficium, modo possim." Erastus repeated this claim regarding his willingness to concede defeat were Weyer willing to publicly correct him in the introduction of the *Repetitio disputationis de lamiis*, fol.):(3^v. See full citation below. See Appendix B, text no. 11 for more of this letter.

> I have received letters from Dr. Johann Weyer, and I have seen others which he had sent to other friends (for they sent two to me) in which he also wants to demonstrate most strongly and copiously his opinion concerning the punishment of witches ..., and meanwhile he endeavors to persuade all that we do not disagree. If this were actually the case, I would truly rejoice. But I fear that we will not be able to reach an understanding.[24]

Although this is a secondhand source, the notion that Weyer thought that Erastus was near his position and could perhaps be won over to his perspective is telling. As I shall relate below, their assumptions about the actual powers of witches and the devil were quite similar; their chief difference was their conclusion about the necessary penalty for witchcraft.

Who were these friends that supplied Erastus with letters from Weyer? Perhaps one was Zwinger, since Erastus had asked him for assistance with the anti-Paracelsian project. The Bremen physician Johann Ewich (1525–1588), who shared Weyer's opinion regarding the punishment of witches, may also have served as the intermediary. Erastus had been in contact with Ewich for some time, and his name often appears in Erastus's correspondence. Another plausible connection between Weyer and Erastus, however, came with the presence of three of Weyer's sons in the Palatinate in the 1570s. Dietrich Weyer apparently entered Palatine service in the late 1560s, and by the mid-1570s, he was a rising star among the Palatine civil servants, taking a position on the high council in 1574.[25] Volker Press regarded Dietrich as a fairly radical Calvinist partisan and characterized him as a "restless spirit, with a marked tendency toward adventure."[26] In fact, Dietrich himself became a key player in the interventionist foreign policy so detested by Erastus and Ursinus. Another son, Johann Weyer II, enrolled in the University of Heidelberg in early 1573 and later also entered the service of the Palatine court.[27] The connection between the elder Weyer and Erastus may have been made through yet a third son,

[24] This remark came in a letter in which Erastus reported having begun the fourth volume of *De medicina nova*. Erastus to J. Camerarius II, Jan. 31, [1573], UB Erlangen (Sammlung Treu), no. 6: "Accepi literas à D. Joh. Wiero, et alias ad amicos alios missas vidi (Miserunt enim mihi duo) in quibus et sententiam suam de strigum poena in quinta libri sui editione copiosius et firmius vult demonstrare: et interim persuadere conatur omnibus nos non dissentire. Quod si ita est, gaudeo equidem pl[urimu]m. At valde vereor ut sit monstraturus consensum."

[25] Schmidt, *Glaube und Skepsis*, 140–142; Press, *Calvinismus und Territorialstaat*, 257. Schmidt infers that Dietrich may have been in the Palatinate as early as 1567.

[26] Press, *Calvinismus und Territorialstaat*, 257.

[27] Toepke, *Die Matrikel der Universitaet Heidelberg*, 2:65.

the physician Heinrich Weyer, who also spent some time in the Palatinate and was closely associated with Erastus's protégé Heinrich Smet.[28]

Given Dietrich Weyer's close association with the pro-disciplinary party and Erastus's rivals Caspar Olevianus and Wenzel Zuleger, we must engage the question of whether Erastus's personal animus against Dietrich's partisans conditioned his antipathy toward Johann Weyer's demonology. The fact that Dietrich Weyer was able to get the disciplinist-dominated state to go along with his father's position on witchcraft suggests that in at least a small way the controversy between Erastus and Johann Weyer mirrored the split between Erastus and Dietrich Weyer's "Calvinist" faction. However, Erastus apparently composed his first disputation against Weyer's demonology prior to Dietrich's assumption of a major role in Palatine politics. Likewise, the basic Palatine governmental position in line with Johann Weyer's views had been determined since the mid-1560s and first defended by the later anti-disciplinist councilor Christoph Prob, who is generally seen as an ally of Erastus.[29] Similarly, the university arts professor Hermann Witekind, who seems to have associated with the ethnic German anti disciplinist faction rather than the largely foreign Calvinist faction during the disciplinary struggle, broke with Erastus and sided with Johann Weyer in the witchcraft debate.[30] Even more ironically, Erastus's close associate Johann Jakob Grynaeus supported allowing the publication of Witekind's book in 1585, whereas Daniel Tossanus, the ardent Calvinist who had been involved in Erastus's excommunication, obstructed its publication.[31] Thus, the church discipline controversy does not seem to have had a decisive impact on the witchcraft debate, beyond perhaps heightening Erastus's own need to associate himself with more conventional intellectual opinions.[32]

Perhaps feeling a little hemmed in with Johann Weyer's opinions in favor in the Palatinate and both Zwinger and Ewich solidly in Weyer's

---

[28] Schmidt, *Glaube und Skepsis*, 142. See Smet, *Miscellanea … medica*. Smet passed a greeting from Heinrich Weyer to Erastus in a letter from March 29, 1571. *Miscellanea … medica*, 244–246.

[29] Schimdt, *Glaube und Skepsis*, 137–143.

[30] Hermann Witekind [alias Augustin Lercheimer], *Christlich Bedencken und Erinnerung von Zauberey*, 3rd ed. (Speyer: Albin, 1597). See Schimdt, *Glaube und Skepsis*, 205–242.

[31] Schmidt, *Glaube und Skepsis*, 211–212. Thus Schmidt also argues that there was not a close association of the theologians and Palatine policy of non-persecution.

[32] Adding to the irony, Clark also noted that "European states with Erastian Protestant churches" tended toward "comparably mild prosecution." *Thinking with Demons*, 517.

camp, Erastus turned to his trusted patron Heinrich Bullinger for support. Also in January of 1573, Erastus wrote to Bullinger:

> Weyer threatens a confutation of our opinion concerning the punishments of witches and has written to many that you agree with him, (I have seen manuscripts of his letters) and for his cause he has many living witnesses. I have replied in a different manner in which you would perhaps not disapprove (I hear [that he is] contaminated by the error of Schwenckfeld) that you would by no means allow that witches should not be punished.[33]

While it might seem that Erastus was being presumptuous to count on Bullinger's backing (he even refers to the matter as "our opinion"), in fact, Bullinger's position was close to Erastus's. Bullinger would also write a demonological tract that defended the proposition that witches merited capital punishment, although the work's primary animus was directed against vestiges of popular magic in the late medieval Catholicism.[34] Erastus's letter is also intriguing for its insinuation that Weyer was "contaminated with the error of Schwenckfeld." Kaspar Schwenckfeld, the Silesian spiritualist reformer, had de-emphasized the importance of outward sacraments in favor of participating in a spiritual inner-communion with Christ. After his falling out with Luther over the Lord's Supper and his unwillingness to establish a firm relationship with the established Protestant church, he was increasingly viewed as a pariah by the magisterial Reformers, both Lutheran and Reformed. Erastus was thus relaying serious accusations to Bullinger, a man who knew the Schwenckfeld "heresy" well. It must be remembered, however, that this was a private disclosure to a close friend; in his publications, Erastus always referred to Weyer as a "most pious man." Erastus may have employed this slur to cover the charge of spiritualism in the mode of Erasmus or Sebastian Castellio in that he questioned whether heretics (in this case witches) should be punished.[35] Perhaps the ambiguity of Weyer's confessional

[33] Erastus added this comment in the postscript of a letter dated Jan. 13, [1573]. Erastus to Bullinger, StAZ, E II 361, fol. 31: "Wierus minatur confutationem sententiae nostrae de Lamiarum pœnis: et te consentire secum scripsit ad diversos: (Vidi literas eius manuscriptas) eiusque rei plures se habere testes vivos. Ego respondi alia te fortasse non improbare (Audio Schvenckfeldii errore contaminatum) hoc de strigibus non puniendis te nequaquam admittere."

[34] Heinrich Bullinger, *Wider die Schwartzen Künst/ Aberglaubigs segnen/ und unwarhafftigs Warsagen/ und andere dergleichen von Gott verbottne Künst: ein kurtzer Tractat auß heiliger Schrifft/ und warhafften guten gründen*, in Abraham Sawr, ed. *Theatrum de Veneficis* (Frankfurt: Nicolaus Basseus, 1586), 298–306. See http://www.rainer-henrich.ch/schwarzkunst.html.

[35] On Erasmus's influence on Weyer, see Midelfort, "Insanity Defense," 238–240.

stance led his contemporaries to ponder whether his equivocation on the punishment of witches betrayed religious sympathies beyond the pale of conventional Protestantism. This accusation of contamination with "error of Schwenckfeld" would prove ironic, since later Erastus himself would be accused of devotion to the spiritualist's writings.[36]

Despite the behind-the-scenes negotiations, Weyer apparently was not interested in Erastus's offer to stage a public debate. He included a barb that appears to refer to Erastus's invitation to debate in the 1577 edition of *De praestigiis daemonum*. He admitted that he "shrinks from debate and constant arguing," but added, "these things I leave freely for those who enjoy them."[37] At any event, the proposed debate never took place, and after the epistolary posturing of 1572–1573, the controversy fell dormant for some years.

The advent of a new edition of *De praestigiis daemonum* in March of 1577 reopened the dispute. The new edition was buttressed by the inclusion of the *Liber Apologeticus*, which reprinted many letters to and from Weyer.[38] At the same time as the printing of the expanded version of *De praestigiis daemonum*, Weyer also published an abridgement of his central arguments entitled *De Lamiis Liber*.[39] Beyond these new publications, Weyer made an addition to the text of *De praestigiis daemonum*, which directly answered many of Erastus's criticisms. This chapter, "A refutation of the objections that have been raised against the preceding chapter," defended his proposition that those accused of witchcraft were deranged women and should be thus spared the death penalty.[40] Weyer ended the chapter by placing his opponents on notice that, as far as he was concerned, the debate was over: "they can expect no further response from me. I say this lest they lay claim to victory on the basis of my silence."[41]

---

[36] Rott, "Neue Quellen für eine Aktenrevision," 5–9; Burchill, *The Heidelberg Antitrinitarians*, 17; idem, "Die Universität zu Heidelberg," 245. Pigafetta alleged that Erastus preferred reading Schwenckfeld at home to hearing sermons in church. Given the animosity that developed between Erastus and the leaders of the Palatine church, it does not seem unlikely that he would have missed a few services.

[37] *De praestigiis daemonum* (1577), book 6, ch. 22 [*sic*], col. 762. Translation from Mora, *Witches, Devils and Doctors*, 557.

[38] Including letters of Zwinger and Ewich. *De praestigiis daemonum* (1577), cols. 901–906.

[39] Johann Weyer, *De Lamiis Liber* (Basel, 1577).

[40] *De praestigiis daemonum*, book 6, ch. 22 [*sic*] in the 1577 edition (cols. 741–763); book 6, ch. 24 in the 1583 edition (cols. 742–762). (N.B. The eighth and ninth chapters in terms of actual succession of the 1577 edition bear the numbers VI and VII.)

[41] Weyer, *De praestigiis daemonum* (1583), col. 763. Translation from Mora, *Witches, Devils and Doctors*, 557. This disclaimer first appeared in the 1577 edition.

Within weeks of the publication of the 1577 edition of *De praestigiis daemonum*, Erastus was at work on a new rebuttal.[42] Erastus indignantly complained that Weyer had not taken his criticisms to heart and simply put forth his old opinions without any alteration. Weyer's compendium of his thoughts on witchcraft, *De Lamiis Liber*, enraged Erastus the most, since he found in it "nothing at all that was of any significance" that he "had not already solidly refuted."[43] Convinced that Weyer's relative silence proved the veracity of his criticisms, Erastus was emboldened to augment his critique. He expanded his original twenty-three page disputatio "De lamiis seu strigibus non inutilia scitu" into the 127-page *Repetitio disputationis de lamiis seu strigibus* (Repetition of the Disputation on Witches).

The *Repetitio disputationis de lamiis seu strigibus* was published by Perna in Basel in 1578 in octavo format without illustrations.[44] Erastus's brother-in-law Johann Jakob Grynaeus arranged the details of its publication.[45] The stated purpose for the book was for the good of Christendom and ended with a prayer for consensus on this contentious issue. Erastus, however, also had a more earthly goal in mind by dedicating the book to members of the Basel city council. With the accession of the Lutheran Elector Ludwig VI, Erastus realized that his days in Heidel-

[42] The book was published in March; Erastus was at work on the refutation by May. Erastus to Grynaeus, May 10, (15)77, Basel UB, G II 4, fol. 207: "Cœpi ... scribere confutationem libri, quem adversus me scripsit Joh. Wierus De Lamiis. Impressit istic successor in Officina Oporiniana. Eius exemplum, si potest seorsum haberi à libro de praestig. Daemonum quintum iam edito, mihi per hunc [Andream] Ruinellam mitti velim. ... Scripsit modeste Wierus, qua in re ne inferior eo sim, sed superior, operam dabo. Rem totam sic explicabo adiuvante Deo, ut porrò neminem aliquid temere desideraturum confidam. Fundamenta totius disputationis feliciter sunt iacta, ut superstructio non videatur operos[a] futura. Turpiter se dedit Wierus, nisi fallor, dum et Mosen et omnium aetatum intelligentes inscitiae et ruditatis accusare non veretur."

[43] *Repetitio disputationis de lamiis seu strigibus: in qua plenè, solidè, & perspicuè, de arte earum, potestate, itemque pœna disceptatur* ... (Basel: Pietro Perna, [1578]), preface, fol.):(3^{v}. "Nihil enim prorsus, quod quidem momenti alicuius esset, deprehendi, quod non antea solide à me confutatum fuisset."

[44] Though the work lacks a date on the title page, its dedicatory letter is dated April 1, 1578, and it appeared at the Lenten Frankfurt fair that year. (*Die Messkatalog Georg Willers*, 2:294.) Robert Muchembled credits what is perhaps the first known illustration of a witch riding a broom to the French edition of Erastus's treatise, but this attribution is manifestly a false citation. *La Sorcière au village (XVe–XVIIIe siècle)* ([Paris]: Archives Gallimard Julliard, 1979), illustration no. 13.

[45] Erastus to Grynaeus, Aug. 18, (15)77, Basel UB, G II 4, fols. 211–212: "Mitto praeterea libellum de Strigib. quem, cum videbis oportunum esse curabis excudi. De dedicatione scripsi tibi, quae mea sit sententia: et literas et nunc accepisse arbitror. Tu praefationis partem posteriorem mutabis pro ratione circumstantiarum."

berg were numbered. Although Erastus entertained a number of career options (see below), relocating to Basel was his preference. The dedication of the *Repetitio disputationis de lamiis seu strigibus* must be seen both as an effort to influence the Basel magistrates on the question of the punishment of witches and as an attempt to further ingratiate himself with the Basel political elite.[46]

Although Erastus was a relative novice in the field of demonology, his treatises on witchcraft proved to be among his most widely read works.[47] Prior to publication of Jean Bodin's refutation of Weyer, Erastus's *Repetitio* and the original disputation from *De medicina nova* were translated into French and published as a complementary addendum to Weyer's work in 1579, which was itself reprinted in 1885.[48] The *Repetitio* was reprinted with the 1581 edition of Nicolaus Jacquier's *Flagellum haereticorum fascinariorum* and again by itself in Amberg in 1606.[49] It was thus a modest publishing success, although the fact that it was never translated into German limited its popular impact. Its popularity does not compare with that of Weyer's *De praaestigiis daemonum* or Bodin's later refutation, *De la demonomanie des sorciers*.[50]

Ironically, Erastus's brief disputation "De lamiis seu strigibus non inutilia scitu," buried in the pages of his *De medicina nova*, elicited a longer response from Weyer than his lengthier *Repetitio* of 1578. I have only been able to uncover one new reference in the 1583 edition of *De praestigiis daemonum* that responds to Erastus's work of 1578.[51] In this section Weyer responded to some of the specific passages from Dioscorides and

---

[46] The ambitions to use this book to garner favor in Basel are obliquely discussed in a letter from Erastus to Grynaeus, Aug. 5, (15)77, Basel UB, G II 4, fols. 203–204.

[47] It likely rates behind his *Explicatio gravissimae questionis utrum excommunicatione* in terms of readership and his anti-Paracelsian disputations in terms of significance. It was not reprinted as frequently as his treatise on the Lord's Supper, the *Gründtlicher bericht*.

[48] "Deux Dialogues de Thomas Erastus, Docteur en Medecine à Heidelberg, touchant le pouvoir des Sorcieres: & de la punition qu'elles meritent," in Iean Wier [Johann Weyer], *Histoires, disputes et discours, des illusions et impostures des diables, des magiciens infames, sorcieres & empoisonneurs*, pp. 757–875 (with its own unpaginated index following the Weyer index) ([Geneva]: Pour Iaques Chouet, 1579 (NLM 4737); reprinted, Paris: Lecrosnier and Delahaye, 1885; reprinted, New York: Arno, 1976).

[49] "Disputatio de Lamiis, seu Strigibus, in qua de earum viribus perspicuè disputatur à Thoma Erasto," reprinted in Nicolas Jacquier's *Flagellum haereticorum fascinariorum*, ed. Heinrich Myntzenberg (Frankfurt, 1581); *Disputatio de lamiis seu strigibus* ... (Amberg: Michael Forster, 1606).

[50] Jean Bodin, *De la demonomanie des sorciers* (Paris, 1580).

[51] This being the insertion from col. 742, line 41 to col. 744 line 33. *De praestigiis daemonum* (1583). See note 20 above and figure 2 below.

Galen that Erastus had assembled against his understanding of the meanings of words from the φαρμακον (pharmakon) family.[52] Aside from this brief treatment of etymological issues, Weyer had basically kept his promise of 1577 that he would not respond to further critiques to his work. Erastus's death in 1583 prevented his response to Weyer's final Latin edition of *De praestigiis daemonum*, although by this time Bodin had already championed Erastus's side of the debate, albeit with much less decorum.

Erastus's Conception of Magic and Witchcraft

A simple definition of magic undergirded Erastus's demonology: magic was the attempt to produce an effect that would have been impossible to achieve using natural powers. In Erastus's scheme, all individuals who sought to produce an outcome exceeding the powers of nature could fairly be called magicians. Almost from the beginning of time individuals had existed who claimed to know more, or to be able to accomplish things, beyond what could be possible through natural means. Erastus believed that any such attempt to produce supernatural effects must necessarily call upon a higher force, since humans could not exceed the powers of nature. In general, magicians employed conjurations, incantations, and other such rites in their attempt to produce magical effects. However, since these physical or verbal acts had no power in themselves, magicians were forced to resort to demonic assistance to accomplish results.[53] Erastus also rejected magical practices on the grounds that the Bible prohibited them. The Pentateuch proscribed all such auguries, enchantments, and divinations. Thus, magical arts suffered a double condemnation in Erastus's mind: they were necessarily demonic and God explicitly forbade them. A person could either seek to improve his condition by natural means, while relying on benevolent providence, or turn to the help of demons. There was no middle ground for white magic.[54]

Although Erastus employed an inclusive definition of magic, he used *magus*, the Latin word for magician, in two distinct senses in his work. In keeping with his broad definition of magic, he often employed it as

[52] Erastus maintained that the words possessed the connotation of enchanting while Weyer argued that they suggested the use of poison. See below.

[53] *Repetitio disputationis de lamiis*, 13–14.

[54] Ibid., 46–47.

a general term denoting all who would seek to exceed natural powers, including learned magicians, enchanters, soothsayers, witches, and so forth. On other occasions he used *magus* to specifically denote a learned magician. In line with the first usage, Erastus conceptualized witches as simply one type of magician. Since Weyer had attempted to drive a wedge between culpable, learned magicians and ignorant, harmless witches, Erastus stressed the point that witches must also be numbered among magicians. His basic argument for including witches in this category remained a simple one: all who sought to exceed the powers of nature were, by definition, magicians.[55]

Since one of Weyer's chief arguments for clemency for accused witches was based on the meaning of Old Testament words for sorcerers, Erastus was very careful to explain the various names of witches. Revealing his own area of expertise as a humanist physician, Erastus spent most of his time on the basic Greek and Latin words for witches. He first addressed terms of the φαϱμαϰον (*pharmakon*) family.[56] This word's basic meaning is that of a drug or poison and is the root of the English word "pharmacy." Most of the words in this family have the second sense of connoting sorcery or enchantment. Erastus explained the etymological link between the differing concepts by noting that because in ancient times many druggists made magical potions or said incantations over their medications, the word came to apply to making spells or incantations. Erastus recognized that the words in the *pharmakon* family have a range of meaning. He did not try to argue that it could not mean poison or poisoner; rather, he sought to demonstrate that the word also could denote sorcery and incantation in writers such as Plato and Aristotle.[57] More importantly for Erastus, the New Testament use of a word of this family, *pharmakeia*, clearly signified magical arts or sorcery, and not poison.[58] Thus, Erastus was able to assert that there was a long heritage for using words of the *pharmakon* family to describe sorcerers or enchantresses.

After treating the most common Greek terms for witches, Erastus discussed the various Latin names. He refused to turn this into a treatise on narrowly defined types of sorcery, but used the exercise to

[55] Ibid., 15, 46. See Clark, *Thinking with Demons*, 201–202.

[56] *Φαϱμαϰεια, φαϱμαϰευτϱια, φαϱμαϰισ*, etc., are some of the forms used by Erastus. When speaking of persons rather than sorcery, in general he used the feminine gender.

[57] *Repetitio disputationis de lamiis*, 6–10.

[58] Ibid., 11. See especially Rev. 18:23, which speaks of the "sorcery" (*φαϱμαϰεια*) of Babylon. Bauer, *A Greek-English Lexicon*, 854.

illustrate the full range of witches' vices while maintaining the underlying commonality of all types of magic. He first answered why witches were called *lamiae*. In antiquity, *lamiae* were thought to be specters or apparitions who appeared in the night in the form of beautiful women. After having intercourse with young men, they would devour their lovers. He was not hesitant to admit that modern witches were not *lamiae* themselves but were merely called that because they claimed to do similar acts. Likewise, modern witches were frequently called *striges* after legendary birds that drank children's blood at night. The name applied since it was popularly thought that witches desired the blood of infants. Another popular name for witches was *venefica*, which, Erastus explained, was similar to the Greek *pharmakeutria*. Like *pharmakeutria*, the root of *venefica* meant poison or venom, and this name could easily be applied to witches since they often made poisons as well as love potions. The Latin *malefica*, (literally, evil doer) picked up another essential characteristic of witches: the almost universal intent to harm others with their magic. Even more to the point was the name *incantatrix*, or enchantress, which stressed their proclivity to use spells and magical songs. Erastus emphasized this category, since its wide range of examples in classical literature helped prove the antiquity of witchcraft. The Old Testament likewise contains numerous prohibitions against enchanters, confirming Erastus's supposition that all magical arts were forbidden by God. Another common name for them was *saga*, a wise woman, suggesting a diviner, which Erastus asserted was appropriate since witches often claimed to know more than was naturally possible. Finally, Erastus concluded with what was perhaps the most apt name for them in his demonological scheme—*praestigiatrix* or trickstress—since he asserted that these witches could not do the things they claimed to do but only elicited demonic illusions.[59]

As previously suggested, it was not Erastus's intent to discriminate between types of magical activity in his analysis of the names of witches, but rather to explain how the apparent variations fit into his theory of magic. All names for witches shared overtones of fraud, deception, and trickery, which were hallmarks of diabolical action. His assumption of diabolical agency was the unifying factor in this scheme. Since the devil was the author of all these magical arts, they naturally shared much

[59] *Repetitio disputationis de lamiis*, 5–29. For *φαϱμακευτϱισ*, see pp. 6–12; *maga*, pp. 12–15; *lamia*, pp. 16–17; *strix*, pp. 17–18; *malefica*, p. 18; *venefica*, p. 18; *incantatrix* (as well as 'επαιοδος), pp. 19–23; *saga*, pp. 23–26; *praestigiatrix*, p. 27.

in common: "There is hardly any type of magical operation," claimed Erastus, "which confines itself within its limits, and which does not, to some degree, borrow a part from the others."[60]

Although his main motif was to stress the commonality of all magical practitioners, Erastus also contrasted the differences between witches and learned magicians. The first dissimilarity was that the satanic dimension of witchcraft was explicit, whereas, this diabolical aspect was often hidden among learned magicians. Erastus asserted that witches knowingly entered a pact with Satan. In contrast, most learned magicians were not fully cognizant of their reliance on demonic powers. The ironic twist here was that ignorant witches were more fully aware of the diabolical nature of their activity than the more gullible learned magicians.[61] Second, Erastus suggested that there was a greater chance that learned magicians would repent upon learning their error, because they may have been unaware that they were serving the devil. On the other hand, witches, being fully aware of their homage to Satan, were already obstinate sinners. The third difference concerned how the magical teachings were spread. Magicians took their knowledge of magical arts from books and teachers; theirs was a learned art. On the other hand, Satan himself instructed the witches. The final difference went to their intent in using magical instruments. Erastus recounted that learned magicians frequently employed their art for some trick or joke or in seeking fame. On the other hand, witches almost always used their powers in an attempt to harm someone. Even though magicians might also use their magic for malevolent purposes, evil intentions were more pervasive among witches. The point of Erastus's comparison of witches with learned magicians was to show that witches were at least as bad as these *magi*, and thus they should not go unpunished. He never forgot the shared characteristics of witches and magicians and suggested that both groups often engaged in activities that were more stereotypically associated with the other. In conclusion, he stressed the commonality of witches and magicians and asserted that one could not draw a hard line between them.[62]

The salient feature of Erastus's conception of witchcraft was that, while he was fundamentally skeptical of the claimed powers of witches, he

[60] Ibid., 24: "Quòd nulla ferè est Magiae Operatricis species, quae intra suos limites se contineat, & partem aliquam ab aliis non mutuetur."

[61] Ibid., 35.

[62] Ibid., 35–38.

vigorously maintained the reality of the pact with the devil. One might question why, in the wake of the Protestant rejection of much of medieval scholasticism, a skeptically minded Protestant would still cling to this extra-biblical idea of the pact with the devil. Although his retention of the pact might seem inappropriate for a Protestant trained in the humanist tradition, Erastus represents a case study of how the idea of the pact could be reinterpreted in a Protestant manner. In fact, his interpretation of the role of the pact in witchcraft can be read as a projection of a Protestant framework of the necessary relations between humans and superior beings onto the learned witchcraft paradigm.

How did Erastus's conception of the diabolical pact relate to his Swiss Reformed heritage? In no other offshoot of the magisterial Reformation was the necessity for correct performance of ritual so thoroughly debunked and emphasis so narrowly placed on faith as with the Swiss Reformed. Of course, the sacraments of the Lord's Supper and Baptism were maintained, but they were now seen as signs of God's covenant with humans, which required faith for true participation, rather than as rituals whose correct performance required God to grant a benefit. Just as proper performance of ritual was devalued in Reformed religion, so Erastus placed little emphasis on the spells and charms of witchcraft. Yes, witches and magicians might practice such things, but the essence of witchcraft could not be found in them. Here we can observe the ambiguous impact of the Reformed conception of a transcendent God on demonology. Even though Erastus was unwilling to grant demons supernatural powers, he still assumed that humans must call upon a higher force to accomplish something impossible through natural means. Just as Christians must place their faith in God if they desired salvation, witches must fully commit themselves to Satan if they desired to see the fruit of evil. In both cases the capacity of the invoked being to fulfill the request was more important than the correct performance of the spell or ritual. Ironically, Erastus offered an example in which Reformed theological assumptions had taken the "magical" dimension out of both religion and magic. Classical sociology and anthropology have seen the primary difference between religion and magic as existing in how the rituals or spells are employed. A magical act seeks to influence the world by the correct performance of its technique, whereas purely religious actions serve only as acts of prayer and worship to their god; all control over divine intervention is necessarily left to the god's providence. In Max Weber's words, religious petitions to the gods are "supplications," whereas magical formulations for intervention in the natural world are "coercions."[63] Bronislaw Malinowski has spoken of magic as "a practical art consisting of acts which are only means to a definite end expected to follow later on."[64] In Erastus's framework, witchcraft has ceased to be magic in the manner in which it has conventionally been characterized by anthropologists and sociologists, and has become primarily anti-religion. Witchcraft was not per se "black magic," in the sense of magic that seeks to harm others, but rather a satanic cult in which the diabolical pact was the covenant sign of the devil's chosen people.

The pact also had a certain self-evident logic for Erastus. If one accepted that there were individuals who sought to use the devil's powers to work wonders, it was reasonable to assume that these individuals must have some special relationship with the devil. It was common sense that not everyone had access to the devil's powers, as Erastus asked, "For why would not everyone be able [to do such things] if no pact were required?"[65] This assumption too was perhaps an inverse projection of Christianity on witchcraft, with witches now seen as the devil's covenant people. In biblical religion, both in the New and Old Testaments, entry into the community was marked by a symbol reflecting the covenant that had been made between God and humans. The Bible contained no specific reference to the devil making such a covenant with witches, but if the relationship between the devil and the witch functioned like the relationship between God and the believer, it would be reasonable to assume that such a pact existed. Erastus believed that the devil used this threshold to tempt people falsely with greater powers after they had committed themselves to him.

The reinterpreted idea of the pact was at the center of Erastus's theological definition of the crime of witchcraft. The apostasy and spiritual fornication of this act implicated witches in a host of spiritual crimes. Witches were not to be punished because of the marvelous things they accomplished, but because they sought to do the work of the devil. Actual harm, *maleficium*, had little place in Erastus's understanding of witchcraft.[66]

[63] Max Weber, *Economy and Society*, trans. Guenther Roth and Claus Wittich, 2 vols. (Berkeley, 1978), 1:422–424. Following Weber, I speak here in terms of ideal types for the purpose of clarity. I do not challenge his caveat that it is perhaps impossible to separate magic and religion completely and, likewise, that most religion retains a measure of magic.

[64] Bronislaw Malinowski, *Magic, Science, and Religion* (New York, 1955), 88.

[65] *Repetitio disputationis de lamiis*, 101: "Cur enim non omnes possunt, si pactio nulla requiritur?"

[66] Ibid., 64–65.

The basic crime of witches was apostasy. Witches were more than simple apostates, however, but heresiarchs, since they spread their cursed heresy of devil worship.[67] If any heretic merited punishment, these superheretics did, and Erastus did not stop to reflect upon the more fundamental question of whether any heretic should be persecuted.

The Powers of Darkness

In Erastus's demonology, the devil started out with a marked disadvantage since he could do nothing that was genuinely miraculous. This was because the power to effect a genuine miracle was the same type of power that acted in the creation of the world. A miracle was, in its essence, a "kind of creation."[68] Indeed, Erastus regarded the miracles that Christ worked in the Gospels as being analogous to God's creation of Eve from Adam's rib.[69] Only God himself had the power to work such miracles; this ability had not been conceded to the devil. This liability did not mean that the devil could produce nothing at all. Erastus followed the traditional line of thought, such as was expressed in the *Malleus Maleficarum*, which maintained that the devil could effect "marvels" but not true miracles.[70] Erastus posited a universe that was not subject to intermediary influences. Unlike the Neo-Platonic chain of being worldview, Erastus's view assumed a transcendent break, characteristic of the Reformed tradition, between the powers of God and the powers of created things. The devil, as a part of the created order, had powers more akin to those of humans than to those of God.

This preliminary liability aside, God had given demonic powers great latitude to work illusions and manipulate nature, all for the purpose of trying the elect. Unlike Weyer, however, Erastus did not outline an encyclopedic treatment of the devil's powers. He also had a tendency, perhaps unconscious, to use *diabolus* and *daemon* interchangeably.[71] The devil/demons had two modes of operating available to them: they could work according to the powers of nature or they could use their special tricks. Like a human being, the devil could produce a change by

[67] Ibid., 106–107.

[68] Ibid., 40.

[69] *De medicina nova*, 1:32–33.

[70] Regarding the similar opinions of Weyer, see *De praestigiis daemonum* (1583), book 1, ch. 14.

[71] His favorite term in the first disputation was *Cacodaemon*.

natural means, although his powers in this realm did not exceed those of humans. Here his ability to manipulate outcomes, as Erastus related, was not superior to those of "a good and diligent farmer."[72] In contrast with this conservative estimation of demonic power, Erastus also suggested that demons were quite skilled in inflicting disease by natural means. Ostensibly because of the devil's incorporeal nature, he could enter the human body and stir up its spirits and humors. Since the spirits and humors that the devil affected were natural, Erastus did not consider this a supernatural ability. The murky state of physiological knowledge in the sixteenth century made it possible for academic physicians to discuss demonic agency in disease as a genuine scientific possibility.[73]

The special talent of demons consisted of making illusions and tricks. Erastus considered this their chief power and took it quite seriously. Demons could create such tangible illusions that they could actually be seen and touched, though these specters were only representations and not the actual items that they portrayed. Using the metaphor of an artist, Erastus explained, "He who draws a man certainly does not make nothing, since he makes a picture of a man, but he can make nothing of an actual man."[74] While God had assigned only meager abilities to demonic forces, the devil exploited these in such a way that made it possible for him to engage in sexual relations with a witch. Satan could assume the form of a body, even if it was not true human flesh. He could also employ natural means at his disposal to titillate the humors and spirits of humans. Thus, the devil was able to have a type of intercourse with humans.[75] While Erastus had a rather philosophically constrained notion of demonic capacity, the devil that he presented was not impotent.

The power of witches, likewise, was limited by the laws of nature and by their dependence on demons. Many witches had an inflated notion of their abilities, imagining themselves able to spread disease, charm

[72] *Repetitio disputationis de lamiis*, 42. "Sed nihilo hic praestantior bono & diligente agricola … fuerit."

[73] Of course, this limited physiological knowledge not only afforded room for speculation regarding supernatural or diabolical activity; the role of vapors and animal spirits in various diseases (such as melancholia and vertigo) was also hotly debated. For a discussion of the role of humors, vapors, and animal spirits in the case of vertigo, see Andrew Wear, "Explorations in renaissance writings on the practice of medicine," in *The Medical Renaissance of the Sixteenth Century*, 118–145, especially, 127–139.

[74] *Repetitio disputationis de lamiis*, 27: "Qui pingit hominem, non facit prorsus nihil, (facit enim pictum hominem) sed veri hominis nihil facit."

[75] Ibid., 61.

lovers, and ruin crops. What they could actually accomplish, however, was severely limited, as Erastus related:

> For beyond the desertion of God and the divine cult, and the flight into the camp of the devil, nearly everything [that they claim to accomplish] are fabrications and fictions or positively uncertain and inconstant, slippery and changeable.[76]

Witches could affect terrestrial life by natural means, as could any human. In using natural powers they had some advantage over demons themselves, since some things were difficult for demons to accomplish because of their incorporeal form. However, unlike demons, witches were unable to enter humans and disturb their humors and spirits.[77] In short, witches had no powers in themselves exceeding other humans. A witch could encourage a demon to action, but the power to act resided in the demon, and not the witch. Nevertheless, Erastus found witches culpable in this regard, since the demon would not have acted without the incitement of the witch. In Erastus's assessment, the fact that demons themselves carried out the action made the witches worse than normal criminals, because they employed such despicable means to accomplish harm.[78]

Erastus's ideas of demonic capacity rested on his interpretation of the two chief instances of sorcery in the Hebrew Scriptures: the stories of Pharaoh's magicians and the famous witch of Endor. In the first of these, Moses and Aaron were sent by God to Pharaoh's court to perform a sign. Aaron cast his staff upon the ground, whereupon it immediately turned into a snake. Pharaoh summoned his own magicians, and likewise they were able to produce snakes "by their enchantments."[79] In an action suggestive of the superiority of the Hebrew God, the snakes of Aaron consumed the snakes of the Egyptian sorcerers. A critical question for Western demonology has been whether or not the snakes of the Egyptians were real snakes or illusions. In the first volume of *De medicina nova*, Erastus entertained the various Patristic interpretations of this story. He conceded that Augustine thought that the snakes were real, whereas Tertullian and Clement considered them to be merely phan-

[76] Ibid., 33–34: "Nam praeter desertionem Dei, cultusque divini, & transfugium in castra Diaboli, omnia ferè sunt vel ementita & ficta, vel certè incerta, inconstantia lubrica mutabilia."

[77] Ibid., 42–43.

[78] Ibid., 111. See Clark, *Thinking with Demons*, 520–521.

[79] Exodus 7:11. The biblical quotations in this chapter are from the KJV. All Latin biblical quotations are from the *Biblia Sacra Iuxta Vulgatam Versionem*, 3rd ed. (Stuttgart: Deutsche Bibelgesellschaft, 1969).

tasms. Erastus accepted the latter interpretation, since he would have been forced to concede too much power to the magicians if they had been able to produce actual snakes. Although the text seemed to imply that the snakes were in fact real, Erastus argued that the image of Aaron's snakes devouring the snakes of Pharaoh's magicians indicated that they were merely illusions.[80] Following this reading of the passage, Erastus drew two important points from the episode. First, magicians could not produce real effects but merely tricks. Second, and more importantly, the passage proved that magicians and witches *could* produce the appearance of a marvel.

The second major biblical proof text was provided by King Saul's visit with the witch of Endor. In this story, Saul, in a moment of desperation, consulted with a medium to communicate with the recently deceased prophet Samuel. He asked the medium to "divine unto me by thy familiar spirit and bring him up whom I shall name."[81] The woman called upon her familiar spirit to bring up Samuel from the dead. Samuel then appeared before Saul and prophesied his impending doom. One can number at least three agents at work in this act of necromancy: the medium, the familiar spirit, and the late Samuel himself. The sense of demonic agency between the medium and Samuel is confirmed by verse 13 when the medium reports seeing "gods ascending out of the earth."[82] As in the case of the snakes produced by the Egyptian magicians, there is nothing in the narrative to suggest that the medium had not been able to conjure up the real Samuel; the prophetic words that he spoke further suggest that it was God's man himself and not a demonic illusion. Erastus avoided this interpretation of the text, however, and suggested that it was not the real Samuel but rather the devil appearing in the likeness of Samuel.[83] It would create problems both for Erastus's theology and his natural philosophy if the familiar spirit could actually produce the dead Samuel. Such power would mean that the devil or a demon

---

[80] *De medicina nova*, 1:39–41.

[81] I Samuel 28:8: "divina mihi in pythone et suscita mihi quem dixero tibi." The Hebrew word for familiar spirit is *'ôwb* [*'ōb*]. The Vulgate translates the Hebrew *'ôwb* with *python*, which is in turn a derivative of the Greek πυθων. There is no simple word for "medium" in the Hebrew or Latin texts, only the compound suggesting a "woman having a familiar spirit." See Ann Jeffers, *Magic and Divination in Ancient Palestine and Syria* (Leiden: Brill, 1996), 176. For the general background regarding this text and its import for the Western witchcraft paradigm, see Charles Zika, "Witch of Endor" in *Encyclopedia of Witchcraft*, 308–310.

[82] I Samuel 28:13b: "et ait mulier ad Saul deos vidi ascendentes de terra."

[83] *Repetitio disputationis de lamiis*, 15.

could produce an authentic miracle, and Erastus had already philosophically ruled out this possibility. Thus, Erastus insisted on the interpretation that the medium "excited a specter and in a specter of demons, but not Samuel."[84] Even though Erastus had to bend the literal sense of the text to understand this episode in terms that fit his natural philosophy, he was again able to draw many positive characterizations of witchcraft from it. He surmised that even the witch of Endor realized that she was committing a capital crime in practicing her art, since she had been initially reluctant to do the king's bidding. She made use of a familiar spirit to work her art, and by this "pythonic spirit," she had been able to produce a fake Samuel, reiterating Erastus's belief that convincing illusions could be made with demonic agency. Erastus also noted that the woman was not delirious or possessed by a demon when she conjured the spirit. She also did not inflict any obvious harm by her actions, which supported his contention that the essence of witchcraft did not lie in actual *maleficium*. Lastly, Erastus asserted that she would not have been able to produce any results if she had not possessed a preexisting relationship with the demon, which Erastus interpreted as being analogous to contemporary witches' pacts with the devil.[85]

Erastus's speculations on sex with the devil and the sexual desires of older women pushed the limits of his inclination to regard the claims of witches skeptically and tended to belie his earlier, more positive statements about the capacities of women. In general, Erastus presented a more positive view of women than Weyer, and yet neither of these men actively undermined the sixteenth century's general assumptions regarding the inferiority of the female sex; both merely had philosophical points to make.[86] Weyer, seeking to save their lives, frequently cited "weakness and credulity of the female sex" to relieve women of culpability for their alleged crimes.[87] Alternatively, Erastus desired that women be viewed as competent enough to be held responsible for their misdeeds.[88] When Erastus sought to make a different point, however, he did not shy away

[84] Ibid., 103: "quod umbram excivit, & in umbra Daemonum, non autem Samuelem: licet opinaretur se Samuelem evocavisse."

[85] Ibid., 103–104.

[86] Regarding the issue of witchcraft and gender in the German context, see Roper, *Oedipus and the Devil* and Sigrid Brauner, *Fearless Wives and Frightened Shrews: The Construction of the Witch in Early Modern Germany* (Amherst: University of Massachusetts Press, 1995).

[87] Weyer, *De praestigiis daemonum* (1583), book 3, ch. 7.

[88] *Repetitio disputationis de lamiis*, 30–31.

from denigrating women. For example, Erastus suggested that the allegation of sex with the devil was made more plausible given the fabled lustfulness of older women. Folk wisdom acknowledged that older women had more inflamed desires than their younger counterparts.[89] Ironically, it seemed Erastus was more inclined to believe these stories of sex with the devil on account of the heightened lusts of women rather than to credit the devil's tempting power. Not satisfied with this squalor, Erastus interpolated a new justification for the death penalty for witches on the grounds of sexual intercourse with the devil. The command "Whoever lies with a beast shall be put to death" immediately follows the injunction "thou shalt not suffer the witch to live" in the book of Exodus.[90] Erastus argued that the proximity of these texts was by no means coincidental. Since the devil was not human, like a beast, it followed that individuals who had sex with him should also be put to death.[91]

In comparison to the author of the *Malleus Maleficarum*, however, Erastus was quite skeptical of the supposed powers of witches and demons. The aforementioned excesses aside, Erastus's writings had none of the misogynistic fervor and were generally devoid of the prurient quality of the *Malleus Maleficarum*. Erastus was no greater a believer in demonic power than Weyer himself. Likewise, he minimized the actual harm or *maleficium* that witches were capable of producing and interpreted Scripture in such a way as to minimize demonic power. It is certainly not fair to say, along with Reginald Scot, the great English champion of clemency for witches, that Erastus was "a principall writer in the behalfe of witches omnipotencie."[92]

Nevertheless, there were two fundamental tensions in Erastus's demonology. On some occasions a strong ambiguity existed between the things that witches attempted to do and what they actually succeeded in accomplishing. Erastus often reeled off lists of things witches *claimed* to do in

[89] Ibid., 113–115.

[90] Exodus 22:18–19: The classic line "thou shalt not suffer the witch to live" is actually Exodus 22:17 in the Masoretic text of the Hebrew Scriptures.

[91] *Repetitio disputationis de lamiis*, 114–115.

[92] Reginald Scot, *The discouerie of witchcraft* (London, 1584; facsimile reprint, New York, 1971), fol. Aiiii^{v}. Scot's characterization of Erastus has something of a rhetorical aim, since he proceeds to comment that even Erastus recognized that most of a witch's so-called powers were nothing other than illusions and tricks. It is quite noteworthy that, already in 1584, Scot picked up on this tension between skepticism and credulity in Erastus's work. His countryman Robert Burton had a similar reading of Erastus. See *The Anatomy of Melancholy*, ed. Thomas C. Faulkner et al. (Oxford: Oxford UP, 1989) pt. 1, section 2, subsection 3 (vol. 1, p. 195). See also Clark, *Thinking with Demons*, 208.

such a fashion that the reader might assume that he meant they *could* actually do these things. At times Erastus himself appeared unsure, as when he argued that witches committed murder, although his earlier statements had implied that they did no harm.[93] Also, there was apparently a measure of change in Erastus's own attitudes. In Erastus's first treatment of witchcraft, he set out ironclad philosophical categories in which witches and demons had no supernatural powers. Although his fundamental philosophical distinctions remained intact in the *Repetitio disputationis de lamiis seu strigibus*, when he probed the specific allegations of witches having sex with the devil and the spread of disease by demonic agency, he strained his philosophical distinctions. It puzzles the modern reader that he could characterize the devil's powers as bound by the laws of nature but simultaneously argue that the devil had sex with humans and created illness by natural means. Nevertheless, these contradictions were no less present in the work of Weyer, and in general Erastus presented a less powerful devil than Weyer.[94]

The Punishment of Witches

As we have seen, Erastus and Weyer inhabited essentially the same worldview regarding what witches could actually accomplish. The controversy between them was focused chiefly on the punishment of witches. Erastus held that witches merited the death penalty according to the scriptural mandate. Since Weyer had endeavored to undercut the biblical foundation of this penalty, Erastus drew upon all possible texts and analogies to support their execution. Thus, Erastus characterized contemporary witchcraft as simply a modern manifestation of forbidden magical arts in order to expand the number of biblical texts that condemned it. Beyond the general prohibition of all magical arts, the Pentateuch included an express commandment to execute witches in Exodus 22:18: "thou shalt not suffer the witch to live." Not only was witchcraft included among the list of forbidden practices meriting the death penalty, God specifically ordered the execution of witches.[95]

Since Erastus did not want to base his case for the death penalty on one verse, he fabricated a list of crimes meriting capital punishment that

[93] *Repetitio disputationis de lamiis*, 52–55.
[94] See Midelfort, "Insanity Defense," 248.
[95] *Repetitio disputationis de lamiis*, 46.

could also be applied to witches. For instance, he argued that witches were guilty of the worst sort of idolatry, since to worship an idol in ignorance was bad enough, but to do homage to the devil knowingly was doubly cursed. Therefore, the Mosaic law requiring the death penalty for idolaters also applied to witches, since they were the worst possible kind of idolater.[96] He also argued that they deserved death because they actively seduced others into their error.[97] They were also guilty of murder and of knowingly practicing proscribed arts. Finally, as discussed above, Erastus proposed his most fantastic accusation in alleging that they merited the death penalty because they engaged in bestial sex.[98]

Weyer had attacked the command of Exodus 22:18 by arguing that the text did not apply to witches or sorcerers at all, but rather that the law was meant to condemn poisoners. He based this assertion on a clever philological analysis of the Old Testament, both of the Hebrew text and Greek and Latin translations, in which he called upon the expertise of Jewish Hebrew scholars.[99] The chief thrust of his argument was to accept the Septuagint's translation of the Hebrew *Mekashshephah* with the Greek *pharmakos* (φαρμακος).[100] Although *pharmakos* could either mean a poisoner or a sorcerer, Weyer stressed the word's etymological root and asserted that it must denote a poisoner in Exodus 22:18. In Weyer's understanding, the passage should read: "thou shalt not suffer the *poisoner* to live." Such an interpretation undercut the only explicit Old Testament law used to mandate capital punishment for witches.

Erastus rejected the notion that the command of Exodus 22:18 was meant to condemn poisoners rather than those practicing magical arts.

---

[96] Ibid., 50–51.

[97] Ibid., 51–52.

[98] Ibid., 60–61.

[99] Weyer, *De praestigiis daemonum* (1583), book 2, ch. 1, cols. 135–143; Mora, *Witches, Devils and Doctors*, 93–98.

[100] The Hebrew word is *mekashshephah* [*mĕkaššēpâ*], whose root idea has the connotation of whispering a spell (i.e., enchanting). The modern scholarly consensus is that the word in Hebrew Scriptures in fact has the connotation of enchantress or sorceress rather than poisoner. Since Exodus 22:17/18 does not include a description of the crimes of the *mekashshephah*, however, it impossible to establish clear definition of the crime of "witchcraft" using this passage. *De praestigiis daemonum* (1583), book 5, col. 26; Mora, *Witches, Devils and Doctors*, 542–547. See Graham Harvey, "The Suffering of Witches and Children: Uses of the Witchcraft Passages in the Bible," in *Words Remembered, Texts Renewed*, ed. Jon Davies et al., *Journal for the Study of the Old Testament*, Supplement Series 195 (1995): 113–134; Jeffers, *Magic and Divination in Ancient Palestine and Syria*, 68; *The Hebrew and Aramaic Lexicon of the Old Testament*, ed. Ludwig Koehler et al. (Leiden: Brill, 1994–2000).

To refute Weyer's interpretation, he was forced to engage in a similar philological study. His effort focused on the meaning of the Greek word *pharmakos*, since it, rather than the Hebrew *mekashshephah*, was the key to Weyer's argument. He established a range of meanings and showed that *pharmakos* had a long heritage of denoting enchanter or sorcerer and not simply poisoner, a position he established by references to authors such as Plato and Galen.[101] With a humanist's acumen, he put forward sound criteria for establishing a word's meaning by first considering the range of meanings possible for the word, but ultimately allowing the context to offer the final determination. In line with this methodology, he suggested that Old Testament meanings were more critical in interpreting the Exodus passage than their extra-biblical usage.[102] In this context he made the point that the translators of the Septuagint had also used a word from the *pharmakon* family to describe Pharaoh's magicians in Exodus 7. Thus, Erastus was able to produce a clear case where *pharmakos* had a connotation of incantation. Alternatively, he argued that Weyer's proposed interpretation was untenable, since he could not produce one biblical example where *pharmakos* meant poisoner. Erastus concluded, on the basis of the range of meaning of *pharmakos* in the Bible, that the traditional understanding of the Exodus 22:18 command to kill the witch remained valid.

Another of Weyer's strategies was to assert that modern witches were unknown in biblical times and, therefore, that the Mosaic law could not be interpreted as pertaining to them since they did not exist at the time of Moses. This challenge was broader than simply exempting them from the direct mandate of Exodus 22:18; if fully accepted, it would have meant that sixteenth-century witches were not liable for the more broadly proscribed arts of divination and incantation. Weyer displayed a measure of that famous Renaissance historical awareness in asserting that the crimes of which modern witches were accused were vastly different from the activities of the Old Testament's enchanters and diviners. Erastus countered this argument by generalizing the conception of a magician and conflating it with the much more common Old Testament notion of an enchanter. Although he had enough literary acumen to perceive the differences among the various groups of magical practitioners, he was theologically constrained to argue that they all were members of the same diabolical family. In Erastus's theory, the specific form of satanic activ-

[101] *Repetitio disputationis de lamiis*, 90–93.
[102] Ibid., 88.

ity might change from time to time, but the devil remained the author of all such arts. This ploy saved Erastus from committing the historical anachronism of asserting that modern witches were one and the same as biblical enchantresses. He maintained that the law of God was flexible enough to treat the general concept of magic and did not limit its relevance by addressing only its ephemeral forms.[103] He admitted that it was possible that there would be new types of magicians; nevertheless, anyone who sought diabolical assistance was by definition a magician. Erastus strengthened his argument for the antiquity of witchcraft by citing numerous texts by classical authors that offered examples of various enchantresses and sorcerers. He was thus able to employ a humanist's knowledge of antiquity, much as Gianfrancesco Pico della Mirandola had done before him, to buttress belief in witchcraft.[104] The dispute between Erastus and Weyer thus yields an example of the ambiguous impact of humanism on the witchcraft debate. Both men displayed a measure of humanist incredulity that would have been uncommon for earlier scholastics.[105] In the case of Weyer, historical criticism was used for the benefit of those accused of witchcraft; with Erastus, knowledge of classical texts was used against the witches. In this example, humanism itself was a neutral factor in the debate on the punishment of witches, depending on how the particular humanist desired to wield the weapon. The impact of humanism on the witchcraft debate was ultimately analogous to its impact on the question of astrology, where we likewise find humanists on both sides of the issue. The combined examples suggest that the humanist method had only a marginal impact as an agent of "disenchantment."

Weyer had also invented a forerunner of the modern insanity defense to win acquittal for those accused of witchcraft. Weyer argued that old women who were incompetent by excesses of *melancholia*—literally, black bile—merely imagined the silly things they confessed. Thus, even

[103] Ibid., 81–83.

[104] Peter Burke, "Witchcraft and Magic in Renaissance Italy: Gianfrancesco Pico and his *Strix*," in *The Damned Art: Essays in the Literature of Witchcraft* (London: Routledge & Kegan Paul, 1977), 32–48.

[105] This is not to suggest that most humanists were skeptics in the mode of David Hume. I follow Kristeller here when he notes that "the humanists did not place much credence in miracles and avoided theological speculations...." Paul Oskar Kristeller, *Renaissance Thought and the Arts* (Princeton, Princeton UP, 1990), 10. Weyer certainly surpassed Erastus as a debunker of alleged stories of witchcraft and miracles. See especially his investigation of the case of Barbara Kremers, a young woman who supposedly lived without eating. Mora, *Witches, Devils and Doctors*, lxvii–lxix.

if they thought they had entered a diabolical pact, they should be treated mercifully by reason of their impaired condition. Erastus countered this argument by first asserting that witchcraft was not a crime limited to old women, since young people and even men became entangled in it. He did not dispute the idea that many practitioners of witchcraft were feeble-minded individuals; however, he rejected the fallacy that *all* who fall under the devil's spell were mentally incompetent. While it might have seemed to befit Christian charity to offer clemency to these women, Erastus argued that such mercy was restricted by the word of God. Thus to forgive them would be damnable rather than praiseworthy.[106] He also attacked the idea that the alleged witches had merely dreamt the things they confessed. He maintained that they were fully cognizant of their decision to ally themselves with the devil; if not, why did they try so hard to cover up their actions?[107]

Weyer's most penetrating critique of the supposed crime of witchcraft had been to attack the legal foundations of the idea of the pact. Weyer undermined the validity of the pact from the perspective of Roman contract theory. Roman law rejected both contracts in which only one party would profit (leonine contracts) and contracts in which one party was not fully aware of the stipulations of the contract. Weyer argued that a witch's pact with the devil violated both of these conditions and was therefore an invalid contract, since only the devil could gain while the witch lost. Furthermore, the devil would not fulfill the extravagant promises he made to the witch to entice her to enter the pact. There were multiple grounds in Roman law to consider the diabolical pact a fraudulent and unenforceable contract.[108]

Ironically, Erastus did not engage Weyer's repudiation of the pact on legal grounds. Despite Erastus's general competence, he admitted that he was not familiar with Roman law and made a plea in the introduction of the *Repetitio disputationis de lamiis seu strigibus* for someone more proficient than himself to challenge Weyer on this issue.[109] Erastus did not think of a witch's contract with the devil in the Roman legal sense as a binding agreement between two good faith individuals; rather, he employed the analogy of the ancient Israelites' covenant with Jehovah.

[106] *Repetitio disputationis de lamiis*, 109.
[107] Ibid., 30–31.
[108] Midelfort, "Insanity Defense," 243–245.
[109] *Repetitio disputationis de lamiis*, fol.):(4^r.

Erastus's conception of the pact was a theologically rather than a legally defined idea.

The fundamental philosophical difference between Erastus and Weyer was that Erastus believed that the pact was possible, whereas Weyer thought that it was as fictitious and imaginary as the other activities witches confessed. Weyer summarized their disagreement as follows:

> These women claim that they fly through the air, are transformed into beasts, excite storms and cause disease by their imprecations.... And yet I have shown, and you admit along with me, that all these things are vain and contrived and tinged with diabolical fiction. And if they are vain, why should the other things that they confess be true.... I know what it is here that deceives the philosopher. He sees that all of the former claims are impossible, and therefore he agrees with me and pronounces them false and meaningless; but he thinks that the latter things have been done because they can be done, and because the *Strigae* themselves confess to doing them.[110]

The title "the philosopher" would appear to be a direct reference to Erastus. With this deft maneuver, Weyer could both compliment Erastus by placing him in the company of Aristotle and chide him on account of his lack of direct experience in sorting out such outrageous claims. Nevertheless, Weyer correctly perceived that he had not been able to prove to Erastus's satisfaction that the pact was actually impossible. Whereas Erastus might not believe witches' outlandish tales, he still believed that it was possible for witches to abandon God and enter the society of the devil. Their confessions of entering a pact with the devil were believable, since they actually could do this. Erastus believed the Scriptures attested to this possibility and asserted that the "experience of all the centuries proves the same."[111] To this belief Weyer could only retort, "Does he not see the devil's fallacy—that he wishes us to conclude the impossible from the possible?"[112] Weyer's argument, however, constructed on an insubstantial logical ploy, could not overturn Erastus's claimed evidence from Scripture and experience. Ironically, Weyer himself had to strengthen his case by emphasizing the cunning of demonic agency.[113]

[110] *De praestigiis daemonum* (1583), book 6, ch. 24, cols. 751–752. Quoted from Mora, *Witches, Devils and Doctors*, 549–550.

[111] *Repetitio disputationis de lamiis*, 100.

[112] *De praestigiis daemonum* (1583), book 6, ch. 24, col. 752. Quoted from Mora, *Witches, Devils and Doctors*, 550.

[113] Such statements from Weyer reinforce Midelfort's insight that Weyer sought to undermine the supposed crime of witchcraft "by affirming that he [the devil] was more powerful than was usually thought." Midelfort, "Insanity Defense," 237.

Conclusion

Erastus's critique revealed the weakness of Weyer's arguments for clemency toward those accused of witchcraft as addressed to a learned, sixteenth-century audience. It was because Weyer argued so boldly that the crime of witchcraft was *impossible* that intellectuals like Erastus found his arguments so implausible. The inadequacy of Weyer's defense of witches was not unlike Galileo's failed argument that the existence of tides proved the earth's movement. Of course, Galileo's theory of diurnal motion was correct, but the specific argument he chose to prove his point missed the mark. Likewise, while Weyer correctly grasped that the entire witch-trial process was a tremendous miscarriage of justice, many of his supporting arguments, while perhaps ingenious, were more than an intellectually honest sixteenth-century scholar could swallow.

Erastus's response to Weyer must be viewed as a humanistically constructed refutation by a man who possessed nearly identical assumptions regarding the operation of the natural world and the devil's role in it. Erastus was neither an avid witch-hunter nor a convinced believer in diabolical power. He was not personally involved in persecuting witches, and his book was neither a program nor a manual for persecuting witches.[114] His writings did not encourage a wholesale persecution in the Palatinate, which remained almost completely untouched by the later waves of witch-hunting.[115] Erastus also made statements to the effect that there had often been abuses in witchcraft trials and that the innocent may have wrongly suffered.[116] Ultimately what distinguished Erastus from Weyer was his limited first-hand familiarity with witch trials, not his belief in the devil. In an academic setting in a principality that had not

[114] Thus I dissent from Anneliese Staff's assertion that "Erastus setzt sich für eine intensive Verfolgung ein." Anneliese Staff, "Von Hexen/ Zauberer/ Unholden/ Schwartkünstler/ und Teufeln ... Bibliographie zu den Beständen der Hexenliteratur der Herzog August Bibliothek Wolfenbüttel," in *Vom Unfug des Hexen-Processes*, 374. Schmidt concurs: "Da Erast kein Verfolgungshandbuch geschreiben hat, sondern prozessferne Thesen im akademischen Rahmen diskutierte, scheint er keine directe Wirkungen auf konkrete Hexenverfolgung gehabt zu haben, sondern nur einem Widerhall in der gelehrten Diskussion." Schimdt, *Glaube und Skepsis*, 168.

[115] The Palatinate had been an early leader in the reception of the learned witchcraft paradigm in Germany. An acute outbreak of disease in Heidelberg had been blamed on witchcraft in 1446–1447, which led to the execution of eight alleged witches. However, the Palatinate saw no major witchcraft trials in the sixteenth century and, after its positive reception of Weyer's views, became one of the most persecution resistant states in the Holy Roman Empire. Schimdt, *Glaube und Skepsis*, passim.

[116] *De medicina nova*, 1:214.

suffered an outbreak of witch trials for approximately seventy years, Erastus remained convinced of the theological possibility of witchcraft. Likewise, he believed in the authenticity of the witches' confessions for the same reasons that convinced the majority of sixteenth-century intellectuals; after all, some men and women had confessed to the crime voluntarily.[117] Since Erastus's skepticism regarding demonic powers was quite strong for a sixteenth-century intellectual, my study supports the conclusions of H.C. Erik Midelfort and Stuart Clark that the eventual lack of faith in the judicial system that extracted the confessions and recriminating accusations was much more important in bringing about the end of witch-hunting than an absence of faith in devil or witchcraft.[118] Unfortunately, Erastus knew far too little about actual witch trials to anticipate this future crisis of faith in the machinery of witchcraft proceedings.

The fundamental message of Erastus was to suggest that, even though there were abuses in witch trials and that witches really could do no harm, Weyer had gone too far when he said that they were all deranged women and that the death penalty should not apply to them. Unfortunately, Erastus's writings probably spread a less subtle message: witches must be killed. That his arguments were later picked up by demonologists across the confessional divide and even reprinted as an accompanying text to Nicolas Jacquier's *Flagellum haereticorum fascinariorum* reveals how useful the witch-hunters found Erastus's critique of Weyer.[119] Although Erastus may have scored some technically correct philological and theological points in his demonological writings, he failed to grasp the human tragedy of the witch-hunt. In the case of witchcraft, which Erastus appears to have addressed solely as an academic question, his lack of experience with the human dimension of the problem allowed him to arrive at an orthodox interpretation of Scripture, if a much less humane conclusion. It was a conclusion with consequences, and Erastus must take his place as one of the figures who defended an intellectual paradigm that allowed approximately fifty thousand women and men to lose their lives

---

[117] *Repetitio disputationis de lamiis*, 98–116, passim, especially 107.

[118] H.C. Erik Midelfort, *Witch-hunting in Southwestern Germany 1562–1684* (Stanford: Stanford UP, 1970), 162–163; Stuart Clark, "Glaube und Skepsis in der deutschen Hexenliteratur von Johann Weyer bis Friedrich von Spee," in *Vom Unfug des Hexen-Processes*, 15–33. On the question of the limits of Weyer's appeal, see Clark, *Thinking with Demons*, 198–209 and Christopher Baxter, "Johann Weyer's *De praestigiis daemonum*: Unsystematic Psychopathology," in *The Damned Art*, 53–75.

[119] Niklaus Paulus, *Hexen und Hexenprozeß vornemlich im 16. Jahrhundert* (Freiburg im Breisgau, 1910), 69.

in the early modern period.[120] Given the magnitude of the tragedy, it is fitting to hear Weyer's prophetic word regarding the irresponsibility of his detractors' arguments:

> Unwittingly these writers provide drawn sword and kindling for the savage executioners, who lack judgment, discretion and any trace of pity.[121]

Erastus's harsh position on witches remains a dual enigma when viewed from the perspective of the rest of his career. Whereas Erastus had adopted a more liberal position in the controversy over church discipline, which had led some of his colleagues to suggest that his ideas would lead to atheism, Erastus supported the conventional wisdom on the question of punishment of witches. In the church discipline controversy, Erastus's experience with arbitrary clerical power made a critical impact on Erastus's reading of scripture. In short, being mindful of the history of ecclesiastical tyranny, he was inclined to interpret the biblical proof texts for church discipline rather differently from his Calvinist brethren. Not unlike Weyer's attack on witchcraft, in the case of excommunication Erastus was able to gaze across centuries of theological tradition and boldly proclaim that the emperor was wearing no clothes. But Erastus lacked the personal experience with witch trials needed to humanize his demonology, and his witches were more theoretical heretics than real ones. The other paradox regards Erastus's own disenchanted outlook, which he appeared to transgress by granting the devil certain *natural* powers to harm humans. On limited occasions, Erastus sounded more like the individuals he had attacked so vigorously in his anti-Paracelsian disputations; for example, Renaissance thinkers who had supported various types of magical practices precisely because they were *natural* or Melanchthon, who wanted to understand the natural influences of the stars on earthly existence. If Erastus allowed that the devil could manipulate such natural powers, one might ask what prevented humans from manipulating these same powers. There is no simple resolution to this contradiction in Erastus's thought. It was real, and it was perceived by Erastus's contemporary Reginald Scot, who proclaimed: "Erastus disagreeth herein with himselfe and his freends" in that Erastus had oth-

[120] The estimate of fifty thousand executions between 1400–1800 is from Wolfgang Behringer, *Witches and Witch-Hunts: A Global History* (Cambridge: Polity, 2004), 156–157. For a regional breakdown of the estimated numbers of trials and executions, see Levack, *Witch-hunt*, 20–24.

[121] *De praestigiis daemonum* (1583), book 2, ch. 1, col. 143. Quoted from Mora, *Witches, Devils and Doctors*, 98.

erwise maintained that all of the witches' wiles were simple tricks and illusions.[122] Erastus's powerful Reformed animus against magic and idolatry apparently won out over his skepticism. It was an extension of his tendency to deny the legitimacy of any claimed natural magic and point to its necessary demonic quality.[123] Particularly in the *Repetitio disputationis de lamiis seu strigibus*, his tendency to emphasize demonic agency took precedence over more empirical arguments. Because of their diabolical perversion of the Christian cultus, Erastus's textbook witch was a heresiarch and super-idolater who deserved death.

Finally, Erastus's demonological treatises must be placed in the context of his history of self-fashioning. In 1570 Erastus's allies had come under deep suspicion of heretical activities. By 1577 Erastus had survived a more serious inquest into his orthodoxy, only to be made a confessional outsider once again with the re-conversion of the Palatinate to Lutheranism. Not unlike his anti-Paracelsian works, his disputations on witchcraft assisted Erastus's attempt to recover a reputation in the cultural and religious mainstream.

Figure 2. Passages from Erastus and Weyer are set in parallel columns for comparison. The identical or nearly identical words and phrases have been placed in italics. The correspondence between the passages is even greater when one takes into account the occasions when Weyer has translated Erastus's Greek text into Latin. The magnitude of direct borrowings from Erastus's text, which Weyer quoted in order to refute him, leave no doubt as to the identity of Weyer's "adversary."

Erastus, *Repetitio disputationis de lamiis*, [1578] pp. 90–92	Weyer, *De praestigiis daemonum*, 1583 col. 742, line 45–col. 744, line 26
Dioscorides cap. de Rhamno	*Dioscorides* velit nolit, *cap. de* Zhamno obtruditur:
ait, *Fertur ramos eius, si pro forib. aut fenestris ponatur* (*αποκρευειν τας των Φαρμακων κακουργειας*) *malefica pharmacorum seu incantamentorum pellere....*	*Fertur, ramos eius, si pro foribus aut fenestris ponatur, αποκρουειν τας των Φαρμακων κακουργειας*. quod adversarius vertit, *Malefica pharmacorum seu incantamentorum pellere....*

[122] Scot, *Discoverie of Witchcraft*, fol. Aiiiiv.

[123] See Walker, *Spiritual and Demonic Magic from Ficino to Campanella*, 156–166; Clark, *Thinking with Demons*, 244.

Galenus raró sic usus est, fateor Causa est in medio posita. Docere enim artem Medicam, non	
Malificia & incantationes voluit: quòd initio	Nec contra nos facit, quod ex
lib. 6. *de Simpl. pharm. Facult.* testatur....	sexto *lib.* Galeni *de Simpl. pharmac. facult.* adducitur de voce Pharmaco: quemadmodum nec
Sic cum	omnino liquet ex Galeni verbis, quod non candidè
Secundo libro de Compositione pharmacorum	objicitur, ubi *lib.* 2
κατατοπους, de περιαπτοις *Archigenis*	*κατατοπους*, de *Archigenis* amuletis
loquitur, de eis se nihil dicturum ait, quia	*loquitur*, ad capitis dolorem ea se relicturum, ut
nullam rationem Medicam	*nullam medicam rationem* habentia, ait:
(ουδενα λογον ιατρικον) habeant, ac sola experientia iudicentur. Vocasse nihilominus talia	...
unà cum aliis, Φαρμακα, licet inania &	
inefficacia iudicaret, ex dictis constat. Sed & *decimo libro* citati prius operis, haec habet.	*libro 10.* de Simplic. adversus me torqueatur, ubi
εγω τοινυν ουτε βασιλισκων, ουτε ελεφαντων,	se basiliscorum aut elephantorum
ουτε ιππων νειλωων, ουτ’ αλλου τινος,	& equorum Nileorum, neq[ue] alterius cuisquam,
ου μη πειραν αυτος εχω, μνηνομε[ ]σω.	cuius ipse periculum non fecerit, mentionem se
των δε καλουμενων φιλτρων,	facere nolle asserit: nec etiam velle meminisse poculorum amatorum,
αγωγιμων ονειροπομπωντε, και μισηθρων,	*αγωγιμων*, *ονειροπομπων* & *μισηθρων*, etiamsi
...	abundè illa expertus esset, sicuti nec lethalium
	medicamentorum, aut, ut ipsi vocant,
καθοποιων.	*παθοποιων*.
...	...
Hippocr. Etiam *libro de morbo sacro*	Quod item *Hippocrates libro de Morbo sacro* in auxilium accersatur, sit potius calumniae exaggerandae causa, quàm veritatis defendendae velut & aliis locis. siquidem
πεφαρμαγμενους υπ ανθρωπων vocare videtur incantatos laesos, cum ibi de curationibus Magicis agat.	*φαρμαγμενους υπ ανθρωπων vocare videtur incantatos laesos, cum ibi de curationibus magicis agat*: ita scribit adversarius.

CHAPTER TEN

EPILOGUE AND CONCLUSION

> And *Erastus*, though a very learned physician, is much less famous for all his elaborate disputations against *Paracelsus*, than for the little tract against particular forms of church government.
>
> Robert Boyle

While the most dynamic period of Erastus's life as it related to church politics ended with the death of Elector Frederick III in 1576, his output of natural philosophical works reached its highest level in the late 1570s and early 1580s. This concluding chapter offers a brief overview of Erastus's later career in Heidelberg and Basel. The biographical treatment is followed by a survey of the reception of Erastus's thought in the sixteenth and seventeenth centuries. Finally, I offer some concluding remarks about Erastus's career and his standing among sixteenth-century intellectuals.

The Lutheran Restoration of Ludwig VI (r. 1576–1583)

The second half of Frederick III's reign had seen the Palatinate emerge as *the* vanguard Calvinist polity in Western Europe, adopting a Genevan-style consistory for the reform of morals and boldly intervening in the French Wars of Religion. Upon the death of his father Frederick the Pious, Elector Ludwig VI became the sovereign of the Palatinate.[1] Unlike Frederick, who had been the chief patron of the Reformed faith in the empire, Ludwig remained a convinced Lutheran. Thus, dynastic succession meant yet another confessional change in the Palatinate. While

[1] Ludwig is styled "Ludwig VI" by modern historians. He was in fact the fourth Ludwig seen exclusively from the perspective of the Palatine Wittelsbach line and was sometimes hailed as such in the sixteenth century. E.g., see Erastus's dedication to the *Disputatio de Putredine* (Basel: Leonard Ostein, 1580), 3.

Ludwig VI had chafed at the high-handed attempt to introduce Reformed practices into the Upper Palatinate while he served as governor there, his antipathy toward specific Reformed practices and preachers had not led him to demonize the movement as a whole. In short, under Ludwig the Palatinate did not become a bastion for Gnesio-Lutheranism but instead returned to a moderate form of Lutheranism such as had been pursued under Ottheinrich. In fact, Ludwig's religious program was in many ways an intentional reprise of his uncle Ottheinrich's in that he recalled a few surviving ministers from the Ottheinrich era and reintroduced a modified version of Ottheinrich's church order.[2]

Ironically, conditions in Heidelberg actually improved for Erastus with Ludwig's ascension. The most zealous disciplinists who had made the last few years of his life so difficult departed the stage in succession. Erastus enjoyed a measure of personal favor with Ludwig that he had once possessed with the prince's father. The tables had quickly turned regarding the relative influence of Erastus and his nemesis Olevianus, and Erastus used his good will with the new administration to lodge a petition to force Olevianus to exonerate him or suffer punishment himself.[3]

While Erastus was safe for the moment in his position at the university, Ludwig did intend to return the church to a Lutheran norm and dismissed the clerics who could not accept the new ecclesiastical regime. Olevianus, against whom Ludwig seems to have harbored something of a grudge, was treated a little more roughly than the rest, first being placed under some form of house arrest and then being expelled from the city. After these preliminary moves, the new elector left Heidelberg in November of 1576 to settle his affairs in the Upper Palatinate. Major changes commenced upon his return in early April 1577.[4] Altars, chal-

[2] For Ludwig's rule, see Press, *Calvinismus und Territorialstaat*, 267–298; Schaab, *Geschichte der Kurpfalz*, 2:50–56.

[3] Erastus to Grynaeus, [Nov. 1576], Basel UB, G II 4, fols. 247, 250: "Quam gratum facerem Electori novo, si nunc peterem, ut Olevianus vel probaret intentatum mihi crimen, vel in locum poenae succederet? Deum oro, ne dem occasionem persecutioni. Nisi hoc metuerem, de capite scelerosi calumniatoris actum iam esset. Non sic ipse mecum egisset." While briefly outlining Olevianus's disfavor and termination, Sudhoff does not discuss this episode. *C. Olevianus und Z. Ursinus*, 421–423. This incident should be viewed from the context of Olevianus's refusal to accept Erastus as a brother a couple months earlier, which Erastus described in a letter to Grynaeus (Sept. 22, 1576, Basel UB, G I 33, fols. 10–11).

[4] Erastus to Grynaeus, April 30, (15)77, Basel UB, G II 4, fol. 205: "... ademit nobis Princeps templum [al]terum: reliquit unum: cuius ereptionem cotidie exspectamus. Caeterea benignum se et clementem erga omnes (et erga me imprimis) gerit Universitati (sic enim vocant) clementer confirmaturum se privilegia dixit, quod hodie futurum

ices, unleavened bread, and organs returned to the Palatine churches. He dismissed the influential Reformed statesmen Count Ludwig von Sayn-Wittgenstein, Baron Johann Philipp von Hohensax, and the Chancellor Christoph Ehem.[5] The instructors at the *Paedagogium* and *Collegium Sapientiae*—including Zacharias Ursinus—who could not accept the doctrinal terms of Luther's Catechism were released in September and October.[6] Even the Calvinist Walloon refuge community was forced to leave its quarters in the Schönau cloister and resettle in the territory of Johann Casimir. Finally, the university's theology faculty were released in January of 1578, though they were allowed to retain their residences until May. Erastus had been intimately involved in the effort to preserve their positions, and then to secure fair compensation after their release. Erastus was briefly back in his position as a leading advocate for the Reformed cause among the Heidelberg intellectual community.[7] However, after the dismissal of the theologians, Reformed academics such as Erastus remained in a state of limbo, anticipating that a Lutheran prince might not long require their services. Erastus's mood toward Ludwig's regime soured, and his letters from 1577 and 1578 narrate the story of the steady erosion of the Reformed community's position in Heidelberg: first being reduced to two churches, then to one, and then having to leave the region to receive the Lord's Supper according to Reformed practice.[8]

The ascension of Ludwig did not mean the absolute end of the Reformed confession in the Palatinate, however, because Frederick had anticipated the problem of his Lutheran heir. Therefore, Frederick had carved a substantial principality out of his dominions, though still legally part of the Electoral Palatinate according to the terms of the Golden

spero." Erastus gives another account of the present and rumored changes in a letter to Gwalther, May 10, 1577, ZBZ, A 49, fols. 306–307. See also Alting, *Historia de ecclesiis Palatinis*, 130 (ch. 71).

[5] Erastus reported Olevianus's release in a letter to Gwalther on Dec. 11, (15)76, StAZ, Ms. E II 345, fols. 724–725. Wenzel Zuleger was released on December 8, 1576. Christoph Ehem was not fired until April 30, 1577 but then was placed under house arrest, and an inquiry was launched into his tenure in office. Press, *Calvinismus und Territorialstaat*, 275–276.

[6] Alting, *Historia de ecclesiis Palatinis*, 133–134 (chs. 72–73).

[7] Alting, *Historia de ecclesiis Palatinis*, 132 (ch. 72); Erastus to Grynaeus, Jan. 15, (15)78, Basel UB, G II 4, fol. 215; Heidelberg, Universitätsarchiv Heidelberg, MS A-160/11, fols. 136–197.

[8] E.g., Erastus to Grynaeus, April 30, (15)77, Basel UB, G II 4, fol. 205; Erastus to Gwalther, May 10, 1577, ZBZ, A 49, fols. 306–307; Erastus to Grynaeus, June 29, (15)77, Basel UB, G II 4, fol. 201; Erastus to Grynaeus, Aug. 5, (15)77, Basel UB, G II 4, fols. 203–204.

Bull, to be administered by his other surviving son Johann Casimir. This principality, with its domains concentrated on the western side of the Rhine, was known as Pfalz-Lautern, after Johann Casimir's principal residence city of Kaiserslautern. Johann Casimir founded something of a shadow academy of the University of Heidelberg dubbed the *Casimirianum* in Neustadt an der Weinstraße.[9] Such luminaries as Girolamo Zanchi, Zacharias Ursinus, Franciscus Junius, and Daniel Tossanus moved to Neustadt. Olevianus, who had never been particularly favored by Johann Casimir, was not invited to join the Neustadt faculty. Instead, he landed an influential pastoral position in Berleburg in the home territory of the recently released Palatine chief steward, Count Ludwig von Wittgenstein, before ultimately crowning what became a distinguished theological career as the first theology professor at the new Reformed academy in Herborn.[10] Ursinus, on the other hand, though he seemed to favor accepting a position in Bernese territory, was not released from Palatine service by Johann Casimir and thus took up a post in Neustadt.[11] Pierre Boquin accepted the Bernese offer and joined the reconstituted Lausanne Academy. While a number of noteworthy intellectuals moved on, a critical mass transferred to Neustadt. As an academic and publishing center, Neustadt was an intellectual bulwark for the Reformed faith in an era of active Lutheran consolidation in the empire. The principality of Pfalz-Lautern proved critical in allowing the Reformed confession to survive the Lutheran restoration.[12]

The accession of Ludwig had left Erastus in an ambiguous if somewhat favored position in the Palatinate. Ludwig seems to have cultivated a genuine affection for Erastus, and he especially prized his medical services. Ludwig offered to make Erastus his personal physician so he could retain his services, but Erastus declined the offer, preferring the independence of his academic position. In addition, Elector Ludwig once displayed

[9] "Neustadt an der Weinstraße" is its current appellation. In the sixteenth century it was distinguished from the other towns of similar names as "Neustadt an der Haardt."

[10] Erastus marveled at a distance, and no doubt with some *Schadenfreude*, as Olevianus experienced difficulty in implementing Reformed liturgical practices into the county of Nassau. Erastus to Gwalther, March 28, 1578, ZBZ, A 49, fols. 316–317.

[11] Erastus's letters with Abraham Musculus and J.J. Grynaeus reveal his affection for Ursinus as well as his frustration with him for his indecision and for stringing the Bernese along.

[12] Press, *Calvinismus und Territorialstaat*, 320–321; Schaab, *Geschichte der Kurpfalz*, 2:53–55. The most active printer in Neustadt was Matthäus Harnisch. Regarding his activities, see Wilhelm Port, "Johann Mayer, Ein Reformierter Drucker des 16. Jahrhunderts," *Zentralblatt für Bibliothekswesen* 59 (1942): 140–155.

his appreciation to Erastus by giving him a wild boar after a successful hunting party. Erastus rather proudly declined payment from the elector, though his generous university salary and his ability to secure release to travel to other lucrative patrons would seem to have been compensation enough. Though Erastus had other career options, he was committed to remaining in Heidelberg as long as circumstances would allow.[13] His professional position was strong, and he kept up a vibrant publishing career in Ludwig's Heidelberg. Erastus's final salvo against Paracelsus, the *Disputation on Potable Gold*, which had been composed in the late days of Frederick's reign, was published in 1578.[14] Likewise, he expanded his critique of Johann Weyer in 1577 and published it the following year. His final work of the Heidelberg era, the *Disputation on Putrefaction*, examined Aristotle's conception of putrefaction and reconciled it with Galen's similar concepts. In the dedication epistle to Elector Ludwig VI, Erastus reflected on his long service to the University of Heidelberg and praised Ludwig as a "prince, patron and father." He likewise defended the art of medicine as one of God's gifts to humans and recognized the physician as the instrument of God.[15]

The first months of Ludwig's reign had brought a welcome respite from the nearly continual strife that had engaged Erastus from 1568 right up until the pious elector's death. A decisive return to a moderate form of Lutheranism in keeping with the Melanchthonian and Upper German heritage of the Palatine Reformation proved to be something of an anachronistic step for Ludwig. The coming of the Heidelberg Catechism as well as the uncovering of a "Crypto-Calvinist" cell in Saxony had added momentum to the movement to consolidate the Lutheran Reformation in the empire and to definitively exclude Sacramentarians. Jakob Andreae and David Chytraeus led the effort which eventually resulted in the drafting of the *Formula of Concord* in the spring of 1577. As in many south German territories, there was a fair measure of debate between the Lutheran theologians of the Palatinate regarding subscribing to the formula. While Ludwig himself was reluctant to sign the *Formula of Concord*, he eventually acceded to political pressure and subscribed.[16]

[13] Erastus to Grynaeus, June 29, (15)77, Basel UB, G II 4, fol. 201; Erastus to A. Musculus, Nov. 23, (15)77, Autograph, Zofingen, no. 1.53.

[14] *De auro potabili* is discussed in chapter 8.

[15] Erastus, *Disputatio de putredine*, 3–8.

[16] Press, *Calvinismus und Territorialstaat*, 287–289. Erastus reported the elector's subscription to Grynaeus on Sept. 9, 1579, Basel UB, G II 4, fol. 241.

One can track the inexorable progress of the *Formula of Concord*—what Erastus and his partisans derided as the "Pandora"—in Erastus's correspondence. He nevertheless drew some satisfaction at the continual Lutheran infighting, particularly the conflict between Andreae and Cyriacus Spangenberg.[17] Indeed, since Erastus no longer had Olevianus and Dathenus to complain about, he now directed his abuse at the leading Lutheran theologians of the region. Beyond a narration of the changing theological climate, his later correspondence from Heidelberg is filled with commentary about unruly students, management of shipments of wine and cheese, and efforts to liquidate his increasingly large investments.

Adherence to the *Formula of Concord* itself did not change the religious landscape of the Palatinate. Ludwig did not impose subscription on his political advisors, and many Reformed councilors served throughout his reign.[18] Although Ludwig was initially inclined to allow the non-theologians among the Reformed academics to keep their posts, in time he acceded to pressure from his advisors and adopted a harder line. The requirement to subscribe to the Lutheran *Formula of Concord* made it impossible for Reformed university faculty to remain. Erastus quit Heidelberg in the fall of 1580.[19]

Erastus's Last Years in Basel 1580–1583

Though he received offers from Bern and later from Marburg, Erastus chose Basel as his place of refuge.[20] While tempted by the Bernese offer, the chance to live near the family of his sister-in-law and to assist in

[17] Erastus to Grynaeus, Oct. 7, (15)78, Basel UB, G II 4, fol. 222. Erastus derided Andreae as "Fabellus" or mockingly referred to him by his given name "Schmidlin" in his correspondence. He dubbed Cyriacus Spangenberg the "Substantialist" for his idiosyncratic approach to the question of original sin.

[18] Press, *Calvinismus und Territorialstaat*, 281, 291.

[19] Wesel-Roth, *Thomas Erastus*, 10, 148.

[20] The interest in Erastus from Bern was long standing. (See Wesel-Roth, *Thomas Erastus*, 81.) He was approached again in 1577 by Abraham Musculus with an invitation to Bern. Erastus to Grynaeus, Nov. 24, (15)77, Basel UB, G II 4, fols. 262–263; Feb. 20, [1578], Basel UB, G II 4, fol. 251. On the later occasion Erastus seems to have slightly favored moving to Bern. In December 1580, Landgrave William IV of Hesse-Kassel commissioned François Hotman to recruit Erastus for Marburg and went as far as to stipulate a salary for his services. François and Jean Hotman, *Francisci et Joannis Hotomanorum Patris Ac Filii, Et Clarorum Virorum Ad Eos Epistolae* (Amsterdam: Apud Georgium Gallet, 1700), 141–142.

the promotion of the Reformed cause stacked the deck in Basel's favor. Of course, returning to Basel was more of a homecoming than an exile. Although Erastus had been away for many decades, through his relations with the Grynaeus clan and his frequent publications with Perna's Basel publishing house, as well as hosting Basel students at the University of Heidelberg, Erastus was a well known person within the city's intellectual community.[21] The Moffett episode, in which the Englishman's theses that defamed Erastus had been censured at the university, had likewise demonstrated that Erastus possessed clout in Basel's academic circles. His wife's desire to be near her sister was likely the decisive factor in the move to Basel. Since Thomas and Isotta had no children of their own, all of their familial affection was lavished on the household of Johann Jakob and Lavinia Grynaeus.

Erastus would thus have the chance to end his academic career where his first exposure to university life had begun. Though the University of Basel was comparable to the University of Heidelberg in quality, it was a more provincial institution. Whereas few of the Heidelberg faculty had been Palatine natives during its recent prominence under Frederick the Pious, the University of Basel was largely staffed by Baslers. For example, Theodor Zwinger and Felix Platter occupied the university's two medical chairs on Erastus's return. The decision of Erastus as well as Simon Grynaeus to return to Basel created potential problems for the talent laden but financially strapped institution. Erastus's financial independence likely facilitated the move; he had already achieved financial security through his generous remuneration at the University of Heidelberg—he had received as much as three times the salary of some of the professors on the arts faculty—and through his private medical practice.[22] The university accommodated its eminent if now unemployed alumnus by bending the rules, though moving Erastus into one of the already occupied medical chairs was out of the question since promotion at the University of Basel was primarily a matter of internal seniority. There had been some discussion of adding a third medical chair in the late 1570s, but the financial crisis brought on by medical professor Isaak Keller's mishandling of the St. Peter's foundation precluded adding

[21] For example he hosted Johann Heinrich Pantaleon and Georg Keller, both sons of prominent Basel intellectuals.

[22] See Christopher Burchill, "Die Universität zu Heidelberg und der 'Fromme' Kurfürst," 239.

an additional position.[23] Although both of the university's medical chairs were filled, Erastus was immediately received into the *consilium medicorum*, a move which deviated from the university's customs.[24] Erastus lectured in the faculty of arts, whose positions were almost always lower in prestige and pay than the higher faculties of law, theology, and medicine in that era, and was formally appointed to the chair of Ethics on January 17, 1582, which may suggest that he had not drawn any income from the university until that point. In fact, he allocated his university salary to the maintenance of Simon Grynaeus's widow.[25] Entering with a chair in the arts faculty was completely in keeping with a Basel university trajectory, and Zwinger had followed a similar path a few years earlier.[26] Basel's faculty was overflowing with medical talent. The elder Jean Bauhin had a position on the arts faculty and likewise belonged to the *consilium medicorum*. His more famous son Caspar Bauhin would join the Basel faculty as a professor of Greek in 1582. With Erastus, Zwinger, Bauhin, and Platter, the medical personnel of the University of Basel during Erastus's brief tenure was far superior to any combination of faculty which had been in residence in Heidelberg during Erastus's stay there, and Basel likely possessed the most illustrious faculty of northern Europe during this period.

Though he was briefly engaged in a diplomatic effort to assist the increasingly isolated Reformed party in Strasbourg, Erastus devoted himself primarily to medical and philosophical interests in his last years.[27] During Erastus's short tenure in Basel he promoted at least seven

[23] Regarding "der Kellerische Handel," which would cramp the finances of the University of Basel for decades, see Thommen, *Geschichte der Universität Basel, 1532–1632*, 214–217. Erastus had been on excellent terms with Keller. In fact, Keller owed Erastus some money, but this was likely for his son's board and general profligacy in Heidelberg, which is abundantly documented in Erastus's correspondence with Gryaneus from 1577. The University of Basel released Keller in 1580.

[24] As Thommen recounts, "Hier wurde er am 10 Januar 1581 in das Kollegium und gegen die Gewohnheit am selben Tag auch noch ins Consilium medicorum 'wegen seiner ausgezeichneten Kenntnisse' aufgenommen," *Geschichte der Universität Basel*, 281. See also Albrecht Burckhardt, *Geschichte der Medizinischen Facultät zu Basel, 1460–1900* (Basel: F. Reinhardt, 1917).

[25] *Athenae rauricae*, 429: "Basileam a. 1580 ad adfinem istum profectus est, ubi d. 17. Jan. 1582. professionem Ethices obtinuit, quam vero is in gratiam viduae Sim, Grynaei, J. Jac. fratris, nonnisi vicario nomine & ea conditione accipere voluit, ut integrum salarium illi viduae cederet." Simon Grynaeus died on Sept. 4, 1582.

[26] Though possessing an M.D. since 1559, Zwinger had occupied the chair of Greek from 1565, the chair of Ethics after 1571, and only received a chair of medicine in 1580 (after the Keller affair). Thommen, *Geschichte der Universität Basel, 1532–1632*, 244–245.

[27] Regarding Erastus's church interests in his last years, see Wesel-Roth, *Thomas Erastus*, 88–89.

students in medicine: a number that may not sound impressive to modern ears, but which represented a bumper crop at a provincial university like Basel with few medical students.[28] Erastus continued to write and publish until his death. He composed two weighty tomes which have received practically no modern scholarly attention. The first was a critique of the Italian physician Conte da Monte's (d. 1587) five-volume interpretation of Galen's conception of disease. In his dedication of the work to the famed diplomat Lazarus von Schwendi, Erastus explained that Da Monte had taken it upon himself to assess the contributions of the great physicians of the century. Since Da Monte reckoned Erastus among these, he was naturally intrigued by the work. On finding many grievous errors in the book, Erastus decided to write a response. Da Monte alleged that German physicians had departed from Galen's concept of disease. Erastus in turn defended the German physicians and alleged that Da Monte accepted Galen's views too uncritically.[29] Da Monte in turn answered Erastus's critique, continuing his assault on Erastus and the other "new physicians" such as Jean Fernel and Girolamo Argenterio, though the response was not published before Erastus's death.[30] In the second book from his Basel period, the final book published in his lifetime, Erastus responded to a critique of his *Disputation on Putrefaction* by Arcangelo Mercenari (d. 1585).[31] Erastus's death in late 1583 left yet another dissatisfied opponent, though Mercenari answered Erastus's retort in hope that other scholars would champion Erastus's side

[28] See the bibliography. These students included Robert Augier, Heinrich Lavater, Theophil Mader, Lazarus Mayenschein, Christian Person, Hieronymus Reussner, and Andreas Ruinella. Regarding the Frenchman Robert Augier, see Bietenholz, *Basle and France*, 71. On the pervasive trend of low medical enrollments, see Malcolm Crystal, "Medicine in Vienna in the Sixteenth and Seventeenth Centuries," (Ph.D. diss., University of Virginia, 1994).

[29] Stübler, *Geschichte der medizinischen Fakultät der Universität Heidelberg 1386–1925*, 50.

[30] Da Monte's original work was titled *De morbis ex Galeni sententia Libri Quinque ... (1580)*. Erastus countered with *Comitis Montani Vincentini Novi Medicorum Censoris, quinque librorum de Morbis nuper editorum Viva Anatome: In qua multa artis medicae capita accuratissimè declarantur a Thoma Erasto Philosopho & Medico* (Basel: Pietro Perna, 1581). Da Monte's response was titled *Defensio Librorum Suorum De Morbis, Adversus Thomam Erastum* (Venice: Franciscus Zilettus, 1584). See Peter H. Niebyl's analysis of the larger background of this controversy: "Sennert, Van Helmont, and Medical Ontology," *Bulletin of the History of Medicine* 45 (1971): 115–137.

[31] *Thomae Erasti ad Archangeli Mercenarii philosophi Patavini Disputationem de putredine responsio* (Response of Thomas Erastus to the disputation concerning putrefaction of Arcangelo Mercenari, philosopher of Padua) (Basel: Konrad Waldkirch, 1583).

of the debate.[32] Though little studied today, both of these controversies continued to resound well into the seventeenth century.[33]

Erastus's health had weakened over the last decade, and he had experienced numerous ailments since the mid-1570s. A bout with pneumonia ended his life. Though apparently not quite sixty, he had enjoyed a full life by sixteenth-century standards. He would not be lacking for companions when he entered the heavenly city. The plague, which had ravaged Basel in the summer 1582, had born away his printer Perna and his close friend Simon Grynaeus.[34] Ursinus passed away the next spring in Neustadt, and Elector Ludwig VI died in November in 1583.[35] Although Erastus was personally fond of Ludwig, in his last days he probably glimpsed the hope that Ludwig's passing meant that the Reformed faith would return to Heidelberg. Two days after Christmas, Count Georg Ernst of Henneberg died, whom Erastus had faithfully served for more than twenty-five years. Four days later, on the last day of 1583, Erastus joined them in death. Erastus was laid to rest on Jan. 2, 1584 in Basel's *Peterskirche*. His monument aptly summed up his career as "not Hermes Trismegistus, but an acute philosopher, an elegant physician, and a sincere theologian."[36] In his testament he endowed foundations at Heidelberg and Basel to enable Reformed students to study medicine. Upon his wife's death, the universities jointly received the handsome bequest of 3,200 fl.—ten times the annual salary of a well-paid professor.[37]

---

[32] Arcangelo Mercenari, *Disputatio de putredine … adversus Thomam Erastum* (Padua: Paulus Meietus, 1583); idem, *Adversus Erasti responsionem, secunda de putredine disputatio, in qua, praeter ea, quae ad exactam putredinis notitiam spectant, plurima philosophi: e medicinaeque studiosis necessaria explicantur …* (Padua: Paulus Meietus, 1585). See Thorndike, *History of Magic and Experimental Science*, 5:666.

[33] E.g., Marco degli Oddi, *Pro sua tutanda de putredine sententia apologia nunc primum in lucem edita, in qua … A. Mecenarii et T. Erasti … disputationes exutiuntur* (Padua, 1585); Caspar Hofmann, *Animadversiones in Com. Montani libros quinque De morbis, et Thomae Erasti anatomen eorundum, nec non ant-Erastica ejusdem Montani* (Amsterdam: Joannes Janssonius, 1641). As discussed below, Caspar Hofmann was a student of Erastus's successor Philipp Scherbe.

[34] See Erastus to Gwalther, Basel, Sept. 7, (15)82, ZBZ (Sim.), Ms. S 140, Nr. 158.

[35] The Jurist Nicolaus Cisner, who had taken over Erastus's house in Heidelberg, passed away on the same day as Ursinus (May 6, 1583). Leopold Löwenstein, "Nicholas Cisner aus Mosbach," *Zeitschrift für die Geschichte des Oberrheins*, Neue Folge 22 (1907): 711–716.

[36] Printed in Adam, *Vitae Germanorum Medicorum* (Heidelberg: Johannes Georg Geyder, 1620), 244–245; Bonnard, *Thomas Éraste*, 206.

[37] The sum was split between the two institutions. The bequest continued to fund two fellowships in Basel until 1715. Wesel-Roth, *Thomas Erastus*, 10; Burckhardt, *Geschichte*

Erastian Legacies

After Erastus's death, five individuals came to the forefront as guardians of his legacy. Johann Jakob Grynaeus continued to represent the theological tradition of Erastus, though from the vantage point of Erastus's death in 1583 one could hardly have imagined how successful he would be in advocating the Reformed faith in Basel and Heidelberg. Erastus's legacy in the field of medicine would be enhanced by his former students Philipp Scherbe (Scherbius; 1555–1605), Heinrich Smet (1535/37–1614), and Theophil Mader (1541–1604). Interestingly, the most important contributor to the Erastian legacy was Erastus's widow's second husband. In this final section, I will review Erastus's intellectual afterlife and make some observations regarding the continued relevance of his work in the late sixteenth and early seventeenth centuries.

In confessional matters the future belonged to Erastus's allies in both Heidelberg and Basel. After Ludwig's death in 1583, Johann Casimir, acting adroitly to exclude his co-regents from the Palatine administration, was able to reestablish the Reformed confession as regent for his young nephew Frederick IV.[38] Johann Casimir called none other than Johann Jakob Grynaeus to aid his reform of the university and appointed him to the theological faculty in 1584. The irony of this turn of events has seldom been recognized. Not only was Johann Jakob Grynaeus in many senses Erastus's intellectual heir, his own brother Simon had once been imprisoned during the height of the Calvinist disciplinary fervor for his alleged role in the Antitrinitarian affair. The restoration of the Reformed faith under Johann Casimir was not only a repudiation of Ludwig's Lutheranism but a tacit repudiation of the extreme Calvinist position typified by Olevianus.

Erastus would also have been pleased with the confessional developments which occurred in Basel after his death. When Simon Sulzer died in 1585, Johann Jakob Grynaeus, whose stay in Heidelberg had been limited by Basel's refusal to accept his permanent resignation, was chosen to succeed him as head of the Basel church.[39] Under Grynaeus's leadership, Basel was brought into accord with the other Swiss Reformed

der Medizinischen Facultät zu Basel, 128; Basel, Staatsarchiv des Kantons Basel-Stadt, Universitätsarchiv Urkunde no. 14; C 12, fol. 22; L 9, fol. 46.

[38] Press, *Calvinismus und Territorialstaat*, 322.

[39] See F. Weiss, "Johann Jakob Grynaeus," 171–180; Guggisberg, *Basel in the Sixteenth Century*, 46–48; Press, *Calvinismus und Territorialstaat*, 331.

churches.[40] Though formal subscription to the *Second Helvetic Confession* would not follow until 1675, Basel's flirtation with Lutheranism was over. Basel became a solid member of the Reformed communion due in large part to the efforts of Grynaeus and his son-in-law Amandus Polanus von Polansdorf. It is also noteworthy that Grynaeus trained that other great internal critic of orthodox Calvinism, Jacobus Arminius, who studied in Basel during the last months of Erastus's life.[41]

As Johann Jakob Grynaeus was restoring Erastus's religious vision in Heidelberg and Basel, Scherbe, Mader, and Smet advanced their deceased mentor's medical reputation. From Bischoffzell in Switzerland, the physician Scherbe had studied with Erastus in Heidelberg. He was Erastus's immediate successor in the chair of Ethics at the University of Basel, before becoming a medical professor at the Altdorf Academy. Through his own work, and through his students Ernst Soner and Caspar Hofmann, he passed along the basic philosophical-medical views of Erastus into the seventeenth century.[42] Smet reprinted Erastus's *De occultis pharmacorum potestatibus* and a few other treatises and letters by Erastus in a collected volume entitled *Miscellanea Medica*. The work grants insight into the reception of Erastus's anti-Paracelsian works as well as Smet's more conciliatory position towards Paracelsian medicine.[43] Mader's edition of Erastus's *Disputations and Medical Letters* paid more direct tribute to Erastus's legacy.[44] Theophil was one of three Mader brothers from Frauenfeld in Thurgau, Switzerland who studied in Heidelberg, and he later joined the Heidelberg University medical faculty himself. The disputations were particularly noteworthy, since they represented the only occasion when a number of the less known members of the Heidelberg

[40] See Max Geiger, *Die Basler Kirche und Theologie im Zeitalter der Hochorthodoxie* (Zollikon: Evangelischer Verlag, 1952), 40–55.

[41] Thommen, *Geschichte der Universität Basel*, 1532–1632, 131–132.

[42] *Athenae rauricae*, 430; Ralf Bröer, "Antiparacelsismus und Dreieinigkeit: Medizinischer Antitrinitarismus von Thomas Erastus (1524–1583) bis Ernst Soner (1572–1605)," *Berichte zur Wissenschaftsgeschichte* 29 (2006): 137–154, especially, 141–148. Caspar Hofmann was also a significant figure in the continental reception of William Harvey's theories regarding the circulation of blood.

[43] Smet, ed., *Miscellanea ... Medica* (see above chapter 8, note 129). He also reprinted Erastus's *Explicatio trium questionum de medicamentis purgantibus*. For more on Smet's conception of Paracelsus, see Külhmann and Telle, "Humanismus und Medizin," 277–281.

[44] *Thomae Erasti Philosophi et Medici celeberrime, Disputationum & Epistolarum Medicinalium volumen doctissimum. Nunc recens in lucem editum, opera et studio Theophili Maderi Philosophiae ac Medicinae doctoris, ac Physices in Academia Heydelbergensi Professoris ordinarij* (Zürich: Johannes Wolf, 1595).

faculty ever made it into print.[45] The letters documented the interaction of the elite physicians of central Europe, similar to Lorenz Scholz von Rosenau's more expansive collections, of which Mader's edition shared some material.[46]

Presbyterianism Triumphant

While Erastus's close associates labored to secure the legacy of the Reformed confession in Basel and the Palatinate, it seemed Erastus's devastating attack on presbyterial church polity by state mandate had been contained and would likely be forgotten. For more than ten years after their deaths, Elector Frederick's and Bullinger's wish for public peace was largely maintained. In the meantime the presbyterial-consistorial model of church organization and discipline seemed to be sweeping the Reformed world. Without a strong sovereign to challenge kirk leaders, Presbyterian hegemony over the Scottish church was relatively unchallenged until James VI came into his majority. In late sixteenth-century France, where the stewardship over the church by a benevolent Protestant sovereign was not in the offing, the Gnesio-Calvinists experienced a challenge from Jean Morély's vision of a more democratic, congregational model of church organization.[47] The French church had been in the process of elaborating a classical-consistorial organizational model since the publication of the *Discipline Ecclésiastique* in 1559, and rejected those who questioned the legitimacy of deploying excommunication as a tool of ecclesiastical discipline at the Synod of La Rochelle in 1571.[48] Similarly the Netherlandish church in exile had taken decisive action to assert the independence of the church consistory to control church discipline, thereby directly repudiating Erastus's views at the 1571 Emden Synod. Since there was significant overlap in the protagonists among the Heidelberg Calvinists and the organizers of the synod—including Petrus

[45] E.g., Hieronymus Niger and Sigismund Melanchthon.

[46] Scholz, *Epistolarum philosophicarum, medicinalium, ac chymicarum a summis nostrae aetatis philosophis ac medicis exaraturum, volumen*. See the bibliography.

[47] See chapter 6, note 22.

[48] Thus Erastus was implicitly, but not explicitly, condemned at La Rochelle, as Beza explained to Bullinger in a letter from Nov. 13, 1571, *CB*, 12: 221–227 (no. 871): "Imo ne in Erastum quidem tale decretum factum esse scio et testor, qui Synodo non tantum interfui, verum etiam praefui." The "doctor" impugned there has been taken by some to be Erastus, though Robert Kingdon has rejected this attribution. Kingdon, *Geneva and the Consolidation of the French Protestant Movement*, 98.

Dathenus and Petrus Colonius—this rejection should come as no surprise.[49] In short, the Calvinist church "under the cross" had made up its mind about Erastianism. England, Hungary, and the German-speaking cantons of Switzerland had not yet fully conformed to this Gnesio-Calvinist model. Yet even in England a vigorous Puritan party led by the likes of Thomas Cartwright and receiving encouragement from abroad from Beza was agitating to install their vision of consistorial-presbyterial discipline by "divine right" in the Anglican church. The international Reformed church was undergoing a process of confessional homogenization not unlike that occurring within German Lutheranism, in both occasions leaving articulate minorities on the sidelines. Might Erastus's theories, and the general Zurich vision of church-state relations, revive when the political conditions were more propitious?

Giacomo Castelvetro and the Explicatio gravissimae quaestionis

That Erastus's name has retained a degree of fame across the centuries is primarily due to the efforts of his widow Isotta's second husband, Giacomo Castelvetro (aka Jacobus Castelvitreus; 1546–1616).[50] From Modena, Castelvetro was likely drawn to Protestantism and radical social thought through the influence of his uncle, famed literary critic Ludovico Castelvetro. Northern Europe offered a measure of intellectual freedom unavailable in his homeland, and Giacomo followed his uncle north. In Basel his path crossed with that of the widowed Isotta de' Canonici. As

[49] The direct connections between Emden and Heidelberg are outlined in J.F. Gerhard Goeters, "Die Emder Synode von 1571," in *Emder Synode. 1571–1971*, ed. Elwin Lomberg (Neukirchen-Vluyn: Neukirchener Verlag, 1973), 183–202; W. Nijenhuis, "The Synod of Emden 1571," in *Ecclesia Reformata: Studies on the Reformation* (Leiden: E.J. Brill, 1994), 2:101–124, especially 113–114. For the Synod's pronouncements on church discipline, see J.F. Gerhard Goeters, ed., *Die Akten der Synode der Niederländischen Kirchen zu Emden vom 4.-13. Oktober 1571* [*BGLRK* 34] (Neukirchen-Vluyn: Neukirchener Verlag, 1971) articles 25–34 (pp. 31–33) and ⟨http://dutchrevolt.leidenuniv.nl/English/Sources%20English/15711004.htm⟩.

[50] What follows is largely based on John Tedeschi, "The Cultural Contributions of Italian Protestant Reformers in the Late Renaissance," 127–151; idem, "Tomasso Sassetti's Account of the St. Bartholomew's Day Massacre," in *The Massacre of St. Bartholomew: Reappraisals and Documents*, ed. Alfred Soman, 99–112 (The Hague: Martinus Nijhoff, 1974). See also Sheila Dimsey, "Giacopo Castelvetro," *The Modern Language Review* 23 (1928): 424–431 and Eleanor Rosenberg, "Giacopo Castelvetro: Italian Publisher in Elizabethan London and His Patrons," *The Huntington Library Quarterly* 6 (1943): 119–148.

Castelvetro was much younger than Isotta, one imagines that monetary considerations must have factored heavily into his decision to marry her in 1587. Castelvetro did not assume possession of Erastus's entire estate, though he certainly obtained a number of Erastus's unpublished manuscripts.[51] The Castelvetros resettled in London, where Giacomo became engaged in a number of noteworthy literary activities. Of Castelvetro's significance in England, John Tedeschi remarked, "with ... John Florio, he may be ranked as a leading champion of Italian culture in Elizabethan and Jacobean England."[52] For our interests, his most important exploit was his publication of Erastus's *Explicatio gravissimae quaestionis* in 1598. Though the book bears the imprint of the fictitious printer "Baocius Sultaceterus" (an anagram of "Iacobus Casteluetrus") at "Pesclavius," we have reliable sources which document that it was in fact printed in London by John Wolfe, the royal printer, with the support, and perhaps even the prompting, of John Whitgift, the Archbishop of Canterbury, and John Aylmer, the Bishop of London, who resisted the Puritan ambition to establish a presbyterian form of church government in England.[53] The next year Castelvetro continued his good services to Erastus's legacy in

---

[51] See the preface of Erastus, *Varia Opuscula Medica*.

[52] Tedeschi, "Tomasso Sassetti's Account of the St. Bartholomew's Day Massacre," 100.

[53] *Explicatio gravissimae quaestionis, utrùm Excommunicatio, quatenùs Religionem intelligentes & amplexantes, à Sacramentorum usu, propter admissum facinus arcet; mandato nitatur Divino, an excogitata sit ab hominibus* (Pesclavius: Apud Baocium Sultaceterum [London: John Wolfe], 1589). Regarding publication of the Explicatio, see Bonnard, *Thomas Éraste*, 186–193; Figgis, "Erastus and Erastianism," 77; K.T. Butler, "Giacomo Castelvetro, 1546–1616," *Italian Studies* 5 (1950): 11–13; Wesel-Roth, *Thomas Erastus*, 149, note 17; Tedeschi, "Tomasso Sassetti's Account of the St. Bartholomew's Day Massacre," 101; Walton, "Der Streit zwischen Thomas Erastus und Caspar Olevian," 239. Whitgift's participation is confirmed by the entry in the Stationer's Register: "20 Junii 1589 A treatise of Thomas Erastus de Excommunicatione. Reported by master ffortescue [*sic*] to be alowed by the Archbishop of Canterbury." Quoted in Dimsey, "Giacopo Castelvetro," 427. Figgis notes a comment from Selden which implied that the printer Wolfe had been rewarded by the Privy Council (p. 77). Beza reported the following to J.J. Grynaeus on Dec. 8, 1589 regarding the publication: "De Libro Erasti, quem mihi significant fratres Londinenses, conscio Londinensi episcopo clam et excussum et magna ex parte in Anglia divenditum, quid tibi faciendum videatur, quaeso ut mihi significes." (*CB*, 30:306–308 (no. 2065); Bonnard, *Thomas Éraste*, 191). The current occupant of the see of London was John Aylmer, someone who, like Whitgift, would have found Erastus's work quite useful in opposing the Puritan faction. Likewise, Daniel Tossanus reported to Grynaeus on Oct. 16, 1589: "Quisquis Autor fuit aut suasor illius editionis, inimicus est pacis Ecclesiarum et male feriatus, cum per Dei gratiam illae controversiae cum Autoribus sint sopitae. Credo aliquem Episcopum Anglum illa scripta fortasse ab illo Italo impetrasse qui viduam D. Erasti duxit." Friedrich W. Cuno, *Daniel Tossanus der Ältere: Professor der Theologie und Pastor (1541–1602)* (Amsterdam: Scheffer, 1898), 2:100.

editing a beautiful folio volume of assorted medical works, issued by the Wechel press of Frankfurt.[54]

Beyond his association with the name of Erastus, Castelvetro led an adventurous life. He entered the service of the Scottish and later the English court. He served as Italian master to King James VI (later James I of England) in Edinburgh from 1592–1594. That Erastus's chief publicist served as the tutor to this future champion of the divine right of kings is particularly noteworthy, and it has been reported that Castelvetro offered to bestow one of Erastus's treatises in his possession as a gift upon the young king.[55] After a stay in Copenhagen and diplomatic activity for the Swedish court, Castelvetro returned to the service of the Stuart monarchy, a status which saved him from the Inquisition's tentacles in 1611.

Castelvetro's publication of the *Explicatio gravissimae quaestionis* finally exposed to the world the major rift on the question of church discipline between the Genevan and Zurich schools of Reformed Protestantism which Bullinger, Beza, and Elector Frederick had hitherto successfully suppressed. The publication was a most unwelcome airing of dirty laundry within the Reformed community, and church leaders in Geneva, Zurich, Heidelberg, and Basel worked collectively to respond to the provocation. Their basic thrust was to exonerate Erastus and blame the entire affair on Erastus's widow and her husband Castelvetro.

The publication of Erastus's work caught Johann Jakob Grynaeus off guard and involved him in a test of loyalties between his deceased relative, patron, and friend Erastus and his current close colleague and collaborator Beza. It was curious on the surface that Grynaeus would not have had a role in publishing Erastus's magnum opus, had it genuinely been authorized, and Grynaeus's first task was to proclaim loudly that he had had nothing to do with it. In his private correspondence with Beza, he uncharitably dubbed his sister-in-law Isotta "Xanthippe," the legendarily shrewish wife of Socrates, and alleged that she had already run through a large chunk of Erastus's estate and thus that the publication was likely motivated by financial gain. Grynaeus also asserted that he was unaware of any explicit dying mandate of Erastus to print the text, as Castelvetro had alleged on the title page of *Explicatio gravissimae quaestionis*.[56] Nevertheless, while distancing himself from Isotta and his new

[54] Erastus, *Varia Opuscula Medica*. See the bibliography.
[55] Butler, "Giacomo Castelvetro," 14.
[56] Grynaeus to Beza, November 4, 1589, *CB*, 30:280–283 (no. 2058).

brother-in-law, Grynaeus did not repudiate Erastus or his views directly, and his timid diplomatic responses to Beza revealed a man awkwardly seeking to remain true to both of his friends and to promote peace in the church.[57]

If Grynaeus was caught in the middle by the publication, Beza was the party injured by Castelvetro's action. Beza was furious and even went so far as to attempt to have the copies of the text which had been sent to the Frankfurt fair seized. The text was particularly galling as from Beza's perspective the only modern theologian who might have agreed with Erastus was Zwingli.[58] He was inclined to defend himself by composing a new repudiation of Erastus's substantive *Confirmatio thesium*, which had offered a frontal assault on Beza's defense of presbyterial discipline. Such a retort would be problematic, however, since Erastus's work had revealed in a salient way the genuine differences of opinion regarding church discipline between Zurich and Geneva. Thus it would be difficult to answer Erastus fully without in some way impugning the Zurich tradition and potentially reigniting the original conflict. Furthermore, church leaders such as Tossanus in Heidelberg argued that a new work was not warranted.[59]

Rather than opposing Erastus with a new text, Beza elected to allow his repudiation of Erastus's original theses, the *Pious and Moderate Tract concerning True Excommunication and the Christian Presbytery* (Tractatus pius et moderatus), stand as his primary answer to the appearance of the *Explicatio gravissimae quaestionis*.[60] This idea had been vetted from Zurich to Heidelberg and had garnered broad consent. Beza's treatise,

[57] See the letters of Grynaeus to Beza from November 24, 1589, *CB*, 30:301–305 (no. 2064) and, especially, from April 5, [1590], *CB*, 31:98–100 (no. 2096).

[58] Beza to Grynaeus, Dec. 8, 1589, *CB*, 30:306–308 (no. 2065): "Scripsi ea de re D. Tussano nostro, ut, si fieri posse ac debere istud posse Illustrissimus Princeps judicabit, Francofurti sequestrentur quae audio adhuc illic latere exemplaria in Paschales nundinas a Castelvetro tardius illuc appulso reservatus, et ad Reginam Angliae aliquid ea de re scribatur.

Cogitabam simpliciter et paucis, nulla prorsus cum ipsius scriptoris notatione, posse ad singulis ipsius objectiones responderi, et libello subjici Patrum ab Ecclesiae christianae constitutae exordio, ac etiam recentiorum insignium aetatis nostrae theologorum, ne D. Zvinglio quidem excepto, hac de re sententiam ipsorum verbis perscriptam subjicere. Nisi tamen nisis ex tuo consilio et ipsorum praesertim Tigurinorum fratrum consensu scribam."

[59] As reported in a letter from Grynaeus to Beza, Dec. 29, 1589, *CB*, 30:322–325 (no. 2070).

[60] Theodore Beza, *Tractatus Pius et Moderatus de vera Excommunicatione, & christiano Presbyterio* … (Geneva: Jean Le Preux, 1590).

though an apt defense of the presbyterial system of church discipline, did not attempt to respond directly to Erastus's theses in their sharpened form and, more importantly, did not contain an answer to Erastus's voluminous *Confirmatio thesium*, which had done so much to buttress the biblical foundations of Erastus's argument. Beza's specific response to the 1589 publication was a long introductory letter which put both Erastus's and his texts in their original contexts and argued—drawing in support from the recollections of Grynaeus and the late Theodor Zwinger—that Erastus had not given a death bed order to his wife to publish the work. An extremely vexing feature of the Castelvetro edition for Beza was the inclusion in an appendix of many letters from Zurich which were fundamentally supportive of Erastus. Beza parried this assault by employing other statements from Gwalther and Bullinger that accepted the concept of excommunication within ecclesiastical discipline. Beza likewise adopted a magnanimous tone and stressed that the Zurich and Genevan traditions had been able to live in harmony and mutual respect on this question. This was rhetorically shrewd in that he neither directly assaulted Erastus nor had to worry about the deceased Bullinger or Gwalther taking offense at his characterization of their positions. Beza was so satisfied with his charitable attitude toward Erastus that he alleged that Erastus himself would have been content with the new preface to the *Tractatus pius et moderatus*.[61] All of the opprobrium was reserved for the malefactors who had published Erastus's work.[62]

The publication of the *Explicatio gravissimae quaestionis* revealed a variety of opinions about Erastus and his legacy within the Reformed community. Beza publicly worked hard to refrain from demonizing Erastus and emphasized how the two men had been reconciled prior to Erastus's death. In fact, Beza recounted that he had visited him in Basel, apparently in 1582, and that the two had embraced and parted as friends.[63]

[61] Beza to [Johann-Rudolf] Stumpf, March 15, 1590, *CB*, 31:70–74 (no. 2087): "usque adeo nisi prorsus fallor, moderatum scriptum, ut ne ipsum quidem D. Erastum, si superstes esset, eo offensum iri putem."

[62] The introductory epistle of the *Tractatus* is expertly annotated in *CB*, 31:40–63 (no. 2085).

[63] Beza to [Johann] Wilhelm Stucki, Dec. 22, 1589, *CB*, 30:319–322 (no. 2069): "Quinetiam Basilae D. Erastum ipsum amicissime compellavi a vobis digressus, et ille me vicissim humanissime est complexus; pollicitus etiam sese, si qui ratione fieri posset, ad nos venturum, et nostra propius inspecturum, ut falso quoque existimem ab istis ipsius morientis voluntatem huic editioni praetexi." See also Beza to [Johann-Rudolf] Stumpf, November 19, 1589, *CB*, 30:297–300 (no. 2063): "et quum postea D. Erastus sese

In his private correspondence, however, Beza vented far and wide about the "tragedy" that Erastus had stirred up and hinted at its diabolical origin. Not surprisingly, Erastus's memory was held in higher regard in Zurich. Unlike Beza's ambivalent view, the Zurich *antistes* Johann-Rudolf Stumpf (1530–1592) spoke of the "most excellent Erastus of blessed memory." In fact, Robert Walton argued that the publication of Erastus's work may have been supported by Stumpf and that the letters included in the appendix of the *Explicatio* were perhaps supplied by the Zurich church leaders.[64] With the publication and analysis of Beza's correspondence from 1589–1590 recently at our disposal, it now seems unlikely that the Zurichers were overly enthused about the Castelvetro project, and thus one may assume that the manuscripts of letters from Bullinger and Gwalther had been among Erastus's papers and were not directly sourced from Zurich. Nevertheless, the Zurich church was not eager to reignite the controversy and thus was satisfied to support Beza's moderate response.

While Beza could publicly assert that the publication of Erastus's theses had not been Erastus's dying wish, and it was helpful for the Reformed community in general to accept this assertion, the weight of evidence suggests that the publication of the *Explicatio gravissimae quaestionis* was consonant with Erastus's wishes. When we recall his earlier tentative effort to publish the theses in 1572 and consider that Erastus had revised the preface to the *Explicatio gravissimae quaestionis* around 1580, it seems obvious that Erastus intended the work to be published. In fact, although Grynaeus could assert that he knew nothing of the death bed oath to print the *Explicatio* specifically, he thought it was plausible that Erastus would have had aspirations to publish more of his works.[65] Thus, rather than taking advantage of Erastus or his widow, Castelvetro had done Erastus a good service securing the publication of his life's work.

Basileam recepisset, ibi quoque amicissime ipsum conveni, et ille me vicissim ut fratrem est complexus." The date of 1582 can be derived from comparing the above comments from Beza with this letter from Grynaeus to Beza, November 24, 1589. *CB*, 30:301–305 (no. 2064).

[64] Walton, "Der Streit zwischen Thomas Erastus und Caspar Olevian," 238.

[65] *CB*, 30:301–305 (no. 2064).

The Netherlands: Erastians, Libertines, and Arminians

In the short run, Erastus's ideas on church-state relations found their greatest resonance in the Netherlands. While exiles from the Low Countries had been a driving force behind the Disciplinist victory in Heidelberg, a large anti-disciplinist or "Libertine" faction found Erastus's ideas a useful weapon to wield against the similar aspirations of Calvinist ecclesiastics in the Netherlands who sought to strengthen consistorial discipline and more definitively establish Calvinist orthodoxy as the official state religion. While less known in the narrative of historical theology than the famous Arminian-Gomarist controversy, this contest between Libertines and Calvinists on the question of church discipline predated, and in many senses prefigured, the controversy over predestination.[66] The social contours of this disagreement were quite similar to the Palatine controversy as well. Both Dutch and French Christians who had experienced living "under the cross" either in exile or as an outlawed minority adhered to the rigorist Calvinist position, while political elites in the provinces of Holland seemed to have inclined to something of an Erastian position, at minimum asserting that the state had a right of oversight in matters of ecclesiastical discipline.[67]

Disagreements concerning discipline and how much influence the magistrate would have over the church were already active in the Netherlands in the 1570s and 1580s. Despite the fact that neither Beza's nor Erastus's texts had yet been published, the debate between them formed part of the background of the controversy in the Netherlands—with both advocates and critics of consistorial discipline applying lessons from their Palatine sojourns to the Dutch scene. A key figure in the early debates over discipline was Caspar Coolhaes, an ethnic German pastor who had worked in parishes in the region of the Rhine Palatinate, where he rather manifestly imbibed the Erastian critique of Calvinist discipline in the early 1570s. Coolhaes vigorously asserted the state's rights vis-à-vis the church in this era and was himself excommunicated in 1582.[68]

[66] See Benjamin J. Kaplan, *Calvinists and Libertines: Confession and Community in Utrecht, 1578–1620* (Oxford: Oxford UP, 1995), 3–5, 229–230.

[67] See Christine Kooi, "Pharisees and Hypocrites: A Public Debate over Church Discipline in Leiden, 1586," *ARG* 88 (1997): 258–278; idem, *Liberty and Religion: Church and State in Leiden's Reformation, 1572–1620* (Leiden: Brill, 2000); Jonathan Israel, *The Dutch Republic: Its Rise, Greatness, and Fall 1477–1806* (Oxford: Oxford UP, 1995).

[68] Ulrich Gäbler, "Zur Verbreitung des Zwinglianismus in den Niederlanden und der Fall Caspar Coolhaes 1581/1582," in *Zwingli und Europa*, ed. Peter Blickle et al. (Zürich:

In the early seventeenth century, influential Libertine and Remonstrant leaders read Erastus and borrowed ideas from him, but did not slavishly follow him and thus create an explicitly Erastian faction, as would later occur in seventeenth century England. The originator of the Remonstrant movement, Arminius—who may have met Erastus in Basel—read Erastus and adopted many similar Erastian positions on church-state relations. Ironically, however, Arminius upheld the notion that excommunication was a valid ecclesiastical censure, though optimally it would only be infrequently employed.[69] Another person arguing along Erastian lines was the Remonstrant Johannes Wtenbogaert/Uytenbogaert.[70] Perhaps the most important Dutch follower of Erastus was the Advocate of Holland Johan van Oldenbarnevelt, whom Simon Groenveld has characterized as "a lifelong Erastian."[71] Discerning the transmission of Erastus's ideas to Oldenbarnevelt is not difficult; Oldenbarnevelt matriculated as a student at the University of Heidelberg in the summer of 1568 just as the church discipline controversy erupted. Oldenbarnevelt was apparently the odd man out in Heidelberg in that most of the Netherlandish students were eager disciplinists and thus sided against Erastus. Erastian ecclesiology also influenced Oldenbarnevelt's famous protégé Hugo Grotius, who took up a similar position to Erastus in his work *De Imperio Summarum Potestatum circa Sacra*. In his recent

Vandenhoeck & Ruprecht, 1985), 217–236. Coolhaes worked in either Münzesheim or Monsheim, neither formally part of Palatine territory, but both ca. fifty kilometers from Heidelberg. The lines of transmission here are murky, but nevertheless, as Gäbler has noted, Coolhaes revealed himself to be an "überzeugten Erastianer" (232–233). See also Andrew Pettegree, "The Calvinist Church of Holland," in *Calvinism in Europe 1540–1620*, 172; Kooi, "Pharisees and Hypocrites," 264–268.

[69] Carl Bangs, "'All the Best Bishoprics and Deaneries': The Enigma of Arminian Politics," *Church History* 42 (1973): 5–16 (especially 8–9).

[70] See Douglas Nobbs, *Theocracy and Toleration: A Study of the Disputes in Dutch Calvinism from 1600 to 1650* (Cambridge: UP, 1938), 25–49. This fine study offers extensive coverage of Erastian theory in the Netherlands without making any concrete connection to the antecedents of these conceptions in the work of Erastus, Bullinger, or Gwalther. He does acknowledge Wtenbogaert's dependence on Erastus (p. 47). Gerrit Jan Hoenderdaal describes Wtenbogaert's *Tractaet van t'Ampt ende Authoriteyt eener Hoogher Christelicker Overheydt, in Kerckelicke Saecken* as possessing "close to Erastian views." "Johannes Wtenbogaert" in *OER*, 4:301–302.

[71] S. Groenveld, "Johan van Oldenbarnevelt," in *OER*, 3:173; Geert H. Janssen, *Het stokje van Oldenbarnevelt* (Hilversum: VerLoren, 2001), 17; Toepke, *Die Matrikel der Universität Heidelberg*, 2:47; Jan den Text, *Oldenbarnevelt* (Cambridge: Cambridge UP, 1973), 1:7–8. Den Text concludes, "In later life Oldenbarnevelt developed a great reverence for the supremacy of the temporal authorities, making him a definite, though not an extreme, Erastian" (8).

critical edition of this work, Harm-Jan van Dam has uncovered Grotius's extensive use of Erastus in *De Imperio*, even quoting passages from Beza via Erastus, though he does not mention Erastus's name explicitly in his text.[72] Thus, to a large degree the Heidelberg controversy over church discipline set the agenda for the later debates in the Netherlands. The Erastian-Libertine faction would generally find itself on the losing side of the contest within the church, although the Dutch Reformed Church itself never secured state sanction to impose its disciplinary regime on the entire populace. Rather, consistorial discipline could only be exercised within a voluntary minority church in the United Provinces. Even after the Synod of Dort (1618–1619), the state wielded tremendous influence over the theology and parameters of action of the Reformed Church.

The Reception of Erastus in England

As much as historians of early modern British Isles like to use the term "Erastianism" and frequently employ it retroactively to the reign of Henry VIII, a full-scale history of Erastus's impact on England has yet to be written. Likewise, there is no scholarly consensus as to how significant Erastus's writings were to Anglicans who opposed presbyterial church polity. Fifty years ago, it was common to completely discount the influence of Erastus himself; Erastus was only important as a label for a theory of church-state relations that seemingly could have been as fairly dubbed "Henricianism" in line with the statist ecclesiology of Henry VIII and his councilors. In historical studies Erastus was in danger of becoming another "Nestorius"—an individual who did not necessarily advocate the ideas for which his name became the eponymous symbol. Anglo-American scholars rarely studied Erastus presumably because there was little need to. One example of this Erastus minimalism can been seen

[72] Figgis, "Erastus and Erastianism," 78; Hugo Grotius, *De Imperio Summarum Potestatum Circa Sacra: Critical Edition with Introduction, English Translation and Commentary* [Studies in the History of Christian Thought 102], ed. Harm-Jan Van Dam, 2 vols. (Leiden: Brill, 2001), 1:131: "This important book [*Explicatio Gravissimae Quaestionis*], in which Erastus sets forth his views on the absolute supremacy of state over church, was in Grotius' library. Whereas he made hardly any use of it in *Ordinum Pietas*, he certainly did in *De imperio*: it is an important source for chapter 11, on elders. Grotius repeatedly quotes Beza from Erastus. Moreover, in 9.17 Luther is quoted from it, and rare information about excommunication and the use of common pastures derives from its Appendix." See also *De imperio*, 1:783. Van Dam also notes that Selden recommended Grotius's *De imperio* for those having difficulty acquiring Erastus's work (*De imperio*, 1:107).

in the dismissive assertion of Charles H. George and Katherine George that "English divines almost never refer to the work of Erastus and when they do it is to reject his only original idea: that the power of excommunication should reside with the civil authorities in a Christian polity."[73] Although this comment betrayed an unsophisticated understanding of Erastus's thought, the Georges' basic point that English theologians rarely mentioned Erastus has some validity for the late sixteenth and early seventeenth centuries. Likewise, in a treatment of the influence of Swiss Reformation on the Anglican state church, Helmut Kressner almost completely discounted Erastus's impact on the English scene—though without apparently knowing much about Erastus or England. In this case, the devaluation was based not so much on an accounting of whom the English divines cited but on Kressner's estimation that there was little to be found in Erastus's work that was not already available in Bullinger or Musculus.[74]

This apparent controversy over Erastus's significance in England dissolves with the realization that there was a time lag in the reception of Erastus's work in the British Isles. While Erastus had only a modest impact there in the late sixteenth century, he was to have a profound impact on English ecclesiastical developments in the mid-seventeenth century.[75] Nevertheless, even prior to the publication of Erastus's theses in 1589, there is evidence that Archbishop Whitgift drew content from Erastus's work to buttress his own *Defense of the Answer to the Admonition*.[76] Whitgift's sponsorship of the publication of the *Explicatio gravissimae quaestionis* is apparently reflected in the wide distribution of the book in England even today.[77] The most prominent figure in England's

[73] Charles H. George and Katherine George, *The Protestant Mind of the English Reformation 1570–1640* (Princeton: Princeton UP, 1961), 188.

[74] Helmut Kressner, *Schweizer Ursprünge des anglikanischen Staatskirchentums* [*SVRG* 170] (Gütersloh: C. Bertelsmann Verlag, 1953). See Walton, "Der Streit zwischen Thomas Erastus und Caspar Olevian," 246.

[75] Walton, "Der Streit zwischen Thomas Erastus und Caspar Olevian," 239–241; William M. Lamont, *Marginal Prynne 1600–1669* (London: Routledge & Kegan Paul, 1963), see especially the chapter "The Erastian Triumph," 149–174; idem, *Godly Rule: Politics and Religion 1603–1660* (London: MacMillan, 1969). See also W.K. Jordan, *The Development of Religious Toleration in England* (Cambridge, Harvard UP, 1936), especially 1:453–492.

[76] Wesel-Roth, *Thomas Erastus*, 93; Sommerville, "Hobbes, Selden, Erastianism, and the History of the Jews," 185; Wesel-Roth's analysis tends to support the supposition that the *pull* of English interest in Erastus's work was as important in its publication as the *push* of Erastus's or Castelvetro's desire to have the theses published.

[77] The English Short Title Catalogue database lists 31 copies in English libraries (15 in Oxford alone, in contrast to only one in Scotland and a handful in the colonies).

early reception of Erastus was Richard Hooker, the great proponent of strong state influence over church affairs. Numerous places in Hooker's *Of the Laws of Ecclesiastical Polity* reveal parallel themes to Erastus and the other leading advocates of the Zurich conception of church-state relations.[78] Other prominent Anglicans who display some measure of sympathy with Erastus's views included Hooker's protégé Richard Field and the early Stuart bishops Richard Bancroft and Thomas Bilson.[79] Another significant individual in the English reception of Erastus was the Puritan Hebrew scholar and theologian Hugh Broughton (1549–1612), who seems to have played a crucial role in disseminating some of Erastus's key concepts, especially his analysis of the role of the Sanhedrin within Judaism at the time of Christ, which may have gone some way to lay the groundwork of the mid-century Erastian revival. He in turn passed these ideas on to William Pynchon (1590–1662), an original member of the Massachusetts Bay Company, who advocated some of Erastus's ideas in New England before his own return to Britain after being convicted of heresy.[80] While Erastus's work had made an impression on some major English divines by the turn of the century, references to Erastus in the writings of English theologians were not common in the late 1500s and into the early decades of the 1600s.[81]

---

http://estc.bl.uk/ accessed September 18, 2009.

[78] Figgis, Crowley, and Baker have all argued for the influence of Erastus on Hooker, and nineteenth-century scholars seem to have taken this influence for granted. Figgis, "Erastus and Erastianism," 77; Weldon S. Crowley, "Erastianism in England to 1640," *Journal of Church and State*, 32 (1990), 558; Baker, "Erastianism in England," 343–346; Richard Hooker, *Of the Laws of Ecclesiastical Polity*, ed. Arthur Stephen McGrade (Cambridge: Cambridge UP, 1989), 10–11.

[79] Figgis, "Erastus and Erastianism," 84; William M. Lamont, "The Rise and Fall of Bishop Bilson," *The Journal of British Studies* 5 (1966): 22–32; Richard Field, *Of the Church* (London, 1606), 201.

[80] Michael P. Winship, "William Pynchon's The Jewes Synagogue," *The New England Quarterly* 71 (1998): 290–297 (especially 293–295). Both Pynchon and Broughton are discussed in this article, though as Winship comments, "Broughton's circle still awaits its scholar" (295).

[81] One example of the limits of Erastus's influence in England ca. 1600 is that there are no references to him in the *General Index of the Publications of the Parker Society* (Cambridge, 1855). Other documented early readers of Erastus included William Harrison and Henry Barrow. See G.J.R. Parry, *A Protestant Vision: William Harrison and the Reformation of Elizabethan England* (Cambridge: Cambridge UP, 2002), 72 and Leland H. Carlson, ed., *Elizabethan Non-Conformist Texts*, vol. 6, *The Writings of John Greenwood and Henry Barrow 1591–1593* (London: George Allen and Unwin, 1970), 186 (in the marginalia of Barrow's "Final Answer to Gifford").

After festering for decades as a significant if surreptitious force within the international Reformed movement, Erastus's ideas resurfaced with a vengeance during the political tumult of the 1640s. The crisis provoked by the Bishops' Wars led Charles I to call the Long Parliament into session, and much of its early debates centered on the question of the proper ordering of the Church of England. The nature of the theological dialogue shifted with the outbreak of the Civil War in 1642. Freed from the king's High Church policies, the Long Parliament commissioned the Westminster Assembly of Divines to establish a new ecclesiastical settlement for England including discipline and church government. As the Parliamentary forces fared poorly in the early stages of the war—due in part to the prowess of the Palatine Wittelsbach Prince Rupert's leadership of the Royalist cause—the Long Parliament found it advantageous to ally with the Presbyterian-led Scots in the Solemn League and Covenant on September 25, 1643. The anticipated outcome of this alliance for both the Scottish and English Presbyterians was the reformation of the English church on a presbyterial basis—the goal sought by English Puritans such as George Withers and Thomas Cartwright from the days of Queen Elizabeth.

As the Westminster Assembly met, it became apparent that there was no consensus on the question of church government. Four factions that took shape: the bishops' party, which generally boycotted the proceedings due to loyalty to King Charles; the Presbyterians, who were the largest grouping and desired a presbyterial-consistorial form of organization; the Independents, likewise a group whose general theological assumptions followed Calvinist lines, but which rejected the need for a regional-national presbyterial hierarchy over local congregations; and, finally what came to be known as the "Erastian" faction, which defended the rights of the magistrate vis-à-vis the church and desired to leave policing of moral offenses in the hands of the state. Regarding the Erastians' impact on the Westminster Assembly, nineteenth-century Scottish theologian William Symington wrote in high style:

> The Erastians were few in number, but by no means contemptible in point of either talent or learning. Generally speaking, they were greatly skilled in oriental literature, of which they did not fail to avail themselves in their attempt to uphold the main positions of Thomas Erastus, the physician of Heidelberg; namely, that the Jewish state and church were one, and that the Christian church is formed on the exact model of the Jewish. This party boasted of only two divines in the Assembly, Dr. John Lightfoot of Ashley, and Mr. Thomas Coleman of Bliton. From among the lay assessors, however, it received great support in the persons more especially of such

> eminent statesmen and lawyers as [John] Selden, [Bulstrode] Whitelocke, and [Oliver] St. John. The champion of the party was Selden, who must be admitted to have been a man deeply skilled in the ancient languages, and in ecclesiastical antiquities, and to have been eminent in sound logic, and a calm, clear, penetrating judgment. The Erastians, in spite of the smallness of their number, were enabled to give the Assembly no little annoyance, and materially to embarrass and retard its proceedings, in consequence not merely of the undeniable superiority of their abilities, but also and principally in consequence of the sympathy and support they obtained from the Houses of Parliament, amongst whose members the theory of Erastus was in high favor.[82]

Symington's eloquent summary concisely assesses the position of the Erastians in the Westminster Assembly. The Erastians, though learned, were a small minority in the Assembly of Divines, and despite some successful delaying tactics, generally came out on the losing end of the debates. Without the necessity for the Long Parliament to implement the program of the Westminster Assembly, the Erastian faction's impact would have been severely limited.

Unlike the Westminster Assembly, which was generally dominated by the Presbyterian faction, men of a more practical Erastian bent held sway in the Long Parliament.[83] Here one must concede that the vast majority of these men were not explicit followers of Erastus, but rather "Erastians" in the mode of Tudor politicians who recognized the state's leadership over the church. Taking a longer view, the willingness of these men to bend English ecclesiastical policy to the conveniences of the alliance with the Scottish Covenanters was an ephemeral phenomenon. The coalescence of Scottish Covenanter and Parliamentary interests did bear enduring fruit in the work of the Westminster Assembly in the Directory of Worship and especially in the Westminster Confession of Faith, Larger and Shorter Catechisms. But making England a genuinely Presbyterian country in structure and practice required additional steps. The Assembly needed the authorization of Parliament to erect presbyteries across the land

---

[82] William Symington, "Historical Sketch of the Westminster Assembly of Divines," in *Commemoration of the Bicentenary of the Westminster Assembly of Divines* (Glasgow, 1843).

[83] Weldon S. Crowley, "Erastianism in the Long Parliament, 1640–1646," *Journal of Church and State* 21 (1979): 451. As Crowley has asserted: "That the Long Parliament was predominantly Erastian there seems to be little doubt." See also Lawrence Kaplan, "English Civil War Politics and the Religious Settlement," *Church History* 41 (1972) 307–325, here 313.

and, furthermore, desired that the presbyteries be fully empowered to excommunicate wayward sinners.

The years 1644–1646 proved to be the Erastian moment par excellence, as the Assembly agitated for more direct control over church discipline. With the signal victory of Parliament's New Model Army over the Royalist forces at Naseby on June 14, 1645, Parliament's dependence on its alliance with the Scottish Covenanters lessened. Likewise, both within the Assembly and in Parliament, resistance was mounting to giving the Presbyterian faction free rein to implement its ecclesiastical vision. The questions of presbyterial organization and excommunication had been hotly debated since the beginning of 1644. In 1645 the "Erastian Conflict" erupted between leading members of the emerging Erastian faction and the Scottish Commissioners in the Assembly. The key propagandist for the Erastian vision of church-state relations was Thomas Coleman (1597/9–1646), who engaged in a heated published controversy with Scottish Presbyterian George Gillespie. Known as "Rabbi Coleman" for his deep knowledge of Jewish antiquities, Coleman used the writings of Erastus to great effect in his debates with the Scottish Presbyterians and was even planning on translating the complete text of Erastus's *Explicatio gravissimae quaestionis* prior to his untimely death in March 1646. Of Coleman, William Lamont has written, "Coleman was an Erastian in the literal, rather than the pejorative, sense: he followed Erastus in an opposition to the clerical disciplinary powers rather than in exaltation of the civil magistrate."[84] Coleman, alongside John Selden (1584–1654), John Lightfoot (1602–1675), Bulstrode Whitelocke (1604–1675), Oliver St. John (ca. 1598–1673), and William Prynne (1600–1669), formed a loose Erastian grouping which frustrated many of the Presbyterians' aims in the Westminster Assembly and Long Parliament.[85]

The prominence of the Erastian faction in mid-1640s Britain can also be measured by the hostility that they encountered from the Scottish Presbyterians. The most manifest artifact of the potency of Erastus's thought was the coining of the pejorative term "Erastian" itself. While it is not impossible that the term arose as a positive designation of the opponents of presbyterial rule, it seems likely that the term was first employed

[84] Lamont, *Marginal Prynne*, 166. See also idem, *Godly Rule*, 115–134; Weldon S. Crowley, "Erastianism in the Westminster Assembly," *Journal of Church and State* 15 (1973): 49–64.

[85] Brief biographies of Whitelocke, Prynne, Selden, and St. John can be found in Ruth Spalding, *Contemporaries of Bulstrode Whitelocke, 1605–1675: Biographies, Illustrated by Letters and Other Documents* (Oxford: British Academy, 1990).

derisively by the Presbyterian faction. Although the *Oxford English Dictionary* places the first documented usage as coming from the pen of Richard Baxter in 1651,[86] we find the term was in print as early as 1645 in the Scottish commissioner George Gillespie's attack on the opinions of Coleman and Erastus; likewise, his fellow Scot Robert Baillie used it frequently in his correspondence from 1645 onward.[87] We can surmise that the expression entered the English language during Westminster Assembly debates, and, as Jeffrey Collins has commented, "it did not take long for it to become a byword for Machiavellian statism in religious affairs."[88] The Scottish Presbyterian theologian Samuel Rutherford also published an exhaustive refutation of Erastus in 1646.[89] One of Rutherford's principal strategies was to divorce Erastus's ideas from Bullinger and Gwalther in order to assault Erastus alone, without seeming to repudiate the home church of the Reformed movement.[90] As Lamont has written of these Scottish Presbyterians, "They might bluster about the Erastians' idolatry of the civil ruler, but they knew that the revival of Erastian sentiments had in fact been fostered by *reading Erastus*."[91] The exasperated, if at times contradictory, musings of Baillie substantiate Lamont's assertion. For example, summing up the influence of the various factions in the Long Parliament, Baillie asserted: "The Erastian partie in the Parliament is stronger than the Independent, and is lyke to work us much woe: Selden is their head."[92] Regarding the Assembly, Baillie commented of Coleman, "he is become their champion, to bring out, in the best way he can, Erastus' arguments against the proposition, for the contentment

[86] *Oxford English Dictionary*, 2nd ed., s.v. "Erastian."

[87] George Gillespie, *Nihil respondes* (London, 1645), 20. "Erastian" also appears on the title page of Gillespie's *Aarons Rod Blossoming* (London, 1646) (See the bibliography); Robert Baillie, *The Letters and Journals of Robert Baillie* ..., ed. David Laing, 3 vols. (Edinburgh: R. Ogle, 1841–1842) 2:277 (see below). See also Crowley, "Erastianism in the Westminster Assembly," 57–62; Figgis, *Erastus and Erastianism*, 77–81.

[88] Jeffrey R. Collins, *The Allegiance of Thomas Hobbes* (Oxford: Oxford UP, 2005), 171.

[89] Samuel Rutherford, *The Divine Right of Church Government and Excommunication* ... (London, 1646). For a perceptive analysis of Rutherford's engagement with the Erastians, see John Coffey, *Politics, Religion and the British Revolutions: The Mind of Samuel Rutherford* (Cambridge: Cambridge UP, 1997), 207–211.

[90] Erastus's sixteenth-century opponents Wenzel Zuleger and Petrus Dathenus had also attempted to separate Bullinger from him.

[91] Lamont, *Godly Rule*, 114.

[92] *The Letters and Journals of Robert Baillie*, 2:277. See also 2:265: "It hath been a mightie neglect that no man hath ansuered Erastus's reply to Beza. The most of the House of Commons are downright Erastians: they are lyke to create us much more woe than all the sectaries of England."

of the Parliament."[93] However, Baillie not only lamented the activity of Selden and Coleman, he also documented the abiding relevance of Erastus's work, asserting: "Erastus is the book that vexes us most. None of the Assemblie, for their life, can doe any thing of moment."[94]

While the Erastian controversy would continue to fester into 1646, the Erastian faction scored a signal triumph in October 1645 when the Long Parliament recognized the right of excommunicated persons to appeal to Parliament.[95] While the legislation established a presbyterial structure of church discipline and authorized suspension from the sacrament as a standard remedy for scandalous persons, the Erastian principle that excommunications could be appealed to the magistrate infuriated the Presbyterians. The Presbyterian-Scottish faction sought to redress this grave undermining of *jure divino* church government, which they saw as inimical to the spirit of the Solemn League and Covenant, but the next round of Parliamentary legislation relating to church discipline in March 1646 likewise maintained a clear role for lay commissioners in the administration of excommunication.[96] Had the Erastian faction

---

[93] Ibid., 2:360.

[94] Ibid., 2:311.

[95] *An ordinance of the Lords and Commons assembled in Parliament Together with rules and directions concerning suspention from the sacrament of the Lords Supper in cases of ignorance and scandall … Die Lunae 20. Octob. 1645* (London, 1645), 7: "If any person suspended from the Lords Supper shall finde himselfe grieved with the proceedings before the Eldership of any Congregation, he shall have liberty to appeale to the Classical Eldership, and from thence to the Pronvinciall Assembly, and thence to the Nationall, and from thence to the Parliament."

[96] *An ordinance of the Lords & Commons assembled in Parliament for keeping of scandalous persons from the sacrament of the Lords supper, the enabling of congregations for the choice of elders, and supplying of defects in former ordinances and directions of Parliament concerning church-government. Die Sabbathi, 14. Martii. 1645* [thus 1646] (London, 1646): 10–11 (article 14): "That in every Province persons shall be chosen by the houses of Parliament, that shall be commissioners to judge of scandalous offences (not enumerated in any Ordinance of Parliament) to them presented. And that the Eldership of that Congregation where the said offence was committed, shall upon examination and proof of such scandalous offence (in like manner as is to be done in the offenses enumerated) certifie the same to the Commissioners, together with the proof taken before them, and before the said certificate, the party accused shall have liberty to make such defense as he shall think fit before the said Eldership and also before the Commissioners, before any certificate shall be made to the Parliament. And if the said Commissioners after examination of all parties, shall determine the offence so presented and proved to be scandalous, and the same shall certifie to the Congregation, the Eldership thereof may suspend such person from the Sacrament of the Lords Supper in like manner as in cases enumerated in any Ordinance of Parliament." The ordinance later maintained a level of Parliamentary oversight over the entire disciplinary regime.

worked alone, its impact would have been muted; however, Erastians and Independents made common cause to obstruct the Presbyterians' aims. Parliament finally sanctioned a compromise Presbyterian settlement in August 1648, envisioning the erection of classes across southern Britain, though its implementation lagged.[97] The remaining history of the Presbyterian faction's failure to establish effectual church discipline in England was caught up in the complex triangulation of power between Parliament, the king, and the Parliamentary Army, which ultimately led to the king's demise and the establishment of a quasi-military dictatorship under Oliver Cromwell. Cromwell's own Independent sympathies and his reliance on more radical religious forces within the New Model Army meant that the endeavor to create a Presbyterian state church in England was lost. As the Scottish Presbyterian Baillie had poignantly prophesied in 1646: "The leaders of the people seem to be inclyned to have no shadow of a King; to have libertie for all religions; to have bot a lame Erastian Presbyterie; to be so injurious to us, as to chase us home with the sword."[98]

Thus the Erastian movement had a decisive impact on Britain at mid century, though this influence is often viewed in a negative light, considering the repugnance of most Christians to accept the claim that the magistrate has the right to settle a nation's religion. Particularly after the totalitarian experiments of the twentieth century, what person of faith would want to give the state carte blanche authority over the church? However, what is not often recognized is how the Presbyterian, Independent, and Erastian factions at the Westminster Assembly were all "Erastian" in the sense that they were participating in a state-sanctioned synod to establish doctrine; furthermore, their decisions would ultimately be approved or rejected by the state.[99] As the nineteenth-century Free Church Presbyterian apologist William Maxwell Hetherington conceded, "It was somewhat ominous of evil, that the very calling of the Assembly was solely the deed of the civil power, and that their deliberations were limited to such matters

[97] *The Form of Church-Government to be used in the Church of England and Ireland: Agreed upon by the Lords and Commons assembled in Parliament, after advice, had with the Assembly of Divines. Die Martis 29 August. 1648* (London, 1648). See Robert S. Paul, *The Assembly of the Lord: Politics and Religion in the Westminster Assembly and the 'Grand Debate'* (Edinburgh: T. & T. Clark, 1985), 517–521; Collins, The Allegiance of Thomas Hobbes, 95–98, 109–110.

[98] March 31, 1646. *The Letters and Journals of Robert Baillie*, 2:362.

[99] Baillie acknowledged this fact and lamented: "You know this is no proper Assemblie, but a meeting called by the Parliament to advyse them in what things they are asked." *The Letters and Journals of Robert Baillie*, 2:186.

as should be proposed to them by the Parliament."[100] In short, the Westminster Assembly, not unlike the Council of Nicaea, to a certain extent, sprang from an Erastian impulse. Neither the Presbyterian nor Erastian factions were really more or less Erastian in this de facto sense of accepting some state authority in determining the confession. Ironically, the bishops who refused to participate in the Assembly, out of what might equally be dubbed an Erastian notion of loyalty to the king of England's rights over the *Ecclesia Anglicana*, appear the least Erastian in practice, in that they rejected parliamentary oversight of the English church.

Rather than seeing the era of the English Civil War as the defining moment of Calvinist-Presbyterian drive to install an essentially clerical regime, recent scholarship has seen the limitation of the unwieldy and unpopular clerical influence of the Laudian era as a driving force behind the religious turmoil. Scholars such as Johann Sommerville, William Lamont, and Weldon Crowley have emphasized the general inclination of the Long Parliament members to curb ecclesiastical power. As Collins aptly quipped, "Securing England's Erastian religious settlement was the chief aim of the Revolution...."[101] Sommerville even more sharply asserted: "Arguably, if there was a revolution in the mid seventeenth century, it was Erastian and not puritan in nature. That is to say, it was a revolution which subordinated the clergy to the laity and the church to the state, and which permanently reversed the clericalism of the Laudian regime."[102]

It would be difficult to overstate the significance of Erastus's thought to the course of mid-seventeenth century British history. Erastus supplied a powerful counter-ideology to what appeared to be the emerging consensus of the English and Scottish Presbyterian factions. When this ideology connected to Parliamentary interest and made common cause with the Independent faction, it had a decisive impact on ecclesiastical developments. In short, the religious life of England reached a "turning point and failed to turn"—to borrow A.J.P. Taylor's famous phrase—in its inability to reach a stable Presbyterian consensus. From the perspective of the international Reformed community, the internal squabbling of these factions—which were all more or less Calvinist in their larger

---

[100] William Maxwell Hetherington, *History of the Westminster Assembly of Divines* (New York, 1843), 201.

[101] Jeffrey R. Collins, "Christian Ecclesiology and the Composition of Leviathan: A Newly Discovered Letter to Thomas Hobbes," *The Historical Journal* 43 (2000): 227.

[102] Sommerville, "Hobbes, Selden, Erastianism, and the History of the Jews," 163.

theological vision—was lamentable and created the context which would make them outsiders *en masse* in the Restoration settlement of 1660. Thus the Erastian success was simultaneously a low point in the history of British Presbyterianism and International Calvinism at large. However, it was also a critical moment in the evolution of a pluralistic confessional atmosphere in Britain and America which would prove to be the nursery of the most successful experiments of religious toleration in the Western world as well as the continuing vitality of religious life in a multi-confessional context. Erastus neither invented nor perfected political Erastianism in England. However, the cogency of his particular formulation with its acid critique of Gnesio-Calvinist ecclesiology helped England's indigenous Erastian heritage meet its greatest challenge, and this development would have no small impact on the evolution of religious liberty in Britain and the colonies.

Transformation of Erastianism

Erastianism in England did not end with its relative success in the Long Parliament. Erastus's greatest advocate and scholar was the great English jurist and polymath John Selden.[103] Selden had been a leading member of the Erastian faction in the Long Parliament and a prominent lay assessor in the Westminster Assembly. After the death of the king, Selden was reasonably close to the Cromwellian regime, and there are even rumors that he and fellow Erastian St. John were approached by Cromwell to write a new constitution for England. Relatively late in life, Selden became a full-blown supporter of Erastus, but when he did, he advocated his ideas with great fervor. In his final work, *Concerning the Sanhedrins and Judicial Prefects of the Ancient Hebrews*, Selden discoursed at great length on many themes drawn directly from Erastus's *Explicatio gravissimae quaestionis*. He offered a positive defense of Erastus and the English Erastian party. Far from eschewing the designation "Erastian," Selden praised Erastus and compared him to Nicolaus Copernicus; both men supported ideas which had tremendous antiquity but found only scorn among their immediate contemporaries. In each case, dubbing their

[103] Regarding Selden, see Reid Barbour, *John Selden: Measures of the Holy Commonwealth in Seventeenth-Century England* (Toronto: University of Toronto Press, 2003) and Jason P. Rosenblatt, *Renaissance England's Chief Rabbi: John Selden* (Oxford: Oxford UP, 2006).

followers "Copernicans" or "Erastians" was rather arbitrary. However, since the "Anti-Erastian" party had actually deviated more from the ancient tradition of church-state relations, Selden thought that they were the ones who should be dubbed innovators.[104]

While the apex of Erastus's influence may have come in the mid-1640s, interest in his thought would remain high through the interregnum into the reign of the Merry Monarch. The *Explicatio gravissimae quaestionis* was itself reprinted in Amsterdam in 1649, the very year Puritan rebels executed Charles I, and the first English translation appeared in 1659, on the eve of the Restoration. A second English translation followed in 1682.[105] At this point, an Erastian party per se no longer existed, though many Erastian ideas had percolated deeply into the English soil. This can be viewed in Erastus's influence on James Harrington's *Oceana*, which contains assertions such as "Excommunication, as not clearly provable out of Scriptures being omitted."[106] The prime literary example of the Independent-Erastian rapprochement is Lewis du Moulin (1605?–80), who drew upon Erastus, Grotius, and Selden for his own distinct statist-congregational theology. Du Moulin possessed a high opinion of Erastus, as revealed by the comment, "For who is not convinced that Erastus was as great a theologian as philosopher, and a most acute investigator into the workings of nature," and likewise noted the points of agreement with Erastus's principles among the English Independents.[107] Erastus's ideas continued to inform the ecclesiastical discourse in Britain into the Restoration and beyond.

If Selden was the seventeenth century's greatest authentic Erastian in the spirit of Thomas Erastus himself, undoubtedly the most well know figure to emerge from the English Erastian milieu was Thomas Hobbes. There is an emerging scholarly consensus that the English Erastian move-

[104] John Selden, *De synedriis & praefecturis iuridicis veterum Ebraeorum*, 3 vols. (London, 1650–1655), 1:529–544, here 544: "Et demum Antierastianus heic novatoris nomen non Erastianus omnino meretur." See Mordechai Feingold, "John Selden and the Nature of Seventeenth-Century Science," in *The Presence of the Past: Essays in Honor of Frank Manuel*, ed. Richard T. Bienvenu and Mordechai Feingold (Kluwer Academic Publishers, 1991), 64; Barbour, *John Selden*, 11–12; 329–336, passim.

[105] *Nullity of Church Censures: Or A Dispute Written by that Illustrious Philosopher, Expert Physician and Pious Divine, Dr. T. Erastus* ... (London, 1659); *A Treatise of Excommunication* (London: for L. Curtis, 1682).

[106] James Harrington, *Oceana* (London: 1656), 65. See also p. 26, where he discusses the Sanhedrin and the origin of excommunication.

[107] Lewis du Moulin, *Paraenesis ad aedificatores imperii in imperio* (London, 1656), Bi^{r}; 628–629. For Du Moulin, see Collins, *The Allegiance of Thomas Hobbes*, 224–241.

ment must be viewed as an essential context for Hobbes's thought. Of course, the genius of Hobbes went beyond his Erastian predecessors, as revealed in Sommerville's comment regarding the English Erastians: "Hobbes endorsed their theoretical premise, and their conclusions, but took his own highly original and idiosyncratic line on history."[108] Interpreting Hobbes through an ecclesiastical and thus Erastian lens has been the major contribution of Collins's study *The Allegiance of Thomas Hobbes*. Collins has argued that it was precisely the same types of anticlerical concerns that drove Erastus to take such an extreme position vis-à-vis church discipline that had a defining impact on shaping the absolutist statist polity of Hobbes's *Leviathan*.[109] Hobbes's influence was titanic, rubbing off on that ultimately more sanguine English political theorist John Locke. Jacqueline Rose recently recovered a strikingly Erastian note—one apparently dependent on Erastus himself—in one of Locke's early political treatises.[110]

This chapter in the Erastian legacy is an instructive episode in the history of ideas, in that we see various concepts advocated by Erastus uncouple and reattach themselves in peculiar combinations, which is further testimony that the English Civil War had been a furnace which produced the amalgamation of many novel political-theological formulations. As we have seen, the failure of the Presbyterian party to achieve a stable, state-mandated presbyterial polity with exclusive jurisdiction over excommunication in the Long Parliament was largely the result of the combined resistance of the Erastians and Independents. In a fascinating turn, some members of the High Church Anglican party, who at earlier junctures had found Erastus's ideas a helpful buttress of their own position against the Presbyterians, rejected the theoretically "Erastian" restoration settlement, and asserted their own *jure divino* authority to head the church.[111] Erastus's influence reverberated in various direc-

[108] Sommerville, "Hobbes, Selden, Erastianism, and the History of the Jews," 174. See also, Johann P. Sommerville, *Thomas Hobbes: Political Ideas in Historical Context* (Basingstoke: Macmillan, 1992), 128–131.

[109] Collins, *The Allegiance of Thomas Hobbes*, passim.

[110] Jacqueline Rose, "John Locke, 'Matters indifferent', and the Restoration of the Church of England," *The Historical Journal* 48 (2005): 601–621, especially pp. 618–619.

[111] Seen, for example, in Henry Hammond and Herbert Thorndike. Of course, Laud's *jure divino* claim to episcopal jurisdiction had been one of the background reasons of the Civil War. Henry Hammond, *Of the power of the keyes, or, Of binding and loosing* (London, 1651); Herbert Thorndike, *The Theological works of Herbert Thorndike* (Oxford, 1856). See also Collins, *The Allegiance of Thomas Hobbes*, 273; idem, "The Restoration Bishops and the Royal Supremacy," *Church History* 68 (1999): 556–557.

tions in the late seventeenth and early eighteenth centuries. His strong assertion that communion should be open influenced English divines, who began to see the Lord's Supper as a "converting sacrament"—very much against the original Zwinglian impulse.[112] Likewise Erastus's conceptions of the essentially civil nature of the Jewish Sanhedrin and the illegitimacy of excommunication as an ecclesiastical censure, as fortified by Selden, became fixtures of theological and political discourse from the second half of the century. Once Erastus's name had become associated with such an important motif in church history—regardless of whether the initial motivation was more from approval or derision—it increased his overall stature as a historical figure. The broad range of references to Erastus by seventeenth-century British authors convincingly attests to this enhanced celebrity.

Perhaps it is here, with this secondary Erastianism, that the final frontier of Erastus's significance lies. Erastus's work, though at times in a stealthy fashion, was a critical element of the intellectual background of figures such as Grotius, Selden, Hobbes, and Locke. Put another way, the individuals who laid the groundwork for modern Western political thought came of age in an era when it seemed a full presbyterial vision of church-state relations might triumph. It would have been difficult for them not to have been influenced by such a trenchant opponent of the *divino juro* claim to presbyterial oversight. Thus they read Erastus and absorbed much of his program, if they did not always cite him frequently. Furthermore, Grotius and Selden created many tertiary Erastians who evince the influence of Erastus mediated through the later authors' writings. Erastus played a pivotal role, to the chagrin of Christian Reconstructionists everywhere, in the rise of the secular modern state which does not use its coercive power to maintain a clerical vision of morality. Should anyone doubt this point, let us remember that some of the refutations of Erastus's conception of church-state relations are still in print and not merely objects for scholarly study.

Erastus must also be seen as an important link between the intense anticlericalism of the late medieval period and the campaign against "priestcraft" which would become such an important part of the Enlightenment era discourse. It is thus with some measure of poetic justice that Pierre Bayle selected quotations from Erastus's school days, which

[112] E. Brooks Holifield, "The Intellectual Sources of Stoddardeanism," *The New England Quarterly* 45 (1972): 372–392.

ridiculed the unreformed pontificate of Julius III and his scandalous romantic liaisons, for inclusion in his *Dictionnaire historique et critique*.[113] Erastus's arguments against excommunication and clerical power in general continued to resound into the late seventeenth- and early eighteenth-century debates concerning religious toleration and echoed in the writings of Deists like Matthew Tindal.[114]

Conclusion

Whereas Erastus's hopes for the restoration of the Reformed faith were realized in Heidelberg and Basel, and his potent critique of the Calvinist vision of discipline would nip at the heels of future generations of would-be presbyterial reformers, his attempt to halt the revival of Paracelsian medicine failed. Here the future belonged to men like Zwinger and Smet, who analyzed the merits of Paracelsian therapy without the polemical heat of Erastus. Erastus's refutation likely served to increase popular interest in Paracelsus and, in stirring up thinkers like Moffett, likely advanced his opponent's cause. Nevertheless, Erastus's unrelenting attack on the magical worldview which pervaded Paracelsianism and especially the pseudo-Paracelsian corpus helped prepare the way for the day when chemistry and alchemy would part company. Likewise, Erastus's analysis of the heretical implications of Paracelsus's philosophy would long be remembered in orthodox Protestant circles.[115]

While Erastus's position in the history of science and medicine has nearly been obscured at times by his repudiation of Paracelsus, it is

[113] *Dictionnaire historique et critique de Pierre Bayle* (Paris, 1820), 8:454–455.

[114] For example, Tindal upheld the unity of political authority in a Christian state and rejected independent clerical jurisdiction over excommunication along lines quite similar to Erastus. M. Tindal, *The rights of the Christian church asserted, against the Romish and all other priests who claim an independent power over it*, 4th ed. (London, 1709), 33–64. See J.A.I. Champion, *The Pillars of Priestcraft Shaken: The Church of England and Its Enemies, 1660–1730* (Cambridge: Cambridge UP, 1992). See also Joris van Eijnatten, "Swiss Anticlericalism in the United Provinces: Jean Barbeyrac's *Oratio de magistratu, forte peccante, e pulpitis sacris non traducendo* (1721)," in *La formazione storica della alterità: Studi di storia della tolleranza nell' età moderna offerti a Antonio Rotondò*, ed. Henri Méchoulan et al. (Florence: Olschki, 2001), 861–886.

[115] For example, no less a divine than Richard Baxter accepted Erastus's characterization of Paracelsus wholesale in "The unreasonableness of infidelity: manifested in four discourses," in *The practical works of the late reverend and pious Mr. Richard Baxter, in four volumes* (London: 1707), 320.

fair to say that Erastus is increasingly recognized as a significant natural philosopher in his own right. He was an acute observer of disease and other natural phenomena, and if he constructed his analysis in an Aristotelian-Galenic framework, he was open to both philosophical and empirical challenges to the received wisdom. Erastus's treatments of topics such as substantial forms, diseases of the total substance, and the occult qualities of drugs were likely his most original intellectual contributions to early modern scientific theory. Erastus's natural philosophical writings continued to elicit comment well into the eighteenth century and influenced the ideas of more definitively "scientific" figures such as Andreas Libavius, Marin Mersenne, and finally Robert Boyle.[116] Given that his works found a quite wide readership, it is perhaps curious that his major works—especially his anti-Paracelsian disputations—were not frequently reprinted in the seventeenth century. The noted physician Guy Patin (1601–1672), who considered Erastus the most learned German of the previous hundred years, mooted the possibility of bringing out a folio edition of the complete works of Erastus but did not complete the task.[117]

While no doubt understudied, Erastus's importance in early modern intellectual history cannot be questioned. Clearly he ranks behind epochal figures such as Luther or Copernicus or individuals who left behind immortal cultural monuments such as Shakespeare or Montaigne.

[116] For the similarity of at least one of Erastus's arguments with those later advanced against the Paracelsian theory by Boyle, see Debus, *English Paracelsians*, 39. The fact that Boyle dubbed an interlocutor who opposed alchemical transmutation "Erastus" in his unpublished *Dialogue on Transmutation* should be sufficient proof that Boyle was well acquainted with Erastus's work, though he clearly disagreed with Erastus's rejection of chrysopoeia. The character "Erastus" shares some similarity with Erastus, as Principe writes, "Boyle does preserve the sneering, declamatory style of the historical figure, and the opinions of the interlocutor Erastus do conform to those of the historical Thomas Erastus." Lawrence Principe, *The Aspiring Adept: Robert Boyle and His Alchemical Quest* (Princeton: Princeton UP, 2000), 75–76. Regarding Mersenne, see above chapter 8, note 208.

[117] Guy Patin, *Lettres de Gui Patin*, ed. J.-H. Reveillé-Parise, 3 vols. (Paris, 1846), 1:109 and 231: "Les Disputes de Thomas Erastus contre Paracelse sont très rares; je suis après à faire imprimer toutes ses œuvres in-folio. Ah! que ce seroit un bon livre!" He also wrote to his son, "While you have a little leisure, read all that Thomas Erastus has written and especially 'De occultis pharmacorum estatibus,' [*sic*] and his four volumes 'Adversus novam medicinam Paracelsi.' " Quoted in, Francis R. Packard, "Guy Patin and The Medical Profession in Paris in the Seventeenth Century," *Annals of Medical History* 4 (1922): 215.

However, Erastus is one of those figures like C.S. Lewis or Locke who forces scholars to confront his legacy because of the multifaceted nature of his contribution. Erastus was a leading figure within the Second Reformation in Germany, the most important opponent of the Paracelsian revival, and a significant natural philosopher in his own right. On top of these achievements, his writings offered the most compelling early modern repudiation of Calvinist ecclesiology and disciplinary theory. In short, he was one of the most important intellectuals of the second half of the sixteenth century, and easily the most important Zwinglian working outside of Switzerland. If he does not rank among luminaries such as Paracelsus or Calvin, due to his wide-ranging contributions his light shines more brightly than contemporaries such as Zacharias Ursinus or Johann Weyer. The broad reach of Erastus's impact puts him on par with figures such as Bodin and Ramus with their similar expansive interests and predilection to meddle in politics.

In the preceding pages, I have attempted to sketch the plot of the Reformation in Heidelberg under Ottheinrich and Frederick III and to tell Erastus's role in that story. The primary goal has been to explore how the Heidelberg context influenced Erastus's thought and action. I conclude with these brief observations on the question of continuity and change in the work of Erastus.

The controversy over church discipline and the closely connected Antitrinitarian affair acted as the primary agent of change and reorientation in Erastus's life. Before the controversy, Erastus was a late Zwinglian expressing irenic views on the meaning of the Lord's Supper. Living among Lutherans and trying to justify the evangelical nature of the Zwinglian position, Erastus constructed a Eucharistic theology which approached the Lutheran and Calvinist belief that the sacrament bestowed grace. Whereas the Heidelberg Catechism had drawn the Philippists, Zwinglians, and Calvinists together, the controversy over church discipline forced Erastus and his friends to realize that there were still issues that divided them. Lacking the disciplinary zeal of the Gnesio-Calvinists and their passion to protect the sanctity of the Lord's Supper, Erastus and his partisans found little need for the Calvinist consistory. The Catholic Mass remained idolatrous to Erastus, but it was not a grave offense for a manifest sinner to receive communion; rather, in Erastus's conception, it was the purpose of communion to offer Christ anew to the sister or brother in need. As far as the Zurich tradition had come in drawing toward a notion of real participation with Christ in the Lord's

Supper as opposed to simple memorialism, a gulf still existed between the Zwinglians and the Gnesio-Calvinists.

In casting about for arguments to undermine the proposed Calvinist disciplinary regime, Erastus became a radical dissenter in the eyes of his opponents. In this role he emphasized three ideas that were revolutionary in their simplicity. First, he contended that excommunication itself was an inherited Catholic practice without any biblical basis. It takes a little imagination to understand how radical this was, but to the Gnesio-Calvinists, he was in effect saying that no discipline should be exercised *within the church*. In their eyes, Erastus was an antinomian whose ideas would lead to atheism. He eagerly jettisoned what his Gnesio-Calvinist colleagues were coming to accept as a defining mark of the true church. From the Calvinist perspective, labeling Erastus a "free thinker" has some validity. Beza suggested his ideas were a program for anarchy. The extremity of Erastus's position was quite comparable to Weyer's contention that the death penalty should not be applied to witches and approached his Antitrinitarian friends' rejection of orthodox Christology. His second contribution, and perhaps the one that most guaranteed his legacy in England, was to build an alternative hermeneutical basis for the Zurich-Bern vision of church-state relations based on the role of the Jewish Sanhedrin in the time of Christ. His third radical assertion, which he shared with predecessors like Musculus, was that there should be no multiplication of jurisdictions within a Christian commonwealth. What was perhaps most dynamic about this notion was its close corollary that, in effect, placed control over church affairs into the hands of the state, though Erastus himself never intended this power to include the determination of correct doctrine. One cannot overemphasize the fact that Erastus's conception of church-state relations assumed a pious sovereign ruling over a state with no major dogmatic conflict. This was the dimension of Erastus's ecclesio-political thought that found more extreme expression in the writings of Thomas Hobbes. What became essential to "Erastianism" in common parlance—that the state should exercise sovereignty over the church—was not essential to Erastus's own thought. From all indications, Erastus was not particularly attached to his own program of church-state relations, since he was willing to accept the compromise solution that the 1570 church discipline order represented. Erastus's program was one of dissent and opposition. He was not nearly so eager to install his own vision as he was to derail the imposition of his opponents' vision. If Erastus's experience had been under less pious sovereigns, it is unlikely that he would have been willing to consign such all-encompassing powers to the magistrate.[118] But in his day, he felt that he had more to fear from the clergy than he did the state, and his later experience in Heidelberg proved his intuition correct.

Looking across the breadth of Erastus's career, continuity was more marked than discontinuity. He remained an active partisan for the Swiss Reformed faith all his adult life, pursuing his own version of the freedom of the Christian, which in the end found itself at loggerheads with the Calvinist attempt to create a godly community on earth. In Erastus's conception, the church was an institution with a limited competence. Its chief function was to present the gospel message through word and sacrament. God had ordained another authority, namely the magistrate, to punish sinners. This limitation of ecclesiastical competence has an analogy in Erastus's thought with the limitation of the role of revelation—be that biblical or personal—in natural philosophy.

He displayed even greater consistency in his long war against superstition and magic in the natural world. He found a new opponent in Paracelsus, but his disenchanted position had been mapped out in advance. Although he was a textually oriented, humanist physician working within the general Aristotelian-Galenic framework, he frequently nipped at the edges of received scientific knowledge. Erastus likewise remained a naturalist throughout his life and made independent observations on topics such as mineral baths, soil science, epilepsy, and zoology, thus making a concrete if modest contribution to the advance of scientific knowledge.

The largest apparent discontinuity in Erastus's career was how the iconoclastic nature of his stance on church discipline contrasted with his harsh refutation of Paracelsus and the fundamental conservatism of his thoughts on the punishment of witches. Thorndike's quip that "his struggle against intolerant Calvinism did not serve to make him tolerant" remains apt.[119] I have argued that the acerbity of his attack on Paracelsus must be viewed at least in part as an attempt by Erastus to restore his own orthodox reputation. Not tolerating dissent was a testimony to a confessional community's orthodoxy, and if anyone had cause to reassert his orthodoxy, it was Erastus. Even if he was attempting subconsciously to justify himself at Paracelsus's expense, however, the intensity of Erastus's repudiation was disproportionate to the task. Thus a

[118] Wesel-Roth, *Thomas Erastus*, 111: "Erast fürchtet den Mißbrauch der staatlichen Befehlsgewalt weniger als den Mißbrauch der Exkommunikation."
[119] Thorndike, *History of Magic and Experimental Science*, 5:653.

parallel exists between Erastus's occasional rage at personal rivals such as Heshusius or Olevianus and his literary feuds with Paracelsus and Weyer.

A related discontinuity is not one of chronology but of the private and public spheres of Erastus's life. Erastus apparently could be more open-minded and gracious in person than his crafted public image implied. Whereas Erastus was orthodox in print, he may not have been so orthodox at his own table. Likewise, while Erastus advocated severity in the punishment of the theoretical crimes of Paracelsus and witches, he appealed for clemency for his friend Johann Sylvan, who was a real-life convicted heretic. In the same manner that his scientific efforts were more constructive when based on phenomena he directly observed, his judgments were more charitable when applied to his culpable friends than to theoretical sinners.

Although the aim of this book has been to place Erastus in historical context, a unified theme is evident in his boundary-crossing career. Erastus fought to establish the independence of the book of nature from the book of revelation. Put another way, for a man whose cosmology began with Genesis, the answer to every question did not have a theological basis and certainly not an ecclesiastical one. In Erastus's conflict with his disciplinary rivals and with Paracelsus, Erastus found that it was not safe to trust those who claimed special revelation or would set themselves up as a special caste to be the guardians of sanctity. Though he did not make the position explicit until pushed to the extreme by his opponents, Erastus possessed a conception of natural knowledge and natural authorities that had been ordained by God to fulfill their own purposes in the world. Medicine was an independent pursuit whose autonomy was sanctioned by the scriptures. To renew science was not to discover new medical revelation or to recover arcane wisdom, but to add to the long heritage of accumulated medical knowledge. The autonomy of medicine as a secular pursuit has an analogy in the autonomy of the Christian magistrate from ecclesiastical authorities. The underlying commonality of Erastus's thought was not that the state or science were fundamentally secular; both were ordained by God. The critical similarity was that religious knowledge or religious authority did not trump the secular. Rather than envisioning an expansive role for religious knowledge and religious authority in the Reformation's wake, Erastus conceptualized reform as a limitation on the competence of religious authorities.

Erastus's aversion to the encroachment of theology and church authorities on science and the state was not a unidirectional phenomenon. His boundary-crossing career reinforced traditional scholastic notions of disciplinary competencies. He blocked Weyer's effort to allow his medical expertise to make an inappropriate legal and theological judgment; i.e., that the death penalty did not apply to witches. Though Erastus himself took part in theological disputes, he did not do so as a "physician" but as a Christian layperson. But since his ecclesiology was so loose and his church's competency so small, speaking as a doctor of Holy Scripture would not have enhanced his authority. He never claimed that his competence as a physician entitled him to definitively treat the church discipline conflict or the Lord's Supper. He did not claim special insight into the "light of nature" which allowed Paracelsus to address *both* theological and scientific matters with presumed authority.

Erastus's significance as a representative of Reformed Protestant natural philosophy is unquestionable. This assertion is not meant to imply that Erastus possessed the best or most progressive answers to the natural philosophical questions of his day. Erastus could be a doggedly straightforward thinker. He would grasp an uncomplicated thesis and hammer it home, often pursuing his line of argumentation to some excess. This characteristic in large part explains Erastus's status as a literary figure; hardly any of his works were ignored, but he never had anything approaching the sixteenth-century equivalent of a bestseller. All of his works clearly expressed a well-defined point of view. If you wanted a response to Weyer, Erastus was competent; the same could be said for his treatments of Paracelsus, the transmutation of metals, or the occult qualities of medicine. His works were good enough to stand as representatives of a particular interpretation of an issue, but none—with the important exception of his writings on excommunication—were so compelling or innovative that they captured the popular imagination or electrified the world of letters.

This brings us to why Erastus's name has come to be linked with church-state relations and not one of his other academic contributions. A cursory overview of Erastus's published corpus would give one the impression that he was chiefly interested in explicating medical topics with a heavy philosophical slant and that theological concerns were peripheral to his career. However, the personal history disclosed by his correspondence reveals a different story. The struggle over excommunication was in fact the defining conflict of his life, and losing this battle left a tremendous impression upon Erastus. This issue festered within Erastus and turned him into an effective and, at times, a mean-spirited opponent of the Gnesio-Calvinists. This existential angst was the furnace which distilled the most compelling work of his career, the *Explicatio Gravissimae Quaestionis*.

In closing, Erastus was a wide-ranging physician much like Paracelsus, Weyer, Ficino, and even Locke, and his career displayed many of the neuralgic points of his age. His thoughtful treatment of numerous subjects elicited commentary for decades long after his passing. An abbreviated list of his readers includes such notables as Boyle, Bayle, Robert Burton, James Ussher, William Harvey, and William Gladstone. On the negative side, his work served to protect and promote the learned witchcraft paradigm for another century. His writings likely had an ambivalent, although perhaps ultimately salutary, impact on the reception of Paracelsus and chemical medicine. More constructively, his actions and writings played a critical role in the foundation of the Reformed Church in the Holy Roman Empire and his influence lives on in the Heidelberg Catechism and in Reformed liturgical practice. Although the Calvinist-presbyterial conception of church discipline went on to dominate the international Reformed communion—and in this manner many Reformed churches became truly "Calvinist"—Erastus's thoughts on church discipline inspired another generation of Reformed Protestants to resist what they conceptualized as the imposition of ecclesiastical tyranny in seventeenth-century England. The success of these seventeenth-century "Erastians" in employing Erastus's ideas helped thwart the effort of Scottish and English Presbyterians to transform the Church of England into a genuinely "Presbyterian" church. It is chiefly to these derisively labeled "Erastians" that Thomas Lüber owes his enduring, and well-merited, fame.

APPENDIX A: FACULTY ROSTERS FROM THE UNIVERSITY OF HEIDELBERG

The Faculty Roster as of 1560:

Theology	Law	Medicine	Arts
1. Petrus Boquinus (Dekan)	Wendolinus Heilmann	Jakob Curio	Balch. Reisner (Dekan)
2. Paul Einhorn (Unicornus)	Dionysius Gravius (Graff)	Petrus Lotichius (Dekan)	Georg Adam
*	Franciscus Balduinus	Thomas Erastus**	Wilhelm Xylander-Aristotle, etc.
	Caspar Agricola		Sigismund Melanchthon
	Nicolaus Cisner		

* Vacancy on the theological faculty due to the dismissal of Heshusius on Sept. 16, 1559.

** We know from other sources that Erastus occupied the second chair rather than the third chair.

UAH MS A. 160/7 fol. 267.

The Faculty Roster as of Dec. 22, 1568:

Theology	Law	Medicine	Arts
1. Petrus Boquinus-NT	1. Caspar Agricola	1. [Jakob Curio]*	1. Victorinus Strigel-Ethics
2. Immanuel Tremellius-OT	2. Berthold Redlich	2. Thomas Erastus	2. Wilhelm Xylander-Aristotle, etc.
3. Girolamo Zanchi-Dogmatics	3. Nicolaus Dobbin	3. Sigismund Melanchthon	3. Hieronymus Niger-Physics
	4. Petrus Alostanus		4. Herman Witekind-Greek
			5. Simon Grynaeus-Math.
			6. Lambertus Ludolphus Pithopoeus [Helm]-Latin

* Curio was not included on the list but must have still held the first chair.

UAH MS A. 160/9 fol. 31.

The Faculty Roster as of Dec., 1573:

Theology	Law	Medicine	Arts
Petrus Boquinus-NT	Hugo Donellus	Thomas Erastus	Ulrich Faber (Dekan)*
Immanuel Tremellius-OT	Caspar Agricola	Albrecht Blaurer	Wilhelm Xylander
Girolamo Zanchi-Dogmatics	Nicolaus Dobbin	Ludwig Gravius (Graff)	Herman Witekind
	Petrus Alostanus		Simon Grynaeus
			Matthaeus Lannoius
			[Lambertus Ludolphus Pithopoeus (Helm)]**

* Faber's association with the faculty at this juncture is uncertain. See Drüll, ed., *Heidelberger Gelehrtenlexikon 1386–1651*, 1:147.

** Pithopoeus was not included on the list but was still a member of the arts faculty since he served as rector that year.

UAH MS A. 160/10 fol. 62.

The Faculty Roster as of April 1577 with Remuneration:

		Stipendia Ordinaria	Stipendia extraordinaria
Theology	Petrus Boquinus	250 fl.	
	Immanuel Tremellius	200 fl.	
	Girolamo Zanchi	160 fl.	120 fl.
Law	Hugo Donellus	200 fl.	200 fl.
	Caspar Agricola	200 fl.	50 fl.
	Nicolaus Dobbin	200 fl.	50 fl.
Medicine	Thomas Erastus	180 fl.	120 fl.
	Albert Blaurer	160 fl.	
	Ludwig Gravius (Graff), Rector	140 fl	
Philosophy and Languages	Herman Witekind	120 fl.	
	Simon Grynaeus	120 fl.	
	Lambertus Ludolphus Pithopoeus (Helm)	120 fl.	30 fl.
	Matthaeus Lannoius	120 fl.	30 fl.
	Johannes Jungnitz	120 fl.	
	Theophil Mader	120 fl.	

UAH MS A. 160/11 fol. 77.

APPENDIX B: EXCERPTS FROM ERASTUS'S CORRESPONDENCE CONCERNING PARACELSUS

Translated by Charles Gunnoe and Jole Shackelford, University of Minnesota

Text No. 1

Erastus to H. Bullinger, Oct. 29, [1570]. StAZ, E II 345. fols. 741–742.[1]

[fol. 741v] Sum iam totus in cogitatione de confutando monstrosiss[imo] et absurdissimo dogmate Paracelsi, et in prima parte (puto libros mihi scribendos fore 4 benè magnos) ea tractare statui, quae ad pietatem attinent, id est de superstitiosa et Magica curatione per verba, characteres, invocationes nescio quorum Angelorum et quicquid huius farinae cacodaemones excogitarunt. Graves hic quaestiones incident quas partim ex philosophia, partim ex Theologia pro virili mea tentabo plane ut solide dissolvere. [...]

[fol. 742r] Cuius causa scripsi illa, haec est: Ille Paracelsus vocat, se Eremitam ab Hohenheim, itemque Bombast. Velim ergo scire, an sit aliqua familia nobilis umb Einseidlen von Hohenheim (oder Bombast) et si quid praeterea sciri de hac re potest. Vehementer te rogo, ut, undecumque aliquid resciscere possis, scisciteris per occasionem. Fuit familiaris aliquando cuidam D[omino] Clausero, Medico Tigurino.

Translation

I am completely absorbed in thinking about how to stem the most monstrous and absurd dogma of Paracelsus, and in the first part[2] (I suppose I will write 4 large volumes) I have resolved to deal with those things which pertain to piety—that is, concerning superstitious and

[1] These extracts come from a much longer letter that is largely about church politics in the Electoral Palatinate.

[2] I.e., *De medicina nova*, 1.

magical healing through words, characters and the invocations of all sorts of angels[3] and whatever else of this nature evil spirits contrive. Here serious questions arise, partly from philosophy, partly from theology, which I will attempt to dispense with clearly and thoroughly to the best of my ability....[4]

The reason for which I have written these things is this: that man Paracelsus calls himself the "Hermit of Hohenheim," also "Bombast." Therefore, I want to know, whether there might be some noble family "von Hohenheim" or "Bombast" in Einsiedeln, and if anything else can be discerned about this matter. I emphatically beg you to investigate thoroughly, at the proper time, anything you can find out from any source whatever.[5] He was once an acquaintance of a certain D. Clauser, a physician in Zurich.[6]

Text No. 2

Erastus to J.J. Grynaeus, Nov. 29, [1570].
Basel UB, Ms. G II 4, fols. 300–301.

[fol. 300v] Fuit superioribus mensibus Spirae Henricus Petri, et cum Joh[anne] Cratone Medico Caesaris collocutus inter alia eidem de Theophrasti vita moribusque notatu digna retulit: quae valde velim exactius cognoscere. Scripsit ad me Crato et vehementer orat, ut incoepto pergam opere, se eiusdem generis quaedam habere quae mihi sit liberaliter communicaturus. Dixit ei inter alia D. Henricus Petri, ut ad

[3] literally, "of I know not what angels."

[4] At this point in the letter Erastus interrupts his discussion of Paracelsus with a brief reference to demonological and astrological questions. In this context he mentions Ludwig Lavater's *De Spectris* (Zürich, 1570) and his own *Defensio libelli Hieronymi Savonarolae*. Before returning to Paracelsus, he comes upon the question of whether witches should be put to death and mentions Weyer's *De praestigiis daemonum*. With this phrase "cuius causa scripsi illa, haec est" Erastus apparently is referring Bullinger to his initial discussion of the anti-Paracelsian project some lines before.

[5] Bullinger fulfilled this request by sending a letter describing his own meeting with Paracelsus. See chapter 8 above (text in note 109). Erastus thanks Bullinger for fulfilling this request for information in text no. 3 below.

[6] Regarding Christoph Clauser (149?-1552), a Zürich Physician, see Gustav Adolf Wehrli, *Der Zürcher Stadtarzt Dr. Christoph Clauser und seine Stellung zur Reformation der Heilkunde im XVI. Jahrhundert, nebst Faksimileausgabe seiner Harnschrift und seiner Kalender* (Zürich: Sedwyla, 1924); Pagel, Paracelsus, 351. Paracelsus's "Begleitbrief an Clauser" from 10 November 1527, is printed in PI, 4:69–74. Erastus mentions this preface again in *De medicina nova*, 2:21.

me ille scripsit, omnes ad unum eodem anno istic interiisse, qui vel ab Erasmo persuasi vel ab aliis Theophr[asticis] remediis ausi fuerint uti. Peto ergo ex te maiorem in modum, ut per occasionem ex viro illo in sua Repub[lica] clariss[imo] mihique meritò colendissimo, intelligas huc pertinentia omnia, et sigillatim ad me scribas. Ego summa cum modestia, sicuti facienda rei cuiuspiam talis mentio fuerit, agam omnia, sicque temperabo, et omnes videant me rem tractare non personam accusare, utque sua cuique laus dubita maneat, nec quisquam praestitae nobis operae fructu defraudetur. [...]

Translation

During the past months, Heinrich Petri[7] has been at Speyer, and having spoken with Johannes Crato,[8] the imperial physician, among other things he related to him some things worth noting concerning the life and customs of Theophrastus, which I greatly desire to learn more precisely. Crato has written to me and vehemently asked that I continue in the work already begun, and that he has certain things of the same sort which he would freely communicate to me. Heinrich Petri told him, among other things, as *he* [Crato] wrote to me, that everyone to a man who had dared to use Theophrastian remedies, whether persuaded by Erasmus [of Rotterdam] or others, perished there [i.e., in Basel] the same year. I ask therefore the best that you can do, that, at the right time, you gather together all pertinent information from that most illustrious and (in my estimation) rightly cultivated man in his republic, and write those things to me one by one.[9] I will undertake all with greatest modesty, just as someone doing this who was of such opinion, and thus I will temper [my treatment]. And all may see that I address the issue and do not attack the person, with the result that his praise remains in doubt for everybody, and nobody is deprived by us of the fruit of a superior work.

[7] Heinrich Petri, a printer from Basel known for publishing the works of Crato and Severinus. See Josef Benzing, *Die Buchdrucker des 16. und 17. Jahrhunderts im deutschen Sprachgebiet* [Beiträge zum Buch- und Bibliothekwesen 12] (Wiesbaden: Otto Harrassowitz, 1963), 33.

[8] Regarding Crato, see Gunnoe and Shackelford, "Johannes Crato von Krafftheim (1519–1585)."

[9] Erastus thanks Grynaeus for fulfilling this task in the bottom of text no. 6.

Text No. 3

Erastus to H. Bullinger, Jan. 3, [1571]. ZBZ, F 62, fol. 204.

[fol. 204ʳ] S[alutem] D[icet] Literas tuas, vir clariss[ime] et colendiss[ime] postremas accepi, et in h[is] quas de Paracelsi rebus ante scripseras, quae mihi ambae valde gratae fuerunt. [...]

Paracelsi doctrina non tantum est in philosophia iniqua, in Medicina monstrosa, verum etiam in Theologia impia et blasphema. Negat creationem à Deo vero perfectam, creatores nostros facit fabros quosdam mortales in astris sedentes, miraculorum potestatem tribuit hominibus, herbis, lapillis, spectris. Futurorum praevissionem à nescio quo Daemone in nos derivat, characteribus, verbis, imaginib[us][10] sub certo syderum positu fabricatis vim tribuit plus quam divinam. Vitam nostram in nostro esse arbitrio, ex De[i] praefinitione nihil esse, posse eam nos ad Iudicium extremum usque prorogare. Caelos nequam homines per errorem fabricari, qui boni esse nullo possint modo [etiam].[11] Monstra his longe absurdiora alia profert. Omnia haec in priora parte confutationis solidè refellere conor, et iam de creatione, miraculis Imaginationibus nostrae viribus demum de fascinationibus pertexui omnia. [...]

[fol. 204ᵛ] Ago ingentes gratias, quod mihi Paracelsum depinxisti. Idem fe[cit] Oporinus, quo usus fuit amanuense per biennium. Pulchrè conven[ti] in omnibus. Magum fuisse et Cacodaemonis confoederatum cer[tum] est. [...]

Translation

Greetings. I received your latest letters, most famous and cultivated man, and in them, the things that you had written before concerning Paracelsus, both of which were very pleasing to me. [...]

The teaching of Paracelsus is not only harmful in Philosophy and monstrous in medicine, but also impious and blasphemous in theology. He denies that creation was in fact completed by God. He asserts that our creators were certain skilled mortal beings residing in stars. He has conceded the power of miracles to humans, herbs, stones and specters.

[10] There is a period in the text after the abbreviated "Imaginib." which makes it difficult to discern whether or not a new sentence is intended to begin with "sub" (which is not clearly capitalized).

[11] The text here is a "7" sign.

He derives a vision of our futures, from I know not what demon. He has ascribed a more than divine power to characters, words and figures made under a certain arrangement of stars. Our life is in our control; nothing is by God's predetermination. We are able to extend it all the way to the final judgment. The heavens form flawed men by mistake, men who are certainly by no means able to be good. He brings forth other monstrosities far more absurd than these. I endeavor to refute all these things solidly in the first part of the confutation,[12] and I have already finished everything concerning creation, our marvelous powers of imagination and finally concerning charms and spells. [...]

I am grateful that you have described Paracelsus to me. [Johannes] Oporinus,[13] who had been his amanuensis for two years, made a similar [account]. They complement each other beautifully in every respect. It is certain that [Paracelsus] was a magician and in league with evil spirits.

Text No. 4

Erastus to J. Camerarius II, Feb. 23, [15]71.
Erlangen UB (Sammlung Trew), No. 1.

[recto] Ego namque constitutum habeo, si Deus vitam concedet, (quod in ipsius sancta voluntate est positum, à me nec petitur anxie, nec reiicitur) quatuor partibus universam Paracelsi doctrinam confutare. Legi libros circiter 120 et ex omnibus mihi, quae visa sunt, annotavi, inque classes partim digessi, partim adhuc digero. In prima remedia superstitiosa Magicasque curationes examino. Et iam absolvi de Creatione disputationem omnem, (in qua, quae bonus et doctus hic vir reprehendit piè, pro meo instituto fusius fortasse, quam par sit, p[er]secutus sum) ac de miraculis. Praeterea de viribus Imaginationis, de fascinatione, et quae huic rei affinia sunt. Quae pars, quia mihi visa est difficilima, ut in quam multae incidant quaestiones, de gravidarum appetitionibus, de menstruatarum visione etc[etera], primo loco periculi faciendi causa suscepta à me fuit. Super est nunc, ut de Magia et Speciebus eius agam, ut coepi, et sic partem primam concludam. In secunda philosophia ipsius expendam. In tertia Medica generatim excutiam. In postrema de particularium morborum curationibus disputabo, quorum ille curationes conscripsit. Vereor autem ne crescant mihi libri nimiu[m]. Pars prima, quam hisce

[12] I.e., *De medicina nova*, 1.
[13] See Benzenhöfer, "Zum Brief des Johannes Oporinus über Paracelsus."

nundinis, ut spero, perfectam Typographo tradam, ut ad alteras exeat, continebit duo fermè alphabeta. Refutare namque me oportuit [verso] Pomponatii librum de incantationibus et Avicennae sententiam, atque alias similes opiniones. Antequam haec excusa sit, spero me secundam quoque perfecturum.[...]

Translation

For I have an agreement, God willing (because it is placed in his holy will, neither anxiously sought out nor rejected by me) to confute the complete doctrine of Paracelsus in four volumes.[14] I have read about 120 books,[15] and from all of those that I have seen, some I have commented on and arranged into categories, and some I am still arranging. In the first volume, I examine his superstitious remedies and his magical cures. I have already finished the whole disputation on creation, and also on miracles, in which I have set forth things that this good and learned man piously condemns,[16] perhaps in greater detail than is appropriate for my purpose. Beyond that, [I treat] the powers of imagination and enchantment and topics that are related to this subject. And that part, because it seemed to me to be most difficult, since in it many questions arise about the passions of pregnant women and the vision of menstruating women, etc., was taken up by me in the first place for the sake of making a test case.[17] Now it remains for me to treat magic and its varieties and, thus, I conclude the first part as I began. In the second volume, I will consider his philosophy. In the third volume, I will investigate his medicine in general. In the last volume I will dispute regarding the treatments of particular diseases, for which he has prescribed cures. But I am very much afraid that the books will not be finished. The first volume—the finished draft

[14] I.e., *De medicina nova*, 1–4.

[15] On the first page of *De medicina nova*, 1, Erastus proclaims that he has read "113 books of Theophrastus." That number, as well as the actual titles Erastus cites in *De medicina nova*, confirms that Erastus had almost every Paracelsian work that had been published by 1571.

[16] In isolation, Erastus's comment, "that this good and learned man piously condemns," is quite ambiguous. In the text of the letter before the extract that has been reproduced here, Erastus discusses a certain little book (libellus) that Camerarius had sent to him without mentioning the title or the author's name. Erastus may be speaking of Bartholomäus Reußner's *Ein kurtze Erklerung und Christliche Widerlegung*.

[17] Pagel comments on these aspects of Erastus's refutation. See Pagel, *Paracelsus*, 316–317.

of which I will give to the printer at this season's fair, as I hope, so that it comes out at the next [i.e., the autumn fair][18]—will contain almost two alphabets. For it seemed appropriate to me to refute Pomponazzi's book *De incantationibus*[19] and Avicenna's opinion, and other similar views. I hope that before this volume has been printed, I will have also finished the second volume.[20]

Text No. 5

Erastus to H. Bullinger, April 9, [15]71. StAZ, E II 361, fols. 18–18ᵃ.

[fol. 18ʳ] Partem primam operis contra Parac[elsum] suscepti, adiuvante Domino, absolvi. Spero proximis nundinis exituram. [. . .] Si Helvetius, (quem tamen fuisse Helvetium nec dum credo) scripsit male, confutavit eundem Helvetius, si non benè, saltem verè. Undique accipio literas, publicante institutum meum D[omino] Joh[anne] Cratone Caes[aris] Medico, quibus ad opus incitor. Et res me ipsa multò magis impellit. Sanctè namque, tibi iuro, nec Arium, nec Photinum, nec Mahometem nec Turcum alium, nec Haereticum vixisse ullum hoc pestilentissimo Mago magis haereticum. Probavi omnia verbis ipsius: et ex vera philosophia solidè sic confutavi, ut in hac re, cum aliàs in paucis mihi satisfaciam, mihi ipse non displiceam. [. . .] Inserui nonnihil ex tuis literis: sed ita inserui, ut tibi non improbatum iri con[si]lium confidam. [. . .]

Translation

With God's help, I have finished the first part of the work against Paracelsus that I have undertaken.[21] I hope it will appear at the next fair[22] [. . .] If a Swiss person wrote evil (however, I do not yet believe that he was Swiss), then a Swiss person has refuted him, if not well, at least truly. I receive letters from all directions, since Johannes Crato, the imperial physician,

[18] Erastus is speaking here of the biannual Frankfurt fair which was held in the spring and in the fall.
[19] Pietro Pomponazzi, *De naturalium effectuum admirandorum causis seu de incantationibus* (Basel, 1556).
[20] Erastus speaks here of *De medicina nova*, 1 and 2.
[21] *De medicina nova*, 1.
[22] I.e., the autumn Frankfurt fair.

is publicizing my intention, by which I am spurred on to the work. But the project itself compels me much more. For I solemnly swear to you, that neither Arius, nor Photinus, nor Muhammad, nor other Turk, nor any heretic who has [ever] lived was more heretical than this most pestilential magician.[23] I have examined all of his words, and I have so solidly confuted them out of true philosophy, that while on most occasions I am seldom satisfied, I am quite pleased with myself in this matter. [...] I have inserted some material from your letters [into *De medicina nova*].[24] However, I have done it in a manner that I trust you would find acceptable.

Text No. 6

Erastus to J.J. Grynaeus, April 17, [1571]. Basel UB, Ms. G II 4, fol. 255.

[fol. 255^r] Paracels[ici] operis partem primam, eamque difficilimam, et omnibus omnium artium studiosis ultissimam, auxiliante Domino absolvi. Editus nunc est alius eiusdem autoris liber, cuius confutationem per appendicem adnectere cogito. Spero me bonis omnibus gratam operam praestitisse. Hoc scio nullam habuisse ullum haeresiarcham opiniones magis blasphemas et pestilentes: quod facilè credent porrò, qui, quae ex eo citavimus, considerabunt. Si [fol. 255^v] potes opera tua nobis adesse, atque ut emendatè politèque edatur curare in Quarto, rogo ne desis. Dedissem Samueli, nisi promisissem Perna iam pridem. Sed potero facere in sequentibus, quod placebit. Indicem velim bonum, qui loca etiam notaret, in quibus eadem repetantur (Saepè enim quae uno in loco concisè, in alio plenius sunt declarta) ut concordantiae cuiusdam simul et indicis muni[a] impleret. Mihi per negocia non licuit contexere.

Pro iis, quae de Paracelso scripsisti, ingentes tibi ago gratias: et oro, ut ex Henrico Petri, quae ante scripsi, exploratius intelligas. [...]

[23] A similar comment is found in *De medicina nova*, 1:25: "Quis porrò negare audebit, Paracelsum cunctis Arianis, Mahometanis, Turcis, Haereticis pestilentiorem haereticum esse?"

[24] I.e., Bullinger's description of Paracelsus that was printed in *De medicina nova*, 1:239–240. See chapter 8 above. I thank Kurt Jakob Rüetschi of the Bullinger-Briefwechsel-Edition for correcting the transcription of this passage.

Translation

The first and the most difficult part of the Paracelsian work,[25] and the most important to all students of all the arts, by the help of God, I have finished. Now another book of the same author has been published,[26] a confutation of which I am considering adding as an appendix. I hope that I have offered a work that is pleasing to all good men. I know that no other heresiarch has had more blasphemous and pestilent opinions; moreover, those who will closely examine what I have cited from him will easily believe that. I ask that you do not fail to help with the work, if you can and see to it that it is published in a quarto edition in a faultless and polished manner. I would have given it to Samuel if I had not already promised it to [Pietro] Perna.[27] If I am able to bring it out in sequential volumes, that will suffice. I desire a good index, which also notes the places, in which the same things are covered again (For often things that are treated concisely in one place have been explained more fully in another) so that it functions as a kind of concordance and index at the same time. Because of my affairs, I am not now able to put it together.

I am grateful for the things which you have written concerning Paracelsus and ask that you discern more exactly from Heinrich Petri, concerning the things that I have written before.

Text No. 7

Erastus to J. Camerarius II, May 30, [1571].
Erlangen UB (Sammlung Trew), No. 2.

[recto] Pars prima tradita fuit Typographo priusquam ult[im]o editum Paracelsi librum viderem. Confutavi tum hunc quoque per appendicem. Negat in hoc, ut caetera sileam, apertè carnis resurrectionem. Negat Virginem ex Adamo propagatum. Negat Christum ex ea aliquid assumsisse.

[25] *De medicina nova*, 1.

[26] Erastus is speaking here of the Michael Toxites's edition of Paracelsus's *Astronomia Magna: oder die gantze Philosophia sagax der grossen und kleinen Welt.*

[27] Perhaps Erastus was speaking of Samuel Apiarius (Biener), who, like Erastus's printers Pietro Perna and Konrad Waldkirch, was also an active printer of Paracelsian writings. On the other hand, Erastus may have been referring to Samuel König. See K. Sudhoff, *Bibliographia Paracelsica*, 704. Regarding Perna, see the titles by Gilly and Rodondò listed above.

Negat denique Patrem omnipotentem esse creatorem. Alia non commemoro, cum fuerint antea confutata. Dedicabo Augusto, quanquam aliud fuerat consilium, ut in praefatione ipsum moneam, quanto à Toxite dedecore infamiaque affectus fuerit illius sceleratiss[imi] libri dedicatione. Apertè, modestè tamen, omnes monebo, quid in talibus facere conveniat Magistratus. [...]

Coniunctus, rogo te, ut ad D[ominum] Cratonem perferri cures. Scripsit is mihi nuper de re eadem, nec minus urget te ipso.

Translation

Part one[28] had been handed over to the printer before I saw the most recently published book of Paracelsus.[29] Then I confuted it too, in an appendix.[30] He openly denies the resurrection of the flesh in this, not to mention others things. He denies that the virgin was propagated from Adam. He denies that Christ had assumed anything from her. And finally, he denies that the Father is an omnipotent creator. Other things I do not bring up, since they were confuted before. I will dedicate it to [Elector] August [of Saxony], although there was another intention, with the result that in the preface I warn him,[31] how much shame and infamy he will have been brought by Toxites with the dedication of that very wicked book of his.[32] Openly and also honestly I will advise all what a Magistrate should do in such situations. [...]

Along with this, I ask you to see to it that this [letter] be delivered to Lord Crato. He wrote me recently concerning that same thing, and no less urges you to the same purpose. [...]

---

[28] *De medicina nova*, 1.

[29] Paracelsus, *Astronomia Magna*.

[30] *De medicina nova*, 1:243–267.

[31] See Erastus's dedicatory preface to *De medicina nova*, 1:aii^{r}-aiv(^{v}). Along with dedicating the first volume of *De medicina nova* to Elector August of Saxony, Erastus also sent him a personal letter (in German) outlining the same errors of Paracelsus that he here describes to Camerarius in greater detail. Erastus to Kurfürst August von Sachsen, Heidelberg, Sept. 9, 1571. Sächsisches Hauptstaatsarchiv (Dresden), Geheim.Rat (Geheim. Archiv), Loc. 8523, Sechs unterschiedliche Bücher, bd. 1; 1570–1574, fols. 186^{r}–187^{v}.

[32] Toxites had dedicated the book to Elector August. See Toxites's preface to the *Astronomia Magna*.

Text No. 8

Erastus to J.J. Grynaeus, June 26, (1571). Basel UB, Ms. G II 4, fol. 291.

[fol. 291^{r}] Si nolle Typographum intelligeres, habeo qui etiam centum Thaleros offerant, cum ipsi gratis dederim. Iam ita increbruit fama huius rei, ut sine mea infamia differi non possit res. Quare te oro, ut, si putes non facturam officium D[ominum] Petrum nostrum, quod mihi de eo promitto, alii tradas. Do enim hac in re tibi plenam potestatem hoc ipso scripto, si vel nolit vel non possit ad proximas nundinas absolvere. Fui ante biduum Francoforti, ubi ea intellexi, quae me vehementer incitant, ad hoc petendum, quod peto. Dixerat mihi D[ominus] Perna se in Bohemiam iturum, et ad mensis Maii finem domi futurum, atque curaturam ut parata interea temporis charta mox procuderetur. Iam à D[omino] Cratone Caes[aris] Medico, qui et ipse urget opus, intellegi eum .12. Maii Pragam nondum appulisse: nec scio adhuc, num redierit domum. Literas eius vidi nullas, nec audivi de eo certi aliquid à quoquam. Rogo igitur ut curae tibi sit. [...]

[fol. 291^{v}] Partem secundam Paracels[icam] aggressus bona ex parte perfeci.

Mitto nunc praefationem et appendicem primae partis: cum citius mittere non licuerit. [...]

Translation

If you think that the printer does not want it,[33] I have some who are offering even 100 thalers, although I would have given it to him for free. Already the talk of the matter has increased to the point that it cannot be postponed without my disgrace. For this reason, if you think our Peter [Perna] will not do the job which I am sending to him, I ask that you give it to someone else. For I give you full power in the affair by this writing, if either he does not want [it] or is not able to finish it by the next fair. A couple days ago I was in Frankfurt, where I have learned certain things, which greatly stimulate me to ask these things that I am

[33] I.e., Pietro Perna.

asking. Perna said to me that he was on his way to Bohemia and would be home at the end of May, and that he would see to it that the text that is readied in the meantime will be produced then. From Lord Crato, the Imperial Physician, who solicited this work, I have heard that he had not yet arrived at Prague as of 12 May. I do not know as yet, whether he will have returned home. I have not seen letters from him nor have I heard anything certain concerning him from anyone. Therefore, I ask that you look into it. [...]

I have to a good extent finished the second part of the Paracelsica.[34]

I am now sending you the preface and appendix for the first part, as I was unable to send them sooner.

Text No. 9

Erastus to H. Bullinger, Aug. 5, [1571]. StAZ, E II 361, fol. 78.

[fol. 78^r] Perna mihi spem facit, fore, ut Paracelsica nostra ad proximas exeant nundinas. Quod si est futurum vehementer cupio de re tota vestra audire libera iudicia. Si peccatum est, locus erit revocationi et emendationi in sequentibus. Quippe dum philosophia tracto in secunda parte, cogar subinde intermiscere theologica, velim, nolim.

Translation

Perna gives me hope that our Paracelsica is coming out at the next fair.[35] But if it is to have a future, I strongly desire to hear your frank opinion of the whole matter. If there is an error, the passage will be removed and corrected in succeeding volumes. Of course, while I handle philosophy in the second part, I am forced from time to time to mix in theology, whether I want to or not.

---

[34] *De medicina nova*, 2.

[35] The autumn fair, 1571.

Text No. 10

Erastus to H. Bullinger, Nov. 2, [1571]. StAZ, E II 361, fol. 74.

[fol. 74r] Accedit hoc, quod partem alterum Paracelsicae confutationis expedire cogor: qua mihi re nulla umquam plus attulit doloris et molestiae. Tam sunt enim prodigiose tum falsa tum impia, ut quid primò suscipiam refellendum plerumque nesciam. Putavi in prima parte me impietatem detexisse, verum, ut video, vix attigi ex plurimis pauca. Non puto sub hoc sole vixisse hominem nequiorem, magisque impium. Et repertus tamen est, qui speciosa oratione impietatem colorando, et absurditatem tegendo, nefario conatu ausus sit librum edere Ideae Medicinae philosophicae et Paracelsiae etc. quo valde multis, imposuit, imponit, imponet. et[cetera].[...]

Translation

As it happens, I am forced to prepare the second part of the Paracelsian confutation; nothing has ever brought me more anguish and annoyance than this. For they are so incredibly deceptive and impious,[36] that I often do not know why I began refuting them in the first place. I thought that I had exposed their impiety in the first part,[37] but as I see, I have scarcely touched on a few of the many points. I do not think that a more evil and impious man has ever lived under this sun.[38] And now there is one who, by coloring [Paracelsus's] impiety with pretty speech and defending [his] absurdity (an abominable endeavor!), has dared to publish a book, the *Idea medicinae philosophicae et Paracelsiae etc.*,[39] by which he has deceived, deceives, and will deceive many people, etc. [...]

36 I.e., Paracelsus's teachings.

37 I.e., *De medicina nova*, 1.

38 For a German translation of this passage, see Gilly, *Zwischen Erfahrung und Spekulation*, 2:182.

39 Severinus, *Idea medicinae philosophicae.*

Text No. 11

Erastus to Th. Zwinger, Heidelberg, Easter, [April 6, 1572]. Basel UB, Fr.Gr. Ms. II 4, no. 93

[verso] Deo est gratia, quod propemodum tertiam quoque parte[m] absolvi: in qua complura non inutilia studiosis Medicinae declarare conor saltem, si non assequor. Mirabuntur boni viri, et miror ips[e]met nonnumquam patientiam meam: quae tamen non semper satis magn[a] est. Illud etiam te rogatum etiam atque etiam velim, ut quae de ha[c] vita moribusque à patruo tuo audivisti, notare mihi velis: imprimis ad curationes spectantia.

Translation

With God's grace, I have also nearly finished the third part,[40] in which at least I endeavor, if I do not succeed, to declare several things that are useful to medicine. Good men will marvel at my patience—even I myself am sometimes amazed—and yet it is not always great enough. I still wish what I have asked you again and again, that you would write down for me those things about this man's life and customs that you have heard from your uncle [Johannes Oporinus], especially regarding his cures.

Text No. 12

Erastus to H. Bullinger, Sept. 24, [1572]. StAZ, E II 361, fol. 32–32[a].

[fol. 32a[r]] Cum obsignaturus essem, duo in mentem venerant. Alterum est quod monere volui ne labores in legendis Antiparac[elsicarum] nostrarum disput[ationum] partibus aliis. Sunt enim secunda et tertia merè phi[losoph]ica et Medica ex sacris literis tamen comprobata. Hoc enim propositum fuit ostendere, verae philosophiae principia à Deo approbari. In tertiae initio confutavi .18. proposit[iones] cuiusdam Paracels[ici] quibus magis impium nihil excogitatum à Cacodaemone arbitror. Filium Dei facit sp[iritu]m in nobis corporeum, quique arte Chemica possit visibilis reddi: imò mortalis qui sit: et alia talia nefanda deliramenta conti-

[40] *De medicina nova*, 3.

nent plurima. Mihi satis est, Si Theologis non displiceant, quae in prima parte disputavimus, ad exterminandas superstitiosas vanitates, quibus irretiti omnium propè, etiam bonorum, animi tenentur.

Translation

Since I have sealed this, two things have come to mind.[41] One is that I wanted to inform you—lest you are troubled in reading the other parts of our Antiparacelsian disputations. For the second and third parts are purely philosophical and medical yet confirmed by Holy Scripture. For it was proposed to show the principles of true philosophy approved by God. In the beginning of the third part, I have refuted "18 Propositions" of a certain Paracelsian,[42] which I judge to be more impious than anything contrived by an evil spirit. He makes the Son of God a corporeal spirit in us, one that can be rendered visible by Chemical art. Indeed, it is even mortal. And most [i.e., the "18 Propositions"] contain other such unspeakable nonsense. It is enough for me, if those things which we have disputed in the first part—for the purpose of banishing superstitious vanities which entangle the minds of almost everyone, even good people—do not displease the theologians.

---

[41] This extract comes from the postscript of the letter. Erastus's second concern was about a family matter, and so it has not been reproduced here.

[42] Erastus is speaking here of Alexander von Suchten. See *De medicina nova*, 3:13–60. Though Suchten is not named in the text, he is named in the index (fol. kkk 2^{r}). See above chapter 8.

CORRESPONDENCE REGISTER

Abbreviations

Cod. Bern.	[Burgerbibliothek Bern] *Catalogus codicum bernensium*. Ed. Hermann Hagen. Bern, 1875.
Crato, *Consiliorum et Epistolarum.*	Crato von Krafftheim, Johannes. *Consiliorum et Epistolarum Medicinalium, Liber....* 5 vols. Frankfurt: Apud Andreae Wecheli haeredes, Claudium Marnium & Joan. Aubrium [Claude de Marne and Jean Aubry], 1591–1594.
DBI	*Dizionario Biografico Italiani*, Rome: Instituto della Enciclopedia Italiana, 1975.
De astrologia.	*De astrologia divinatrice epistolae....* Basel: Pietro Perna, 1580.
De causa morborum.	"De causa morborum continente, tractatus." In *Disputationum de nova Philippi Paracelsi Medicina Pars Tertia*. Basel: Pietro Perna, 1572.
Disp. et Epist.	*Thomae Erasti Philosophi et Medici celeberrime, Disputationum & Epistolarum Medicinalium volumen doctissimum. ...* Zürich: Johannes Wolf, 1595.
Explicatio Gravissimae Quaestionis.	*Explicatio Gravissimae Quaestionis, utrum Excommunicatio....* [London: J. Wolfe], 1589.
Goldast	Melchior Goldast, ed. *Philologicarum Epistolarum Centuria Una Diversorum A Renatis Literis Doctissimorum Virorum....* Leipzig, 1674.
Hagen	Hermann Hagen, *Briefe von Heidelberger Professoren und Studenten*. Bern, 1886.
Hot.	Thesaurus Hottingerianus, letter collection in the Zentralbibliothek Zürich.

Koch	Ernst Koch, "Die Badereisen des Grafen Georg Ernst zu Henneberg." *Zeitschrift des Vereins für hennebergische Geschichte und Landeskunde in Schmalkalden* 15 (1905): 1–45.
Miscellanea Medica.	Smet, Heinrich., ed. *Miscellanea ... Medica.* Frankfurt: Jonas Rhodius, 1611.
Rott	Hans Rott, ed. "Neue Quellen für eine Aktenrevision des Processes gegen Sylvan und seine Genossen." *Neues Archiv für die Geschichte der Stadt Heidelberg und der rheinischen Pfalz* 8 & 9 (1910 & 1911): 184–259, 1–70.
Sim.	Simmlersche Sammlung, letter collection in the Zentralbibliothek Zürich (mostly copies).
Scholz	*Epistolarum Philosophicarum: medicinalium, ac chymicarum a summis nostrae aetatis philosophis ac medicis exaraturum, volumen ... Nunc primum labore, ac industria, Laurentii Scholzii a Rozenaw ... foras datum.* Frankfurt: Apud Andreae Wecheli haeredes, Claudium Marnium & Joan. Aubrium [Claude de Marne and Jean Aubry], 1598.
U-F	Uffenbach-Wolfschen Briefsammlung, Hamburg.
Vulcanius	*Correspondance de Bonaventura Vulcanius pendant son séjour à Cologne, Genèvé et Bâle* (1573–1577). H. de Vries de Heekelingen, ed. La Haye: Nijhoff, 1923.
Zedler	C.G. Ludovici, *Grosses vollständiges Universal-Lexicon aller Wissenschaften und Künste ...* (Halle: J.H. Zedler, 1732–1750).
Zofingen	Staatsbibliothek und Stadtarchiv, Zofingen.

Johannes Acronius (alias Frisius) Arts Professor in Basel (1526–1564) *NDB*, 1:39.

1. Erastus to an unnamed mathematician [Acronius],[1] Frankfurt Fair, April 2, 1558. Printed in *De astrologia*, 129–158 (no. 10).
2. Erastus to an unnamed mathematician [Acronius], Heidelberg, 1558. Printed in *De astrologia*, 159–166 (no. 11).
3. Erastus to an unnamed mathematician [Acronius], Heidelberg, Oct. 7, 1558. Printed in *De astrologia*, 166–189 (no. 12).

Basilius Amerbach, Basel Jurist, Professor, and Magistrate (1533–1591) *NDB*, 1:246–247.

1. Erastus to Amerbach, Heidelberg, May 1, 1564. Basel UB, MS G II 16, fol. 295.

Bonifacius Amerbach, Basel Humanist and Jurist (1495–1562) *NDB*, 1:246–247.

1. Erastus to Amerbach, Maßfeld (Henneberg), July 29, 1557. Basel UB, MS Ki.Ar. 18a, 177–178.

Guillaume Arragos (Arragosius) (1513–1610)
see Erastus to Zwinger

Valentin Ampelander (Rebmann) Theologian and Humanist in Bern (d. 1587)

1. Erastus to Ampelander, Heidelberg, Nov. 29, n.y. Cod. Bern, A. 27, 4. Printed in Hagen, 33.

Elector August of Saxony (1526–1586) *NDB*, 1:448.

1. Erastus to August, Heidelberg, Sept. 9, 1571. Sächsisches Hauptstaatsarchiv (Dresden), Geheim.Rat (Geheim Archiv), Loc. 8523, Sechs unterschiedliche Bücher, bd. 1; 1570–1574, fols. 186r–187v. Excerpt printed in Kühlmann and Telle, eds. *Corpus Paracelsisticum*, 2:227–228.

"Lord Baron" (*Domino Baro*), cf. Lazarus von Schwendi (also possibly Johann Philipp Freiherr von Hohensax)

Basel Magistrate (not named)

1. Erastus to [a Basel magistrate; Heinrich Petri, Lucas Gebhard, or Balthasar Hanius?] [likely 1577/78]. Basel UB, MS G II 4, fol. 268 (included with the letters addressed to J.J. Grynaeus in the Basel UB).

Theodore Beza (Théodore de Bèze) Theologian in Geneva (1519–1605)

1. Erastus to Beza, Heidelberg, April 17, [1568]. Gotha, Forschungsbibliothek, cod. chart. A 405, fol. 274. Printed in *CB*, 11:344–345 (Addendum to vol. 9, no. 601bis).
2. Erastus to Beza, Heidelberg, January, 1570. First fragment, BL, Add. MS 28571, fols. 62–63 (copy); second fragment M.H.R., Archives Tronchin, Geneva, vol. 5, fol. 112. Printed in *CB*, 11:29–35 (no. 732).

[1] Stefano Dall'Aglio, "Da Girolamo Savonarola a Tommaso Erasto: Itinerari di una polemica astrologica tra Firenze e Heidelberg," in *Armando Saitta, Scritti in ricordo di*

1. Beza to [Erastus], Geneva, [1568]. Printed in Beza, *Epistolarum theologicarum liber unus* (Geneva: E. Vignon, 1573), 182–188 (no. 29). Reprinted in Goldast, 268–275 (falsely described as a letter of Camillus Franchinus to Erastus). Reprinted in *CB*, 9:208–214 (no. 651).
2. Beza to Erastus, Geneva, Dec. 18, 1569. Oxford, Bodleian Library, MS lat misc. c 17, fol. 10. Printed in *CB*, 10:245–247 (no. 723).

Albrecht Blaurer, Medical Professor in Heidelberg; City Physician in St. Gallen (1543–1592)

1. Erastus to Blaurer, n.d. St. Gallen, Vadianische Sammlung, MS 41 (Tom. XII), fol. 166. (Copy ZBZ (Hot.), MS F 43, fol. 471).

Martin Borrhaus (alias Cellarius) Theologian in Basel (1499–1564) *NDB*, 2:474.

1. Erastus to M. Borrhaus, Sept. 20, 1561 (copy). Landesbibliothek und Murhardsche Bibliothek der Stadt Kassel, Universitätsbibliothek Kassel, 4° MS Hass. 101 [2.

Heinrich Brucaeus, Medical Professor in Rostock (1530/31–93) Zedler, 4, col. 1495.

1. Erastus to Brucaeus, Heidelberg, Oct. 14, 1577. Printed in *Miscellanea Medica*, 308–312 (Liber VI; no. VI).

Christoph Bullinger, Son of Heinrich Bullinger (1537–1568/69)

1. C. Bullinger to Erastus, Sept. 10, (15)60. ZBZ (Hot.), MS F 37, fol. 534.

Heinrich Bullinger, Theologian and *Antistes* in Zürich (1504–1575) *NDB*, 3:12.[2]

1. Erastus to Bullinger, Oct. 8, (1560). StAZ, MS E II 361, fols. 7 & 83–83[a].
2. Erastus to Bullinger, Oct. 8, [1560]. StAZ, MS E II 361, fol. 8.
3. Erastus to Bullinger, Oct. 30, [1560]. StAZ, MS E II 361, fols. 85–85[a].
4. Erastus to Bullinger, Heidelberg, Jan. 1, [1561]. StAZ, MS E II 361, fols. 63–63[a].
5. Erastus to Bullinger, Schleusingen and Frankfurt, March 18 & March 25, (1561). ZBZ (Hot.) F 38, fols. 264–265. (fragment).
6. Erastus to Bullinger, May 19, [1561]. StAZ, MS E II 345, fol. 736 & E II 361, 85[b].
7. Erastus to Bullinger, July 16, [1561]. StAZ, MS E II 361, fol. 62.
8. Erastus to Bullinger, Sept. 18, (15)61. StAZ, MS E II 345, fol. 491.
9. Erastus to Bullinger, Oct. 6, [1561]. StAZ, MS E II 345, fol. 734.
10. Erastus to Bullinger, Heidelberg, Nov. 21, [1561]. StAZ, MS E II 361, fol. 29.
11. Erastus to Bullinger, Heidelberg, Dec. 10, [1561]. StAZ, MS E II 361, fols. 64[v]&[r].

[11B. [Erastus] to [Bullinger], [ca. Jan. 1562]. ZBZ, S 103, 69.][3]

Armando Saitta (Milan: FrancoAngeli, 2002), 63–65. The connection of letters in this collection to Acronius is confirmed by Erastus to Grynaeus, Dec. 29, (15)79, Basel UB, MS G II 4, fols. 285–286.

[2] This list of the Bullinger-Erastus correspondences retains the numeration of Benrath with a few corrections and augmentations. Benrath, "Die Korrespondenz zwischen Bullinger und Thomas Erastus," 131–141.

[3] This letter fragment in the ZBZ is likely from Erastus to Bullinger. See Janse, *Albert Hardenberg als Theologe*, 406, note 352.

12. Erastus to Bullinger, Heidelberg, Feb. 11, (15)62. StAZ, MS E II 361, fol. 83^{b} (fragment).
13. Erastus to Bullinger, Heidelberg, March 26, [1562]. StAZ, MS E II 361, fol. 26.
14. Erastus to Bullinger, Heidelberg, April 6, [1562]. StAZ, MS E II 361, fol. 65.
15. Erastus to Bullinger, Heidelberg, April 16, [1562]. StAZ, MS E II 361, fol. 82.
16. Erastus to Bullinger, Heidelberg, May 25, [1562]. StAZ, MS E II 345, fols. 732–733.
17. Erastus to Bullinger, Heidelberg, June 24, [1562]. StAZ, MS E II 345, fol. 739.
18. Erastus to Bullinger, Heidelberg, Dec. 5, [1562]. StAZ, MS E II 361, fol. 27.
19. Erastus to Bullinger, Heidelberg, Jan. 30, [1563]. StAZ, MS E II 361, fol. 86.
20. Erastus to Bullinger, Feb. 26, [1563]. StAZ, MS E II 345, fol. 735.
21. Erastus to Bullinger, March 9, [1563]. StAZ, MS E II 361, fol. 25.
22. Erastus to Bullinger, April 29, [1563]. StAZ, MS E II 345, fols. 738 & 740.
23. Erastus to Bullinger, June 11, [1563]. StAZ, MS E II 345, fol. 745.
24. Erastus to Bullinger, July 2, (15)63. StAZ, MS E II 361, fol. 88.
25. Erastus to Bullinger, Heidelberg, July 14, [1563]. StAZ, MS E II 361, fol. 89.
26. Erastus to Bullinger, [Sept./Oct., 1563]. StAZ, MS E II 361, fol. 28.
27. Erastus to Bullinger, April 4, [1564]. StAZ, MS E II 361, fols. 84–84^{b}.
28. Erastus to Bullinger, Maulbronn, April 12, [1564]. StAZ, MS E II 345, fols. 648^{v} & 649.
29. Erastus to Bullinger, April 20, [1564]. StAZ, MS E II 345, fol. 731.
30. Erastus to Bullinger, May 26, [1564]. StAZ, MS E II 361, fol. 87.
31. Erastus to Bullinger, July 29, [1564]. StAZ, MS E II 361, fol. 66.
32. Erastus to Bullinger, August 25, [1564]. StAZ, MS E II 361, fol. 81.
33. Erastus to Bullinger, Oct. 13 [1564]. StAZ, MS E II 361, fol. 68.
34. Erastus to Bullinger, Heidelberg, Jan. 13, 1565. StAZ, MS E II 361, fol. 9.
35. Erastus to Bullinger, Heidelberg, Jan. 24, [1565]. StAZ, MS E II 361, fol. 50.
36. Erastus to Bullinger, March 11, [1565]. StAZ, MS E II 361, fol. 48.
37. Erastus to Bullinger, April 24, [1565]. StAZ, MS E II 361, fol. 52.
38. Erastus to Bullinger, Heidelberg, May 25, [1565]. StAZ, MS E II 361, fol. 40.
39. Erastus to Bullinger, Heidelberg, Sept. 26, [1565]. StAZ, MS E II 361, fol. 41.
40. Erastus to Bullinger, Oct. 24 [1565]. StAZ, MS E II 361, fol. 39.
41. Erastus to Bullinger, Nov. 23, 1565. StAZ, MS E II 371, fol. 1012.
42. Erastus to Bullinger, Heidelberg, Jan. 1, 1566. StAZ, MS E II 361, fol. 10.
43. Erastus to Bullinger, Heidelberg, Feb. 14, 1566. StAZ, MS E II 371, fol. 1065.
44. Erastus to Bullinger, Heidelberg, April 5, 1566. StAZ, MS E II 361, fol. 4.
45. Erastus to Bullinger, April 12, [1566]. StAZ, MS E II 361, fol. 49.
46. Erastus to Bullinger, May 5, 1566. StAZ, MS E II 361, fol. 2.
47. Erastus to Bullinger, June 30, 1566. StAZ, MS E II 371, fols. 1108–1109.
48. Erastus to Bullinger, August 7, [1566]. StAZ, MS E II 371, fol. 1130.
49. Erastus to Bullinger, August 9, [1566]. StAZ, MS E II 361, fol. 73.
50. Erastus to Bullinger, Sept. 24, [1566]. StAZ, MS E II 361, fol. 43.
51. Erastus to Bullinger, Roth bei Nürnberg, Oct. 26, [1566]. StAZ, MS E II 361, fol. 36.
52. Erastus to Bullinger, Jan. 4, 1567. StAZ, MS E II 361, fol. 13.
53. Erastus to Bullinger, March 28, [1567]. StAZ, MS E II 361, fol. 67.
54. Erastus to Bullinger, April 10, [1567]. StAZ, MS E II 350, fol. 95.
55. Erastus to Bullinger, Heidelberg, April 17, [1567]. StAZ, MS E II 350, fol. 89.
56. Erastus to Bullinger, [1567]. StAZ, MS E II 361, fol. 37.
57. Erastus to Bullinger, July 13, 1567. StAZ, MS E II 361, fol. 11.
58. Erastus to Bullinger, July 31, [1567]. StAZ, MS E II 361, fol. 46.

59. Erastus to Bullinger, Sept. 21, [1567]. StAZ, MS E II 361, fol. 75.
60. Erastus to Bullinger, Feb, 29, [1568]. StAZ, MS E II 361, fol. 54.
61. Erastus to Bullinger, April 17 & 18, [1568]. StAZ, MS E II 361, fol. 42.
62. Erastus to Bullinger, May 27, 1568. StAZ, MS E II 361, fol. 12.
63. Erastus to Bullinger, July 18, [1568]. StAZ, MS E II 361, fol. 35.
64. Erastus to Bullinger, August 21, [1568]. StAZ, MS E I 25, 8, fol. 52.
65. Erastus to Bullinger, Oct. 25, [1568]. StAZ, MS E II 361, fol. 71.
66. Erastus to [Bullinger ?], Dec. 12, 1568. StAZ, MS E I 25, 8, fol. 87^a (fragment).
67. Erastus to Bullinger, Feb. 2, 1569. StAZ, MS E II 346a, fols. 549–550.
68. Erastus to Bullinger, March 6, 1569. StAZ, MS E II 361, fol. 14.
69. Erastus to Bullinger, [April, 1569]. StAZ, MS E II 361, fol. 70.
70. Erastus to Bullinger, April 13, [1569]. ZBZ F 62, fol. 203.
71. Erastus to Bullinger, May 3, [1569]. StAZ, MS E II 361, fol. 15.
72. Erastus to Bullinger, May 22, [1569]. StAZ, MS E II 361, fol. 38.
73. Erastus to Bullinger, July 8, (15)69. StAZ, MS E II 346a, fol. 551.
74. Erastus to Bullinger, Oct. 10, 1569. StAZ, MS E II 361, fols. 16–16a.
75. Erastus to Bullinger, Nov. 21, [1569]. StAZ, MS E II 361, fol. 77.
76. Erastus to Bullinger, Jan. 1, (15)70. StAZ, MS E II 361, fol. 17.
77. Erastus to Bullinger, Jan. 24, [1570]. StAZ, MS E II 361, fol. 33.
78. Erastus to Bullinger, Feb. 4, [1570]. StAZ, MS E II 361, fol. 76.
79. Erastus to Bullinger, March 21, [1570]. StAZ, MS E II 361, fol. 57.
80. Erastus to Bullinger, April 1, [1570]. StAZ, MS E II 361, fol. 59.
81. Erastus to Bullinger, n.d. [After June 5, 1570]. StAZ, MS E II 345, fols. 743–744.
82. Erastus to Bullinger, July 18, [1570]. StAZ, MS E II 345. fol. 730.
83. Erastus to Bullinger, August 8, 1570. StAZ, MS E II 345. fol. 691.
84. Erastus to Bullinger, Sept. 21, [1570]. StAZ, MS E II 361, fol. 61.
85. Erastus to Bullinger, Oct. 29, [1570]. StAZ, MS E II 345. fols. 741–742.
86. Erastus to Bullinger, Jan. 3, 1571. ZBZ, F 62, fol. 204.
87. Erastus to Bullinger, Feb. 2, [1571]. StAZ, MS E II 361, fol. 72.
88. Erastus to Bullinger, April 9 & 18, (15)71. StAZ, MS E II 361, fols. 18–18^a.
89. Erastus to Bullinger, [Easter, April 15, 1571]. StAZ, MS E II 361, fol. 45.
90. Erastus to Bullinger, April 22, [1571]. StAZ, MS E II 361, fol. 69.
91. Erastus to Bullinger, May 27, (15)71. StAZ, MS E II 361, fol. 19.
92. Erastus to Bullinger, Aug. 5, [1571]. StAZ, MS E II 361, fol. 78.
93. Erastus to Bullinger, Nov. 2, [1571]. StAZ, MS E II 361, fol. 74.
93b. Erastus to [Bullinger], [ca. March 1, 1572]. StAZ, MS E II 361, fol. 44.[4]
94. Erastus to Bullinger, April 24, [Bn.: 1572]. StAZ, MS E II 361, fol. 3.
95. Erastus to Bullinger, [ca. April/June 1572]. StAZ, MS E II 361, fol. 34.
96. Erastus to Bullinger, August 18, [1572]. StAZ, MS E II 342, fol. 693.
97. Erastus to Bullinger, n.d., [1572]. StAZ, MS E II 361, fol. 79.

[4] This letter is in fact addressed to Johann Jakob Grynaeus and not Bullinger. Benrath omitted the letter from his list, and it is included in the StAZ catalog as a letter to Grynaeus. However, the Basel UB catalog has the letter's equivalent, which is a letter actually written to Grynaeus but addressed to Bullinger (viz. Erastus to [J.J. Grynaeus], March 1, (15)72, Basel UB, Ms. G II 4, fol. 180). In comparing the letters it is apparent that Erastus has falsely addressed the letters. This is confirmed by the fact that he refers to the addressee as his relative ("affinis") in the letter falsely addressed to Bullinger. Grynaeus seems to have sorted the false addresses out, kept his letter, and sent the one addressed to "Grynaeus" on to Bullinger in Zurich.

98. Erastus to Bullinger, Sept. 7, [1572]. StAZ, MS E II 361, fol. 80.
99. Erastus to Bullinger, Sept. 24, [1572]. StAZ, MS E II 361, fols. 32–32[a].
100. Erastus to Bullinger and Rudolf Gwalther, Dec. 21, 1572. StAZ, MS E II 361, fol. 20.
101. Erastus to Bullinger, Jan. 13, [1573]. StAZ, MS E II 361, fol. 31.
102. Erastus to Bullinger, March 23, 1573. StAZ, MS E II 361, fol. 55.
103. Erastus to Bullinger, April 24, (1573). StAZ, MS E II 361, fol. 53.
104. Erastus to Bullinger, July 31, 15(73). StAZ, MS E II 345, fol. 697.
105. Erastus to Bullinger, Aug. 21, 15(73). StAZ, MS E II 345, fol. 698.
106. Erastus to Bullinger, Sept. 21, [1573]. StAZ, MS E II 361, fol. 60.
107. Erastus to Bullinger, Nov. 6, 15(73). StAZ, MS E II 345, fol. 699.
108. Erastus to Bullinger, Nov. 20, [1573]. StAZ, MS E II 361, fol. 30.
109. Erastus to Bullinger, Dec. 17 & 27, [1573]. StAZ, MS E II 361, fol. 58.
110. Erastus to Bullinger, Jan. 1, (15)74. StAZ, MS E II 361, fol. 21.
111. Erastus to Bullinger, Jan. 24, 1574. StAZ, MS E II 381, fol. 1370.
112. Erastus to Bullinger, May 10, [1574]. StAZ, MS E II 361, fol. 47.
113. Erastus to Bullinger, [May 20, 1574]. StAZ, MS E II 361, fol. 1.
114. Erastus to Bullinger, June 16, [1574]. StAZ, MS E II 361, fol. 51.
115. Erastus to Bullinger, Sept. 30, 1574. StAZ, MS E II 361, fol. 22.
115[b]. Erastus to Bullinger, Oct. 11, 1574. StAZ, MS E II 361, fol. 23.
116. Erastus to Bullinger, Nov. 28, 1574. StAZ, MS E II 361, fol. 24.
117. Erastus to Bullinger, Dec. 8, 1574. StAZ, MS E II 378, fols. 1965–1968.

1. Bullinger to Erastus, Dec. 12, 1565. StAZ, MS E II 371, fols. 1013–1014.
2. Bullinger to Erastus, Zürich, Oct. 17, 1568. London, British Museum, Add. MSS no. 28,571, fol. 54. Printed in *Explicatio Gravissimae Quaestionis*, 350–351.
3. Bullinger to Erastus, Zürich, Oct. 29, 1568. Printed in *Explicatio Gravissimae Quaestionis*, 351–353.
4. Bullinger to Erastus, Zürich, Feb. 20, 1569. Printed in *Explicatio Gravissimae Quaestionis*, 353–354.
5. Bullinger to Erastus, [March 14, 1569]. [Partially] printed in Explicatio Gravissimae Quaestionis, 354–355.
6. Bullinger to Erastus, Zürich, August, 1, 1569. StAZ, MS E II 342, fol. 557. Printed in *Explicatio Gravissimae Quaestionis*, 367–370.
7. Bullinger to Erastus, Zürich, August 23, 1569. Printed in *Explicatio Gravissimae Quaestionis*, 371–372.
8. Bullinger to Erastus, Zürich, Nov. 5, 1569. Printed in *Explicatio Gravissimae Quaestionis*, 372–374.
9. Bullinger to Erastus, [Dec. 15, 1569; MS falsely dated to Nov. 1557]. StAZ, MS E II 342, fol. 359.
10. Bullinger to Erastus, Sept. 3, 1572. StAZ, MS E II 342, fol. 693.
11. Bullinger to Erastus, Zürich, Jan. 11, 1574. Printed in *Explicatio Gravissimae Quaestionis*, 388–389.

Daniel von Büren II, Bürgermeister in Bremen (1512–1593) *NDB*, 2:742.[5]

1. Erastus to von Büren, June 26, [1561]. SUB Bremen, MS 10, no. 64, fols. 113^r–114^v.
2. Erastus to von Büren, Dec. 26, 1563. SUB Bremen, MS 10, no. 40, fols. 72^r–73^v.

[5] Commonly known as "Daniel von Büren der Jüngere." All such designations have been rendered with "II" instead of "junior," "the younger," etc.

3. Erastus to von Büren, Jan. 22 [1566]. SUB Bremen, MS 10, no. 62, fols. 111^{r}–111^{v}.
4. Erastus to von Büren, Heidelberg, June 3, [1566]. SUB Bremen, MS 10, no. 46, fols. 82^{r}–82^{v}.
5. Erastus to von Büren, [ca. April /May 1569]. SUB Bremen, MS 10, no. 47, fols. 83^{r}–83^{v}.

Joachim Camerarius II, Physician and Naturalist in Nuremberg (1534–1598) [*NDB*, 3:105]

1. Erastus to Camerarius, Feb. 23, (15)71. Er.UB (Sammlung Trew).
2. Erastus to Camerarius, May 30, [1571]. Er.UB (Sammlung Trew).
3. Erastus to Camerarius, April, 20, (1572). Er.UB (Sammlung Trew).
4. Erastus to Camerarius, Sept. 14, (1572). Er.UB (Sammlung Trew).
5. Erastus to Camerarius, Dec. 26, (15)72. Er.UB (Sammlung Trew).
6. Erastus to Camerarius, Jan. 31, [1573]. Er.UB (Sammlung Trew).
7. Erastus to Camerarius, Feb. 17, 1574. Er.UB (Sammlung Trew).
8. Erastus to Camerarius, Sept. 11, 1577. Er.UB (Sammlung Trew).
9. Erastus to Camerarius, May 11, (1578). Er.UB (Sammlung Trew).
10. Erastus to Camerarius, July 7, (15)78. Er.UB (Sammlung Trew).
11. Erastus to Camerarius, Nov. 24, (15)78. Er.UB (Sammlung Trew).
12. Erastus to Camerarius, Jan. 16, (15)79. Er.UB (Sammlung Trew).
13. Erastus to Camerarius, Feb. 10, (1579). Er.UB (Sammlung Trew).
14. Erastus to Camerarius, Aug. 22, (15)79. Er.UB (Sammlung Trew).
15. Erastus to Camerarius, Nov. 5, (15)79. Er.UB (Sammlung Trew).
16. Erastus to Camerarius, Nov. 17, (15)79. Er.UB (Sammlung Trew).
17. Erastus to Camerarius, Basel, Feb. 8, (15)81. Er.UB (Sammlung Trew).
18. Erastus to Camerarius, Basel, Oct. 19, (15)81. Er.UB (Sammlung Trew).
19. Erastus to Camerarius, Basel, Feb. 7 (1582). Er.UB (Sammlung Trew).

Girolamo Capivaccio (Capodivacca, Capiavaccio, Capiavaciceus) Medical Professor in Padua (1523–1589) *DBI*, 18:649–651.

1. Erastus to Capivaccio, Sept. 23, 1574. Printed in *Disp. & Epist.*, fols. 50^{r}–54^{v} (no. 17).
2. Erastus to Capiavaccio, Feb. 8, 1575. Printed in *Disp. & Epist.*, fols. 65^{r}–70^{r} (no. 20).

[2a. Erastus to Capivaccio, Sept. 8, 1575. Printed in *Scholz*, cols. 482–503 (no. 269). This is the same letter as Erastus to Crato, Sept. 8, 1575. Printed in *Disp. et Epist.*, fols. 76^{v}–88^{v} (no. 23).]

3. Erastus to Capivaccio, Jan. 26, 1576. Printed in *Disp. & Epist.*, fols. 70^{r}–73^{r} (no. 21). Abbreviated version printed in *Scholz*, cols. 503–508 (no. 270).

1. Capiavaccio to Erastus, Padua, 1576. Printed in Scholz, cols. 121–126 (no. 83).

Stephan Cirler (Zirler) Palatine Bureaucrat (c. 1520–1568)[6]

1. Erastus to Cirler, Feb. 26, 1559. UAH, A/7, fols. 337^{r}–338^{r}.

1. Cirler to Erastus, ca. early April, 1559. UAH, A/7, fols. 339^{r}–339^{v}.

[6] The letters to Cirler were composed in Erastus's capacity as university rector.

Volcher Coiter (Folckerus Coiterus) Anatomist and Physician in Nuremberg (1534–1576) *NDB*, 3:317.

1. Erastus to Coiter, n.d. Germanisches National Museum, K. 5.
2. Erastus to Coiter, March 7, [1572]. Private collection.
3. Erastus to Coiter, Aug. 28, n.y. [ca. 1572–1574]. Basel UB, MS G2 II 37, fol. 11.

Johannes Crato von Krafftheim (Crafftheim) Imperial Physician (1519–1585) *NDB*, 3:402.[7]

1. Erastus to Crato, Feb. 7, 1565. Printed in *Varia Opuscula Medica* (Frankfurt: A. Wechel, 1590), 86–87. Reprinted in *Disp. et Epist.*, fols. 88^{v}–90^{r} (no. 24).
2. Erastus to Crato, Heidelberg, July 11, 1572. Printed in *De causa morborum*, fols. Aaa 2^{r}–2^{v}.
3. Erastus to Crato, Sept. 8, 1575. Printed in *Disp. et Epist.*, fols. 76^{v}–88^{v} (no. 23).
4. Erastus to Crato, April 29, 1576. Hd.UB, MS 3604, 44, photograph.
5. Erastus to Crato and Christoph Schilling, July 11, 1577. Hd.UB, MS 3604, 45, photograph. Printed in *Disp. & Epist.*, fols. 20^{r}–22^{r} (no. 8). [Crato and Schilling are not mentioned by name in the printed version.]
6. Erastus to Crato, June 22, 1578. Hd.UB, MS 3604, 46, photograph. Printed in *Disp. & Epist.*, fols. 17^{r}–20^{r} (no. 7) [without Erastus's addendum; Crato not named in the printed version].
7. Erastus to Crato, Nov. 27, 1578. Hd.UB, MS 3604, 47, photograph.

Jakob Curio (alias Hofenius, Hoffmann, Hoffmenius, etc.) Mathematics and Medical Professor in Heidelberg (1497–1572), Zedler, 6, col. 1875.

1. Erastus to [Curio], Jan. 16, 1559. Printed in *De astrologia*, 202–207 (no. 14).[8]
2. Erastus to [Curio], Feb. 1559. Printed in *De astrologia*, 207–236 (no. 15).

Celio Secondo Curione (Coelius Secundus Curio) Arts Professor in Basel (1503–1569) *NDB*, 3:442.

1. Erastus to Curione, Bologna, Sept. 6, 1552. Printed in *Coelii Secundi Curionis Selectarum Epistolarum libri duo* (Basel: Johannes Oporinus, 1553), 58–59. (http://www.uni-mannheim.de/mateo/cera/curio1/jpg/s058.html). Reprinted in *Olympiae Fulviae Moratae … opera omnia: … cum eruditorum testimoniis / Quibus praeter C.S. Curionis epistolas selectas …* (Basel: Pietro Perna, 1580), 318.
2. Erastus to Curione, April 21, n.y. [ca. 1563]. Basel UB, MS G I 66, fol. 94. (Copy U-F, 59, 60.)
3. Erastus to Curione, n.d. (copy). Basel UB, MS G2 II 40, fols. 161–165.

Conrad Dasypodius (Hasenfratz) Mathematician and Clockmaker in Strasbourg (c. 1531–1601) *NDB* 3:520.

1. Dasypodius to Erastus, Jan. 10, 1581. StAZ, MS E II 382, fols. 1026–1028^{a}.
2. Dasypodius to Erastus, Strasbourg, Jan. 27, 1581. StAZ, MS E II 382, fol. 1029.

[7] The letters preserved as photographs in Heidelberg UB are from originals from the Stadtbibliothek in Wrocław/Breslau which apparently did not survive the Second World War.

[8] The connection of letters in this collection to Curio is confirmed by Erastus to Grynaeus, Dec. 29, (15)79, Basel UB, MS G II 4, fols. 285–286.

Toussaint Ducret, Huguenot Physician (d. 1584)

1. Duret to Erastus, Dedicatory epistle. Printed in Toussaint Ducret, *De Arthritide vera assertio, eiusque curandae methodus, adversus Paracelsistas* (Lyon: Bartholomaeus Vincentius, 1575), Aii-Av.

Andreas Dudith (Dudić, Duditus, Dudich) Humanist, Imperial emissary, Bishop of Knin, later Pécs (1533–1589)

1. Erastus to Dudith, Sept. 14, 1577. Printed in Crato, *Consiliorum et Epistolarum* (1592), 3:318–320. Reprinted in Scholz, cols. 481–482 (no. 268).

1. Dudith to Erastus, Paskov, Moravia, Feb. 1, 1579. Printed in *De Cometis dissertationes novae clariss. vivorum Thom. Erasti, Andr. Dudithij, Marc. Squacialupi, Symon. Grynaei* (Basel: Leonhard Ostein, 1580), 23–26.

Thaddaeus Dunus (Taddeo Duni) City Physician in Zürich (1523–1613)

1. Erastus to Dunus, April 9, 1571. Printed in *Disp. et Epist.*, fols. 106^{r}–106^{v} (no. 27).

Elizabeth von Braunschweig-Lüneburg, Countess of Henneberg (1510–1558) *NDB*, 4:443–444

1. Erastus to Gräfin Elizabeth, Heidelberg, Oct. 12, (15)61. GHA, Sekt. I, 1103.

1. Gräfin Elizabeth to Erastus, Maßfeld, 1561. GHA, Sekt. I, 1103.
2. Gräfin Elizabeth to Erastus, Schleusingen, [Oct. 8], 1561. GHA, Sekt. I, 1103.
3. Gräfin Elizabeth to Erastus, Schleusingen, April 12, 1563. GHA, Sekt. I, 1103.
4. Gräfin Elizabeth to Erastus, July 28, 1565. GHA, Sekt. I, 5637.

Johann Ewich, Physician in Bremen (1525–1588)
Cf. Dedicatory epistle of *Theses de Morbis totius substantiae* … (Heidelberg: Johann Meyer, 1575), fol. A2.

Camillus Franchinus, Physician in Bologna

1. Erastus to Franchinus, n.d. Printed in *Disp. et Epist.*, 38^{v}–43^{r} (no. 14).
2. Erastus to Franchinus, Heidelberg, January, 1560. Printed in *De causa Morborum*, 1–80.

* Franchinus to Erastus, n.d. SUB Bremen, MS 7, fols. 248^{r}–249^{v}.
[Franchinus [*sic*] to Erastus. Printed in Goldast, 268–275. See *CB*, 9:208–214 (no. 651).]

Frederick III the Pious (Friedrich III. der Fromme) Elector of the Palatinate (1515–1576) *NDB*, 5:530–532.

1. Erastus to Friedrich, Oct. 6, [1568 ?]. Hd.UB, Cod. Pal. germ. 839, fols. 62–63 (copy); General-Landesarchiv Karlsruhe, Kopialbuch 961, fols. 108–114 (copy).

Count Georg Ernst of Henneberg (1511–1583) *ADB*, 8:671–673.[9]

1. Erastus to Georg Ernst, Heidelberg, April 28, [c. 1562]. GHA, Sekt. I, 5810.
2. Erastus to Georg Ernst, March 27, 1564. Excerpts printed in Koch, 5–7.

[9] A full investigation of Erastus's correspondence with the Henneberg court remains

3. Erastus to Georg Ernst, July 10, [pre-June 1565]. GHA, Sekt. I, 5810.
4. Erastus to [Georg Ernst], March 11, [1569]. Cambridge, Harvard University, Houghton Library, Autographfile.
5. Erastus to Georg Ernst, March 5, 1572. Printed in Koch, 10–13.
6. Erastus to Georg Ernst, April 18, 1572. Partially printed in Koch, 14–15.
7. Erastus to Georg Ernst, April 2, (1573). GHA, Sekt. I, 5720. Partially printed in Koch, 17.
8. Erastus to Georg Ernst, May 13, (1573). GHA, Sekt. I, 5720. Largely printed in Koch, 17–19.
9. Erastus to Georg Ernst, July 24, (15)73. GHA, Sekt. I, 5720.
10. Erastus to Georg Ernst, Heidelberg, Feb. 7, (15)75. GHA, Sekt. I, 261.
11. Erastus to [Georg Ernst], April 21, 1575. Berlin, Staatsbibliothek PKB, Autographensammlung Darmstaedter, G 1 1572 (1).
12. Erastus to Georg Ernst, Oct. 17, n.y. GHA, Sekt. I, 5810.
13. Erastus to Georg Ernst, June 11, n.y. Germanisches National Museum, K. 5. Listed under the name "Lieber."

1. Georg Ernst to Erastus, [1560]. GHA, Sekt. I, 5599.
2. Georg Ernst to Erastus [and Elector Frederick III], May 6, 1567. GHA, Sekt. I, [5684 ?]
3. Georg Ernst to Erastus, Zillbach, Jan. 27, 1568. GHA, Sekt. I, 1103.
4. Georg Ernst to Erastus, Feb. 22, 1568. GHA, Sekt. I, 1103.
5. Georg Ernst to Erastus, April 5, 1570. GHA, Sekt. I, 5681.
6. Georg Ernst to Erastus, Feb. 23, 1572. GHA, Sekt. I, [5684 ?].
7. Georg Ernst to Erastus, April 1, 1572. GHA, Sekt. I, [5684 ?]. Partially printed in Koch, 13–14.
8. Georg Ernst to Erastus, [Wildbad,] May 29, 1572. GHA, Sekt. I, [5684 ?]. Partially printed in Koch, 15.
9. Georg Ernst to Erastus, [Wildbad,] June 7, 1572. GHA, Sekt. I, [5684 ?]. Partially printed in Koch, 15.
10. Georg Ernst to Erastus, Schleusingen, Aug. 26, (15)72. GHA, Sekt. I, 5711.
11. Georg Ernst to Erastus, Zillbach, Sept. 22, (15)72. GHA, Sekt. I, 5711.
12. Georg Ernst to Erastus, Schleusingen, March 26, 1573. GHA, Sekt. I, 5720.
13. Georg Ernst to Erastus, Schleusingen, May 25, 1573. GHA, Sekt. I, 5720. Partially printed in Koch, 19.
14. Georg Ernst to Erastus, Schleusingen, July 12, 1573. GHA, Sekt. I, 5720.
15. Georg Ernst to Erastus, Maßfeld, Jan. 31, (15)75. GHA, Sekt. I, 261.

Konrad Gessner, Natural Historian and Bibliographer in Zürich (1516–1565) *NDB* 6:342–345.

1. Erastus to Gessner, April 11, (1557). StAZ, MS E II 361, fol. 56.
2. Erastus to Gessner, Heidelberg, Sept. 17, 1564. ZBZ, MS Z VIII 119, fols. 2–18. Printed in *Varia Opuscula Medica* (Frankfurt: A. Wechel, 1590), 88–101. Reprinted in *Disp. et Epist.*, fols. 90^r–105^v (no. 25).
3. Erastus to Gessner, n.d., ZBZ, MS Z VIII 119, fol. 1.

---

a desideratum. This provisional list is based on the data and manuscripts supplied by the Thüringishes Staatsarchiv Meiningen and Ernst Koch's analysis (op. cit.).

Johann Jakob Grynaeus, Pastor in Rötteln, Baden; Theologian [and later *Antistes*] in Basel (1540–1617) *NDB* 7:241.

1. Erastus to Grynaeus, Jan. 24, [1570]. Basel UB, MS G II 4, fol. 278.
2. Erastus to Grynaeus, March 20, [1570]. Basel UB, MS G II 4, fols. 279–280.
3. Erastus to Grynaeus, June 26, [ca. 1570]. Basel UB, MS G II 4, fol. 284.
4. Erastus to Grynaeus, June 26, [ca. 1570]. Basel UB, MS G II 4, fol. 249.
5. Erastus to Grynaeus, Aug. 16, [ca. 1570]. Basel UB, MS G II 4, fol. 261.
6. Erastus to Grynaeus, Oct. 16, [1570]. Basel UB, MS G II 4, fol. 287.
7. Erastus to Grynaeus, Nov. 29, [1570]. Basel UB, MS G II 4, fols. 300–301.
8. Erastus to Grynaeus, Dec. 18, 1570. Basel UB, MS G II 4, fol. 176.
9. Erastus to Grynaeus, Feb. 2, [1571]. Basel UB, MS G II 4, fol. 282.
10. Erastus to Grynaeus, April 17, [1571]. Basel, MS G II 4, fol. 255.
11. Erastus to Grynaeus, April 19, [ca. 1571]. Basel UB, MS G II 4, fol. 252.
12. Erastus to Grynaeus, June 26, (1571). Basel, MS G II 4, fol. 291.
13. Erastus to Grynaeus, Oct. 19, [1571]. Basel UB, MS G II 4, fol. 295, (291[a].)
14. Erastus to [J.J. Grynaeus] March 1, (15)72. Basel UB, MS G II 4, fol. 180.
15. Erastus to Grynaeus, Oct. 12, [ca. 1572]. Basel UB, MS G II 4, fol. 296.
16. Erastus to Grynaeus, Sept. 30, (15)72. Basel UB, MS G II 4, fol. 177.
17. Erastus to Grynaeus, Dec. 3, [1572]. Basel UB, MS G II 4, fols. 276–277.
18. Erastus to Grynaeus, Feb. 22, (15)73. Basel UB, MS G II 4, fol. 181.
19. Erastus to Grynaeus, [June, 1573]. Basel UB, MS G II 4, fol. 275.
20. Erastus to Grynaeus, [July/August 1573]. Basel UB, MS G II 4, fol. 298.
21. Erastus to Grynaeus, August 8, [1570–1575, likely 1573]. Basel UB, MS G II 4, fol. 298[a].
22. Erastus to Grynaeus, Sept. 18, [ca. 1573]. Basel UB, MS G II 4, fols. 289–290.
23. Erastus to Grynaeus, Nov. 29, (15)73. Basel UB, Autographen Slg. Erastus.
24. Erastus to Grynaeus, Feb. 5, (15)74. Basel UB, MS G II 4, fols. 183–184.
25. Erastus to Grynaeus, Sept. 21, (15)74. Basel UB, MS G II 4, fol. 185.
26. Erastus to Grynaeus, Sept. 30, (15)74. Basel UB, MS G II 4, fol. 182.
27. Erastus to Grynaeus, Oct. 4, [1574 ?]. Basel UB, MS G II 4, fols. 292–293.
28. Erastus to Grynaeus, Oct. 19, (15)74. Basel UB, MS G II 4, fol. 188.
29. Erastus to Grynaeus, Nov. 13 & 15, 1574. Basel UB, MS G II 4, fols. 186–187.
30. Erastus to Grynaeus, Nov. 16 (15)74. Basel UB, MS G II 4, fol. 190.
31. Erastus to Grynaeus, Nov. 17, (15)74. Basel UB, MS G II 4, fol. 189.
32. Erastus to Grynaeus, Jan. 4, (15)75. Basel UB, MS G II 4, fol. 206.
33. Erastus to Grynaeus, April 25, [1575 ?]. Basel, MS G II 4, fol. 267.
34. Erastus to Grynaeus, July 24, (15)75. Basel UB, MS G II 4, fol. 191.
35. Erastus to Grynaeus, Sept. 20, [1575]. Basel UB, MS G II 4, fols. 273–274.
36. Erastus to Grynaeus, Oct. 2, (15)75. Basel UB, MS G II 4, fols. 429–430.
37. Erastus to Grynaeus, Dec. 11, (15)75. Basel UB, MS G II 4, fol. 192.
38. Erastus to Grynaeus, Jan. 12, [ca. 1575–1577]. Basel UB, MS G II 4, fol. 248.
39. Erastus to Grynaeus, Jan. 27, (15)76. Basel UB, MS G II 4, fol. 195.
40. Erastus to Grynaeus, Feb. 3, (15)76. Basel UB, MS G II 4, fol. 196.
41. Erastus to Grynaeus, March 7 (15)76. Basel UB, MS G II 4, fol. 194.
42. Erastus to Grynaeus, [ca. March, 1576]. Basel UB, MS G II 4, fol. 264.
43. Erastus to Grynaeus, Pentecost [June 10], (15)76. Basel UB, MS G II 4, fol. 197.
44. Erastus to Grynaeus, June 21, (15)76. Basel UB, MS G II 4, fol. 197[a].
45. Erastus to Grynaeus, June 24, (15)76. Basel UB, MS G II 4, fol. 269.
46. Erastus to Grynaeus, Aug. 15, (15)76. Basel UB, MS G II 4, fol. 198.
47. Erastus to Grynaeus, August 19, [1576]. Basel UB, MS G II 4, fol. 272.
48. Erastus to Grynaeus, Sept. 22, 1576. Basel UB, MS G I 33, fols. 10–11.

49. Erastus to Grynaeus, Oct. 29. (15)76. Basel UB, MS G II 4, fol. 193.
50. Erastus to Grynaeus, [Nov. 1576]. Basel UB, MS G II 4, fols. 250, (247).
51. Erastus to Grynaeus, Dec. 6, [1576]. Basel UB, MS G II 10, fols. 603–604.
52. Erastus to Grynaeus, Dec. 27 / 28, (15)76. Basel UB, MS G II 4, fol. 199.
53. Erastus to Grynaeus, [ca. December 28, 1576]. Basel UB, MS G II 4, fol. 265.
54. Erastus to Grynaeus, Dec. 29, [ca. 1576]. Basel UB, MS G II 4, fol. 303.
55. Erastus to Grynaeus, March 4, [1577]. Basel UB, MS G II 4, fol. 299.
56. Erastus to Grynaeus, March 15, (15)77. Basel UB, MS G II 4, fol. 210.
57. Erastus to Grynaeus, April, 12, (15)77. Basel UB, MS G II 4, fol. 208.
58. Erastus to Grynaeus, April, 30, (15)77. Basel UB, MS G II 4, fol. 205.
59. Erastus to Grynaeus, May 10, (15)77. Basel UB, MS G II 4, fol. 207.
60. Erastus to Grynaeus, June 29, [1577]. Basel UB, MS G II 4, fol. 283.
61. Erastus to Grynaeus, June 29, (15)77. Basel UB, MS G II 4, fol. 201.
62. Erastus to Grynaeus, Aug. 5, (15)77. Basel UB, MS G II 4, fols. 203–204.
63. Erastus to Grynaeus, Aug. 18, (15)77. Basel UB, MS G II 4, fols. 211–212.
64. Erastus to Grynaeus, Aug. 19, (15)77. Basel UB, MS G II 4, fol. 202.
65. Erastus to Grynaeus, [mid-Sept., ca. 1577]. Basel UB, MS G II 4, fol. 271[a].
66. Erastus to Grynaeus, Sept. 14, (15)77. Basel UB, MS G II 4, fol. 200.
67. Erastus to Grynaeus, Sept. 14, (15)77. Basel UB, MS G II 4, fol. 209.
68. Erastus to Grynaeus, Sept. 20, (15)77. Basel UB, MS G II 4, fol. 213.
69. Erastus to Grynaeus, Nov. 24, (15)77. Basel UB, MS G II 4, fols. 262–263.
70. Erastus to Grynaeus, Jan. 15, (15)78. Basel UB, MS G II 4, fol. 215.
71. Erastus to Grynaeus, Jan. 23, [1578]. Basel UB, MS G II 4, fol. 253.
72. Erastus to Grynaeus, Jan. 29, (1578). Basel UB, MS G II 4, fol. 260.
73. Erastus to Grynaeus, Feb. 20, [1578]. Basel UB, MS G II 4, fol. 251.
74. Erastus to Grynaeus, March 18, (15)78. Basel UB, MS G II 4, fol. 217.
75. Erastus to Grynaeus, March 25, [1578]. Basel UB, MS G II 4, fol. 297.
76. Erastus to Grynaeus, April 3, (15)78. Basel UB, MS G II 4, fol. 223.
77. Erastus to Grynaeus, April 13, (15)78. Basel UB, MS G II 4, fol. 219.
78. Erastus to Grynaeus, April 23, (15)78. Basel UB, MS G II 4, fol. 227.
79. Erastus to Grynaeus, April 23, [1578]. Basel UB, MS G II 4, fol. 270.
80. Erastus to Grynaeus, May 5, (15)78. Basel UB, MS G II 4, fol. 218.
81. Erastus to Grynaeus, May 6, [1578]. Basel UB, MS G II 4, fol. 271.
82. Erastus to Grynaeus, May 21, (15)78. Basel UB, MS G II 4, fol. 229.
83. Erastus to Grynaeus, June 23, (15)78. Basel UB, MS G II 4, fol. 220.
84. Erastus to Grynaeus, June 25, (15)78. Basel UB, MS G II 4, fol. 216.
85. Erastus to Grynaeus, June 29, (15)78. Basel UB, MS G II 4, fols. 225–225[a].
86. Erastus to Grynaeus, Aug. 10, (15)78. Basel UB, MS G II 4, fol. 224.
87. Erastus to Grynaeus, Oct. 7, (15)78. Basel UB, MS G II 4, fol. 222.
88. Erastus to Grynaeus, Nov. 8, (15)78. Basel UB, MS G II 4, fol. 226.
89. Erastus to Grynaeus, Dec. 8, (15)78. Basel UB, MS G II 4, fol. 228.
90. Erastus to Grynaeus, Dec. 20, (15)78. Basel UB, MS G II 4, fol. 214.
91. Erastus to Grynaeus, Dec. 24, (15)78. Basel UB, MS G II 4, fol. 221.
92. Erastus to Grynaeus, Jan. 3, (15)79. Basel UB, MS G II 4, fol. 245.
93. Erastus to Grynaeus, Jan. 5, (15)79. Basel UB, MS G II 4, fol. 236.
94. Erastus to Grynaeus, Jan. 14, (15)79. Basel UB, MS G II 4, fol. 238.
95. Erastus to Grynaeus, Feb. 1, (15)79. Basel UB, MS G II 4, fol. 239.
96. Erastus to Grynaeus, March 27, (15)79. Basel UB, MS G II 4, fols. 242–243.
97. Erastus to Grynaeus, April 22, (15)79. Basel UB, MS G II 4, fol. 237.
98. Erastus to Grynaeus, [Heidelberg] and Speyer, May 15 & 16, (15)79. Basel UB, MS G II 4, fol. 233.

99. Erastus to Grynaeus, July 13, (15)79. Basel UB, MS G II 4, fol. 246.
100. Erastus to Grynaeus, [late July, 1579]. Basel UB, MS G II 4, fol. 294.
101. Erastus to Grynaeus, Aug. 18, (15)79. Basel UB, MS G II 4, fol. 240.
102. Erastus to Grynaeus, Sept. 9, (15)79. Basel UB, MS G II 4, fol. 241.
103. Erastus to Grynaeus, Sept. 14, (15)79. Basel UB, MS G II 4, fol. 230.
104. Erastus to Grynaeus, Oct. 31 & Dec. 1, (15)79. Basel UB, MS G II 4, fols. 231–232.
105. Erastus to Grynaeus, Dec. 29, (15)79. Basel UB, MS G II 4, fols. 285–286.
106. Erastus to Grynaeus, Jan. 19, (15)80. Basel UB, MS G II 4, fol. 312.
107. Erastus to Grynaeus, Feb. 14, (15)80. Basel UB, MS G II 4, fol. 307.
108. Erastus to Grynaeus, Feb. 25, (15)80. Basel UB, MS G II 4, fol. 302.
109. Erastus to Grynaeus, March 2, [1578–1580; likely 1580]. Basel UB, MS G II 4, fol. 254.
110. Erastus to Grynaeus, April 14, (15)80. Basel UB, MS G II 4, fol. 308.
111. Erastus to Grynaeus, Heidelberg, April 24, (15)80. Basel UB, MS G II 4, fol. 311.
112. Erastus to Grynaeus, May 29, [ca. 1580 ?]. Basel UB, MS G II 4, fol. 288.
113. Erastus to Grynaeus, Aug. 20, [1580]. Basel UB, MS G II 4, fol. 281.
114. Erastus to Grynaeus, Sept. 2, (15)80. Basel UB, MS G II 4, fols. 304–305.
115. Erastus to Grynaeus, Sept. 7, (15)80. Basel UB, MS G II 4, fol. 309.
116. Erastus to Grynaeus, Sept. 24, (15)80. Basel UB, MS G II 4, fol. 306.

1. Grynaeus to Erastus, Rötteln, Sept. 2, 1571. Dedicatory forward from Origin, *Adamantii magni illius et vetusti scripturarum interpretis Opera quae quidem extant omnia doctiss. virorum studio iam olim translata & recognita*, ed. Johann Johannes Grynaeus (Basel: Per Eusebium Episcopium, et Nicolai Fr. Haeredes, 1571).

Simon Grynaeus, Arts and Medical Professor in Heidelberg and Basel (1539–1582)
See below under "Unnamed Mathematician"

1. Erastus to S. Grynaeus. Heidelberg, June 5, 1564. Printed in *Ratio Formandorum Syllogismorum* ... (Basel: Johannes Oporinus, 1565), 75–163.

Thomas Grynaeus, Paster in Rötteln, Margravate of Baden (1512–1564)

1. Erastus to T. Grynaeus, Heidelberg. April 4, [ca. 1562]. Basel UB, MS G II 4, fol. 266.
2. Erastus to [Thomas ?] Grynaeus, Heidelberg. Sept. 11, (15)62. Basel UB, MS G II 4, fol. 175.

1. T. Grynaeus to Erastus, Rötteln, Aug. 29, (15)62. Basel UB, MS G II 10, fols. 703–704.

Rudolf Gwalther, Theologian and *Antistes* in Zürich (1519–1586) *NDB*, 7:360–361.

1. Erastus to Gwalther, Oct. 31, [1560]. ZBZ (Hot.), MS F 38, fol. 271.
2. Erastus to Gwalther, Heidelberg, Dec. 5, [1560]. ZBZ (Hot.), MS F 38, fol. 269.
3. Erastus to Gwalther, Heideberg, April 6, [ca. 1561 / 1562]. ZBZ (Hot.), MS F 38, fol. 270.
4. Erastus to Gwalther, Heidelberg, Nov. 21, [1561]. ZBZ (Hot.), MS F 38, fol. 268.
5. Erastus to Gwalther, July 7, [1562]. ZBZ (Hot.), MS F 38, fol. 267.
6. Erastus to Gwalther, Heidelberg, Sept. 26, [1565]. ZBZ (Hot.), MS F 59, fol. 490.
7. Erastus to Gwalther, March 24, (15)70. StAZ, MS E II 345, fols. 689–690.

8. Erastus to Gwalther, May 10, [1570]. ZBZ (Sim.), MS S 122, no. 31.
9. Erastus to Gwalther, Oct. 29, (1570). ZBZ (Hot.), MS F 38, fol. 277.
10. Erastus to Gwalther, June 27, (15)71. ZBZ (Hot.), MS F 38, fol. 276.
11. Erastus to Gwalther, April 24, (1572). ZBZ (Sim.), MS S 126, no. 96.
12. Erastus to Gwalther and Bullinger, Dec. 21, 1572. StAZ, MS E II 361, fol. 20.
13. Erastus to Gwalther, Sept. 24, (1573). ZBZ (Hot.), MS F 38, fol. 274.
14. Erastus to Gwalther, May 18, (15)74. ZBZ (Hot.), MS F 38, fol. 275.
15. Erastus to Gwalther, Sept. 30, (15)74. StAZ, MS E II 345, fol. 714.
16. Erastus to Gwalther, Oct. 11, (15)74. ZBZ (Hot.), MS F 38, fol. 278.
17. Erastus to Gwalther, Oct. 30, (1575). ZBZ, MS A 49, 297–298.
18. Erastus to Gwalther, Feb. 7, (15)76. ZBZ, MS A 49, 299–300 (address 305).
19. Erastus to Gwalther, April 19, (15)76. ZBZ, MS A 49, 301–303 (address 304).
20. Erastus to Gwalther, Dec. 11, (15)76. StAZ, MS E II 345, fol. 724–725.
21. Erastus to Gwalther, May 10, 1577. ZBZ, MS A 49, 306–307 (address 313).
22. Erastus to Gwalther, Sept. 19, (1577). ZBZ, MS A 49, 308–309
23. Erastus to Gwalther, Nov. 15, 1577. ZBZ, MS A 49, 310–311.
24. Erastus to Gwalther, Feb. 11 & 21, 1578. ZBZ, MS A 49, 314–315.
25. Erastus to Gwalther, March 28, 1578. ZBZ, MS A 49, 316–317.
26. Erastus to Gwalther, May 21, (15)78. ZBZ, MS A 49, 318–319.
27. Erastus to Gwalther, June 23, 1578. ZBZ, MS A 49, 320–321.
28. Erastus to Gwalther, Sept. 20 (1578). ZBZ, MS A 49, 322–323.
29. Erastus to Gwalther, Jan. 31, (15)79. ZBZ, MS A 49, 324–325.
30. Erastus to Gwalther, Sept. 21, (15)79. ZBZ (Sim.), MS S 138, no. 5.
31. Erastus to Gwalther, April 6, (15)80. ZBZ (Sim.), MS S 138, no. 102.
32. Erastus to Gwalther, Dec. 3, (1580). ZBZ (Sim.), MS S 139, no. 63.
33. Erastus to Gwalther, Jan. 9 (1581). ZBZ (Sim.), MS S 139, no. 84.
34. Erastus to Gwalther, Jan. 16, (15)81. ZBZ (Sim.), MS S 139, no. 85.
35. Erastus to Gwalther, Jan. 30, (15)81. StAZ, MS E II 382, fol. 1028[b].
36. Erastus to Gwalther, Feb. 24, (1581). StAZ, MS E II 382, fol. 1025.
37. Erastus to Gwalther, Basel, May 7, (15)81. ZBZ (Sim.), MS S 139, no. 156.
38. Erastus to Gwalther, Baden [CH], July 27, (15)81. ZBZ (Sim.), MS S 140, no. 2.
39. Erastus to Gwalther, Dec. 7, (15)81. ZBZ, MS A 49, 326–329.
40. Erastus to Gwalther, March 21, [1582]. ZBZ (Sim.), MS S 140, no. 83.
41. Erastus to Gwalther, Basel, Sept. 7, (15)82. ZBZ (Sim.), MS S 140, no. 158.

Rudolf Gwalther II, Theologian in Zürich (1552–1577)

1. Erastus to Rudolf Gwalther [II] and Rudolf Zwingli, Jan. 24, 1572. ZBZ (Hot.), MS F 42, fol. 74.

Johannes Haller II, Chief pastor in Bern (1523–1575) *NDB* 7:549.

1. Erastus to Haller, Heidelberg, Sept. 22, 1566 (copy). ZBZ (Hot.) MS F 46, 618.
2. Erastus to Haller, Heidelberg, Sept. 12, 1567. Zofingen, no. 2.34. (Copy Cod. Bern. A. 30, 45; also Basel UB & Sim. copies). Printed in Hagen, 31–32.
3. Erastus to Haller, Heidelberg, Sept. 17, 1568 (copy). ZBZ (Hot.) MS F 46, 618.
4. Erastus to Haller, Heidelberg, April 17, [1569] (copy). ZBZ (Hot.) MS F 46, 617–618.

Albert Hardenberg (alias Rizaeus) Theologian in Bremen and Emden (1510–1574) *NDB*, 7:663.

1. Erastus to Hardenberg, Heidelberg, Feb. 4, 1560. SUB Bremen MS 10, no. 41, fols. 74^r–76^v. Defectively printed in L.C. Mieg, *Monumenta Pietatis* (Frankfurt, 1701), 1:345–349.

2. Erastus to Hardenberg, [October, 1560]. SUB Bremen MS 10, no. 65, fol. 115.
3. Erastus to Hardenberg, Heidelberg, Nov. 11, 1560. SUB Bremen MS 10, no. 49, fols. 87^r–87^v.
4. Erastus to Hardenberg, Heidelberg, Sept. 11, 1561. SUB Bremen MS 10, no. 54, fol. 95.
5. Erastus to Hardenberg, Heidelberg, March 23, (15)62. SUB Bremen MS 10, no. 58, fol. 103.
6. Erastus to Hardenberg, Easter [April 22], 1565. SUB Bremen MS 10, no. 63, fol. 112.
7. Erastus to Hardenberg, Sept. 8, 1565. SUB Bremen MS 10, no. 66, fol. 116.
8. Erastus to Hardenberg, Dec. 10, [1565 ?]. SUB Bremen MS 10, no. 56, fol. 100.
9. Erastus to Hardenberg, [ca. mid 1570-Jan. 1572]. London, Lambeth Palace Library, MS 2010, fols. 152^r–153^v.

1. Hardenberg to [Erastus], Oct. 30, 1560 (copy). StAZ, MS E II 346a, fols. 426^r–427^r (copy).[10]

Johann Philipp Freiherr von Hohensax, Statesman (1550–1596) *ADB*, 13:516. Possible recipient of letters addressed to "Lord Baron" (*Domino Baro*)

Peter Hybner (Hübner, Hibner, Hühner) Arts Professor in Bern; Schoolmaster in Burgdorf

1. Erastus to Hybner, Basel, 1582. Cod. Bern. A. 27, 5. Printed in Hagen, 33–34.

Jean Lalamant (Lalemant, Lalamantius) Physician in Autun, Burgundy (1525–1550)

1. Lalamantius to Erastus, Dec. 5 & Dec. 11, 1576. SUB Bremen, 8, fols. 255–256. Printed in Goldast, 263–267 (no. 66).

Johannes (Hans) Lange, Court Physician in Heidelberg (1485–1565) *ADB*, 17:637–638.

* Johann Lange to Theodoric Pamphilus.[11] Printed in Johannes Lange, *Epistolarum Medicinalium Volumen Tripartium* … (Frankfurt: Apud heredes Andreae Wecheli, 1589), 586–621.

Ludwig Lavater, Theologian, Naturalist, [and later *Antistes*] in Zürich; (1527–1586) *ADB*, 18:83–84.

1. Erastus to Lavater, March 25, 1578. Dibner Library, Smithsonian Institution, Washington, D.C. No. 19831128.

[10] Janse, *Albert Hardenberg als Theologe*, 529.

[11] Vivian Nutton has suggested that Lange's frequent correspondent "Theodoric Pamphilus" may be a pseudonym for Erastus. The tentative identification comes from the similarity of names, Nutton's identification of Theodoric as Swiss (which I have not confirmed), and Theodoric's interest in the causes of sterility. Erastus's own fertility problems might have prompted the discourses and could also offer a justification for using the pseudonym. See Nutton, "The Reception of Fracastoro's Theory of Contagion: The Seed That Fell among Thorns?" *Osiris* (1990): 217.

Jan Lasicki (Johannes Lasitius) Polish Reformed Theologian (1534 – ca. 1600)

1. Lasicki to Erastus, Strasbourg, Oct. 16, 1580 (copy). Basel UB, MS G I 69, no. 91, fols. 92^{v}–93^{v}.

Peter Lotichius (Secundus) Medical Professor and Poet in Heidelberg (1528–1560) *NDB*, 15:238–241.

1. Erastus to Lotichius, 1558. Printed in *De astrologia*, 190–201 (no. 13).

Ludwig VI, Elector of the Palatinate (1539–1583) *NDB*, 15:414.

1. Erastus and Ludwig Grave (Gravius) to Ludwig, n.d. Hd.UB, Cod. Pal. germ. 807, fols. 177–181.

Theophil Mader, Physician in Frauenfeld and Zürich (c. 1532–1604) Zedler, 19, cols. 133–134.

1. Erastus to Mader, Basel, August 29, 1582. Printed In *Disp. et Epist.*, fols. 49^{v}–50^{r} (no. 16).
2. Erastus to Mader, Jan. 12, 1583. SUB Bremen MS 8, fol. 253.
3. Erastus to Mader, n.d. SUB Bremen MS 8, fol. 254.

Ortholph Maroldt (Maroldus) Henneberg Court Physician, Zedler, 19, col. 1641.
All of the following fragments are printed in Ortholph Maroldt, *Domini Ortholphi Maroldi ... Practica Medica ...* (Frankfurt: Johannes Beyer, 1650).

1. Erastus to Maroldt, n.d. *Practica Medica*, 98–99.
2. Erastus to Maroldt, 1573. *Practica Medica*, 135.
3. Erastus to Maroldt, 1580. *Practica Medica*, 107.

Arcangelo Mercenario, Italian Physician (d. 1585)
Cf. bibliography

Girolamo Mercuriale (Mercurialis) Medical Professor in Padua; Imperial Physician (1530–1606)

1. Erastus to 'H.M.' [Hieronymus Mercurialis], Heidelberg, 1560. *De astrologia*, 89–106 (no. 8).
2. Erastus to 'H.M.' [Hieronymus Mercurialis], Heidelberg, n.d. *De astrologia*, 107–128 (no. 9).
3. Erastus to 'Doct. G.M.' [i.e., "Girolamo Mercuriale"], Heidelberg, July 19, 1561. Printed in *De causa morborum*, 117–145.

1. Mercuriale to Erastus, n.d. SUB Bremen MS 8, fols. 272–274.

Jakob Friedrich Meurer (Jacobus Fridericus Meurerus) Jurist of the Landgrave of Hesse

1. Erastus to Meurerus, n.d. Printed in *Cista Medica*, ed. Johannes Hornung (Nuremberg: Halbmayr, 1625), 329–331 (no. 149).

Peter Monau (Monavius) Imperial Physician (1551–1588) *ADB*, 22:168.

1. Erastus to Monau, August 27, 1578. Printed in Crato, *Consiliorum et Epistolarum* (1591), 1:289–299. Reprinted in Scholz, cols. 508–512 (no. 271). Abbreviated version printed in *Disp. et Epist.*, fols. 4^{r}–6^{v} (no. 3) and dated August 23, 1578.

2. Erastus to Monau, ca. beginning of Jan. 1579. Printed in Crato, *Consiliorum et Epistolarum* (1591) 1:299–320. Reprinted in Scholz, cols. 512–520 (no. 272). Abbreviated version printed in *Disp. et Epist.*, fols. 6^{v}–11^{v} (no. 4).
3. Erastus to Monau, Sept. 4 & 9, 1579. Printed in Crato, *Consiliorum et Epistolarum* (1591), 1:320–330. Reprinted in Scholz, cols. 521–525 (no. 273). Printed in *Disp. et Epist.*, fols. 11^{r}–13^{v} (no. 5) [without the Sept. 9 postscript].
4. Erastus to Monau, Nov. 16, 1579. Printed in Crato, *Consiliorum et Epistolarum* (1592), 3:321–322. Reprinted in Scholz, col. 525 (no. 274).
5. Erastus to Monau, Feb. 23, 1580. Printed in Crato, *Consiliorum et Epistolarum* (1592), 3:322–334. Reprinted in Scholz, cols. 525–528 (no. 275); *Disp. et Epist.*, fols. 13^{v}–16^{v} (no. 6). [The *Disp. et Epist.*, version is a little longer but lacks the date of the month.]
6. Erastus to Monau, Basel, April 18, 1581. Printed in Crato, *Consiliorum et Epistolarum* (1592), 3:334–336. Reprinted in Scholz, col. 528–529 (no. 276).

1. Monau to Erastus, Padua, March 17, 1578. Printed in Scholz, cols. 374–376 (no. 217). Reprinted in Crato, *Consiliorum et Epistolarum* (1671), 5:419–422.
2. Monau to Erastus, Breslau, July 30, 1578. Printed in Scholz, cols. 376–379 (no. 218). Reprinted in *Crato, Consiliorum et Epistolarum* (1671), 5:422–428.
3. Monau to Erastus, Nov. 4, 1578. Printed in Scholz, cols. 379–382 (no. 219). Reprinted in Crato, *Consiliorum et Epistolarum* (1671), 5:428–434.
4. Monau to Erastus, June 8, 1579. Printed in Scholz, cols. 382–386 (no. 220). Reprinted in Crato, *Consiliorum et Epistolarum* (1671), 5:434–440.
5. Monau to Erastus, Aug. 18, 1579. Reprinted in Scholz, cols. 386–387 (no. 221). Reprinted in Crato, *Consiliorum et Epistolarum* (1671), 5:441.
6. Monau to Erastus, Dec. 17, 1579. Reprinted in Scholz, cols. 387–391 (no. 223). Reprinted in Crato, *Consiliorum et Epistolarum* (1671), 5:442–449.

Abraham Musculus, Theologian in Bern (1534–1591)

1. Erastus to A. Musculus, (copy) March 27 & April 2, 1576. Basel UB Ms G I 68, fols. 67^{v}–68.
2. Erastus to A. Musculus, Nov. 23, (15)77. Autograph, Zofingen, no. 1.53. (Copy Basel UB Ms G I 68, fols. 60^{v}–64, no. 52). Printed in Carl Büttinghausen, *Ergözlichkeiten aus der Pfälzischen und Schweizerischen Geschichte und Literatur* (Zürich, 1766–1768), 3:8–15. The printed version is incorrectly dated. Transcription: http://www.heidelberg-fruehe-neuzeit.uni-hd.de/themen/uni/quellen/erastus_quelle01-01.html.
3. Erastus to A. Musculus, April 2, (15)78. Zofingen, no. 2.58.
4. Erastus to A. Musculus, Sept. 10, (15)79. Zofingen, no. 2.36. (Copies Cod. Bern A. 30, 25; Basel UB Ms G I 69, fols. 47–48, no. 36). Printed in Hagen, 32.
5. Erastus to A. Musculus. Oct. 22, [1579 ?]. Zofingen, no. 1.54. (Copy Basel UB Ms G I 68, fol. 63^{v}–64, no. 58).
6. Erastus to A. Musculus, Dec. 25, (15)79. Zofingen, no. 2.118. (Copy Basel UB Ms G I 69, fol. 113, no. 118).
7. Erastus to A. Musculus, Dec. 8, 1581. Cod. Bern A 30, 15.
8. Erastus to A. Musculus, Basel, July 27, (15)82. Zofingen, no. 2.67. (Copies Cod. Bern A 30, 28; Basel UB Ms G I 69, fol. 74^{v}, no. 67).

Wolfgang Musculus (Müslin, Mäuslin, etc.) Theologian in Augsburg and Bern (1497–1563) *NDB*, 18:627.

1. Erastus to W. Musculus, Heidelberg, March 11, 1560 (copy). Burgerbibliothek Bern, Cod. 689, No. 12, fols. 28^r–29^v. Printed in Reinhard Bodenmann, *Wolfgang Musculus (1497–1563)* (Geneva: Droz, 2000), 444–446.
2. Erastus to W. Musculus, Heidelberg, Sept. 25, (15)61. Zofingen, no. 2.62. (Copies Cod. Bern A. 30, 34; Basel UB). Printed in Hagen, 30.

1. W. Musculus to Erastus, Bern, March 22, 1560 (copy). Burgerbibliothek Bern, Cod. 689, No. 12, fols. 30^r–31^v. Printed in Reinhard Bodenmann, *Wolfgang Musculus (1497–1563)* (Geneva: Droz, 2000), 447–449.

Oswald Myconius (Geisshaüsler) Theologian and *Antistes* in Basel (1488–1552) *NDB*, 18:662.

1. Erastus to Oswald Myconius, (Bologna) Dec. 31, 1544 (copy). ZBZ (Sim), MS S 56, fol. 166.

Bernardino Paterno (Bernardus Paternus) Medical Professor at Padua (d. 1592)

1. Erastus to Paterno, Sept. 24, 1574. Printed In *Disp. et Epist.*, 54^v–59^v (no. 18).
2. Erastus to Paterno, Feb. 4, 1575. Printed In *Disp. et Epist.*, 59^v–65^r (no. 19).

Konrad Pellikan, Humanist and Hebrew Scholar in Zürich (1478–1556) *ADB*, 25:334–338.[12]

1. Erastus to Pellikan, May 17, 1546. StAZ, MS E II 361, fol. 120. (Copy ZBZ (Sim.), MS S 60, no. 92).
2. Erastus to Pellikan, June 21, [ca. 1546]. ZBZ (Hot.), MS F 47, fol. 300. (Copy ZBZ (Sim.), MS S 60, no. 93).
3. Erastus to Pellikan, July 9, 1549. ZBZ (Hot.), MS F 47, fol. 181. (Copy ZBZ (Sim.), MS S 70, no. 168).
4. [Erastus] to Pellikan, [Winter, 1550]. ZBZ (Hot.), MS F 47, fols. 304–305. (Copy ZBZ (Sim.), Ms.S. 72, no. 64). Partially printed in Johann Heinrich Hottinger, *Historia ecclesiastica novi testamenti* (Zurich, 1651–1667), 5:571–574. Excerpts from Hottinger printed in *Dictionnaire historique et critique de Pierre Bayle* (Paris, 1820), 8:454–455.
5. Erastus to Pellikan, [Early year, 1551]. ZBZ (Hot.), MS F 47, fol. 302. (Copy ZBZ (Sim.) Ms.S. 75, no. 4). Brief excerpt printed in Johann Heinrich Hottinger, *Historia ecclesiastica novi testamenti* (Zurich, 1651–1667), 5:574–575.
6. Erastus to Pellikan, May 4, 1552. ZBZ (Hot.), MS F 47, fol. 224. (Copy Sim. Ms.S. 77, no. 157).
7. Erastus to Pellikan, June 12, 1552. ZBZ (Hot.), MS F 47, fol. 232. (Copy Sim. Ms.S. 78, no. 4).

* Erastus to Pellikan, copy of a fragment, n.d., U-F, 5, 453.

[12] The attribution of the autographs in the ZBZ of letters 2, 3, & 5 from Erastus to Pellikan is based on the reconstruction of Christoph Zürcher, *Konrad Pellikans Wirken in Zürich, 1526–1556* (Zurich: Theologischer Verlag, 1975), 290.

Samuel Pellikan

1. Erastus to Samuel Pellikan, Bologna, March 29, [1551]. ZBZ (Hot.), MS F 47, fol. 223.

Antonio Francesco Pigafetta, Physician and Anatomist in Heidelberg

1. Erastus to Pigafetta, Heidelberg, March 5, 1572. Printed In *Disp. et Epist.*, 2^v–4^r (no. 2).

Johannes Pontanus, Ducal Physician, Königsberg and Gotha, Saxony, Zedler, 28, cols. 1459–1460.

1. Erastus to Pontanus, Schleusingen, 1556. Printed in *De causa morborum*, 83–116.
2. Erastus to Pontanus, Heidelberg, July 15, 1572. Printed in *De causa morborum*, 81–82.

Christoph Schilling, Silesian Physician and Humanist (d. 1583) *ADB*, 31:253–255.

1. Fragment, Erastus to Schilling, Feb. 8, 1579. Printed in *Disp. et Epist.*, 43^r–49^v (no. 15). See also Crato and unnamed.

Lazarus von Schwendi, Baron of Hohenlandsberg, Imperial Minister (1522–1583) *ADB* 30:382–401.

1. Erastus to Baron [von Schwendi], March 9, 1581. Hd.UB Hs. 3604, 48 (copy).
2. Erastus to von Schwendi, Basel, August 27, 1581. Dedicatory Epistle of *Comitis Montani Vicentini …* (Basel: Pietro Perna, 1581), ()2–()3.

Josias Simmler, Theologian and Humanist Scholar in Zürich (1530–1576) *ADB*, 34:355–358.

1. Erastus to Simmler, Sept. 30, (15)74. ZBZ (Hot.), MS F 59, fol. 482.
2. Erastus to Simmler, Oct. 11, (15)74. ZBZ (Hot.), MS F 59, fol. 483.
3. Erastus to Simmler, April 2, (15)75. ZBZ (Hot.), MS F 59, fol. 484.
4. Erastus to Simmler, Sept. 29, (15)75. ZBZ (Hot.), MS F 59, fol. 485.
5. Erastus to Simmler, Dec. 23, [1575]. ZBZ (Hot.), MS F 59, fols. 488–489.
6. Erastus to Simmler, April 19, [1576]. ZBZ (Hot.), MS F 59, fol. 487.
7. Erastus to Simmler, April 28, (15)76. ZBZ (Hot.), MS F 59, fol. 486.

Heinrich Smet (Hendrik Smet, Henri de Smet, Henricus Smetius à Leda) Physician in Lemgo; Court Physician and Professor in Heidelberg (1537–1614) BN, 5: 762.

1. Erastus to Smet, Heidelberg, April 20, 1571. Printed in *Miscellanea Medica*, 246–247 (Liber 5, no. 5).
2. Erastus to Smet, Heidelberg, April 18, 1572. Printed in *Miscellanea Medica*, 256–257 (Liber 5, no. 11).
3. Erastus to Smet, Heidelberg, Aug. 1, 1575. Printed in *Disp. & Epist.*, fols. 24^r–29^r (no. 10; Smet not named). Printed in *Miscellanea Medica*, 273–282 (Liber 5, no. 16).

1. Smet to Erastus, Lemgo, March 29, 1571. Printed in *Miscellanea Medica*, 244–246 (Liber 5, no. 4).
2. Smet to Erastus, Lemgo, March 17, 1572. Printed in *Miscellanea Medica*, 251–252 (Liber 5, no. 9).

3. Smet to Erastus, Lemgo, August 29, 1572. Printed in *Miscellanea Medica*, 257–258 (Liber 5, no. 12).

Lukas Stenglin (Lucas Stengel or Stenglius) Physician in Augsburg (1523–1587).

1. Erastus to Stenglin, Jan. 10, 1575. Printed in *Disp. et Epist.*, fols. 73ʳ–76ᵛ (no. 22).

Christoph Stathmion (Maß) City Physician in Coburg (1508/9–85).

1. Erastus to Stathmion, Maßfeld, August 2, [1557]. *De astrologia*, 5–10 (no. 1).
2. Erastus to Stathmion, Maßfeld, August 17, [1557?]. *De astrologia*, 11–18 (no. 2).
3. Erastus to Stathmion, Maßfeld, Nov. 5, [1557?]. *De astrologia*, 18–29 (no. 3).
4. Erastus to Stathmion, Maßfeld, Jan. 6, [1558?]. *De astrologia*, 30–41 (no. 4).
5. Erastus to Stathmion, Maßfeld, Feb. 18, [1558?]. *De astrologia*, 41–50 (no. 5).
6. Erastus to Stathmion, Maßfeld, March 17, [1558?]. *De astrologia*, 51–58 (no. 6).
7. Erastus to Stathmion, Heidelberg, [ca. 1558–1559]. *De astrologia*, 58–88 (no. 7).

Victorinus Strigel, Philippist Theologian in Leipzig and Heidelberg (1524–1569) *ADB* 36:590–594.

1. Strigel to Erastus, Amberg, April 8, 1567. ZBZ (Sim.) Ms.S 115, no. 131.
2. Strigel to Erastus, Amberg, May 14, 1567. ZBZ (Sim.) Ms.S 115, no. 132.

Johannes Wilhelm Stucki, Theologian in Zürich (1542–1607) *ADB*, 36:717–720.

1. Erastus to Stucki, Sept. 20, 1578. Printed in *Disp. et Epist.*, fol. 105ᵛ (no. 26).

Johannes Sturm, Humanist Pedagogue in Strasbourg (1507–1589) *ADB* 37:21–38.

1. Erastus to Sturm, May 16, 1579. Archives St. Thomas, Strasbourg, 155, no. 209. (Copies ZBZ (Sim.) MS S 137, no. 145; Strasbourg, Bibliothèque Nationale et Universitaire, Schmidt, MS 3881, no. 170).

1. Sturm to Erastus, Nordheim, Feb. 24, 1582. Copies ZBZ (Sim.) MS S 140, no. 71; Basel G I 69, no. 83, fols. 85ᵛ–87ᵛ; Strasbourg, Bibliothèque Nationale et Universitaire, Schmidt, MS 3881, no. 580, fol. 247.

Johann Sylvan (Sylvanus) Palatine Theologian and Antitrinitarian (d. 1572) *ADB* 37:285–286.

1. Erastus to Sylvan, June 21, (1569). Staatsarchiv Amberg, Religions-und Reformationswesen, no. 67, fol. 130. Printed in *Rott*, 61.
2. Erastus to Sylvan, Jan. 19, (1570). Staatsarchiv Amberg, Religions-und Reformationswesen, no. 67, fol. 89. Printed in *Rott*, 61–62.

1. Sylvan to Erastus, Heidelberg, [Oct.], 1570. UAH, A/10, fol. 179. Printed in D.L. Wundt, *Magazin für Kirchengschichte*, Bd. 1 (Heidelberg 1789): 148–150; K. Sudhoff, *C. Olevianus und Z. Ursinus, Leben und ausgewählte Schriften* (Elberfeld: R.L. Friedrichs, 1857), 507–508; *Rott*, 14–16.

Daniel Tossanus (Toussain) Theologian in Heidelberg and Neustadt (1541–1602) *ADB* 38:469–474.

1. Tossanus to Erastus, September 14, (1580). Autograph ZBZ. Printed in Friedrich W. Cuno, *Daniel Tossanus der Ältere: Professor der Theologie und Pastor (1541–1602)* (Amsterdam: Scheffer, 1898), 2:162.

Johann Konrad Ulmer, Theologian in Schaffhausen (1519–1600) *ADB* 39:209–210.

1. Erastus to Ulmer, March 29, (1567). Stadtbibliothek Schaffhausen, Ministerialbibliothek, Min. 128 (Ulmeriana IV), no. 132.
2. Erastus to Ulmer, Dec. 9, 1568. Stadtbibliothek Schaffhausen, Ministerialbibliothek, Min. 128 (Ulmeriana IV), no. 156.
3. Erastus to Ulmer, March 6, (15)69. Stadtbibliothek Schaffhausen, Ministerialbibliothek, Min. 128 (Ulmeriana IV), no. 136. (Copy ? ZBZ (Sim.) Ms.S 119, no. 137).
4. Erastus to Ulmer, May 22, [1569; 1568 or later]. Stadtbibliothek Schaffhausen, Ministerialbibliothek, Min. 128 (Ulmeriana IV), no. 190.
5. Erastus to Ulmer and Schaffhausen Scholarchs, Heidelberg, March 19, (15)70. Stadtbibliothek Schaffhausen, Ministerialbibliothek, Min. 128 (Ulmeriana IV), no. 157 (Copy ZBZ (Sim.) Ms.S 121, no. 178).
6. Erastus to Ulmer, April 8, (15)72. Stadtbibliothek Schaffhausen, Ministerialbibliothek, Min. 128 (Ulmeriana IV), no. 200.
7. Erastus to Ulmer, March 20, (15)78. Stadtbibliothek Schaffhausen, Ministerialbibliothek, Min. 128 (Ulmeriana IV), no. 168.

1. Ulmer to Erastus, March 10, 1578. Stadtbibliothek Schaffhausen, Ministerialbibliothek, Min. 125 (Ulmeriana I), no. 115.
2. Ulmer to Erastus, [July 19 ?], 1578. Stadtbibliothek Schaffhausen, Ministerialbibliothek, Min 125 (Ulmeriana I), no. 101.

Bonaventura Vulcanius, Netherlandish Humanist (1538–1614) BN, 5:754–759.

1. Erastus to Vulcanius, (Heidelberg) July 10, 1576. Leiden UB, Cod. Vulc. 105III. Printed in *Vulcanius*, 361–362 (no. 175).
2. Erastus to Vulcanius, Heidelberg, Nov. 21, 1576. Leiden UB, Cod. Vulc. 105III. Printed in *Vulcanius*, 399–401 (no. 194).

1. Vulcanius to Erastus, Basel, between May 9 and 25, 1576. Leiden UB, Cod. Vulc. 36, fols. 60^{v}–61^{r}. Printed in *Vulcanius*, 152–153 (no. 64).
2. Vulcanius to Erastus, Basel, Sept. 4, 1576. Leiden UB, Cod. Vulc. 36, fols. 71^{r} & ^{v}. Printed in *Vulcanius*, 177–180 (no. 78).
3. Vulcanius to Erastus, Basel, Sept. 13, 1576. Leiden UB, Cod. Vulc. 36, fols. 75^{v}–76^{r}. Printed in *Vulcanius*, 191–193 (no. 86).
4. Vulcanius to Erastus, Basel, Jan. 6, 1577. Leiden UB, Cod. Vulc. 36, fol. 88^{v}. Printed in *Vulcanius*, 225–226 (no. 104).

Johannes Wolf, Theologian in Zürich (1521–1571)

1. Erastus to Wolf, Feb. 11 & 12, [1561]. ZBZ (Hot.), MS F 38, fol. 266.
2. Erastus to Wolf, Heidelberg, Sept. 29, (15)61. ZBZ (Hot.), MS F 38, fol. 272.
3. Erastus to Wolf, n.d. [1561/62]. ZBZ (Hot.), MS F 38, fol. 273.
4. Erastus to Wolf, Heidelberg, Jan. 13, 1565. ZBZ (Hot.), MS F 59, fol. 481.

5. Erastus to Wolf, July 30, 1570 (copy). StAZ, MS MS E II 345, fol. 688.

1. [Wolf] to Erastus, n.d. ZBZ (Hot), MS F 41, fol. 303.
2. Wolf to Erastus, Zürich, n.d. (copy ?). ZBZ (Hot), MS F 41, fol. 508.
3. [Wolf] to [Erastus], Zürich, n.d. ZBZ (Hot), MS F 41, fol. 461.
4. Wolf to Erastus, Zürich, Feb. [5],1561. ZBZ (Hot), MS F 41, fol. 205.
5. Wolf to Erastus, Zürich, Aug. 24, 1561. ZBZ (Hot), MS F 41, fols. 370–371.
6. Wolf to Erastus, Zürich, May 5, 1562. ZBZ (Hot), MS F 41, fols. 203–204.
7. Wolf to Erastus, Zürich, Oct. 15, 1562. ZBZ (Hot), MS F 41, fol. 219.
8. [Wolf] to Erastus, Zürich, May 16, 1566. ZBZ (Hot), MS F 41, fol. 459.
9. Wolf to Erastus, Zürich, April 23, 1566. ZBZ (Hot), MS F 41, fol. 455.
10. Wolf to Erastus, Zürich, Oct. 29, 1568. ZBZ (Hot), MS F 41, fol. 197.
11. Wolf to Erastus, Zürich, May 24, 1569. ZBZ (Hot), MS F 41, fol. 421.
12a. [Wolf] to Erastus, Zürich, July 25, 1569. ZBZ (Hot), MS F 41, fol. 304.
12b. Wolf to Erastus, July 25, 1569. ZBZ (Hot), MS F 41, fol. 454.
12c. Wolf to Erastus, Zürich, July 25, 1569. ZBZ (Hot), MS F 41, fol. 500.
13. Wolf to Erastus, March 2, 1572. ZBZ (Hot), MS F 41, fol. 175.

Girolamo Zanchi, Italian Reformed Theologian in Strasbourg and Heidelberg (1516–1590)

1. Erastus to Zanchi, Heidelberg, Oct. 21, [1560 ?]. Printed in Girolamo Zanchi. *Epistolarum Libri Duo* … (Hanau: Guiliemus Antonius, 1609), 2:418–420.

1. Zanchi to Erastus, [ca. 1570]. Printed in Girolamo Zanchi. *Epistolarum Libri Duo* … (Hanau: Guiliemus Antonius, 1609), 1:203–204. Reprinted in *Epistolarum Libri Duo*, in *Operum Theologicorum*. 8 vols. (Geneva, 1613), col. 153.

Theodor Zwinger, Physician and Professor in Basel (1533–1588) *ADB* 45:543–544.

1. Erastus to Zwinger, Heidelberg, Sept. 20, n.y. Basel UB, Fr.Gr. MS II 4, no. 95.
2. Erastus to Zwinger and Guillaume Arragos (Aragosius), n.d. Basel UB, Fr.Gr.Ms. II 23, no. 182.
3. Erastus to Theodor Zwinger, Heidelberg, Easter [April 6, 1572]. Basel UB, Fr.Gr. MS II 4, no. 93. Excerpts printed in Kühlmann and Telle, eds. *Corpus Paracelsisticum*, 2:756–757.
4. Erastus to Zwinger, April 23, (15)78. Basel UB, Fr.Gr. MS II 4, no. 94.

* Erastus to Zwinger, Cf. Dedicatory epistle of Thomas Erastus, *Ad Archangeli Mercenarii philosophi Patavini Disputationem de putredine responsio* (Basel: Conrad Waldkirch, 1583).

1. Zwinger to Erastus, Basel, May 15, 1578, Basel UB, Fr. Gr. MS II 23 no. 507.

Rudolf Zwingli (1551–1571), see Erastus to Rudolph Gwalther II.

Unidentified Recipients

1. Erastus to unnamed [Christoph Schilling?; Theophil Mader?], Heidelberg, March 26, 1577. SUB Bremen MS 8, fols. 250–252. Partially printed (without the first three paragraphs) in *Disp. & Epist.*, fols. 1^r–2^v (no. 1). Partially printed in J. Beverwijk, *Joh. Beveronicii Epistolica Quaestio, de vitae termino, Fatali an Mobili? … Pars Tertia, et Ultima* (Leiden, Joannis Maire, 1639). Full reprint in Goldast, 291–299.

2. Erastus to unnamed, Sept. 15, (15)77. *Disp. & Epist.*, fols. 22^r–24^r (no. 9).
3. Erastus to unnamed, April 15, 1578 (copy). Er.UB (Sammlung Trew).
4. Erastus to unnamed, Dec. 29, n.y. London, Lambeth Palace Library, MS 2010, fols. 158^r–161^r.

Unknown Jurist

1. Unknown Jurist to Erastus, January 10, 1581, StAZ, MS E II 341, fol. 557

Other Probable Correspondents

Johannes Fabricius
Achilles Pirmin Gasser[13]
Hubert Languet
Gerhard de Mortaigne
Johannes Oporinus
Jakob Schegk
Simon Simoni
Christoph Thretius
Georg Vetter
Johann Weyer

Other Manuscript Sources

Bern, Staatsarchiv des Kantons Bern

2 copies of *De Excommunicatione Domini Thomae Erasti Theses, gravissimae quaestiones....* MS B III 69 and B III 111. Both copies include Erastus's response to Beza's critique of his theses and various letters concerning the church discipline controversy.

Bologna, Biblioteca Universitaria di Bologna

"Graecae linguae rudimenta authore Thoma Erasto" (58 folios), MS 1072 (lat. 579), vol. II, fascicle 15. From the papers of Ulysse Aldrovandi [Aldrovandus]

Erlangen UB

"Volget ein Consilium wie man sich zur holz legen soll...." MS B 321, fols. 12–20. Medical consilium for Count Georg Ernst concerning the use of wood cure.

"Volget ein von eiusdem Erasti consilium de usu termarium...." MS B 321, fols. 20–22. A consilium concerning thermal baths.

Gdansk, Biblioteka Gdanska Polskiej Akademii Nauk

Ms. 2319. Perscriptions of Erastus.

[13] Cf. Karl-Heinz Burmeister, *Achilles Pirmin Gasser, 1505–1577: Arzt und Naturforscher, Historiker und Humanist*, 2 vols. (Wiesbaden: Guido Pressler, 1970). See also Inventario dei Libri Stampati Palatino-Vaticani, 1:292. Erastus gave Gasser a copy of *De occultis pharmacorum potestatibus* in Oct. of 1574.

Heidelberg, UB, Codices Palatini germanici[14]

"Ein pulver fur gifft Doctor Thomas Erasti." Cod. Pal. germ. 182, fol. 27^{r}. http://digi.ub.uni-heidelberg.de/diglit/cpg182/0075

"Preservatieff fur denn steinn unnd Griess" [in another hand: "Dockter Erasten Wasser"]. Cod. Pal. germ. 187, fol. 85^{r}. http://digi.ub.uni-heidelberg.de/diglit/cpg187/0187

"Ein Infusio Rosarum Doctor Thomas Erastus." Cod. Pal. germ. 192, fol. 183^{v}. http://digi.ub.uni-heidelberg.de/diglit/cpg192/0402

"Doctor Erastus Recept unnd Experimenta vor die Schwindtsucht an der Hoheneckerin nicht allein gebraucht sonder auch sonst gantz gerecht erfunden, ist mir von ime selbst uff mein ansprechen uberliffert vnd inn geheim vertrauet worden Anno e[t]c. 79." May 10, 1579. Cod. Pal. germ. 192, fols. 281^{r}–281^{v}. http://digi.ub.uni-heidelberg.de/diglit/cpg192/0633

[Cod. Pal. germ. 193 is named as the consilia of "Johann Kraus, Thomas Erastus, Johann Lange, Marx Rechklau," however none of the manuscripts are specifically attributed to Erastus.]

"Docter Erastus Rath wie Mann ein Menschen Haltten soll da mann sich des usatz besorgt." Cod. Pal. germ. 236, fols. 58^{v}–59^{r}. http://digi.ub.uni-heidelberg.de/cpg236/0124

"Wie man die welschen wurst machen soll Doct: Thomas Erastus" [Sausage Recipe]. Cod. Pal. germ., 239, fols. 70^{v}–71^{r}. http://digi.ub.uni-heidelberg.de/cpg239/0146

"Doctoris Thomasen Erasti Bedencken und Rxcept Vor Meinen Genedigen Hern Anno 1563 gemacht." Cod. Pal. germ. 239, fols. 73^{r}–76^{r}. http://digi.ub.uni-heidelberg.de/diglit/cpg239/0151

"Docter Tomas waßer fur denn Schlag." Cod. Pal. germ. 250, fol. 25^{v}.[15] http://digi.ub.uni-heidelberg.de/diglit/cpg250/0054

"Docter Arastes waßer fur denn Schlag." Cod. Pal. germ. 250, fol. 34^{r}. http://digi.ub.uni-heidelberg.de/cpg250/0071

"Doctor Thomas wasser fur den Schlag." Cod. Pal. germ. 256, fol. 108^{r}.[16] http://digi.ub.uni-heidelberg.de/cpg256/0219

"Doctor Erasti wasser fur den Schlag." Cod. Pal. germ. 256, fols. 116^{v}–117^{r}. http://digi.ub.uni-heidelberg.de/cpg256/0236

"Doctor Erasti Lieblich unnd kräfftig wasser fur den Schlag Aqua Epileptica genennt" [Nota. Ein Apotecker pfundt ist vier unnd zwantzig Loth.] Cod. Pal. germ. 256, fols. 128^{v}–129^{r}. http://digi.ub.uni-heidelberg.de/cpg256/0260

---

[14] The following list is largely drawn from Matthias Miller and Karin Zimmermann, *Die medizinischen Handschriften unter den Codices Palatini germanici derUniversitätsbibliothek Heidelberg* (http://www.ub.uni-heidelberg.de/archiv/5709/). Digitized editions of the manuscripts can be accessed at http://www.ub.uni-heidelberg.de/helios/digi/codpalgerm.html.

[15] Attributed to Erastus in Miller and Zimmermann, *Die medizinischen Handschriften unter den Codices Palatini germanici*, 490.

[16] Attributed to Erastus in Miller and Zimmermann, *Die medizinischen Handschriften unter den Codices Palatini germanici*, 562.

"Doctor Erasti wasser unnd preservatieff fur den Stein und griess." Cod. Pal. germ. 256, fol. 353^{r}. http://digi.ub.uni-heidelberg.de/cpg256/0719
"Doctor Erasti wasser guet fur Bose Augen." Cod. Pal. germ. 256, fol. 522^{v}. http://digi.ub.uni-heidelberg.de/cpg256/1066
Anonymous prescription. Cod. Pal. germ. 264, fol. 43^{v}.
Anonymous prescriptions. Cod. Pal. germ. 278, fols. 131^{r}, 136^{r}, 149^{v}, 175^{r}.
"Pulver vor Giefft D. Thomae Erasti." Cod. Pal. germ. 282, fols. 131^{r}–131^{v}. http://digi.ub.uni-heidelberg.de/cpg282/0267
"Ein pulver wie mirs Doctor Thomas undt Reichart geordnet hat." Cod. Pal. germ. 282, fols. 136^{r}–136^{v}. http://digi.ub.uni-heidelberg.de/cpg282/0277
"Ein Trisinet oder puluer vor das hertzbochenn wie es Doctor Thomas Erastus vor Freulein Sophien geordnet hatt." Cod. Pal. germ. 282, fols. 149^{v}–150^{r}. http://digi.ub.uni-heidelberg.de/cpg282/0304
"Ein kunst zum angesicht vonn Doctor Thomasen." Cod. Pal. germ. 282, fols. 175^{r}–175^{v}. http://digi.ub.uni-heidelberg.de/cpg282/0355

Kassel, Landesbibliothek und Murhardsche Bibliothek der Stadt Kassel
Consilium II from Dec. 21, 1564, for the Heidelberg Pharmacist Philipp Stephan Springer. 40 MS med. 11, fols. 10^{r}–16^{v}.

Oxford, Bodleian Library
"Quaestio de excommunicatione, 'a Thoma Erasto Heidelbergensi proposita.'" Selden MSS 1659, 3432, fol. 91.

Wolfenbüttel, Herzog-August-Bibliothek
Arthritis Treatment for B. Gephardt. Codex Guelf. 66.1 Aug.° fols. 200^{v}–212^{r}.

Zürich, Zentralbibliothek
Defensio Quarundam Thesium de aëris intemperie ad disputandum propositarum, in qua cum aliis rebus, tum de natura, causis, differentiis, et modis generationes pestis plurima scitu utilissima disputatur. Autore Thoma Erasto Medico, Schola Heidelbergensis publico professore (Sept. 8, 1563). ZBZ MS B 238, fols. 1–51.
Copy of the forward and part of the text of *Explicatio gravissimae quaestionis....* ZBZ MS F 207. fols. 75–84.
"Sint ne sagae supplicio Capitis afficiendae." ZBZ, MS F 154.

Zürich, Staatsarchiv des Kantons Zürich
Quaestio nunc orta motaque est disciplina ecclesiastica ... Heidelberg, July 23, 1568. MS E II 437a, pp. 541–629. Erastus's 103 Theses concerning excommunication.
"[W]ere Zeitungen." MS E II 350, pp. 43–50. Report in German of political affairs around Europe written in Erastus's own hand.

BIBLIOGRAPHY

Thomas Erastus: Theological Works

Bestendige Ableinung der ungegründten beschuldigung/ damit D. Johann Marbach/ das büchlein Thomae Erasti Medici, vom verstand der wort CHRisti/ Das ist mein Leib/ etc. unterstehet verdechtig zu machen. Heidelberg: Johann Mayer, 1565 (VD 16 E 3670).[1]

Declaratio eorum, quae in libello D.D. Iacobi Scheckij, summi & clarissimi Philosophi, De una Persona & duabus Naturis Christi nunnullis obscuriora, et Ubiquitati corporis Christi patrocinari sunt visa. Geneva: Jean Crespin (Joannes Crispinus), 1566 (WLB exemplar). This book appeared anonymously with a preface by Simon Simoni.[2]

Erzelung Etlicher vrsachen/ warumb das hochwirdig Sacrament des Nachtmals vnsers Herrn/ vnd Heylandts Jhesu Christi/ nicht solle ohne das brodbrechen gehalten werden. Heidelberg: Johann Mayer, 1563 (VD 16 E 3914; http://daten.digitale-sammlungen.de/bsb00035956/image_3). Reprint with the title *Erzelung Etlicher Ursachen/ warumb das Hochwirdige Sacrament des Nachtmals unsers HErren unnd Heylands Jesu Christi/ nichts solle ohne das brotbrechen gehalten werden*. Heidelberg, Johann Meyer, 1565 (exemplar Universiteitsbibliotheek Utrecht). Commonly refered to as *Das Büchlein vom Brotbrechen*; Erastus's name does not appear on the title page.

Explicatio Gravissimae Quaestionis utrùm Excommunicatio, quatenùs Religionem intelligentes & amplexantes, à Sacramentorum usu, propter admissum facinus arcet; mandato nitatur Divino, an excogitata sit ab hominibus. Pesclavius: Baocius Sultaceterus [London: John Wolfe], 1589 (STC (2nd ed.), 10511). Reprint with the title: *Explicatio quaestionis gravissimae....* Amsterdam: Apud Georgium Trigg, 1649. Contains Erastus's 75 theses regarding excommunication (the *Explicatio Gravissimae Quaestionis* per se, pp. 1–63); "Thesium (Quae de excommunicatione positae fuerant) Confirmatio" (pp. 65–349) and numerous letters outlining the history of the controversy (pp. 350–389).

Gründtlicher bericht/ wie die wort Christi/ Das ist mein leib/ etc. zuverstehen seien/ auß den worten der einsetzung und der erclärung Christi selbst genommen: darauß ain ieder leicht lernen mag/ wessen er sich in disem zanck verhalten solle. Heidelberg: Ludwig Lück, 1562 (VD 16 G 3575). Reprint, (same

[1] Appeared at the autumn Frankfurt fair, 1565. *Die Messkatalog Georg Willers* (Hildesheim: Olms, 1972–173), 1:67.

[2] Appeared at the autumn Frankfurt fair, 1566. *Die Messkatalog Georg Willers*, 1:78.

title and publisher) in 1562 (VD 16 G 3576). See below under reprints within other titles.

Responsio Thomae Erasti, ad Libellum D. Iacobi Schegkii, quo nuper Anonymo libro sui, de una persona & duabus in Christo naturis interpreti respondit: in qua mox ab inititio demonstratur, Theologos Heydelbergenses et Vvirtebergicos in disputatione de praesentia carnis Christi in omnibus locis, ac in ipsa quoque coena Dominica, non dissentire amplius. Geneva: Apud Io. Crispinum [Jean Crespin], 1567 (HAB exemplar).

Thomas Erastus: Scientific and Medical Writings, etc.

Thomae Erasti ad Archangeli Mercenarii philosophi Patavini Disputationem de putredine responsio. Adiunximua eam, cui respondetur, Dissertationem, bona fide. (Archangeli Mercenarii, Philosophiae in Gymnasio Patauino Interpretis Ordinarii. de putredine disputatio aduersus Thomam Erastum ...). Basel: Conrad Waldkirch, 1583 (VD 16 E 3668). Reprints: Leipzig: Hans Steinmann, 1590; Frankfurt: Apud Danielem & Davidem Aubrios & Clementem Schleichium [David & Daniel Aubry & Clemens Schleich], 1626.

Astrologia Confutata. Ein wahrhafte Gegründte Unwidersprechliche Confutation/ der falschen Astrologei oder abgottischen warsagung aus des himels und der gestirnen lauff/ der warheit zu steuer/ unnd dem gemeinen man zur warnung/ aus welsher und Lateinischer sprach/ wie volgend zu sehen/ von neuem ins deutsch gebracht. Schleusingen: Hermann Hamsing, 1557 (VD 16 S 2040). This book is Erastus's translation of Girolamo Savonarola's *Contra gli astrologi* (Florence, ca. 1497) along with original materials by Erastus on astrology. http://opacplus.bsb-muenchen.de/search?oclcno=165533159.

Comitis Montani Vicentini Novi Medicorum Censoris, quinque librorum de Morbis nuper editorum Viva Anatome: In qua multa artis medicae capita accuratissimè declarantur a Thoma Erasto Philosopho & Medico. Basel: Ex Officina Petri Pernae, 1581 (VD 16 E 3672). http://digital.slub-dresden.de/ppn274506343.

De astrologia divinatrice epistolae D. Thomae Erasti, iam olim ab eodem ad diversos scriptae, & in duos libros digestae, ac nunc demum in gratiam veritatis studiosorum in lucem aeditiae, opera et studio Ioannis Iacobi Grynaei. Basel: Pietro Perna, 1580 (VD 16 E 3669).[3] http://digital.slub-dresden.de/ppn273543210; http://diglib.hab.de/wdb.php?dir=drucke/64–12-quod-1.

De Causa Morborum Continente, Tractatus. In quo integra, perfecta & dilucida huius quaestionis, & ad eam pertinentium rerum explanatio continetur. Basel: Pietro Perna, 1572 (VD 16 E 3696). Published with *Disputationum de nova Philippi Paracelsi Medicina Pars Tertia.* [Basel]: Pietro Perna, 1572 (VD 16 E 3679).[4]

---

[3] Appeared at the Lenten Frankfurt fair, 1580. *Die Messkatalog Georg Willers*, 2:441.

[4] Published with its own title page, pagination and index. It is mentioned on the title page of *De nova*, 3.

"De cometarum ortu, natura et causis tractatus: in quo Aristot. sententia explicatur, & contra D. Marcellum Squarcialupum Plumbinensem defenditur." In *De Cometis dissertationes novae clariss. vivorum Thom. Erasti, Andr. Dudithij, Marc. Squacialupi, Symon. Grynaei*, 103–166. Basel: Ex officina Leonardi Ostenii, sumptibus Petri Pernae [Leonhard Ostein], 1580 (VD 16 E 3671).

"De cometarum significationibus iudicium Thomae Erasti Medicinae in Schola Heidelbergensi Professoris." In *De Cometis dissertationes novae clariss. vivorum Thom. Erasti, Andr. Dudithij, Marc. Squacialupi, Symon. Grynaei*, 1–23. Basel: Leonhard Ostein, 1580 (VD 16 E 3671). This work is a revised version of the similar title ("De cometarum significationibus sententia ...") first printed in *Disputatio de auro potabili* ... (VD 16 E 3674).

"De cometarum significationibus sententia Thomae Erasti, veris ac certis ex ipsa rei natura petitis argumentis probata" [Initial title page: *Iudicium de indicatione cometarum*] (VD16 E 3685). In *Disputatio de auro potabili, in qua accurate admodum disquiritur, num ex metallis opera chemiae, concinnata pharmaca tute utiliterque bibi possint*. Basel: Pietro Perna, 1578 (VD 16 E 3674).

[Erastus, Thomas, Andreas Dudith, Marco Squacialupi, and Simon Grynaeus] *De Cometis dissertationes novae clariss. vivorum Thom. Erasti, Andr. Dudithij, Marc. Squacialupi, Symon. Grynaei*, 103–166. Basel: Ex officina Leonardi Ostenii, sumptibus Petri Pernae [Leonhard Ostein], 1580 (VD 16 E 3671).[5] http://digital.slub-dresden.de/ppn273541927.

De occultis pharmacorum potestatibus: quid, et quotuplices eae sint: quibus in morbis, quomodo, quando, quem in curationibus usum habeant ... accessit huic tractatui disputatio alia ejusdem ferè argumenti, de medicamentorum purgantium facultate, tribus absoluta quaestionibus, in qua tota propè horum pharmacorum natura declaratur. Basel: Pietro Perna, 1574 (VD 16 E 3691).[6] http://digital.slub-dresden.de/ppn273579770.

Defensio libelli Hieronymi Savonarolae de astrologia divinatrice, adversus Christophorum Stathmionem, Medicum Coburgensem: in qua simul declaratur, quae sit ista Divinatio: quae eius partes: ad quam praenotionis speciem pèrtineat: quomodo à licitis Divinationibus differat. Accessit huic alia eiusdem argumenti disputatio, qua 178. Theses pro divinatione Astrologica scriptae solidissimè confutantur. [Geneva ?]: Apud Ioannem Le Preux and Ioannem Parvum [Jean Le Preux & Jean Petit], 1569 (Basel UB exemplar).[7]

Disputatio de auro potabili, in qua accurate admodum disquiritur, num ex metallis opera chemiae, concinnata pharmaca tutè utiliterque bibi possint. Basel: Pietro Perna, 1578 (VD E 3674).[8] Reprinted with a different order of contents, Basel: Conrad Waldkirch, 1584 (VD E 3675).

[5] Appeared at the Lenten Frankfurt fair, 1580. *Die Messkatalog Georg Willers*, 2:441.

[6] Appeared at the autumn Frankfurt fair, 1574. *Die Messkatalog Georg Willers*, 2:43.

[7] Appeared at the Lenten Frankfurt fair, 1569. Die Messkatalog Georg Willers, 1:217. Cf. Hans Joachim Bremme, *Buchdrücker und Buchhändler zue Zeit der Glaubenskämpfe: Studien zur Genfer Druckgeschichte 1565–1580* (Geneva: Droz, 1969), 195 & 248.

[8] Appeared at the Lenten Frankfurt fair, 1578. *Die Messkatalog Georg Willers*, 2:288–289.

"Disputatio de Febribus Putridis: in qua tria de febribus paradoxa, D. Laurentii Juberti, Galli, secundum scilicet, tertium, & quartum Decadis secundae, diligenter excutiuntur." In *Disputatio de putredine: in qua natura, differentiae, et causa putredinis, ex Aristotele, & ipsa rerum evidentia, clare exponitur, consensio inter philosophos & Medicos declarantur, omnia denique ad perfectam eius notitiam necessaria, deligenter explicantur*,133–245. Basel: Leonhard Ostein, 1580 (VD 16 E 3676).

"Disputatio ... de medicamentorum purgantium facultate ..." Cf. "Explicatio Trium Quaestionum...."

Disputatio de putredine: in qua natura, differentiae, et causa putredinis, ex Aristotele, & ipsa rerum evidentia, clarè exponitur, consensio inter Philosophos & Medicos declaratur, omnia denique ad perfectam eius notitiam necessaria, diligenter explicantur, à Thoma Erasto, medicina in Schola Heidelbergensi professore. Basel: Apud Leonardum Ostenium, sumptibus Oporinianorum [Leonhard Ostein], 1580 (VD 16 E 3677);[9] reprint, Leipzig: Hans Steinmann, 1590 (see below). Reprint, Frankfurt: D.& D. Aubrius & C. Schleichius [David and Daniel Aubry and Clemens Schleich], 1626 (Basel UB).

Disputationum de medicina nova de Philippi Paracelsi Pars Prima: In qua, quae de remediis superstitiosis & Magicis curationibus ille prodidit, praecipuè examinantur. Basel: Pietro Perna, [1571] (VD 16 E 3679).[10]

Disputationum de nova Philippi Paracelsi medicina Pars Altera: In qua Philosophiae Paracelsicae Principia & Elementa explorantur. [Basel], Pietro Perna, 1572 (VD 16 E 3679).[11]

Disputationum de nova Philippi Paracelsi Medicina Pars Tertia. [Basel]: Pietro Perna, 1572 (VD 16 E 3679).[12]

Disputationum de nova medicina Philippi Paracelsi Pars Quarta et Ultima. Basel: Pietro Perna, 1573 (VD 16 E 3679).[13]

Thomae Erasti Philosophi et Medici celeberrime, Disputationum & Epistolarum Medicinalium volumen doctissimum. Nunc recens in lucem editum, opera et studio Theophili Maderi Philosophiae ac Medicinae doctoris, ac Physices in Academia Heydelbergensi Professoris ordinarij. Zürich: Apud Johannen Wolphium, Typis Frosch. [Johannes Wolf], 1595 (VD 16 E 3680) http://opacplus.bsb-muenchen.de/search?oclcno=214415614. Reprint, Zurich: [Johannes] Wolf, 1605 (B.Pal., E843/E844).

"Epistola eiusdem ad M. Symonem Grynaeum...." Cf. *Ratio Formandorum Syllogismorum.*

"Epistola de natura, materia, ortu atque usu lapidis sabulosi, qui in Palatinatu ad Rhenum reperitur" (VD16 E 3681). In *Explicatio Quaestionis famosae illius, utrum ex metalis ignobilibus aurum verum & naturale arte conflari possit.* Basel: Pietro Perna, 1572 (VD 16 E 3684). Published with *Disputationum de*

[9] Appeared at the Lenten Frankfurt fair, 1580. *Die Messkatalog Georg Willers*, 2:431.
[10] Appeared at the autumn Frankfurt fair, 1571. *Die Messkatalog Georg Willers*, 1:382.
[11] Appeared at the Lenten Frankfurt fair, 1572. *Die Messkatalog Georg Willers*, 1:421.
[12] Appeared at the autumn Frankfurt fair, 1572. *Die Messkatalog Georg Willers*, 1:457.
[13] Appeared at the autumn Frankfurt fair, 1573. *Die Messkatalog Georg Willers*, 1:518.

nova Philippi Paracelsi medicina Pars Altera: In qua Philosophiae Paracelsicae Principia & Elementa explorantur. Basel: Pietro Perna, 1572 (VD 16 E 3679).

Examen de simplicibus, quae ad compositionem Theriacae Andromachi requiruntur ... una cum Conradi Hoffmani, ... analysi ejusdem compositionis ... primo in lucem datum. Lyon, 1607 (HAB exemplar).

Explicatio Quaestionis famosae illius, utrum ex metalis ignobilibus aurum verum & naturale arte conflari possit. Basel: Pietro Perna, 1572 (VD 16 E 3684). Published with *Disputationum de nova Philippi Paracelsi medicina Pars Altera: In qua Philosophiae Paracelsicae Principia & Elementa explorantur*. [Basel]: Pietro Perna, 1572 (VD 16 E 3679).

"Explicatio trium quaestionum de medicamentorum purgantium facultatibus: Quibus tota ferè natura eorum declaratur" [title page: *Disputatio de medicamentorum purgantium facultate*]. (VD 16 E 3688).[14] In *De occultis pharmacorum potestatibus*,130–194. Basel: Pietro Perna, 1574 (VD 16 E 3691).

Kurtzer Bericht für den gemeinen Mann/ wie er sich in disen sterbenden leuffen/ ohne sondern kosten mit Preservativen unnd Remedien verwaren und halten soll. Heidelberg: Johann Mayer, 1563 (VD 16 ZV 20849; B.Pal. Stamp. IV 263: ted.761e). Note: VD 16 references a 1574 edition printed without Erastus's name which instead reads "gestelt durch die Medicos zu Heidelberg" (VD 16 K 2727).[15]

Ratio Formandorum Syllogismorum brevissima & facilima, non tam ex arte usum, quam ex usu artem docens: illustri Comiti Hieronymo Fuggero, et Mathiae Gerhardo à Castelan nobili Tyrolensi conscripta à Thoma Erasto Medico. Huic accessit, Epistola eiusdem ad M. Symonem Grynaeum, de discrimine Logicae, Dialecticae, et Scientiae Demonstrativiae: quod non minus est scitu tum necessarium, tum utile, quàm est à multis hucusque vel neglectum, vel ignoratum. Basel: Johannes Oporinus, 1565 (ZV 5332). Reprint, Amberg: Ex Typographeio Forsteriano, 1602 (VD17 1:064612Y). Reprint, Lübeck: Typis Albinianis, sumtu Samuelis Jauchii, Bibliopolae, 1612 (VD 17 23:282004B; this reprint does not contain the "Epistola eiusdem ad M. Symonem Grynaeum").

Repetitio disputationis de lamiis seu strigibus: in qua plenè, solidè, & perspicuè, de arte earum, potestate, itemque poena disceptatur.... Basel: Pietro Perna, [1578] (VD 16 E 3692);[16] reprint, Amberg: Michael Forster, 1606 (BSB exem-

[14] This work does not have its own title page and is described with a different sequence of terms (though with more or less the same larger sense) on the title page of *De occultis pharmacorum potestatibus* (see above).

[15] Appeared at the Lenten Frankfurt fair, 1574. *Die Messkatalog Georg Willers*, 2:26. This work apparently had an afterlife as modified by physicians in Amberg: *Kurtzer Bericht Für den gemeinen Mann, Wie er sich in disen sterbenden läufften verhalten, vnd was er im fall der not gebrauchen sol. Erstlich gestellet Durch die Medicos zu Heydelberg, Anjetz aber Vff Churf. befelch von den Medicis zu Amberg revidirt, vnnd vff selbige Statt, auch hieobige Landschafft gerichtet* (Amberg, 1597; reprint Amberg, 1598). (See the catalog of the Bibliotheksverbundes Bayern.)

[16] Appeared at the Lenten Frankfurt fair, 1578. *Die Messkatalog Georg Willers*, 2:294.

plar; VD17 12:633273X). Cf. also below "Disputatio de lamiis seu strigibus ..."

Varia Opuscula Medica Th. Erasti D. Medici celeberrimi; quae cum ipse studiosis communicare statuisset, morte praeventus, in lucem edere non potuit, Quorum feriem sequens pagina indicabit. Ed. Giacomo Castelvetro [Jacobus Castelvetrius]. Frankfurt: Johannes Wechel, 1590 (VD 16 E 3689).

Contents:

1. De Medicina laudibus oratio.
2. Medicina methodus brevissima.
3. Disputatio de Saporibus, quatenus hi utiles sunt ad pervestigandas medicamentorum vires, in qua etiam aliae quaedam utiles scitu quaestiones declarantur.
4. Epistola de natura, & ortu lapidis Sabulosi, qui in Palatinatu ad Rhenum reperitur, ac de usu eiusdem.
5. De Vapore disputatio ad D. Matth. Stoium Medicum.
6. Epistola de quibusdam quaestionibus ad curationem pestilentiae pertinentibus, ad Conradum Gesnerum Medicum Tigurinum.
7. Anatome librorum quinque Comitis Montani.
8. In aliquot primi libri Aphorismos praelectiones.
9. In primum & secundum Hippocratis prognosticum praelectiones.
10. Expositio primi Aphoris. sect. 5.lib.6 Epidem. Hippocra. (Morborum naturae medicatrices.)
11. Varia ad morbos varios consilia.

Thomas Erastus: Treatises, Reprints, and Consilia within Other Titles

"Libellus utilissimus de conformatione Syllogismi...." In *Valentini Rasci Regiomontani Borussi Institutionum Logicarum libri IV: Accessit Ad Calcem Thomae Erasti libellus utilissimus de conformatione Syllogismi aliquoties desideratus.* Lübeck: Impensa Samuelis Iauchii, 1612 (VD17 23:286219Z). Presumably a reprint of *Ratio Formandorum Syllogismorum.*

"De cometarum significationibus sententia...." (VD16 E 3686). In Andreas Dudith, *Andreae Duditii Viri Clarissimi De Cometarum Significatione Commentariolus. In quo non minùs eleganter, quàm doctè & verè, Mathematicorum quorundam in ea re vanitas refutatur. Addidimus D. Thomae Erasti eadem de re sententiam.* Basel: Ex Officina Petri Pernae, 1579 (VD 16 D 2846). Reprinted with the title, *De Cometarum Significatione Cl. Virorum Andreae Duditii Commentariolus, & D. Thomae Erasti sententia.* Wrocław (Breslau): Typis Baumannianis, Impensis Davidis Mülleri, Bibliopolae Vratisl., 1619 (VD 17 23:278929Z).

"De cometarum significationibus iudicium." In Johann Andreas Bose, ed. *De Significatu Cometarum Dissertationes Et Iudicia Doctorum Hominum collecta, emendata, & Cometomanticae nostri temporis opposita a Jo. Andrea Bosio.* Jena: Georg Sengenwald, 1665 (VD 17 39:122988M).

"De occultis medicamentorum proprietatibus: quid, et quotuplices eae sint: quibus in morbis, quomodo, quando, quem usum habeant." In *Miscellanea ... medica, cum praestantissimis quinque medicis D. Thoma Erasto ... Henrico*

Brucaeo … Levino Batto … Joanne Weyero … Henr. Weyero … communicata, et in libros XII. digesta … Ed. Heinrich Smet. Frankfurt: Jonas Rhodius, 1611 (NLM exemplar). Reprint of the first part of *De Occultis Pharmacorum Potestatibus ….*

Defensio Libelli Hieronymi Savonarolae, De Astrologia Divina Trice, Adversus Christophorum Stathmionem, medicum Cobugensem …. In Girolamo Zanchi, *De Divinatione tam artificiosa …* Hanau: Guilielmus Antonius [Wilhelm Antonius], 1610 (HAB exemplar; VD17 23:295245N).

"Disputatio de Lamiis, seu Strigibus, in qua de earum viribus perspicuè disputatur à Thoma Erasto." In Nicolas Jacquier, *Flagellum haereticorum fascinariorum*, ed. Heinrich Myntzenberg, 500–604. Frankfurt: Bassaeus, 1581 (HAB exemplar). Reprint of Erastus's *Repetitio disputationis de lamiis seu strigibus.*

Disputatio de Putretine … and *Thomae Erasti ad Archangeli Mercenarii … Disputationem de putredine responsio.* In *Archangeli Mercenari à Monte Santo, Dilucidationes Obscuriorum Locorum et Quaestionem philosophiae naturalis Aristotelis eiusque interpretum….* Leipzig: Hans Steinmann, 1590 (VD 16 ZV 10886; HAB exemplar).

Gründtlicher bericht/ wie die wort Christi/ Das ist mein leib/ etc. zuverstehen seien. In *Christliche, und allein auff Gottes wort gegründete Glaubensbekanntnus / Mit Bericht von Thom. Erastus.* Herborn: Christoph Rab [Rabe; Raben], 1603. (VD17 23:648456T). Reprint, (each version with slightly altered title) Herborn: Christoph Rab, 1605 (VD17 1:076736K). Reprint, Herborn: Christoph Rab, 1610 (VD17 1:081611K). Reprint, Herborn: Christoph Rab, 1619 (Basel UB exemplar).

"Utrum artis Medicae sit necessitas: quandoquidem suae cuique vitae terminus ita praefinitus, ut ulla arte ea, neque prolongari, neque ante tempus abrumpi possit." In *Joh. Beveronicii Epistolica Quaestio, de vitae termino, Fatali an Mobili? … Pars Tertia, et Ultima …*, Jan Beverwijk, 133–136. Leiden: Joannis Maire, 1639. Printed version of letter to [Christoph Schilling or Theophil Mader?] from March 26, 1577 (see Correspondence Register).

Thomas Erastus: Early Modern Translations

"Deux Dialogues de Thomas Erastus, Professeur en Medecine à Heidelberg, touchant le pouvoir des Sorcieres: & de la punition qu'elles meritent."[17] In Johann Weyer (Iean Wier), *Histoires, disputes et discours, des illusions et impostures des diables, des magiciens infames, sorcieres & empoisonneurs: Des ensorcelez & demoniaques, & de la guerison d'iceux. Item de la punition que meritent les magiciens, les empoisonneurs, & les sorcieres. Le tout compris en six livres (augmentez de moitié en ceste derniere edition) par Iean Wier*

[17] The title on the internal title page is: "Deux Dialogues de Thomas Erastus, Docteur en Medecine à Heidelberg, touchant le pouvoir des Sorcieres: & de la punition qu'elles meritent."

medecin du Duc du Cleves, pp. 757–875. [Geneva]:[18] Pour Iaques Chouet, 1579 (NLM 2297040R). French translation of both Erastus's "De Lamiis seu Strigibus non inutilia scitu" from within the *Disputationum de medicina nova de Philippi Paracelsi Pars Prima* (pp. 193–215) and the *Repetitio disputationis de lamiis*.

The Nullity of Church Censures: or A DISPUTE Written by that Illustrious Philosopher, Expert Physician and Pious Divine Dr. Thomas Erastus, Publick Professor in the University of Heidelberge, and Basil. Wherein is proved by the holy Scriptures and sound Reason; that Excommunication and Church-Senates or Members, exercising the same, are not of Divine Institution; But a meere humane Invention. London: Printed for G.L., 1659. (Wing (2nd ed.), E3217; BL E.1783.(2.)). English translation of the 75 theses of *Explicatio Gravissimae Quaestionis*.

A Treatise of Excommunication: wherein 'tis Fully, Learnedly, and Modestly Demonstrated that there is no Warrant, Precept, or President, either in the Old or New Testament, for Excommunicating any Persons, or Debarring them the Sacraments, whilst they make an outward Profession of the true Christian Faith / written originally in Latine, by the famous and pious Thomas Erastus Doctor in Physick, about the year 1568. London: for L. Curtis, 1682 (Wing (2nd ed.), E3218). English translation of the 75 theses of *Explicatio Gravissimae Quaestionis*.

[*The true Understanding of those Words: This is my Bodie*. London: 1578. English translation of *Gründtlicher bericht/ wie die wort Christi/ Das ist mein leib/ etc. zuverstehen seien*.][19]

Vraye & droite intelligence de ces paroles de la Saincte Cene de Iesus Christ, CECY EST MON CORPS, &c. TRAITTE CLAIR ET UTILE COMposé premierement en Allemand par M. THOMAS ERASTUS Docteur: Et nouuellement traduit en François par M. PIERRE DE COLOGNE … AUTRE bref Traitté des Sacramens en general, fait en Latin par M. THEODORE DE BEZE, & nouuellement traduit en François par M. LOVIS DES MASVRES. Trans. Pierre de Cologne [aka Petrus Colonius, Pieter van Keulen]. Metz: Iean d'Arras & Odinet Basset, 1564 (FVB 18454; B.Pal. Stamp. V 1634 (franc. 8)). Reprint ?, Lyon: Par Ian d'Ogerolles, 1564 (FVB 18453; Oxford, Magdalen College Q.5.14.(1)). Reprint, [Orleans: Eloi Gibier ?], 1564 (FVB 18455). Reprint, [Orleans: Eloi Gibier ?] "Suivant l'exemplaire imprimé à Lyon, par Jean D'ogerolles," 1565 (FVB 18456; Bodleian Library 8° I 13(2) Th. BS). French translation of *Gründtlicher bericht/ wie die wort Christi/ Das ist mein leib/ etc. zuverstehen seien*.

[18] Bremme, *Buchdrücker und Buchhändler*, 135.

[19] William Thomas Lowndes, *The Bibliographer's Manual of English Literature* (London, 1834), 1:676. Lowndes's full reference is: "Erastus, Thomas. The true Understanding of those Words: This is my Bodie. Also Beza's Treatise of the Sacraments in generall, translated by John Shutt. London, 1578. 16mo." I have not been able to confirm the existence of this book.

Theses and Disputations Presided over by Erastus (Disputants Names Underlined)

"Ad has de natura et causis epilepsiae theses praes. D.T. Erasto, respondebit … J. Seidelius [Jakob Seidel], etc." Heidelberg, 1573 (BL 7306.f.6.(4.)). Reprinted in *Disp. et Epist.*, fols. 16^r–17^v.

"An occultae medicamentorum, in quorum numero & cibos ponimus, potestates, methodo investigari possint, vel per solam experientiam in subiectis rebus deprehendere & observare necesse habeamus." Simon Grynaeus. In *Disp. et Epist.*, fols. 3^r–4^r.

"De Amuletis" (no disputant named). In *Disp. et Epist.*, fols. 95–115^v.

"De Constitutione hyemis praeteritae anni 1559." Heinrychus Smetius [Heinrich Smet] ("1560 in scholis medicis"). In *Disp. et Epist.*, fols. 1^r–1^v.

"De Dentibus." Simon Grynaeus. In *Disp. et Epist.*, fols. 5^v–7^r.

"De Febrium definitione." Sebastianus Caesar, Themarensis. In *Disp. et Epist.*, fols. 8^v–10^v.

"De Humoribus." Sigismund Melanchthon. In *Disp. et Epist.*, fols. 2^r–2^v.

"De hydrope theses, etc. Praes. T. Erastus." Sebastianus Caesar, Themarensis. Heidelberg: Excudebat I. Maier, 1572 (BL 7306.f.6.(16.)). Reprinted in *Disp. et Epist.*, fols. 12^v–16^r.

"De Lethargo theses: … respondebit Heinricus Lavaterus Tigurinus, ad VIII. diem Augusti, hora & loco consuetis." Basel: Ex Officina Oporiniana, 1582 (VD 16 ZV 20330; WLB exemplar).

"De melancholia, ad disputandum propositae, … ad diem 5. Octobris, anno 1577. …" Leo Wolfhardt. In *Comitis Montani Vincentini Novi Medicorum Censoris …*, 240–256. Reprinted in *Disp. et Epist.*, fols. 43^v–51^v.

"De Renum calculis [1567]." Peter Turner, Anglus. In *Disp. et Epist.*, fols. 7^r–8^v.

"De Saporibus." Hieronymus Niger. In *Disp. et Epist.*, fols. 2^v–3^r.

"De Tumoribus praeter naturam." Sigismund Melanchthon. In *Disp. et Epist.*, fols. 1^v–2^r.

Disputationes duae: prior, de somno et vigilia: posterior, de comate seu cataphora: Habitae in Auditorio Medicorum Basiliensivm ab Andrea Christiano Ripensi. (de somno et vigilia theses, ad disputandum propositae, praeside Cl. V.D. Thoma Erasto, philosopho et medico …) (de Comate, sive cataphora, theses, Publicè … supremam in Arte Medica Lauream consequendi causa, 7. Febr. disputatae.) Adiuncta est Quaestio ab eodem in publico Promotionis Actu discussa: Sit'ne pestis morbus contagiosus? Basel, 1583 (VD 16 ZV 5335).

"Resp. De dolore colico theses … Praes. T. Erasto, etc." Franciscus Faber, Freibergensis. Heidelberg, 1570 (BL 7306.f.6.(21.)).

"Resp. Theses de destillatione. Praes. T. Erasto, etc." Bernhartus Grock. Heidelberg, 1570 (BL 7306.f.6.(7.)).

"Resp. Theses de Revulsione … Praes. T. Erasto, etc." Timotheus Mader. Heidelberg, 1571 (BL 7306.f.6.(35.)). Reprinted in *Disp. et Epist.*, fols. 10^v–12^v [disputant named as "Matthaeus Maderus"].

"Resp. Theses de singultu … Praes. T. Erasto, etc." Jeremias Eysenmenger [Bretten]. Heidelberg, 1574 (BL 7306.f.6.(18.)). Reprinted in *Disp. et Epist.*, fols. 24^v–25^v.

"Theses de Catarrhis seu destillationibus, ..." Kaspar Peucer. Heidelberg: Jakob Müller (Jacobus Mylius), 1577 (NLM exemplar).

"Theses de canitie ad quas praeside Thoma Erasto ... respondebit Andreas Ruinella Praegallus Rhaetus." Pridie Non. Novembr. Basil: Leonhard Ostein, 1581.

"Theses de Convulsione ..." (no disputant named). In Erastus, *Comitis Montani Vincentini Novi Medicorum Censoris* ..., 280–316. Reprinted in *Disp. et Epist.*, fols. 78[r]–95[r].

"Theses de Contagio ad disputandum propositae ..." Timotheus Mader. Heidelberg: Michael Schiratius, 1574 (B.Pal. Stamp. IV 531.3; lat. 2219c). Reprinted in *Disp. et Epist.*, fols. 18[r]–24[r]. Reprinted in Heinrich Smet, *Miscellanea Medica*, 260–271.

"Theses de Lienteria (ex Galeni Sententia) specimen prouectus sui editurus publicum, defendere conabitur M. Christianus Person Witebergensis: cal. octobris." Basel, 1583 (VD 16 ZV 5336; SBB exemplar).

"Theses de Morbis Totius Substantiae ad disputandum propositae ..." Theophil Mader. Heidelberg: Johannes Mayer, 1575 (B.Pal. Stamp.IV.531.4; lat. 2220d). Reprinted in *Comitis Montani Vincentini Novi Medicorum Censoris* ..., 257–280. Reprinted in *Disp. et Epist.*, fols. 25[v]–36[r].

"Theses de Pinguedinis in Animalibus Generatione et Concretione ... tutabitur M. Michael Schenckius Heydelbergensis. Disputabuntur in Auditorio Medicorum 4. Calend. Martii." Heidelberg: Jakob Müller (Jacobus Mylius), 1580 (VD ZV 5334; SBB, ZBZ exemplars). Reprinted in *Disp. et Epist.*, fols. 67[r]–77[v]. Reprinted in Fabianus Hippius, ed. *Problemata Physica Et Logica Peripatetica.* Wittenberg: Clemens Berger, 1604 (VD 17 39:113614V).

"Theses de Pleuritide ... respondebit M. Lazarus Mayenschein Noribergensis. ad xiiii. Diem Septembris...." Basel: Leonhard Ostein, 1583 (VD ZV 5337; SBB exemplar).

"Theses de Putredine ad disputandum propositae: ad quas, praeside ... respo[n]debit ... Leo Wolfhardus Memmingensis, ad X. Calend. Aprilis ... in auditorio Medicorum." Heidelberg: Jakob Müller, 1577 (VD 16 ZV 21760). Reprinted in *Disputatio de putredine* ..., 115–131. Basel: Leonhard Ostein, 1580 (VD 16 E 3676). Reprinted in *Disp. et Epist.*, fols. 36[r]–43[v]. Reprinted in Fabianus Hippius, ed. *Problemata Physica Et Logica Peripatetica.* Wittenberg, Clemens Berger, 1604 (VD 17 39:113614V).

"Theses de sudore agitandae XVI. die Novembris ... Quas moderatore Thoma Erasto, asseret Hieronymus Reusnerus Leorinus." Basel: Leonhard Ostein, 1581 (Disputationum Medicarum Basiliensium, part 1, no. 49).

"Theses de Somno ..." Johannes Beatus Humelius. Heidelberg: Jacobus Mylius [Jakob Müller], 1578 (NLM exemplar). Reprinted in *Disp. et Epist.*, fols. 51[r]–58[v]. Reprinted in Fabianus Hippius, ed. *Problemata Physica Et Logica Peripatetica.* Wittenberg, Clemens Berger, 1604 (VD 17 39:113614V).

"Theses Physiologicae, de animae facultatibus ..." Robertus Augerius. Basel: Leonhard Ostein, 1583 (ZBZ exemplar).

"Theses ... subsequentes de artis medicae definitione & divisione / praeside Thoma Erasto, ... defendere conabitur Theophilus Maderus, A.D. VI. Kal. Sextil." Basil: Ex Officina Oporiniana, 1583 (Basel UB exemplar).

"Utrum Humores alii à sanquine, scilicet Pituita, Bilis flava & suecus Melancholicus, Corporis integrè sani partes aliquas nutriant?" Daniel Obrecht, 1579. In *Disp. et Epist.*, fols. 58v–67r.

Thomas Erastus: Modern Editions and Translations

"Antwurt uff die Censur des Biechleins vom Brodtbrechen im Nachtmal Cristi." In M.A. Gooszen. *De Heidelbergsche Catechismus en het Boekje van de Breking des Broods, in het Jaar 1563–1564 bestreden en verdedigd*, 139–165. Leiden: Brill, 1892. Unpublished response to the attacks upon *Das Büchlein vom Brotbrechen*. Edited from the manuscript in the Sächsisches Hauptstaatsarchiv Dresden.

Das Büchlein vom Brotbrechen. Ed. J.I. Doedes. Utrecht: Kemink & Zoon, 1891. Reprint of *Erzelung Etlicher ursachen/ warumb das hochwirdig Sacrament des Nachtmals unsers Herrn/ und Heylandts Jhesu Christi/ nicht solle ohne das brodbrechen gehalten werden*. [Doedes was unaware of Erastus's authorship of this treatise.]

"Deux Dialogues de Thomas Erastus, Professeur en Medecine à Heidelberg, touchant le pouvoir des Sorcières: et de la punition qu'elles méritent." In Johann Weyer (Jean Wier). *Histoires, disputes et discours ...*, pp. 399–553 (indices pp. 601–608). Paris. Lecrosnier and Delahaye, 1885 (http://gallica.bnf.fr/ark:/12148/bpt6k73076c.notice); Reprint, New York: Arno, 1976. Reprint of the 1579 French translation.

Disputationen über die neue Medizin des Philippus Paracelsus. Trans. and ed. Franz Josef Schmidt. Hamm: self-published, 1978 (Institut für Geschichte der Medizin, Universität Heidelberg exemplar). German translation of *Disputationum de medicina nova de Philippi Paracelsi Pars Prima*.

Epistola de natura, materia, ortu atque usu lapidis sabulosi qui in Palatinatu ad Rhenum reperitur. Als Beitrag zur Geschichte der Bodenkunde zum 400. Todestage von Thomas Erastus im Faksimile neu herausgegeben, übersetzt, mit Anmerkungen versehen, eingeleitet von Wolfgang Ziehen. Aalen: Scientia Verlag, 1984. Latin facsimile edition with German translation and notes.

"Fontis Kissingensis vires a D. Thoma Erasto descriptae." In L. Heffner. "Kissingen, seine Salz- und Mineralquellen." In *Archiv des historischen Vereins von Unterfranken und Aschaffenburg* 13 (Würzburg, 1854): 322–323. German translation in Hedwig Pfister. *Bad Kissingen vor vierhundert Jahren* [Mainfränkische Hefte 19]. Würzburg, 1954. pp. 25–26. Description of the medicinal powers of Bad Kissingen for Joachim Camerarius.

The Theses of Erastus Touching Excommunication. Trans. Robert Lee. Edinburgh: Myles MacPhail, 1844. English translation of the 75 theses of *Explicatio Gravissimae Quaestionis*.

"Thomas Erasts Disputation über die Zähne." Ed. Curt G. Lorber. *Ruperto Carola* 15, bd. 34 (1963): 200–205.

Sources Printed Before 1750

Agricola, Johann Georg. *Cervi Excoriati Et Dissecti In Medicina Usus. Das ist: Kurtze Beschreibung Welcher gestalt deß zu gewisser zeit gefangenen Hirschens fürnembste Glieder in der Artzney zugebrauchen* ... Amberg: Michael Forster, 1603.

Alting, [Johann] Heinrich. *Historia de ecclesiis Palatinis....* / In Menso Alting, *Mensonis Altingii ... Vita descripta per Ubbonem Emmium*. Groningen, 1728.

Adam, Melchior. *Vitae Germanorum Medicorum*. Heidelberg: Johann Georg Geyder, 1620.

Baxter, Richard. *The unreasonableness of infidelity: manifested in four discourses*. In *The practical works of the late reverend and pious Mr. Richard Baxter, in four volumes*. London, 1707.

Beza, Theodore. *Epistolarum theologicarum Theodori Bezae Vezelii, liber unus*. Geneva: E. Vignon, 1573.

——. *Tractatus Pius et Moderatus de vera Excommunicatione, & christiano Presbyterio, iampridem pacis conciliand[ae] causa, CL. V. Th. Erasti D. Medici centum manuscriptis thesibus oppositus, & nunc primum, cogente necessitate, editus*. Geneva: Jean Le Preux, 1590; Reprint, London: Impensis Ioan. Norton, 1590.

Bodin, Jean. *De la demonomanie des sorciers*. Paris, 1580 (NLM exemplar).

Boyle, Robert. *The Skeptical Chymist*. London, 1661.

Brenz, Johannes. *Warhafftiger, und Gründtlicher Bericht, Von dem Gesprech zwischen deß Churfürstenn Pfaltzgraffen, und deß Hertzogen zu Wirtemberg Theologen, von deß Herrn Nachtmal zu Maulbronn gehalten*. [Frankfurt am Main], 1564 (VD16 B 7937).

Christliche Gebet/ die man daheim in heusern/ und in der Kirchen brauchen mag. Heidelberg: Johann Mayer, 1563 (WLB exemplar).

Crato von Krafftheim, Johannes. *Consiliorum et Epistolarum Medicinalium, Liber, Ex collectaneis clariss. viri Dn. Petri Monavii Uratisl. quondam Medici Caesarei, selectus, Et nunc in primùm à Laurentio Scholzio Sil. medico Uratislaviensi in lucem editus*. 5 vols. Frankfurt: Apud Andreae Wecheli haeredes, Claudium Marnium & Joan. Au [Claude de Marne and Jean Aubry], 1591–1594 (NLM exemplar).

——. *Consiliorum et epistolarum medicinalium libri septem*. Frankfurt: Sumptibus Johannis Petri Zubrodt, 1671 (NLM exemplar).

Cyprian, Ern[st] Sal[oman]. *Catalogus Codicum Manuscriptorum Bibliothecae Gothanae*. Leipzig: Apud Io. Frieder. Gleditsch et Filium, 1714.

Dessen von Kronenburg, Bernhard. *Medicinae Veteris Et Rationalis, Adversus Oberronis Cuiusdam Mendacissimi Atque Impudentissimi Georgii Fedronis, ac universae Sectae Paracelsiae imposturas, defensio*. Cologne: Johann Gymnich, 1573.

Dorn, Gerhard. *De Naturae Luce Physica, ex Genesi desumta, Iuxta sententiam Theophrasti Paracelsi, Germani Philosophi ac Medici prae cunctis excellentissimi, TRACTATUS. Cui annexa est modesta quaedam admonitio ad Thomam Erastum, Germanum etiam Philosophum atque Medicum, de retractandis calumnijs, & convitijs in Paracelsum & suos perperam ac imeritò datis in lucem per quator tomos, de Nova medicina*. Frankfurt: Christoph Rab [Christophorus Corvinus], 1583 (VD 16 D 2408). Reprinted in *Theatrum Chemicum*. Ed. Lazarus Zetzner. Strasbourg, 1659–1661.

DuClo, Gaston [aka Gaston le Doux; Gasto Claveus]. *Apologia Chrysopoeiae et Argyropoeiae, adversus Thomam Erastum, Doctorem et Professorem Medicinae*. Reprint, Oberursel (Ursellis): Cornelius Sutor, 1602 (NLM exemplar). (First edition 1598). Reprinted in L. Zetzner, *Theatrum Chemicum*.

———. *Claveus Germanicus: Das ist, Ein köstlichess Büchlein von dem Stein der Weisen … aus Latein ins Teutsch versetzt, durch einen Leibhaber der uhralten … kunst Chymiae*. Halle ("Hall in Sachsen"): Peter Schmidt, 1617 (NLM exemplar). German translation of entry below.

———. *Philosophia chymica tribus tractatibus comprehensa Opus doctissimum, et nunc in primum integrum in lucem editum…*. Lyon, 1612 (NLM exemplar). Contains a reprint of *Apologia Crysopoeiae et Argyropoeiae adversus Thomam Erastum*.

Ducret, Toussaint. *De Arthritide vera assertio, eiusque curandae methodus, adversus Paracelsistas*. Lyon: Bartholomaeus Vincentius, 1575 (NLM exemplar). Dedicatory epistle to Erastus (pp. Aii-Av).

Fecht, Johannes, ed. *Historiae Ecclesiasticae a.n.c. XVI. Supplementum*. Frankfurt and Speyer: Christoph Olffen, 1684.

Fenot, Jean Antoine. *Alexipharmacum, Sive Antidotus Apologetica, ad virulentias Iosephi cuiusdam Quercetani Armeniaci, evomitas in libellum Jacobi Auberti, de ortu & causis Metallorum contra Chymistas*. Basil: [Pietro Perna], 1575.

Figulus, Benedictus [aka Benedikt Töpfer]. *Pandora Magnalium Naturalium Aurea Et Benedicta, De Benedicto Lapidis Philosoph. Mysterio*. Strasbourg: Lazarus Zetzner, 1608.

Gessner, Konrad. *Epistolarum Medicinalium Conradi Gesneri, philosophi et medici tigurini, libri III*. Zurich: Christoph Froschauer, 1577. Cf. *Opera Omnia* [Microform], Zug: IDC, 1985.

———. *Historiae animalium liber III qui est de Avium natura*. Zurich: Christoph Froschauer, 1555.

———. *Historiae animalium liber IIII qui est de Piscium et Aquatilium animantium natura*. Zurich: Christoph Froschauer, 1558.

Gilbert, William. *De Magnete*. London: Petrus Short, 1600.

Gillespie, George. *Aarons Rod Blossoming. Or, the Divine Ordinance of Church-Government Vindicated, So as the present Erastian Controversy concerning the distinction of Civill and Ecclesiasticall Government, Excommunication, and Suspension, is fully debated and discussed, from the holy Scriptures, from the Jewish and Christian Antiquities, from the consent of latter Writers, from the true nature and rights of Magistracy, and from the groundlessnesse of the chief Objections made against the Presbyteriall Government in point of a domineering arbitrary unlimited power*. London: Printed by E.G. for Richard Whitaker, 1646 (Wing (2nd ed.), G743).

———. *Nihil respondes: or, A discovery of the extream unsatisfactorinesse of Master Colemans peece, published last weeke under the title of A brotherly examination re-examined*. London: for Robert Bostock, 1645 (Wing (2nd ed.) G755).

Goldast, Melchior, ed. *Philologicarum Epistolarum Centuria Una Diversorum A Renatis Literis Doctissimorum Virorum....* Leipzig: Impensis Joh. Bart. Oeleri, Literis Colerianis, 1674.

Grynaeus, Johann Jakob. *Epistolae familiares LXVI ad Christophor. Andr. Iulium scriptae quas una cum vita Grynaei ... in lucem ed. et variis scholiis illustravit Sigism. Iac. Apinus.* Nuremberg: Apud haeredes Io. Dan. Tauberi, 1720.

Grynaeus, Simon. *Commentarii Duo, de ignitis meteoris unus: alter de cometarum causis atque significationibus ... Accessit eiusdem Observatio Cometae, qui anno superiore 77. ab initio 78 fulsit. Et disputatio de invsitata magnitudine & figura veneris conspecta in fine anni 1578, & ad initium [1579].* In *De Cometis dissertationes novae clariss. Vivorum Thom. Erasti, Andr. Dudithij, Marc. Squacialupi, Symon. Grynaei.* Basel: Ex officina Leonardi Ostenii, sumptibus Petri Pernae [Leonhard Ostein], 1580.[20]

Guibert, Nicolas. *Alchymia ratione et experientia ita demum viriliter impugnata & expugnata, una cum suis fallaciis & deliramentis, quibus homines imbubinârat: ut nunquam imposterum se erigere valeat.* Strasbourg: Lazarus Zetzner, 1603 (Tü UB exemplar).

Hofmann, Caspar. *Animadversiones in Com. Montani libros quinque De morbis, et Thomae Erasti anatomen eorundum, nec non ant-Erastica ejusdem Montani. Cum auctario de causa continente.* Amsterdam. Joannes Janssonius, 1641 (NLM exemplar).

Hottinger, Johann Heinrich. *Historia ecclesiastica novi testamenti....* Zurich, 1651–1667.

Hornung, Johannes, ed. *Cista Medica.* Nuremberg: Halbmayr, 1625.

Klebitz, Wilhelm. *Victoria Veritatis, Ac Ruina Papatus Saxonici: Responsio Wilhelmi Klebitii Necessaria ad Argumenta Doct. Tilemanni Heshusii; Pro Defensione Ivsta I. Causae christianae, & Verae. II. Illustrissimi Electoris Palatini, III. Philippi Melanthonis. IIII. Senatus Ecclesiastici.* Freiburg: Daniel Delenus, 1561.

Lange, Johannes. *Epistolarum Medicinalium Volumen Tripartium* ... Frankfurt: Apud heredes Andreae Wecheli, 1589.

Lercheimer, Augustin. Cf. Herman Witekind.

Libavius, Andreas. *D.O.M.A. Defensio et declaratio perspicua alchymiae transmutatoriae, opposita Nicolai Guiperti Lotharingi Ph. Med. expugnationi virili: Et Gastonis Clavei Iurisconsulti Nivernatis Apologia contra Erastum malé sartae & pravae....* Oberursel (Ursellis): Ex officina Cornelii Sutorii: sumptibus Petri Kopffii Bibliopolae, 1604 (VD17 12:655902X).

Luchten, Adam. *Disputatio De Facultate Medicamentorum Purgantium: In qua doctrina Hippocratis & Galeni confirmatur, & contra Philosophos & Medicos clarissimos Jacobum Schegkium & Thomam Erastum defenditur. Proposita ab Adamo Luchtenio ... Ad quam respondebit publice M. Samuel Satlerus.* Helmstedt: Ex officina Iacobi Lucii, 1606 (VD17 3:016764U).

[20] While clearly published with *De Cometis dissertationes novae* and mentioned on its title page and list of contents, this work of Grynaeus has its own title page and pagination (pp. 1–88).

——. *Disputatio Medica, De Natura, Essentia, Subiecto & causis Convulsionis/ Ad mentem Clarissimi Philosophi Thomae Erasti in illustri Iulia ad disputandum proposita, ab Adamo Luchtenio, Phil. & Med. Doctore & Professore Physiologiae. Ad quam publice respondebit Laurentius Conerdingius.* Helmstedt: Jakob Lucius, 1610 (VD 17 70:676222H).

Magirus, Johann. *Ioannis Magiri physiologiae peripateticae libri sex cum commentariis, in quibus praecepta illius perspicue, eruditeque explicantur, & ex optimis quibusuis peripateticae philosophiae interpretibus, Platone, Aristotele, Zabarella, Archangelo Mercenario, Thoma Erasto …: accessit Caspari Bartholoini malmogij Dani Enchiridion metaphysicum, ex philosphorum coryphaei Aristotelis, optimorumque eius interpretum monumentis adornatum.* London: Apud Ioannem Billium, 1619.

Marbach, Johannes. *Christlicher und warhafftiger Vnderricht/ von den Worten der Einsatzung des heyligen Abentmals Jhesu Christi/ … sampt gründlicher widerlegung der Sacramentierer hieuon jrrigen Lehr/ und meynung.* Strasbourg: Christian Müller, 1565 (VD 16 M 902; Basel UB exemplar printed in 1566).

Marius, Georg. *Etlicher Gelehrten Bedencken vonn dem heylsamen Salzbronnen zu Offenauw …* Heidelberg: Johann Spieß, 1584 (Hd UB exemplar). The third 'Bedencken' is by Erastus. Cf. fols. Aivr & v.

Marolt, Ortolph. *Domini Ortholphi Maroldi Med. Doct. et quodam apud Schmalcaldius practici eminentissimi, Practica Medica ad omnis generis morbos feliciter curandos accomadata.* Frankfurt: Johannes Beyer, 1650 (BSB, NLM exemplars). Contains over 20 of Erastus's medical consultations (*consilia*) and prescriptions.

Mercenari, Arcangelo. *Adversus Erasti responsionem, secunda de putredine disputatio, in qua, praeter ea, quae ad exactam putredinis notitiam spectant, plurima philosophi: e medicinaeque studiosis necessaria explicantur.…* Padua: Paulus Meietus, 1585.

——. *Archangeli Mercenarii … Dilucidationes obscuriorum locorum & quaestionum Philosophiae naturalis Aristotelis, extrema ipsius recognitione emendatae. Additae sunt Disputationes de putredine contra Tomam Erastum … Tertia editio, etc.* Venice: Apud Paulum Meietum, 1588 (BL 004071170).

——. *Disputatio de putredine … adversus Thomam Erastum.…* Padua: Paulus Meietus, 1583.

Mersenne, Marin. *Quaestiones celeberrime in Genesim.…* Paris, 1623.

Meier, Georg. *Etlicher Gelehrten Bedencken Vonn dem heylsamen Saltzbronnen zu Offenauw nechst vnder der Reichsstatt Wimpffen gelegen. Sampt kurtzer Beschreibung auch etlicher anderer dero Gegendt nützlichen Bronnen/ als zu Denig/ S. Menardt/ Bachstainach zu Eberbach/&c. … Durch … Georgium Marium, der Artzney Doctorn/&c.* Heidelberg, Johann Spies, 1584 (VD 16 M 2218).

——. *In Iudaeorum medicastrorum calumnias & homicidia; pro Christianis pia exhortatio. Ex Theologorum & Iureconsultorum Decretis.* [Speyer,] 1570.[21]

[21] Erastus was given a copy of this book by "Doctor Struppius," which was in turn

Moffet, Thomas. *De Anodinis Medicamentis eorumque causis et usibus Physica & Medica consideratio in Theses aliquot digesta*. Basel: Ex Officina Brylingeriana, 1578 (Basel UB, Med. Conv. 293 No. 167).

——. *De jure et praesentia chemicorum medicamentorum dialogus apologeticus*. Frankfurt: Apud haeredes Andreae Wecheli, 1584 (NLN exemplar). Reprinted in Lazarus Zetzner. *Theatrum Chemicum*. Includes a dialogue between "Philerastus" (a representative of traditional Galenic medicine) and "Chemista."

Monte, Conte da (Montanus). *Defensio Librorum Suorum De Morbis, Adversus Thomam Erastum*. Venice: Apud Franciscum Zilettum, 1584 (NLM exemplar).

——. *De morbis ex Galeni sententia Libri Quinque....* Venice: Joannes Guerilius, 1591 (NLM exemplar; first edition 1580).

Musculus, Wolfgang. *Common Places of Christian Religion....* London, 1563.

——. *Loci communes in usus sacrae theologiae candidatorum parati*. Basil: Off[icina] Hervagiana, 1560.

Oddi, Marco degli. *Pro sua tutanda de putredine sententia apologia nunc primum in lucem edita, in qua ... A. Mercenarii et T. Erasti ... disputationes excutiuntur. Cui addita est altera epistola olim adversus Argenterium promulgata pro Aristotolis et Galeni placitis defendendis*. Padua: Paulus Meietus, 1585 (BL 1179.h.5.(2.))

Pantaleon, Heinrich. *Prosopographia Heroum Atque Illustrium Virorum Totius Germaniae*. 3 vols. Basel: In Officina Haeredum Nicolai Brylingeri, 1565–1566.

Paracelsus [Theophrastus von Hohenheim]. *Astronomia Magna: oder die gantze Philosophia sagax der grossen und kleinen Welt*. Ed. Michael Toxites. Frankfurt: Sigmund Feyrabend, 1571.

Protocoll Das ist/ Acta oder Handlungen des Gesprechs zwischen den Pfältzischen und Wirtembergischen Theologen/ von der Ubiquitet oder Allenthalbenheit des Leibs Christi/ und von dem buchstäblischen verstand der wort Christi/ Das ist mein Leib/ &c. Im April des Iars 1564. zü Maulbrun gehalten. Heidelberg: Johann Mayer, 1565.

Protocoll Des Gesprächs zwischen den Pfältzischen und Würtenbergischen Theologen/ im Aprill des 1564. Jars zü Maulbrunn gehalten. Tübingen, printer not named, 1565.

Protocollum, hoc est, Acta colloquii inter Palatinos et Vvirtebergicos theologos, de Ubiquitate sive Omnipraesentia corporis Christi, Et de sensu verborum Christi, Hoc est corpus meum, &c. Anno M.D.LXVIII. Mulbrunnae habiti. Item Vvirtembergicorum Theologorum de hoc ipso Colloquio eodem anno edita Epitome. Cui addita est Palatinorum Theologorum vera et constans Responsio, ... a quodam Theologiae studiose Latinè reddita. Heidelberg: Michael Schirat 1566.

given to Gabriel Harvey by Erastus's widow. Erastus's copy is in the British Library (BL C.60.h.18.). Virginia F. Stern, "The Bibliotheca of Gabriel Harvey," *Renaissance Quarterly* 25 (1972): 40.

R.B. [Richard Bostocke; Rychard Bostok]. *The difference betwene the auncient Phisicke, first taught by the godly forfathers, consisting in unitie peace and concord: and the later Phisicke proceding from Idolaters, Ethnickes, and Heathen: as Gallen, and such other consisting in dualitie, discord and contrarietie. And wherein the naturall Philosophie of Aristotle doth differ from the trueth of Gods worde, and is iniurous to Christianitie and sounde doctrine....* London: for Robert Walley, 1585.

Reußner, Bartholmäus. *Ein kurtze Erklerung und Christliche Widerlegung/Der unerhörten Gotteslesterungen und Lügen/ welche Paracelsus in den dreyen Büchern Philosophiae ad Athenienses hat wider Gott/ sein Wort und die löbliche Kunst der Artzney außgeschüttet.* Görlitz: Ambrosius Fritsch, 1570.

Rutherford, Samuel. *The Divine Right Of Church-Government And Excommunication: Or A peaceable Dispute for the perfection of the holy Scripture in point of Ceremonies and Church-Government; In Which The removal of the Service-book is justifi'd. The six Books of Tho: Erastus against Excommunication are briefly examin'd; with a Vindication of that eminent Divine Theod: Beza against the Aspersions of Erastus, The Arguments of Mr. William Pryn, Rich: Hooker, Dr. Morton, Dr. Jackson, Dr. John Forbes, and The Doctors of Aberdeen; Touching Will-Worship, Ceremonies, Imagery, Idolatry, Things Indifferent, An Ambulatory Government; The due and just Power of the Magistrate in matters of Religion, and The Arguments of Mr. Pryn, in so far as they side with Erastus, are modestly discussed....* London: John Field for Christopher Meridith, 1646.

[Sawr, Abraham, ed.] *Theatrum de Veneficis. Das ist: Von Teuffelsgespenst Zauberern und Gifftbereitern/ Schwartzkünstlern/ Hexen und Undholden/ vieler fürnemmen Historien und Exempel/ bewärten/ glaubwirdigen/ Alten und Newen Scribenten/ was von solchen jeder zeit disputiert und gehalten worden/ mit sorderm fleiß (derer Verzeichnuß am folgenden Blat zu finden) an Tag geben* Frankfurt: Nicolaus Basseus, 1586.

Schegk, Jakob. *De una persona, & duabus Naturis Christi, Sententia Iacobi Schegkij....* Frankfurt: Peter Braubach, 1565 (VD 16 S 2493).[22]

———. *Disputationum Physicarum et Medicarum Libri VIII.* Frankfurt: Johannes Wechel, 1590 (Tü UB exemplar).

———. *Hyperaspistes Responsi, ad quator Epistolas Petri Rami contra se aeditas.* Tübingen, 1570.

———. *Responsio Iacobi Schegkii Schorndorffensis, ad libellum Anonymi interpretis libri sui de una persona & duabus naturis in Christo.* Tübingen: Ulrich Morhart, 1566 (ZBZ exemplar).[23]

———. *Responsum Iacobi Schegkii Schorndorffensis, ad Simonis Simonii libellum vanissimum, quo conatus est veritatem libri de una persona & duabus naturis in Christo refellere ... Breve Responsum ad Scriptum D. Thomae Erasti, quo explicatur hactenus non consentire Schegkium cum Erasto.* Tübingen: Ulrich Morhart, 1568 (VD 16 S 2491).[24]

[22] Appeared at the autumn Frankfurt fair, 1565. *Die Messkatalog Georg Willers*, 1:59.
[23] Appeared at the autumn Frankfurt fair, 1566. *Die Messkatalog Georg Willers*, 1:78.
[24] Appeared at the Lenten Frankfurt fair, 1568. *Die Messkatalog Georg Willers*, 1:143.

Schenck von Grafenberg, Johannes. *Observationem Medicarum rariorum, libri VIII*. Lyons: Sumptibus Joannis-Antonii Huguetan, 1644 (NLM exemplar). Selections from Erastus regarding epilepsy reprinted on pp. 102–103.

Scholz, Lorenz, ed. *Consiliorum Medicinalium, conscriptum a praestantiss. atque exercitatiss. nostrorum temporum medicis, liber singulis.... Nunc primum studio & opera, Laurentii Scholzii a Rozenaw med. Vratisl. hoc modo in lucem editus*. Frankfurt: Apud Andreae Wecheli haeredes, Claudium Marnium & Joan. Aubrium [Claude de Marne and Jean Aubry], 1598. Includes the medical consilia of Erastus:
"In cordis palpitatione, pro quodam Comite," cols. 275–279 (no. 103)
"In epilepsia nocturna, pro alio quodam Nobili iuvene" cols. 124–127 (no. 43)
"Pro phthisicis," cols. 231–233 (no. 89).

——. *Epistolarum Philosophicarum: medicinalium, ac chymicarum a summis nostrae aetatis philosophis ac medicis exaraturum, volumen ... Nunc primum labore, ac industria, Laurentii Scholzii a Rozenaw ... foras datum*. Frankfurt: Apud Andreae Wecheli haeredes, Claudium Marnium & Joan. Aubrium [Claude de Marne and Jean Aubry], 1598. Includes letters of Erastus to Andreas Dudith, Girolamo Capivaccio, and Peter Monau.

Scot, Reginald. *The discouerie of witchcraft*. London: William Brome, 1584; facsimile reprint, New York: Da Capo, 1971.

Selden, John. *De synedriis & praefecturis iuridicis veterum Ebraeorum*. 3 vols. London, 1650–1655.

Smet, Heinrich (Henricus Smetius a Leda), ed. *Miscellanea Henrici Smetii a Leda Rub. F. Alostani Flandri in Acad. Heidelbergensi Med. Professoris ordinarii, Medica. Cum praestantissimis quinque medicis D. Thoma Erasto ... Henrico Brucaeo ... Levino Batto ... Joanne Weyero ... Henr. Weyero.... Communicata, et in libros XII. digesta*. Frankfurt: Jonas Rhodius, 1611 (NLM exemplar; VD 17 23:290916S).

Stathmion, Christoph. *Astrologia Asserta. Oder ein kurtze unnd gründliche verlegung/ der langen unnd ungegründten schrifft D. Thome Erasti/ Darinne er sich unterstehet/ die Kunst/ so auß der Sternen lauff natürlich urteylet/ zu vernichten*. Nuremberg: Valentin Neuber, 1558 (VD 16 S 8644).

Stenglin, Lukas. *Apologia Adversus Stibii Spongiam, non ita dudum a Michaele Toxite....* Augsburg: Matthäus Frank, 1569.[25]

——. *Lucae Stenglii Augustani Quaestiones III. Quarum primus est. An Stimmi seu Antimonium aergrotantibus citra noxam exhiberi possit....* Augsburg: Philipp Ulhart, 1566.

Ursinus, Zacharias. *Opera Theologica*. Ed. Quirinus Reuter. 3 vols. Heidelberg: Johann Lancelot, 1612.

[Ursinus, Zacharias]. *Verantwortung Wider die ungegründten aufflagen unnd verkerungen/ mit welchen der Catechismus Christlicher lere/ zu Heidelberg im Jar M.D.LXIII. außgangen/ von etlichen unbillicher weise beschweret ist. Geschrieben Durch die Theologen der Uniuersitet Heidelberg. Item/ D. Mar-*

[25] Appeared at the Lenten Frankfurt fair, 1569. *Die Messkatalog Georg Willers*, 1:212.

tin Luthers meinung vom Brotbrechen im H. Abendmal. Heidelberg: Johann Meyer, 1564 (VD16 H 1284).

Weyer, Johann. *De Lamiis Liber*. Basel: Oporinus, 1577.

——. *Ioannis VVieri de Praestigiis Daemonum, et incantationibus ac veneficiis Libri sex, auti & recogniti*. Basel: Ex Officiana Oporiniana, 1568.

——. *Ioannis VVieri de Praestigiis Daemonum, et incantationibus ac veneficiis Libri sex, postrema editione quinta aucti & recogniti. Accessit Liber Apologeticus, et Pseudomonarchia Daemonum*. Basel: Ex Officiana Oporiniana, 1577.

——. *Ioannis VVieri de Praestigiis Daemonum, et incantationibus ac veneficiis Libri sex, postrema editione sexta aucti & recogniti. Accessit Liber Apologeticus, et pseudomonarchia Daemonum*. Basel: Ex Officiana Oporiniana, 1583.

Witekind, Hermann (alias Augustin Lercheimer). *Christlich Bedencken und Erinnerung von Zauberey*. 3rd ed. Speyer: Albin, 1597 (Hd UB exemplar).

Zanchi, Girolamo. *Hieronymi Zanchii Bergomatis, Theologi Clarissimi, Epistolarum Libri Duo....* Hanau: Antonius, 1609. Includes one letter to and another from Erastus.

——. *Operum theologicorum*. 8 vols. [Geneva?]: Stephanus Gamonetus, 1605.

Zedler, J.H., ed. *Grosses vollständiges Universal-Lexicon aller Wissenschafften und Künste*. Halle, 1732–1750. Prints a prescription of Erastus for a "Syrupus Antiphthisicus" in vol. 41, cols. 1126–1127.

Zetzner, Lazarus, ed. *Theatrum Chemicum*. Strasbourg: Sumptibus heredem Eberh. Zetzneri, 1659–1661 (NLM exemplar).

Ziegler, Jacob. *D. Jacobo Laterensi Tigurino, Viro ad unguem facto, ... Insignibus artis Medicae, a Viro Clariss. Doctore Joan. Nicolao Stupano, sub merito exornando: primum quidem Conradi Gesneri ... Thomae Erasti ... Theodori Zvingeri, ... Felicis quinetiam Plateri....* Basel: Typis Ioan. Iacobi Genathi, 1615 (VD17 23:624408B).

Other Primary Sources

Baillie, Robert. *The Letters and Journals of Robert Baillie....* Ed. David Laing. 3 vols. Edinburgh: R. Ogle, 1841–1842.

Beza, Theodore. *Correspondance de Théodore de Bèze* [*THR*]. Ed. Hippolyte Aubert, et al. Geneva: Droz, 1960–.

Bromiley, G.W., ed. *Zwingli and Bullinger*. Philadelphia: Westminster Press, 1953.

Bullinger, Heinrich. *The Decades of Henry Bullinger*. Ed. Thomas Harding. Cambridge, 1849.

——. *Heinrich Bullinger Werke*. Ed. Fritz Büsser, et al. Zürich: Theologischer Verlag, 1972–.

[Heinrich Bullinger], *Stimmen aus dem Schweizerischen Reformationszeitalter über die Exkommunikation oder den Kirchenbann*. Bern: Hallersche Buchdruckerei, 1839.

Burton, Robert. *The Anatomy of Melancholy*. Ed. Thomas C. Faulkner, et al. Oxford: Oxford UP, 1989.

Büttinghausen, Carl. *Ergözlichkeiten aus der Pfälzischen und Schweizerischen Geschichte und Literatur*. Zürich, 1766–1768.

Calvin, John. *Commentaries on the Book of the Prophet Jeremiah and the Lamentations*. Trans. John Owen. 5 vols. Grand Rapids: William B. Eerdman, 1950.

——. *Ioannis Calvini Opera Quae Supersunt Omnia*. Corpus Reformatorum, vols. 29–87. Ed. Wilhelm Baum, Eduard Cunitz and Eduard Reuss. Brunswick and Berlin, 1863–1900.

——. *John Calvin: Institutes of the Christian Religion*. Ed. John T. McNeill, trans. Ford Lewis Battles. Philadelphia: Westminster Press, 1960.

Friedländer, Gottlieb. *Beiträge zur Reformationsgeschichte*. Berlin, 1837.

Gessner, Konrad. *Das dritte Buch der medizinischen Briefe des Zürcher Philosophen und Arztes Konrad Gesner*. Trans. Josef Peine. Düsseldorf: Michael Triltsch, 1941.

——. *Die Briefe Konrad Gesners an Crato von Krafftheim nach der Briefsammlung von 1566*. Ed. Egon Helmich. Düsseldorf: G.H. Nolte, 1938.

Green, Lowell C. *Melanchthon in English*. St. Louis: Center for Reformation Research: 1982.

Grotius, Hugo. *De Imperio Summarum Potestatum Circa Sacra: Critical Edition with Introduction, English Translation and Commentary* [Studies in the History of Christian Thought 102]. Ed. Harm-Jan Van Dam. 2 vols. Leiden: Brill, 2001.

Hagen, Hermann. *Briefe von Heidelberger Professoren und Studenten*. Bern, 1886.

The Heidelberg Catechism in German, Latin and English: with an Historical Introduction. New York: Charles Scribner, 1863.

Hooker, Richard. *Of the Laws of Ecclesiastical Polity*. Ed. Arthur Stephen McGrade. Cambridge: Cambridge UP, 1989.

Kirk, G.S., et al. *The Presocratic Philosophers*. 2nd ed. Cambridge: Cambridge UP, 1983.

Kluckhohn, August, ed. *Briefe Friedrich des Frommen Kurfürsten von der Pfalz mit verwandten Schriftstücken*. 2 vols. Braunschweig, 1868–1872.

Kühlmann, Wilhelm and Joachim Telle, eds. *Corpus Paracelsisticum: Dokumente frühneuzeitlicher Naturphilosophie in Deutschland*. Tübingen: Max Niemeyer, 2001–.

Lawson, George. *Politica sacra et civilis*. Ed. Conal Condren. Cambridge: Cambridge UP, 1992.

Melanchthon, Philipp, *Philippi Melanthonis Opera quae supersunt omnia*. Corpus Reformatorum, vols. 1–28. Ed. K.G. Bretschneider and H.E. Bindseil. Halle and Brunswick, 1834–1860.

Olevianus, Caspar. *A Firm Foundation*. Ed. and trans. Lyle D. Bierma. Baker: Grand Rapids, 1995.

——. *Der Gnadenbund Gottes 1590: Faksimile-Edition mit einem Kommentar*. Ed. Gunther Franz, J.F. Gerhard Goeters and Wilhelm Holtmann. Cologne: Rheinland-Verlag, 1994.

Paracelsus [Theophrastus von Hohenheim]. *Theophrast von Hohenheim gen. Paracelsus, Sämtliche Werke. I. Abteilung: Medizinische, naturwissenschaftliche und philosophische Schriften*. 14 vols. Ed. Karl Sudhoff. Munich: Oldenbourg, 1922–1933.

——. *Four Treatises*. Ed. Henry E. Sigerist. Baltimore: Johns Hopkins UP, 1941. Paperback ed., 1996.
Patin, Guy. *Lettres de Gui Patin*. Ed. J -H. Reveillé-Parise. 3 vols. Paris, 1846.
Robinson, Hastings, trans. *The Zurich Letters*. Cambridge, 1842 & 1845.
Rott, Hans, ed. "Neue Quellen für eine Aktenrevision des Prozesses gegen Sylvan und seine Genossen." *Neues Archiv für die Geschichte der Stadt Heidelberg und der rheinischen Pfalz* 8 & 9 (1910 & 1911): 184–259; 1–70.
Savonarola, Girolamo. *Scritti filosofici*. Ed. Gian Carlo Garfagnini and Eugenio Garin. Rome: A. Belardetti, 1982–1988.
Sehling, Emil, ed. *Die evangelischen Kirchenordnungen des XVI. Jahrhunderts*. Band 14, Kurpfalz, [ed. J.F. Gerhard Goeters]. Tübingen: J.C.B. Mohr (Paul Siebeck), 1969.
Selden, John. *The Table Talk of John Selden*. Ed. Samuel Harvey Reynolds. Oxford, 1892.
Socinus, Laelius. *Opere* [Studi e testi per la storia religiosa del Cinquecento 1]. Ed. Antonio Rotondò. Florence: L.S. Olschki, 1986.
Sudhoff, Karl. *C. Olevianus und Z. Ursinus, Leben und ausgewählte Schriften der Väter und Begründer der reformierten Kirche*, vol. 8. Elberfeld: R.L. Friedrichs, 1857.
Thorbecke, August. *Statuten und Reformationen der Heidelberg Universität vom 16. bis 18. Jahrhundert*. Leipzig: Dunkler & Humblot, 1891.
Toepke, Gustav. *Die Matrikel der Universität Heidelberg*. Heidelberg: self published, 1886. http://digi.ub.uni-heidelberg.de/diglit/matrikelregister/0219.
Ursinus, Zacharias. "Briefe des Heidelberger Theologen Zacharias Ursinus aus Heidelberg und Neustadt a.H." Ed. Hans Rott. *NHJ* 14 (1906): 39–172.
——. "Briefe des Heidelberger Theologen Zacharias Ursinus (1534–1583)." Ed. Gustav Adolf Benrath, *NHJ* 8 (1964): 93–141.
——. "Briefe des Heidelberger Theologen Zacharias Ursinus aus Wittenberg und Zürich (1560/61)." Ed. Erdmann Sturm. *Heidelberger Jahrbücher* 14 (1970): 85–119.
——. *The Commentary of Dr. Zacharias Ursinus on the Heidelberg Catechism*. Trans. G.W. Willard. Columbus, 1852.
Vulcanius, Bonaventura. *Correspondance de Bonaventura Vulcanius pendant son séjour à Cologne, Genève et Bâle* (1573–1577). Ed. H. de Vries de Heekelingen. La Haye: Nijhoff, 1923.
Wackernagel, Hans Georg. *Die Matrikel der Universität Basel*. Basel: Verlag der Universitätsbibliothek, 1956.
Weyer, Johann. *Witches, Devils and Doctors in the Renaissance: Johann Weyer, De praestigiis daemonum*. Ed. George Mora, et al. Binghamton, N.Y.: Center for Medieval and Early Renaissance Studies, 1991.
Wiesert, Hermann. "Die Rektoren und die Dekane der Ruperto Carola zu Heidelberg 1386–1985." In *Semper Apertus: Sechshundert Jahre Ruprecht-Karls-Universität Heidelberg 1386–1986*, ed. Wilhelm Doerr et al., 4:299–417. Berlin: Springer, 1985.
Willers, Georg. *Die Messkatalog Georg Willers*. 2 vols. Hildesheim: Olms, 1972–1973.
Winkelmann, Eduard. *Urkundenbuch der Universität Heidelberg*. 2 vols. Hei-

delberg: Carl Winter's Universitätsbuchhandlung, 1886. http://digi.ub.uni-heidelberg.de/diglit/winkelmann1886bd2.
Zwingli, Ulrich. *Huldrych Zwingli Writings*, Trans. E.J. Furcha and H. Wayne Pipkin. 2 vols. Pittsburgh: Pickwick, 1984.
——. *Huldreich Zwinglis sämtliche Werke*. Corpus Reformatorum, vols. 88–101. Ed. Emil Egli, et al Leipzig: Verlag von Martin Henius Nachfolger, 1905–1968.

Fiction

Hausrath, Adolf D. [Pseudonym "George Taylor"] *Klytia [historischer Roman aus dem 16. Jahrhundert.]* Berlin, 1875. English translation: *Klytia: A Story of Heidelberg Castle*, trans. Sutton Fraser Corkran. Leipzig, 1883. Historical novel by the noted Heidelberg theologian.

Secondary Sources

Political and Church History

Allgemeine Deutsche Biographie. 56 vols. Leipzig, 1875–1912.
Ardolino, Frank. "Erastianism in Peele's *Old Wives' Tale*." *Discoveries* 22.2 (2005). http://cstl-cla.semo.edu/reinheimer/discoveries/archives/222/ ardolino222pf .htm.
Athenae rauricae sive catalogus professorum Academiae Basiliensis ab anno 1460 ad annum 1778. Basel, 1778.
Austin, Kenneth. *From Judaism to Calvinism: The Life and Writings of Immanuel Tremellius, C. 1510–1580* [St Andrews Studies in Reformation History]. Aldershot, England: Ashgate, 2007.
Baker, J. Wayne. "Calvin's Discipline and the Early Reformed Tradition: Bullinger and Calvin." In *Calviniana: Ideas and Influence of Jean Calvin* [*SCE&S* 10], ed. Robert V. Schnucker, 107–119. Kirksville, Mo., 1988.
——. "Church Discipline or Civil Punishment: On the Origins of the Reformed Schism, 1528–1531." *Andrews University Studies* 23 (1985): 3–18.
——. "Church, State and Dissent: The Crisis of the Swiss Reformation, 1531–1536." *Church History* 57 (1988): 135–152.
——. "Erastianism in England: The Zürich Connection." In *Die Zürcher Reformation: Ausstrahlungen und Rückwirkungen* [*ZBRG* 18], ed. Alfred Schindler and Hans Stickelberger, 327–349. Bern: Peter Lang, 2001.
——. *Heinrich Bullinger and the Covenant: The Other Reformed Tradition*. Athens: Ohio UP, 1980.
——. "In Defense of Magisterial Discipline: Bullinger's 'Tractatus de Excommunicatione' of 1568." In *Heinrich Bullinger 1504–1575: Gesammelte Aufsätze zum 400. Todestag* [*ZBRG* 7], vol., I, ed. Ulrich Gäbler and Erland Herkenrath, 141–159. Zürich: Theologischer Verlag, 1975.
Barton, Peter F. *Um Luthers Erbe: Studien und Texte zur Spätreformation Tilemann Heshusius (1527–1559)*. Witten: Luther Verlag 1972.

Benedict, Philip. *Christ's Churches Purely Reformed: A Social History of Calvinism*. New Haven: Yale UP, 2002.

Benrath, Gustav Adolf. "Die Eigenart der der pfälzischen Reformation und die Vorgeschichte des Heidelberger Katechismus." In *Heidelberger Jahrbücher* 7 (1963): 13–32.

——. "Die Korrespondenz zwischen Bullinger und Thomas Erastus." In *Heinrich Bullinger 1504–1575: Gesammelte Aufsätze zum 400. Todestag*, vol. 2 [*ZBRG* 8], ed. Ulrich Gäbler and Erland Herkenrath, 87–141. Zürich: Theologischer Verlag, 1975.

——. "Die kurpfälzischen Kirchenvisitationen im 16. Jahrhundert." *Blätter für Pfälzische Kirchengeschichte und religiöse Volkskunde* 42 (1975): 17–24.

Biegger, Katharina. *De invocatione beatae Mariae virginis: Paracelsus und die Marienverehrung* [Kosmosophie 6]. Stuttgart: Franz Steiner Verlag, 1990.

Biel. Pamela. *Doorkeepers at the House of Righteousness: Heinrich Bullinger and the Zurich Clergy 1535–1575* [*ZBRG* 15]. Bern: Peter Lang, 1991.

Bierma, Lyle D. *German Calvinism in the Confessional Age: The Covenant Theology of Caspar Olevianus*. Grand Rapids: Baker, 1997.

——. "Olevianus and the Authorship of the Heidelberg Catechism: Another Look." *SCJ* 13 (1982): 17–27.

——. *The Doctrine of the Sacraments in the Heidelberg Catechism: Melanchthonian, Calvinist, or Zwinglian?* [Studies in Reformed Theology and History, New Series, 4] Princeton: Princeton Theological Seminary, 1999.

Bierma, Lyle D. with Charles D. Gunnoe Jr., Karin Y. Maag and Paul W. Fields, *An Introduction to the Heidelberg Catechism: Sources, History, and Theology*. Grand Rapids: Baker, 2005.

Bietenholz, Peter G. *Basle and France in the Sixteenth Century: The Basle Humanists and Printers in their Contacts with Francophone Culture* [*THR* 112]. Geneva: Droz, 1971.

——. "Limits to Intolerance: The Two Editions of Beza's *Epistolae Theologicae*." *Bibliothèque d'Humanisme et Renaissance* 35 (1973): 311–313.

Bizer, Ernst. *Studien zur Geschichte des Abendmahlsstreits im 16. Jahrhundert*. Gütersloh: Gerd Mohn, 1940; reprint, Darmstadt: Wissenschaftliche Buchgesellschaft, 1962.

Blickle, Peter, et al. eds. *Zwingli und Europa: Referate und Protokoll des Internationalen Kongresses aus Anlass des 500. Geburtstages von Huldrych Zwingli, vom 26. bis 30. März 1984*. Zürich: Vandenhoeck & Ruprecht, 1985.

Bodenmann, Reinhard. *Wolfgang Musculus (1497–1563): Destin d'un autodidacte lorrain au siècle des réformes. Etude basée sur la biographie établie par son fils, la correspondance personnelle et de nombreux autres documents d'époque* [*THR* 343]. Geneva: Droz, 2000.

Bonjour, Edgar. *Die Universität Basel 1460–1960*. Basel: Verlag Helbing & Lichtenhahn, 1971.

Bonnard, Auguste. *Thomas Éraste (1524–1583) et la Discipline Ecclésiastique*. Lausanne: Georges Bridel, 1894.

Bruening, Michael W. *Calvinism's First Battleground: Conflict and Reform in the Pays de Vaud, 1528–1559*. Heidelberg: Springer, 2005.

Burchill, Christopher J. "Girolomo Zanchi: Portrait of a Reformed Theologian and his Work." *SCJ* 15 (1984): 185–205.

——. *The Heidelberg Antitrinitarians* [Bibliotheca Dissidentium 11, ed. André Séguenny]. Baden-Baden: Editions Valentin Koerner, 1989.

——. "On the Consolation of a Christian Scholar: Zacharias Ursinus (1534–1583) and the Reformation in Heidelberg." *Journal of Ecclesiastical History* 37 (1986): 565–583.

——. "Die Universität zu Heidelberg und der 'Fromme' Kurfürst." In *Semper Apertus: Sechshundert Jahre Ruprecht-Karls-Universität Heidelberg 1386–1986*, ed. Wilhelm Doerr, et al., 1:231–254. Berlin: Springer, 1985.

Burnett, Amy Nelson. "Simon Sulzer and the Consequences of the 1563 Strasbourg Consensus in Switzerland." *ARG* 83 (1992): 154–179.

——. *Teaching the Reformation: Ministers and Their Message in Basel, 1529–1629*. Oxford: Oxford UP, 2006.

——. *The Yoke of Christ: Martin Bucer and Christian Discipline* [*SCE&S* 26]. Kirksville, Mo., 1994.

Butler, K.T. "Giacomo Castelvetro, 1546–1616." *Italian Studies* 5 (1950): 1–42.

Campi, Emidio. "Bullinger und Beza im Lichte ihrer Korrespondenz." In *Théodore de Bèze (1519–1605). Actes du Colloque de Genève (septembre 2005)* [*THR* 424]. Geneva: Droz, 2007.

Carsten, F.L. *Princes and Parliaments in Germany*. Oxford: Oxford UP, Clarendon Press, 1959.

Chadwick, Owen. "The Making of a Reforming Prince: Frederick III, Elector Palatine." In *Reformation, Conformity and Dissent*, ed. R. Buick Knox, 44–69. London: Epworth, 1977.

Clasen, Claus-Peter. *The Palatinate in European History 1559–1618*. Oxford: Basil Blackwell, 1963.

Cohn, Henry, J. *The Government of the Rhine Palatinate in the Fifteenth Century*. Oxford: Oxford UP, 1965.

——. "The Early Renaissance Court in Heidelberg." *European Studies Review* 1 (1971): 295–322.

——. "Territorial Princes in Germany's Second Reformation, 1559–1622." In *International Calvinism 1541–1715*, ed. Menna Prestwich, 135–166. Oxford: Oxford UP, 1985.

Cuno, Friedrich Wilhelm. *Daniel Tossanus der Ältere: Professor der Theologie und Pastor (1541–1602)*. 2 vols. Amsterdam: Scheffer, 1898.

Dán, Robert. *Matthias Vehe-Glirius: Life and Work of a Radical Antitrinitarian with his Collected Writings* [Studia Humanitatis 4]. Leiden: Brill; Budapest: Akadémiai Kiadó, 1982.

Davies, J[ohn] Llewelyn. "Erastus and Excommunication." *The Contemporary Review* 18 (1871): 527–546. Reprinted in J.L. Davies, *Theology and Morality*, 198–243. London, 1873.

Denis, Philippe, and Jean Rott. *Jean Morély (ca. 1524 – ca. 1594) et l'utopie d'une démocratie dans l'Eglise* [THR 278]. Geneva: Droz, 1993.

Doerr, Wilhelm, et al. *Semper Apertus: Sechshundert Jahre Ruprecht-Karls-Universität Heidelberg 1386–1986*, 6 vols. Berlin: Springer, 1985.

Drüll, Dagmar. *Heidelberger Gelehrtenlexikon 1386–1651*. Berlin: Springer, 2002.

Edel, Andreas. *Der Kaiser und Kurpfalz. Eine Studie zu den Grundelementen politischen Handelns bei Maximilian II. (1564–1576)* [Schriftenreihe der His-

torischen Kommission bei der Bayerischen Akademie der Wissenschaften 58]. Göttingen: Vandenhoek & Ruprecht, 1995.
Eire, Carlos. *War Against the Idols: The Reformation of Worship from Erasmus to Calvin*. Cambridge: Cambridge UP, 1986.
Figgis, J. Neville. "Erastus and Erastianism." *Journal of Theological Studies* 2 (1901): 66–101. Slightly abbreviated version printed in idem. *The Divine Right of Kings*, 267–316. New York: Harper and Row, 1965.
——. *Political Thought from Gerson to Grotius, 1414–1625*. New York: Harper, 1960.
Ford, James Thomas. "Wolfgang Musculus on the Office of the Christian Magistrate." *ARG* 91 (2000): 149–167.
Geiger, Max. *Die Basler Kirche und Theologie im Zeitalter der Hochorthodoxie*. Zollikon: Evangelischer Verlag, 1952.
Gerrish, B.A. *The Old Protestantism and the New: Essays on the Reformation Heritage*. Chicago: University of Chicago Press, 1982.
Goeters, J.F. Gerhard. *Die Akten der Synode der Niederländischen Kirchen zu Emden vom 4.-13. Oktober 1571. Im lateinischen Grundtext mitsamt den alten niederländischen, französischen und deutschen Übersetzungen* [*BGLRK* 34]. [Neukirchen-Vluyn]: Neukirchener Verlag, 1971.
——. "Bibliographia Oleviana." *Monatshefte für Evangelische Kirchengeschichte des Rheinlandes* 37–38 (1988–1989): 320–337.
——. "Caspar Olevianus als Theologe." *Monatshefte für Evangelische Kirchengeschichte des Rheinlandes* 37–38 (1988–1989): 287–319.
——. "Entstehung und Frühgeschichte des Katechismus." In *Handbuch zum Heidelberger Katechismus*, ed. Lothar Coenen, 3–23. Neukirch: Neukirchener Verlag des Erziehungsvereins, 1963.
——. "Genesis, Formen und Hauptthemen des reformierten Bekenntnisses in Deutschland. Eine Übersicht." In *Die reformierte Konfessionalisierung in Deutschland* [*SVRG* 195], ed. Heinz Schilling, 44–59. Gütersloh: Gerd Mohn, 1986.
Gooszen, M.A. *De Heidelbergsche Catechismus en Het Boekje van de Breking des Broods, in het jaar 1563–1564 bestreden en verdedigd*. Leiden: Brill, 1892.
Gordon, Bruce. *Clerical Discipline and the Rural Reformation: The Synod in Zurich, 1532–1580* [*ZBRG* 16]. Bern: Peter Lang, 1992.
Gordon, Bruce and Emidio Campi, eds. *Architect of Reformation: An Introduction To Heinrich Bullinger, 1504–1575*. Grand Rapids, Baker, 2004.
Graham, Michael F. *The Uses of Reform: "Godly Discipline" and Popular Behavior in Scotland and Beyond, 1560–1610* [*SMRT* 58]. Leiden: Brill, 1996.
Graham, W. Fred, ed. *Later Calvinism: International Perspectives* [*SCE&S* 22]. Kirksville, Mo., 1994.
Guggisberg, Hans R. *Basel in the Sixteenth Century*. St. Louis: Center for Reformation Research, 1982.
——. "Pietro Perna, Fausto Sozzini und die Dialogi quatuor Sebastian Castellios." In *Studia bibliographica in Honorem Herman de la Fontaine Verwey*, ed Menno Hertzberger, 171–201. Amsterdam, 1967.
Hartvelt, G.P. "De Avondmaalsleer van de Heidelbergse Catechismus en haar Toepassing in de Prediking." *Homiletica en Biblica* 20 (1964): 121–140.

——. "Petrus Boquinus," *Gereformeerd theologisch tijdschrift* 62 (1962): 49–77.

Hautz, J.G. *Die erste Gelehrtenschule Reformirten Glaubensbekenntnisses in Deutschland oder Geschichte des Pädagogiums zu Heidelberg unter dem Kurfürsten Friedrich III. von der Pfalz in den Jahren 1565–1577*. Heidelberg, 1855.

——. *Geschichte der Universität Heidelberg*. 2 vols. Mannheim, 1864.

Heckel, Johannes, "Cura religionis, Ius in Sacra, Ius circa Sacra." In *Festschrift Ulrich Stutz zum siebzigsten Geburtstag* [Kirchenrechtliche Abhandlungen 117–118], 224–298. Stuttgart: Ferdinand Enke, 1938.

Henss, Walter. *Der Heidelberger Katechismus im konfessionspolitischen Kräftespiel seiner Frühzeit*. Zürich: Theologischer Verlag, 1983.

——. "Frühe Spuren der Reformation in der Kurpfalz." *Blätter für pfälzische Kirchengeschichte und religiöse Volkskunde* 50 (1983): 5–42.

Henson, H. Hensley. "Erastianism." In *Studies in English Religion in the Seventeenth Century: St. Margaret's Lectures 1903*, 125–170. New York: E.P. Dutton, 1903.

Hermann, Rudolf. *Die Problem der Exkommunikation bei Luther und Thomas Erastus*. Berlin: Verlag Alfred Töpelmann, 1955.

Hillerbrand, Hans J., ed. *The Oxford Encyclopedia of the Reformation*. New York: Oxford UP, 1996.

Hollweg, Walter. *Der Augsburger Reichstag von 1566 und seine Bedeutung für die Entstehung der Reformierten Kirche und ihres Bekenntnisses* [*BGLRK* 17]. Neukirchen-Vluyn: Neukirchener Verlag des Erziehungsvereins, 1964.

——. *Heinrich Bullingers Hausbuch: Eine Untersuchung über die Anfänge der reformierten Predigtliteratur* [*BGLRK* 8]. Neukirchen-Vluyn: Verlag der Buchhandlung des Erziehungsvereins, 1956.

——. *Neue Untersuchungen zur Geschichte und Lehre des Heidelberger Katechismus* [*BGLRK* 13 & 28]. 2 vols. Neukirchen-Vluyn: Neukirchener Verlag des Erziehungsvereins, 1961–1968.

Horn, Curt. "Johann Sylvan und die Anfänge des Heidelberger Antitrinitarismus." *NHJ* 17 (1913): 219–310.

Hutter, Ulrich. "Zacharias Ursinus und der Heidelberg Katechismus." In *Martin Luther und die Reformation in Ostdeutschland und Südosteuropa*, ed. Ulrich Hutter, 79–105. Sigmaringen: Jan Thorbecke, 1991.

Janse, Wim. *Albert Hardenberg als Theologe: Profil eines Bucers-Schülers* [Studies in the History of Christian Thought 57]. Leiden: Brill, 1994.

——. "Calvin's Eucharistic Theology: Three Dogma-Historical Observations." In *Calvinus sacrarum literarum interpres: Papers of the International Congress on Calvin Research* [Reformed Historical Theology 5] ed. Herman J. Selderhuis, 37–69. Göttingen: Vandenhoeck & Ruprecht, 2008.

——. "Die Melanchthonrezeption des Nonkonformisten Wilhelm Klebitz (ca. 1533–1568)." In *Melanchthon und der Calvinismus* [Melanchthon-Schriften der Stadt Bretten 9], ed. Günter Frank and Hermann J. Selderhuis, 257–290. Stuttgart-Bad Cannstatt: Frommann-Holzboog, 2005.

——. "Non-conformist Eucharistic Theology: The Case of the Alleged 'Zwinglian Polemicist' Wilhelm Klebitz (c. 1533–1568)." *Nederlands Archief voor Kerkgeschiedenis/Dutch Review of Church History* 81 (2001), 5–25

——. "Wittenberg Calvinizans: The Involvement of Melanchthon, Peucer, and

Eber in the Bremen Sacramentarian Controversy, 1560." In *Ordentlich und Fruchtbar: Festschrift für Willem van't Spijker*, ed. Wilhelm Neuser and Herman J. Selderhuis, 53–68. Leiden: J.J. Groen en Zoon, 1997.

Lessing, Gotthold Ephraim. "Von Adam Neusern, einige authentische Nachrichten," in *Lessings Werke*, ed. R. Boxberger, vol. 11, part. 2, 203–259. Berlin: W. Spemann, n.d.

Kingdon, Robert M. *Geneva and the Consolidation of the French Protestant Movement 1564–1572* [*THR* 92]. Geneva: Droz, 1967.

Kittelson, James. "Marbach vs. Zanchi: The Resolution of Controversy in Later Reformation Strasbourg." *SCJ* 7 (1977): 31–44.

Kluckhohn, August. *Friedrich der Fromme, Kurfürst von der Pfalz, der Schützer der reformirten Kirche, 1559–1576*. Nördlingen, 1879.

——. "Wie ist Kurfürst Friedrich III. von der Pfalz Calvinist geworden?" *Münchener Historisches Jahrbuch für 1866* (1866): 421–520.

Köhler, Walther. *Zürcher Ehegericht und Genfer Konsistorium* [Quellen und Abhandlungen zur schweizerischen Reformationsgeschichte 7 & 10]. 2 vols. Leipzig: N. Heinsius Nachfolger, 1932, 1942.

Koch, Walther. "Johann Marbach in seiner Bedeutung für die Pfälzische Kirchengeschichte." *Blätter für Pfälzische Kirchengeschichte und religiöse Volkskunde* 22 (1962): 119–129.

Kooi, Christine. "Pharisees and Hypocrites: A Public Debate over Church Discipline in Leiden, 1586," *ARG* 88 (1997): 258–278.

Kressner, Helmut. *Schweizer Ursprünge des anglikanischen Staatskirchentums* [*SVRG* 170]. Gütersloh: C. Bertelsmann Verlag, 1953.

Kutter, Markus. *Celio Secondo Curione: Sein Leben und sein Werk (1503–1569)* [*BBG* 54]. Basel: Helbing und Lichtenhahn, 1955.

Linder, Gottlieb. *Simon Sulzer und sein Antheil in der Reformation im Lande Baden sowie an den Unionbestrebungen*. Heidelberg: Carl Winter's Universitätsbuchhandlung, 1890.

Luttenberger, Albrecht Pius. *Glaubenseinheit und Reichsfriede: Konzeptionen und Wege konfessionsneutraler Reichspolitik 1530–1552 (Kurpfalz, Jülich, Kurbrandenburg)* [Schriftenreihe der Historischen Kommission bei der Bayerischen Akademie der Wissenschaften 20]. Göttingen: Vandenhoek & Ruprecht, 1982.

Maag, Karin. *Seminary or University? The Geneva Academy and Reformed Higher Education, 1560–1620*. Aldershot, England: Scolar Press, 1995.

Maruyama, Tadataka. *The Ecclesiology of Theodore Beza: The Reform of the True Church* [*THR* 166]. Geneva: Droz, 1978.

Merz, Johannes. "Calvinismus im Territorialstaat: Zur Begriffs- und Traditionsbildung in der deutschen Historiographie." *Zeitschrift für bayerische Landesgeschichte* 57 (1994): 45–68.

Mentzer, Raymond, ed. *Sin and the Calvinists: Morals Control and the Consistory in the Reformed Tradition* [*SCE&S* 32] Kirksville, Mo., 1994.

Migliorato, Giuseppe. "Erasto ed erastianismo: Problematica di un giurisdizionalismo confessionista." *Critica storica* 16 (1979): 185–223.

Miller, Perry. *The New England Mind: The Seventeenth Century*. New York: MacMillan, 1939; reprint, Boston: Beacon Press, 1961.

Moeller, Bernd. *Imperial Cities and the Reformation*. Trans. H.C.E. Midelfort and M.U. Edwards. Philadelphia: Fortress, 1972.

Mühling, Andreas. *Caspar Olevian 1536–1587: Christ, Kirchenpolitiker und Theologe*. Zug: Achius Verlag, 2008.

——. "Der Heidelberger Katechismus im 16. Jahrhundert: Entstehung, Zielsetzung, Rezeption." *Monatshefte für Evangelische Kirchengeschichte des Rheinlandes* 58 (2009) 1–11.

——. *Heinrich Bullingers europäische Kirchenpolitik*. Bern: Lang, 2001.

Münch, Paul. *Zucht und Ordnung: Reformierte Kirchenverfassungen im 16. und 17. Jahrhundert (Nassau-Dillenburg, Kurpfalz, Hessen-Kassel)* [Spätmittelalter und Frühe Neuzeit Tübinger Beiträge zur Geschichtsforschung 3]. Stuttgart: Klett-Cotta, 1978.

Naphy, William. *Calvin and the Consolidation of the Genevan Reformation*. Manchester, Manchester UP, 1994. Reprint Louisville: Westminster John Knox, 2003.

Neue Deutsche Biographie. Berlin, 1953–.

Neuser, Wilhem. "Die Väter des Heidelberger Katechismus." *Theologische Zeitschrift* 35 (1979): 177–194.

Nijenhuis, W. *Ecclesia Reformata: Studies on the Reformation* [Kerkhistorische Bijdragen 3] 2 vols. Leiden: Brill, 1994.

Nischan, Bodo. "The 'Fractio Panis': A Reformed Communion Practice in Late Reformation Germany." *Church History* 53 (1984): 17–29.

Nobbs, Douglas. *Theocracy and Toleration: A Study of the Disputes in Dutch Calvinism from 1600 to 1650*. Cambridge: Cambridge UP, 1938.

Pelikan, Jaroslav. *The Christian Tradition: A History of the Development of Doctrine*. vol. 4, *Reformation of Church and Dogma (1300–1700)*. Chicago: University of Chicago Press, 1984.

——. "Creation and Causality in Christian Thought." *Journal of Religion* 40 (1960): 246–255.

Perini, Leandro. *La vita e i tempi di Pietro Perna* [Studi e testi del Rinascimento europeo 17]. Roma: Edizioni di Storia e Letteratura, 2002.

Pettegree, Andrew, Alistair Duke and Gillian Lewis, eds. *Calvinism in Europe, 1540–1620*. Cambridge: Cambridge UP, 1994.

Poensgen, Georg, ed. *Ottheinrich: Gedenkschrift zur vierhundertjährigen Wiederkehr seiner Kurfürstenzeit in der Pfalz (1556–1559), Ruperto Carola Sonderband*, 1956.

Port, Wilhelm, "Johann Mayer, Ein Reformierter Drucker des 16. Jahrhunderts." *Zentralblatt für Bibliothekswesen* 59 (1942): 140–155.

Potter, G.R. "Church and State, 1528: A Letter from Zwingli to Ambrosius Blarer (4 May 1528)." *Occasional Papers of the American Society for Reformation Research* (1977): 110–122.

Press, Volker. "Bayerns wittelsbachische Gegenspieler—Die Heidelberger Kurfürsten 1505–1685." In *Um Glauben und Reich: Kurfürst Maximilian I*, ed. Hubert Glaser, 24–48. Munich: Hirmer, 1980.

——. *Calvinismus und Territorialstaat. Regierung und Zentralbehörden der Kurpfalz 1559–1619*. Stuttgart: Ernst Klett Verlag, 1970.

——. "Die Grafen von Erbach und die Anfänge des reformierten Bekenntnisses in Deutschland." In *Aus Geschichte und ihren Hilfswissenschaften*, eds. Hermann Bannasch and Hans-Peter Lachmann, 653–685. Marburg: Elwert, 1979.

——. "Die Grundlagen der kurpfälzischen Herrschaft in der Oberpfalz 1499–1621." In *Verhandlungen des Historischen Vereins für Oberpfalz und Regensburg*, 31–67. Regensburg: Verlag des Historischen Vereins, 1977.

——. "Hof, Stadt und Territorium." In *Die Geschichte der Universität Heidelberg*, 45–68. Heidelberg: Heidelberger Verlagsanstalt, 1986.

——. "Die 'Zweite Reformation' in der Kurpfalz." In *Die reformierte Konfessionalisierung in Deutschland* [*SVRG* 195], ed. Heinz Schilling, 104–129. Gütersloh: Gerd Mohn, 1986.

Raitt, Jill, ed., *Shapers of the Religious Tradition of Germany, Switzerland and Poland, 1560–1600*. New Haven: Yale UP, 1981.

Rorem, Paul. *Calvin and Bullinger on the Lord's Supper*. Bramcote, Nottingham: Grove Books Limited, 1989.

Roth, Carl. "Stammtafeln einiger ausgestorbener Basler Gelehrtenfamilien." *Basler Zeitschrift für Geschichte und Altertumskunde* (1917): 393–403.

Rotondò, Antonio. *Calvin and the Italian Anti-Trinitarians* [Reformation Essays & Studies 2]. Trans. John and Anne Tedeschi. St. Louis: Foundation for Reformation Research, 1968.

——. "Pietro Perna e la vita culturale e religiosa di Basilca fra il 1570 e il 1580." In *Studi e ricerche di storia ereticale italiana del' Cinquecento*, vol. 1, 273–394. Turin: Giappichelli, 1974.

Rott, Hans. *Friedrich II. von der Pfalz und die Reformation*. Heidelberg: Carl Winter's Universitätsbuchhandlung, 1904.

——. "Kirchen- und Bildersturm bei der Einführung der Reformation in der Pfalz." *Neues Archiv für die Geschichte der Stadt Heidelberg* 6 (1905): 229–254.

Rudolf, Friedrich. "Die Kirche in Heidelberg nach den letzten Briefen Bullinger-Beza." *Zwingliana* 8 (1944): 96–107.

Schaab, Meinrad. *Geschichte der Kurpfalz*. 2 vols. Stuttgart: W. Kohlhammer, 1988–1992.

——. ed. *Territorialstaat und Calvinismus*. Stuttgart: W. Kolhammer, 1993.

Schindler, Alfred and Hans Stickelberger, eds. *Die Zürcher Reformation: Ausstrahlungen und Rückwirkungen* [*ZBRG* 18]. New York: Peter Lang, 2001.

Schmidt, C[arl]. *Der Antheil der Strassburger an der Reformation in Churpfalz. Drei Schriften Johann Marbach's mit einer geschichtlichen Einleitung*. Strasbourg, 1856.

Seeling, Werner. "Johannes Sylvan: Neue Erkenntnisse über die Hinrichtung eines kurpfälzischen Theologen im Jahre 1572." *Blätter für pfälzische Kirchengeschichte und religiöse Volkskunde* 40 (1973): 86–99.

——. *Johannes Willing (1525–1572): ein Schicksal zwischen Luthertum und Calvinismus. Versuch einer Biographie* [*Veröffentlichungen des Vereins für Pfälzische Kirchengeschichte* 11] Otterbach: Argobast, 1972.

Seiler, Christophe and Andreas Steigmeier. *Geschichte des Aargaus: Illustrierter Überblick von der Urzeit bis zur Gegenwart*. Aarau: AT Verlag, 1991.

Seisen, J.D. *Geschichte der Reformation zu Heidelberg von ihren ersten Anfängen bis zur Abfassung des Heidelberger Catechismus*. Heidelberg: J.C.B. Mohr, 1846.

Skalnik, James Veazie. *Ramus and Reform: University and Church at the End of the Renaissance* [*SCE&S* 60]. Kirksville, Mo.: Truman State UP, 2002.

Staedtke, Joachim, ed. *Glauben und Bekennen: Vierhundert Jahre Confessio Helvetica Posterior*. Zürich: Zwingli Verlag, 1966.

Steinmetz, David. *Calvin in Context*. Oxford: Oxford UP, 1995.

——. *Luther in Context*. Bloomington: Indiana UP, 1986.

Stephens, W.P. *The Theology of Huldrych Zwingli*. Oxford: Oxford UP, Clarendon Press, 1986.

Strohm, Christoph, et al., eds. *Späthumanismus und reformierte Konfession: Theologie, Jurisprudenz und Philosophie in Heidelberg an der Wende zum 17. Jahrhundert* [Spätmittelalter und Reformation 31]. Tübingen: Mohr Siebeck, 2006.

Sturm, Erdmann K. *Der junge Zacharias Ursin: Sein Weg vom Philippismus zum Calvinismus (1534–1562)* [*BGLRK* 33]. Neuenkirchen-Vluyn: Neukirchener Verlag, 1972.

Sunshine, Glenn S. *Reforming French Protestantism: The Development of Huguenot Ecclesiastical Institutions, 1557–1572* [*SCE&S* 66]. Kirksville, Mo.: Truman State UP, 2003.

Tedeschi. John. "The Cultural Contributions of Italian Protestant Reformers in the Late Renaissance." In *Schifanoia: notizie dell' Istituto di studi rinascimentali de Ferrara* (Modena: Panini, 1986): 127–151.

——. "Tomasso Sassetti's Account of the St. Bartholomew's Day Massacre." In *The Massacre of St. Bartholomew: Reappraisals and Documents*, ed. Alfred Soman, 99–112. The Hague: Martinus Nijhoff, 1974.

Thompson, Bard. "An Historical Reconstruction of Melanchthonianism in the German Reformed Church based on Liturgical Evidence." Ph.D. diss., Columbia University, 1953.

——. "The Palatinate Church Order of 1563." *Church History* 23 (1954): 339–354.

Vierordt, Karl Friedrich. *Geschichte der evangelischen Kirche in dem Großherzogtum Baden*. 2 vols. Karlsruhe, 1847–1856.

Visser, Derk, ed. *Controversy and Conciliation: The Reformation in the Palatinate 1559–1583*. Allison Park, Pennsylvania: Pickwick, 1986.

——. *Zacharias Ursinus: The Reluctant Reformer*. New York: United Church Press, 1983.

Vogler, Bernard. "Die Entstehung der protestantischen Volksfrömmigkeit in der rheinischen Pfalz zwischen 1555 und 1619." *ARG* 72 (1981): 158–196.

——. *Vie religieuse en pays rhénan: dans la seconde moitié du XVIe siècle (1556–1619)*. Lille, 1974.

Walton, Robert C. "Heinrich Bullinger, Repräsentant der reichen Bauern und seine Beziehungen zur städtischen Oligarchie." In *Reform Reformation Revolution*, ed. Siegfried Hoyer, 132–142. Leipzig: Karl-Marx-Universität, 1980.

——. "The Institutionalization of the Reformation at Zurich." *Zwingliana* 13 (Heft 8, 1972): 497–515.

——. "Der Streit zwischen Thomas Erastus und Caspar Olevian über die Kirchenzucht in der Kurpfalz in seiner Bedeutung für die internationale reformierte Bewegung." *Monatshefte für Evangelische Kirchengeschichte des Rheinlandes* 37–38 (1988–1989): 205–246.
——. *Zwingli's Theocracy*. Toronto: University of Toronto Press, 1967.
Weiss. F. "Johann Jakob Grynaeus." In *Basler Biographien*, 159–200. Basel: B. Schwabe, 1900.
Wesel-Roth, Ruth. *Thomas Erastus: Ein Beitrag zur Geschichte der reformierten Kirche und zur Lehre von der Staatssouveränität*. Lahr/Baden: Moritz Schauenberg, 1954.
——. "Thomas Erast." In *Neue Deutsche Biographie*, bd. 4, (1955), 560.
Wilbur, Earl Morse. *A History of Unitarianism: Socinianism and its Antecedents*. Cambridge: Harvard UP, 1947.
Williams, George Huntston. *The Radical Reformation* [*SCE&S* 15] 3rd ed. Kirksville, Mo., 1992.
Wolgast, Eike. *Reformierte Konfession und Politik im 16. Jahrhundert: Studien zur Geschichte der Kurpfalz im Reformationszeitalter*. Heidelberg: Universitätsverlag C. Winter, 1998.
——. *Die Universität Heidelberg 1386–1986*. Berlin: Springer, 1986.
Wotschke, Theodor. "Christoph Thretius: Ein Beitrag zur Geschichte des Kampfes der reformierten Kirche gegen den Antitrinitarismus in Polen." *Altpreussische Monatsschrift* 44, Heft 2 (1907): 152–210.
Wundt, Daniel Ludwig. *Magazin für die Kirchen- und Gelehrten-Geschichte des Kurfürstenthums Pfalz*. 2 vols. Heidelberg, 1789–1790.

English Erastianism and Anti-Erastianism

Bangs, Carl. "'All the Best Bishoprics and Deaneries': The Enigma of Arminian Politics." *Church History* 42 (1973): 5–16.
Barbour, Reid. *John Selden: Measures of the Holy Commonwealth in Seventeenth-Century England*. Toronto: University of Toronto Press, 2003.
Bicentenary of the Assembly of Divines at Westminster. Edinburgh, 1843.
Coffey, John. *Politics, Religion and the British Revolutions: The Mind of Samuel Rutherford*. Cambridge: Cambridge UP, 1997.
Collins, Jeffrey R. *The Allegiance of Thomas Hobbes*. Oxford: Oxford UP, 2005.
——. "The Restoration Bishops and the Royal Supremacy." *Church History* 68 (1999): 549–580.
Collinson, Patrick. *The Elizabethan Puritan Movement*. Berkeley: University of California Press, 1967.
Crowley, Weldon S. "Erastianism in England to 1640." *Journal of Church and State* 32 (1990): 549–566.
——. "Erastianism in the Long Parliament, 1640–1646." *Journal of Church and State* 21 (1979): 451–467.
——. "Erastianism in the Westminster Assembly." *Journal of Church and State* 15 (1973): 49–64.
Feingold, Mordechai. "John Selden and the Nature of Seventeenth-Century Science." In *In the Presence of the Past: Essays in Honor of Frank Manuel*

[International Archives of the History of Ideas 118], ed. Richard T. Bienvenu and Mordacai Feingold, 55–78. Dordrecht: Kluwer, 1991.

Gladstone, W[illiam] E[wart]. "The Theses of Erastus, and the Scottish Church Establishment." *New Quarterly Review* (1844). Reprint in idem, *Gleanings of Past Years, 1843–1878*, vol. 3, pp. 1–40. London, 1879.

Higgs, Laquita M. *Godliness and Governance in Tudor Colchester*. Ann Arbor: University of Michigan Press, 1998.

Holifield, E. Brooks. "The Intellectual Sources of Stoddardeanism." *The New England Quarterly* 45 (1972): 372–392.

Jenkins, Gary W. *John Jewel and the English National Church: The Dilemmas of an Erastian Reformer*. Aldershot, England: Ashgate, 2006.

Kaplan, Lawrence. "English Civil War Politics and the Religious Settlement." *Church History* 41 (1972): 307–325.

Lamont, William M. *Godly Rule: Politics and Religion 1603–1660*. London: MacMillan, 1969.

——. *Marginal Prynne, 1600–1669*. London: Routledge & Kegan Paul, 1963.

——. "The Rise and Fall of Bishop Bilson" *The Journal of British Studies* 5 (1966): 22–32.

Matthew, H.C.G. and Brian Howard Harrison, eds. *Oxford Dictionary of National Biography*. Oxford: Oxford UP, 2004.

Parry. G.J.R. *A Protestant Vision: William Harrison and the Reformation of Elizabethan England*. Cambridge: Cambridge UP, 2002.

Rosenblatt, Jason P. *Renaissance England's Chief Rabbi: John Selden*. Oxford: Oxford UP, 2006.

Sommerville, Johann P. "Hobbes, Selden, Erastianism, and the History of the Jews." In *Hobbes and History*, ed. G.A.J. Rogers and Tom Sorell, 160–188. London: Routledge, 2000.

Spalding, Ruth. *Contemporaries of Bulstrode Whitelocke, 1605–1675: Biographies, Illustrated by Letters and Other Documents*. Oxford: British Academy, 1990.

Winship, Michael P. "William Pynchon's The Jewes Synagogue." *The New England Quarterly* 71 (1998): 290–297.

Wojcik, J.W. "'Behold the fear of the Lord': The Erastianism of Stillingfleet, Wolseley, and Tillotson" *Archives internationales d'histoire des idées* 148 (1996): 357–374.

Wright, George. *Religion, Politics and Thomas Hobbes*. Dordrecht: Springer, 2006.

Medical and Natural Philosophical Works

Allen, Don Cameron. *The Star-Crossed Renaissance: The Quarrel about Astrology and Its Influence in England*. Durham, Duke UP, 1941. reprint, London: Cass and Company, 1966.

Dall'Aglio, Stefano. "Da Girolamo Savonarola a Tommaso Erasto: Itinerari di una polemica astrologica tra Firenze e Heidelberg." In Armando Saitta, *Scritti in ricordo di Armando Saitta*, 42–71. Milan: FrancoAngeli, 2002.

Ball, Philip. *The Devil's Doctor: Paracelsus and the World of Renaissance Magic and Science*. New York: Farrar, Straus and Giroux, 2006.

Barnes, Robin Bruce. "Hope and Despair in Sixteenth Century German Almanacs." In *Die Reformation in Deutschland und Europa: Interpretationen und Debatten*, [ARG Sonderband Washington]. Gütersloh: Gütersloher Verlagshaus, 1993.

Benzenhöfer, Udo. *Paracelsus*. Reinbek bei Hamburg: Rowohlt, 1997.

Blaser, Robert-Henri. "Un rare témoignage de fidélité envers Paracelse à Bâle: Les 'Theses de anodinis medicamentis' du médicin anglais Thomas Moffet (1578)." In *Current Problems in History of Medicine*, eds. R. Blaser and H. Buess, 502–512. Basel: Karger, 1966. German Version in Blaser R.-H. *Paracelsus in Basel*, 200–210. Muttenz /Basel: St. Argobast Verlag, 1979.

Bono, James J. *The Word of God and the Languages of Man: Interpreting Nature in Early Modern Science and Medicine*. Madison: University of Wisconsin Press, 1995.

Bröer, Ralf. "Antiparacelsismus und Dreieinigkeit: Medizinischer Antitrinitarismus von Thomas Erastus (1524–1583) bis Ernst Soner (1572–1605)." *Berichte zur Wissenschaftsgeschichte* 29 (2006): 137–154.

——. "Blutkreislauf und Dreieinigkeit: Medizinischer Antitrinitarismus von Michael Servet (1511–1553) bis Giorgio Biandrata (1515–1588)." *Berichte zur Wissenschaftsgeschichte* 29 (2006): 21–37.

——. "Friedenspolitik durch Verketzerung: Johannes Crato (1519–1585) und die Denunziation der Paracelsisten als Arianer." *Medizinhistorisches Journal* 37 (2002): 139–182.

Brooke, John Hedley. *Science and Religion: Some Historical Perspectives*. Cambridge: Cambridge UP, 1991.

Brosseder, Claudia. "The Writing in the Wittenberg Sky: Astrology in Sixteenth-Century Germany." *Journal of the History of Ideas* 66 (2005): 557–576.

Burckhardt, Albrecht. *Geschichte der Medizinischen Fakultät zu Basel, 1460–1900*. Basel: F. Reinhardt, 1917

Bylebyl, Jerome J. "The School of Padua: Humanistic Medicine in the Sixteenth Century." In *Health, Medicine and Mortality in the Sixteenth Century*, ed. Charles Webster, 335–370. Cambridge: Cambridge UP, 1979.

Caroti, Stefano. "Melanchthon's Astrology." In *'Astrologi hallucinati': Stars and the End of the World in Luther's Time*, ed. Paola Zambelli, 109–121. Berlin: de Gruyter, 1986.

Chapman, Allan. "Astrological Medicine." In *Health, Medicine and Mortality in the Sixteenth Century*, ed. Charles Webster, 275–300. Cambridge: Cambridge UP, 1979.

Conrad, Lawrence I., et al., eds. *The Western Medical Tradition 800 BC to AD 1800*. Cambridge: Cambridge UP, 1995.

Costil, Pierre. *André Dudith Humaniste Hongrois 1533–1589: Sa Vie, son Oeuvre et ses Manuscrits Grecs*. Paris: Société D'édition "Les Belles Lettres," 1935.

Crystal, Malcolm. "Medicine in Vienna in the Sixteenth and Seventeenth Centuries." Ph.D. diss., University of Virginia, 1994.

Debus, Allen G., ed. *The Chemical Philosophy: Paracelsian Science and Medicine in the Sixteenth and Seventeenth Centuries*. 2 vols. New York: Science History Publications, 1977.

——. *The English Paracelsians*. New York: Franklin Watts, 1966.

——. *The French Paracelsians*. Cambridge: Cambridge UP, 1991.
——. *Man and Nature in the Renaissance*. Cambridge: Cambridge UP, 1978.
——. ed. *Science, Medicine and Society in the Renaissance: Essays to honor Walter Pagel*. 2 vols. New York: Science History Publications, 1972.
Debus, Allen G. and Michael Walton, eds. *Reading the Book of Nature: The Other Side of the Scientific Revolution* [*SCE&S* 41]. Kirksville, Mo., 1998.
Dilg, Peter and Hartmut Rudolf, eds. *Resultate und Desiderate der Paracelsus-Forschung* [Sudhoffs Archiv Beihefte 31]. Stuttgart: Franz Steiner Verlag, 1993.
Emberger-Wandel, Gudrun. "Ein Professorleben im 16. Jahrhundert: Jakob Schegk gen. Degan aus Schorndorf." *Heimatblätter, Jahrbuch für Schorndorf und Umgebung* 5 (1987): 16–29.
Evans, R.J.W. *Rudolf II and his World*. Oxford: Oxford UP, 1973.
——. *The Wechel Presses: Humanism and Calvinism in Central Europe, 1572–1627*. Oxford: Past and Present, 1975.
Garin, Euginio. *Astrology in the Renaissance: The Zodiac of Life*. Trans. Carolyn Jackson et al. London: Routledge, 1983.
Gause, Ute. *Paracelsus: Genese und Entfaltung seiner frühen Theologie*. Stuttgart: J.C.B. Mohr (Paul Siebeck), 1993.
Gillet, J.F.A. *Crato von Crafftheim und seine Freunde*. 2 vols. Frankfurt: H.L. Brönner, 1860–1861.
Gilly, Carlos. "Die Bekenntnis zur Gnosis von Paracelsus bis auf die Schüler Jacob Böhmes." In *De Hermetische Gnosis in de loop der eeuwen*, ed. G. Quispel, 401–442. The Hague, Gegevens Koninklijke Bibliotheek, 1992.
——. "Zwischen Erfahrung und Spekulation: Theodor Zwinger und die religiöse und kulturelle Krise seiner Zeit." *Basler Zeitschrift für Geschichte und Altertumskunde* 77 (1977): 57–137 & 79 (1979): 125–233.
Gilly, Carlos and Cis van Heertum, eds. *Magia, alchimia, scienza dal '400 al '700. L'influsso di Ermete Trismegisto/Magic, Alchemy and Science 15th–18th centuries. The Influence of Hermes Trismegistus*. Florence, Centro Di, 2002.
Gillispie, Charles Coulston, ed. *Dictionary of Scientific Biography*. New York: Scribner, [1970–1980].
Goldammer, Kurt. *Paracelsus in neuen Horizonten: Gesammelte Aufsätze* [*SBPF* 24] Vienna: Verband der wissenschaftlichen Gesellschaften Österreichs, 1986.
Grell, Ole Peter and Andrew Cunningham, eds. *Medicine and the Reformation*. London: Routledge, 1993.
Gunnoe, Charles D. "The Debate between Johann Weyer and Thomas Erastus on the Punishment of Witches." In *Cultures of Communication from Reformation to Enlightenment: Constructing Publics in the Early Modern German Lands*, ed. James Van Horn Melton, 257–285. Aldershot, England: Ashgate Press, 2002.
——. "German Protestantism and Astrology: The Debate between Thomas Erastus and the Melanchthon Circle." In *Religion und Naturwissenschaften im 16. und 17. Jahrhundert* [*SVRG* 210] ed. Kaspar von Greyerz, Thomas Kaufmann, Kim Siebenhüner, and Roberto Zaugg, 86–101. Gütersloh: Gütersloher Verlagshaus, 2010.
——. "Thomas Erastus and his Circle of Anti-Paracelsians." In *Analecta Paracelsica*, ed. Joachim Telle, 127–148. Stuttgart: Franz Steiner Verlag, 1994.

Gunnoe, Charles D., and Jole Shackelford, "Johannes Crato von Krafftheim (1519–1585): Imperial Physician, Irenicist, and Anti-Paracelsian." In *Ideas and Cultural Margins in Early Modern Germany: Essays in Honor of H.C. Erik Midelfort*, ed. Elizabeth Plummer and Robin Barnes, 201–216. Aldershot, England: Ashgate, 2009.

Harley, David. "Rychard Bostok of Tandridge, Surrey (C. 1530–1605), M.P., Paracelsian Propagandist and Friend of John Dee." *Ambix* 47 (2000): 29–36.

Hellman, C. Doris. *The Comet of 1577*. New York: Columbia, 1944.

Hemleben, Johannes. *Paracelsus: Revolutionär, Arzt und Christ*. 2nd ed. Frauenfeld and Stuttgart: Verlag Huber, 1974.

Hooykaas, R[eijer]. *Religion and the Rise of Modern Science*. Grand Rapids: Eerdmans, 1972.

Kahn, Didier. *Alchimie et paracelsisme en France à la fin de la Renaissance (1567–1625)* [Cahiers d'Humanisme et Renaissance 80]. Geneva: Droz, 2007.

——. "Cinquante-neuf thèses de Paracelse censurées par la Faculte de theologie de Paris, le 9 octobre 1578." In *Documents oubliés sur l'alchimie, la kabbale et Guillaume Postel: offerts, à l'occasion de son 90e anniversaire, à François Secret par ses élèves et amis* [*THR* 353], ed. François Secret and Matton Sylvain, 161–178. Geneva: Droz, 2001.

Karcher, J. "Thomas Erastus (1524–1583), der unversöhnliche Gegner des Theophrastus Paracelsus." *Gesnerus* 14 (1957): 1–13.

Koch, Ernst. "Die Badereisen des Grafen Georg Ernst zu Henneberg." *Zeitschrift des Vereins für hennebergische Geschichte und Landeskunde in Schmalkalden* 15 (1905): 1–45.

Kühlmann, Wilhelm and Joachim Telle. "Humanismus und Medizin an der Universität Heidelberg im 16. Jahrhundert." In *Semper Apertus: Sechshundert Jahre Ruprecht-Karls-Universität Heidelberg 1386–1986*, ed. Wilhelm Doerr et al., 1:255–289. Berlin: Springer, 1985.

Kusukawa, Sachiko. *The Transformation of Natural Philosophy: The Case of Philip Melanchthon*. Cambridge: Cambridge UP, 1995.

LeNoble, Robert. *Mersenne ou Naissance du Mécanisme*. Paris: Librairie Philosophique J. Vrin, 1943.

Lindberg, David C. *The Beginnings of Western Science*. Chicago: University of Chicago Press, 1992.

Lindberg, David C., and Ronald L. Numbers. *God and Nature: Historical Essays on the Encounter between Christianity and Science*. Berkeley: University of California Press, 1986.

Lloyd, G.E.R. *Aristotle: The Growth and Structure of his Thought*. Cambridge: Cambridge UP, 1968.

Matthäus, Klaus. "Zur Geschichte des Nürnberger Kalenderwesens: Die Entwicklung der Nürnberg gedruckten Jahreskalender in Buchform." *Archiv der Geschichte des Buchwesens* 9 (1969): 965–1396.

Midelfort, H.C. Erik. "The Anthropological Roots of Paracelsus' Psychiatry." In *Kreatur und Kosmos*, ed. Rosemarie Dilg-Frank, 67–77. Stuttgart: Fischer, 1981.

Millen, Ron. "The Manifestation of Occult Qualities in the Scientific Revolution." In *Religion, Science, and Worldview*, eds. M.J. Osler and P.L. Farber, 185–216. Cambridge: Cambridge UP, 1985.

Milt, Bernhard. “Conrad Gessner und Paracelsus.” *Schweizerische medizinische Wochenschrift* 59 (1929): 486–509.

——. “Paracelsus and Zürich.” *Vierteljahrsschrift der Naturforschenden Gesellschaft in Zürich* 86 (1941): 321–354.

Moran, Bruce T. “Paracelsus, Religion, and Dissent: The Case of Philipp Homagius and Georg Zimmermann.” *Ambix* 43 (1996): 65–79.

Müller, Konrad. “Ph. Melanchthon und das kopernikanische Weltsystem.” *Centaurus* 9 (1963): 16–28.

Müller-Janke, Wolf-Dieter. *Astrologisch-Magische Theorie und Praxis in der Heilkunde der frühen Neuzeit.* Sudhoffs Archiv Beiheft, 25. Stuttgart: Franz Steiner Verlag Wiesbaden, 1985.

Newman, William R. *Atoms and Alchemy: Chymistry and the Experimental Origins of the Scientific Revolution.* Chicago: University of Chicago Press, 2006.

——. *Promethean Ambitions: Alchemy and the Quest to Perfect Nature.* Chicago: University of Chicago Press, 2005.

Niebyl, Peter H. “Sennert, Van Helmont, and Medical Ontology.” *Bulletin of the History of Medicine* 45 (1971): 115–137.

Nutton, Vivian. “Humanist Surgery.” In *The Medical Renaissance of the Sixteenth Century*, eds. A. Wear, R.K. French, and I.M. Lonie, 75–99. Cambridge: Cambridge UP, 1985.

——. “John Caius und Johannes Lange: Medizinischer Humanismus zur Zeit Vesals.” *NTM* 21 (1984): 81–87.

——. ed. *Medicine at the Courts of Europe, 1500–1837.* London: Routledge, 1990.

——. “The Reception of Fracastoro’s Theory of Contagion: The Seed That Fell among Thorns?” *Osiris*, 2nd Series, vol. 6, *Renaissance Medical Learning: Evolution of a Tradition* (1990): 196–234.

——. “The Seeds of Disease: An Explanation of Contagion and Infection from the Greeks to the Renaissance.” *Medical History* 27 (1983): 1–34.

Pagel, Walter. *Paracelsus: An Introduction to Philosophical Medicine in the Era of the Renaissance.* 2nd ed. Basel: Karger, 1982.

——. “Paracelsus in the Neoplatonic and Gnostic Tradition,” *Ambix* 8 (1960): 125–166.

——. “The Prime Matter of Paracelsus,” *Ambix* 9 (1961): 117–135; reprint, in *Religion and Neoplatonism in Renaissance Medicine*, VII, 117–135. London. Variorum Reprints, 1985.

——. *The Smiling Spleen: Paracelsianism in Storm and Stress.* Basel: Karger, 1984.

——. “Thomas Erastus.” In *DSB* 4:386–388.

Pagel, Walter and Marianne Winder. “The Higher Elements and Prime Matter in Renaissance Naturalism and in Paracelsus.” *Ambix* 21 (1974): 94–127.

Park, Katherine and Lorraine Daston, eds. *The Cambridge History of Science.* Vol. 3, *Early Modern Science.* Cambridge: Cambridge UP, 2006.

Pfister, Hedwig. *Bad Kissingen vor vierhundert Jahren* [Mainfrankische Hefte, 19]. Würzburg, 1954.

Pisa, Karl. *Paracelsus in Österreich: Eine Spurensuche.* St. Pölten/Vienna: Niederösterreichisches Pressehaus, 1991.

Principe, Lawrence. *The Aspiring Adept: Robert Boyle and His Alchemical Quest.* Princeton: Princeton UP, 2000.

Puschmann, Theodor. *A History of Medical Education from the Most Remote to the Most Recent Times.* Trans. Evan H. Hare. London, 1891.

Rath, Gernot. "Die Briefe Konrad Geßners aus der Trewschen Sammlung." *Gesnerus* 7 (1950): 140–170; 8 (1951): 195–215.

Richardson, Linda Deer. "The Generation of Disease: Occult Causes and Diseases of the Total Substance." In *The Medical Renaissance of the Sixteenth Century*, eds. A. Wear, R.K. French, and I.M. Lonie, 175–194. Cambridge: Cambridge UP, 1985.

Rudolf, Hartmut. "Kosmosspekulation und Trinitätslehre: Ein Beitrag zur Beziehung zwischen Weltbild und Theologie bei Paracelsus." In *Paracelsus in der Tradition* [Salzbürger Beiträge zur Paracelsusforschung 21], ed. Sepp Domandl, 32–47. Vienna: Verband der wissenschaftlichen Gesellschaften Österreichs, 1980.

Schmidt, C. *Michael Schütz genannt Toxites.* Strasbourg, 1888.

Schmitt, Charles. "Aristotle among the Physicians." In *The Medical Renaissance of the Sixteenth Century*, eds. A. Wear, R.K. French, and I.M. Lonie, 1–15. Cambridge: Cambridge UP, 1985.

——. *Aristotle and the Renaissance.* Cambridge: Harvard UP, 1983.

——. "Philosophy and Science in Sixteenth Century Italian Universities." In *The Aristotelian Tradition and Renaissance Universities.* London: Variorum Reprints, 1984.

Shackelford, Jole. "Early Reception of Paracelsian Theory: Severinus and Erastus." *SCJ* 26 (1995): 123–135.

——. *A Philosophical Path for Paracelsian Medicine. The Ideas, Intellectual Context, and Influence of Petrus Severinus (1540/2–1602).* Copenhagen: Museum Tusculanum Press, 2004.

Sigwart, Christoph. "Jacob Schegk, Professor der Philosophie und Medizin." In *Kleine Schriften*, 2nd ed., 256–291. Freiburg, 1889.

Schreiner, Susan, *The Theater of his Glory: Nature and the Natural Order in the Thought of John Calvin.* Durham: Labyrinth Press, 1991.

Siraisi, Nancy G. *Medieval and Early Renaissance Medicine: An Introduction to Knowledge and Practice.* Chicago: University of Chicago Press, 1990.

——. "Oratory and Rhetoric in Renaissance Medicine." *Journal of the History of Ideas* (2004): 191–211.

——. "Philosophy and Science in a Medical Milieu." In *Avicenna in Renaissance Italy: The Canon and Medical Teaching in Italian Universities after 1500*, 221–293. Princeton: Princeton UP, 1987.

Steinmann, Martin. *Johannes Oporinus, Ein Basler Buchdrucker um die Mitte des 16. Jahrhunderts* [*BBG* 105]. Basel: Helbing & Lichtenhahn, 1967.

Sticker, Georg. "Ein Gespräch des Königs Ferdinand mit Paracelsus." *Nova Acta Leopoldina* 10 (1941): 267–279.

Stübler, Eberhard. *Geschichte der medizinischen Fakultät der Universität Heidelberg 1386–1925.* Heidelberg: Carl Winter's Universitätsbuchhandlung, 1926.

Sudhoff, Karl. *Bibliographia Paracelsica: Besprechung der unter Hohenheims Namen 1527–1893 erschienenen Druckschriften.* Berlin, 1894; reprint, Graz: Akademische Druck- und Verlagsanstalt, 1958.

Telle, Joachim, ed. *Analecta Paracelsica: Studien zum Nachleben Theophrast von Hohenheims im deutschen Kulturgebiet der frühen Neuzeit* [Heidelberger Studien zur Naturkunde der frühen Neuzeit 4] Stuttgart: Franz Steiner Verlag, 1994.

——. "Kurfürst Ottheinrich, Hans Kilian und Paracelsus: Zum pfälzischen Paracelsismus im 16. Jahrhundert." In *Von Paracelsus zu Goethe und Wilhelm von Humboldt* [*SBPF* 22], pp. 130–146. Vienna: Verband der wissenschaftlichen Gesellschaften Österreichs, 1981.

Temkin, Owsei. *The Falling Sickness: A History of Epilepsy from the Greeks to the Beginning of Modern Neurology*. Baltimore, 1945. Rev. ed. Baltimore: Johns Hopkins UP, 1971.

——. "Fernel, Joubert, and Erastus on the Specificity of Cathartic Drugs." In *Science, Medicine and Society in the Renaissance*, ed. Allen Debus, 1:61–68. New York: Science History Publications, 1972.

——. *Galenism: Rise and Decline of a Medical Philosophy*. Ithaca: Cornell UP, 1973.

Thommen, Rudolf. *Geschichte der Universität Basel 1532–1632*. Basel, 1889.

Thorndike, Lynn. *A History of Magic and Experimental Science*. 8 vols. New York: Columbia UP, 1923–1958.

Trevor-Roper, H.R. "The Paracelsian Movement." In *Renaissance Essays*, 149–199. Chicago: University of Chicago Press, 1985.

Tschinkel, Augustin. "Paracelsus bei König Ferdinand I." In *Paracelsus—Werk und Wirkung* [*SBPF* 13], ed. Sepp Domandl, 335–343. Vienna: Verband der wissenschaftlichen Gesellschaften Österreichs, 1975.

Walker, D.P. *Spiritual and Demonic Magic from Ficino to Campanella*. London: Warburg Institute, 1958.

Walter, Tilmann. "Paracelsuskritische Haltungen oder "Antiparacelsismus"?, 1570–1630." *Würzburger medizinhistorische Mitteilungen* 27 (2008): 381–408.

Wear, Andrew. "Explorations in Renaissance Writings on the Practice of Medicine." In *The Medical Renaissance of the Sixteenth Century*, eds. A. Wear, R.K. French, and I.M. Lonie, 118–145. Cambridge: Cambridge UP, 1985.

——. "Galen in the Renaissance." In *Galen: Problems and Prospects*, ed. Vivian Nutton, 229–262. London: Wellcome Institute, 1981.

Webster, Charles. "Alchemical and Paracelsian Medicine." In *Health, Medicine and Mortality in the 16th Century*, ed. Charles Webster, 301–334. Cambridge: Cambridge UP, 1979.

——. "Conrad Gessner and the Infidelity of Paracelsus." In *New Perspectives on Renaissance Thought*, eds. J. Henry and S. Hutton, 13–23. London: Duckworth, 1990.

——. *From Paracelsus to Newton: Magic and the Making of Modern Science*. Cambridge: Cambridge UP, 1982.

——. *Paracelsus: Medicine, Magic and Mission at the End of Time*. New Haven: Yale UP, 2008.

Weeks, Andrew. *Paracelsus: Speculative Theory and the Crisis of the Early Reformation*. Albany: State University of New York, Press, 1997.

White, Andrew Dickson. *A History of the Warfare of Science with Theology in Christendom*. 2 vols. New York, 1896.

Williams, Gerhild Scholz and Charles D. Gunnoe, eds. *Paracelsian Moments: Science, Medicine, and Astrology in Early Modern Europe* [*SCE&S* 64]. Kirksville, Mo.: Truman State UP, 2002.

Zapletal, Vladimir. "Paracelsus-Tradition in der Tschechoslowakei." In *Gestalten und Ideen um Paracelsus* [*SBPF* 11], ed. Sepp Domandl, 157–169. Vienna: Verlag Notring, 1972.

Zaunick, Rudolf. "Michael Toxites (Schütz) und Kurfürst August von Sachsen." *Sudhoffs Archiv* 36 (1943): 90–99.

Zimmermann, Volker, ed. *Paracelsus: Das Werk—die Rezeption*. Stuttgart: Steiner Verlag, 1995.

Demonology

Anglo, Sydney, ed. *The Damned Art: Essays in the Literature of Witchcraft*. London: Routledge & Kegan Paul, 1977.

Barry, Jonathan, et al. *Witchcraft in early modern Europe: Studies in culture and belief*. Cambridge: Cambridge UP, 1996.

Behringer, Wolfgang. *Witchcraft Persecutions in Bavaria: Popular Magic, Religious Zealotry, and Reason of State in Early Modern Europe*. Cambridge: Cambridge UP, 1997.

Binz, Carl. *Doctor Johann Weyer, ein rheinischer Arzt, der erste Bekämpfer des Hexenwahns*. 2nd ed. Berlin, 1896; reprint, New York: Arno, 1976.

Briggs, Robin. *Witches & Neighbors: The Social and Cultural Context of European Witchcraft*. New York: Viking, 1996.

Clark, Stuart, *Thinking with Demons: The Idea of Witchcraft in Early Modern Europe*. Oxford: Clarendon Press, 1997.

Ginzburg, Carlo. *Ecstasies: Deciphering the Witches' Sabbath*. New York: Pantheon, 1991

——. *The Night Battles*. Baltimore: Johns Hopkins UP, 1983.

Golden, Richard M., ed. *Encyclopedia of Witchcraft: The Western Tradition*. Santa Barbara: ABC-CLIO, 2006.

Kieckhefer, Richard. *European Witch Trials*. Berkeley: University of California, 1976.

——. *Magic in the Middle Ages*. Cambridge: Cambridge UP, 1990.

Lehmann, Hartmut and Otto Ulbricht, eds. *Vom Unfug des Hexen-Processes: Gegner der Hexenverfolgung von Johann Weyer bis Friedrich Spee* [Wolfenbüttler Forschungen 55]. Wiesbaden: Otto Harrassowitz, 1992.

Levack, Brian. *The Witch-Hunt in Early Modern Europe*, 3rd ed. Harlow: Pearson Longman, 2006.

——. ed. *Articles on Witchcraft, Magic and Demonology*. 12 vols. New York: Garland, 1992.

Midelfort, H.C. Erik. "Johann Weyer and Transformation of the Insanity Defense." In *The German People and the Reformation*, ed. R. Po-Chia Hsia, 234–261. Ithaca: Cornell UP, 1988.

——. "Were There Really Witches." In *Transition and Revolution*, ed. Robert Kingdon, 189–233. Minneapolis: Burgess Publishing Co., 1974.

——. *Witch Hunting in Southwestern Germany 1562–1684: Social and Intellectual Foundations*. Stanford: Stanford UP, 1972.

Monter, E. William. *European Witchcraft*. New York: Wiley, 1969.

——. "Inflation and Witchcraft: The Case of Jean Bodin." In *Action and Conviction in Early Modern Europe*, ed. Theodore Rabb and Jerold E. Siegel, 371–389. Princeton: Princeton UP, 1969.

——. *Witchcraft in France and Switzerland: The Borderlands during the Reformation*. Ithaca: Cornell UP, 1976.

Paulus, Niklaus. *Hexen und Hexenprozeß vornehmlich im 16. Jahrhundert*. Freiburg: Herdersche Verlagshandlung, 1910.

Roper, Lyndal. *Oedipus and the Devil: witchcraft, sexuality, and religion in early modern Europe*. London: Routledge, 1994.

——. *Witch Craze: Terror and Fantasy in Baroque Germany*. New Haven: Yale UP, 2004.

Schmidt, Jürgen Michael. *Glaube und Skepsis: die Kurpfalz und die abendländische Hexenverfolgung, 1446–1685*. Bielefeld: Verlag für Regionalgeschichte, 2000.

——. "Thomas Erast." In *Lexikon zur Geschichte der Hexenverfolgung*, ed. Gudrun Gersmann, Katrin Moeller and Jürgen-Michael Schmidt, in historicum.net, http://www.historicum.net/no_cache/persistent/artikel/6102/.

Teale, John L. "Witchcraft and Calvinism in Elizabethan England: Divine Power and Human Agency." *Journal of the History of Ideas* 23 (1962): 21–36.

Thomas, Keith. *Religion and the Decline of Magic*. New York: Scribner's, 1971.

Valente, Michaela. *Johann Wier: agli albori della critica razionale dell'occulto e del demoniaco nell'Europa del Cinquecento*. Florence: Leo S. Olschki, 2003.

Walker, D.P. "The Cessation of Miracles." In *Hermeticism and the Renaissance: Intellectual History and the Occult in Early Modern Europe*, ed., Ingrid Merkel and Allen G. Debus, 111–124. Washington: Folger, 1988.

——. *Spiritual and Demonic Magic from Ficino to Campanella*. London: Warburg Institute, 1958.

INDEX